Nursing Assisting
A Foundation in Caregiving

Diana L. Dugan, RN

THIRD EDITION

hartmanonline.com

Hartman

Credits

Managing Editor
Susan Alvare Hedman

Designer
Kirsten Browne

Cover Illustrator
Jo Tronc

Production
Thad Castillo
Tak Minagawa

Photography
Art Clifton/Dick Ruddy/Pat Berrett

Proofreaders
Kristin Calderon
Kristin Cartwright
Eliza Martin
Lupe Garcia Ortiz

Sales/Marketing
Deborah Rinker
Kendra Robertson
Erika Walker
Belinda Midyette

Customer Service
Fran Desmond
Thomas Noble
Angela Storey
Eliza Martin
Jeff Brown

Warehouse Coordinator
Chris Midyette

Copyright Information

© 2012 by Diana L. Dugan
Hartman Publishing, Inc.
1313 Iron Ave SW
Albuquerque, New Mexico 87102
(505) 291-1274
web: hartmanonline.com
e-mail: orders@hartmanonline.com
Twitter: @HartmanPub

ISBN 978-1-60425-030-5
ISBN 978-1-60425-033-6 (Hardcover)

PRINTED IN THE USA

Third Printing, 2014

Notice to Readers

Though the guidelines and procedures contained in this text are based on consultations with healthcare professionals, they should not be considered absolute recommendations. The instructor and readers should follow employer, local, state, and federal guidelines concerning healthcare practices. These guidelines change, and it is the reader's responsibility to be aware of these changes and of the policies and procedures of her or his healthcare facility.

The publisher, author, editors, and reviewers cannot accept any responsibility for errors or omissions or for any consequences from application of the information in this book and make no warranty, expressed or implied, with respect to the contents of the book. The Publisher does not warrant or guarantee any of the products described herein or perform any analysis in connection with any of the product information contained herein.

Special Thanks

A heartfelt thank you to our insightful and wonderful reviewers:

Jill Holmes Long, MA, RN-BC
Hayesville, NC

Katherine Howard, MS, RN-BC
Middlesex County College, NJ

Charles Illian, BSN, RN
Orlando, FL

Wendy Pickard-Tanios, RN, BS
Round Rock, TX

Christine Smith, MSN, RN
Poquoson, VA

Anne L. Varljen, BSN, CIC, RN
Austin, TX

Gender Usage

This textbook utilizes the pronouns "he," "his," "she," and "hers" interchangeably to denote healthcare team members and residents.

Permissions

Excerpt from *Falling into Life* by Leonard Kriegel from *The American Scholar*, Volume 57, Number 3, Summer 1988. Copyright © 1988 by Leonard Kriegel. Reprinted with permission of Leonard Kriegel.

Excerpt on The Great Chicago Fire adapted from *To Be a Nurse* by Susan M. Sacharski. Copyright © 1990. Reprinted with permission of Susan M. Sacharski.

Dedication

This book is dedicated to my dad, Robert, and my late mom, Margaret, the two most loving parents on the face of the earth. Thank you for your tremendous love and guidance over all these years and for always telling me I could do anything. Thank you for showing others a path of responsibility, honesty, and love.

To my dearest John, for your incredible love and devotion, thank you for your constant efforts on behalf of our entire family. I give you my undying gratitude for your dedication, encouragement, help, and support. All who know you have the greatest respect for you. Without you, these books would never have been possible.

> THE SEA HAS ITS PEARLS,
> THE HEAVEN ITS STARS,
> BUT MY HEART, MY HEART,
> MY HEART HAS ITS LOVE.
> —Heinrich Heine, [1797-1856], *Das Meer hat seine Perlen. Stanza 1*

For our dear children, Mark and Carrie, and Marissa and Jon, thank you for your love, tremendous efforts, and encouragement. We are so very proud of each one of you. We wish you the very best in all of your ventures in the medical field. It is incredibly exciting to watch all of you soar!

To my family and John's family, including his mom, Mary Alice, and his dad, Thomas, who has passed away, and George E. Barrett for all of your love and support. Thank you to all of our brothers and sisters and their families, especially Paul and Paula, and Mary Kay and Barry, for your love and your efforts on behalf of our families. And to Cassie, our puppy who has passed away, for your companionship all those years.

For family and our good friends, thank you for your encouragement, help, and love, especially Mary and Ron, Kathy and Roy, Lorri and Paul, Linda and Robert, Tina S., Ruth Darling, Barbara J. Ramutkowski, and David and Marita.

To Mark T. Hartman, the best publisher who ever lived, thank you for your constancy, vision, and dedication. Wishing you the very best and sending our good wishes to Elliott and Warren for much success in their exciting futures.

To Susan Alvare Hedman, simply the most talented editor in the world. I wouldn't work with anyone but you! With sincere love and appreciation for your tireless efforts and your nonstop hard work on behalf of our books. Thank you to Mark Hedman for his support and love of Susan and Isa.

For all of the people affiliated with Hartman Publishing: Thad Castillo, Kirsten Browne, Deborah Rinker, Fran Desmond, Thomas Noble, Angela Storey, Kendra Robertson, Erika Walker, Eliza Martin, Belinda Midyette, Chris Midyette, Jeff Brown, Kristin Cartwright, Kristin Calderon, and Jo Tronc, thank you for everything. To our discerning reviewers, thank you for working so diligently to make this book the best it can be.

To the instructors, thank you for your dedication to quality care. To the students, I am sending you my sincere good wishes for your success in the world of health care. I want to hear great things about you!

My best to all,

Diana L. Dugan

Contents

5 Diversity and Human Needs and Development

6 Infection Prevention

7 Safety and Body Mechanics

Procedures

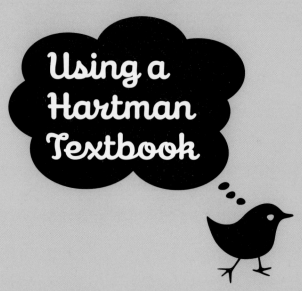

Using a Hartman Textbook

Understanding how your book is organized and what its special features are will help you make the most of this resource!

look!

Carefully-chosen quotes begin each chapter and may be used for discussion. Additional information highlights how health care has changed over the years by detailing interesting events in medicine from the past.

We have assigned each chapter its own colored tab. Each colored tab contains the chapter number and title, and you'll see them on the side of every page.

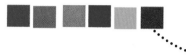

1. Explain HIPAA and related terms

Everything in this book, the student workbook, and the instructor's teaching material is organized around learning objectives. A learning objective is a very specific piece of knowledge or a very specific skill. After reading the text, if you can do what the learning objective says, you know you have mastered the material.

bloodborne pathogens

You'll find bold key terms at the beginning of each chapter and then again throughout the text. These terms are defined in the text and in the glossary at the back of this book.

Making an occupied bed

All care procedures are highlighted by the same black bar for easy recognition.

Guidelines: Accurate Documentation

Guidelines and Observing and Reporting are colored green for easy reference.

Residents' Rights

Take your time when feeding residents
dangerous

Residents' Rights boxes teach important information about abuse and neglect and how to recognize and prevent both. Ways to support and promote Residents' Rights are also included. Tip and Trivia boxes show interesting and educational tidbits that you can use inside and outside of work.

Chapter Review

Chapter-ending questions test your knowledge of the information found in the chapter. We have included the textbook's learning objective numbers to make it easier for you to go back and reread a section if you need to refresh your memory. When you see this notation after a question—(LO 3)—it refers to that particular learning objective number in the chapter on which you are working. If you have trouble answering a question, you can return to the text and reread the material.

See the Appendix at the end of the book for additional information.

Beginning and ending steps in care procedures

For most care procedures, these steps should be performed. Understanding why they are important will help you remember to perform each step every time care is provided.

Beginning Steps

Identify yourself by name.

Identify the resident.

Greet the resident by name.

A resident's room is his home. Residents have a right to privacy. Before any procedure, knock and wait for permission to enter the resident's room. Upon entering his room, identify yourself and state your title. Residents have the right to know who is providing their care. Identify and greet the resident. This shows courtesy and respect. It also establishes correct identification. This prevents care from being performed on the wrong person.

Wash your hands.

Handwashing provides for infection prevention. Nothing fights infection in facilities like performing consistent, proper hand hygiene. Handwashing may need to be done more than once during a procedure. Practice Standard Precautions with every resident.

Explain procedure to resident.

Speak clearly, slowly, and directly.

Maintain face-to-face contact whenever possible.

Residents have a right to know exactly what care you will provide. It promotes understanding, cooperation, and independence. Residents are able to do more for themselves if they know what needs to happen.

Provide for the resident's privacy with a curtain, screen, or door.

Doing this maintains residents' right to privacy and dignity. Providing for privacy in a facility is not simply a courtesy; it is a legal right.

Adjust the bed to a safe level, usually waist high.

Lock the bed wheels.

Locking the bed wheels is an important safety measure. It ensures that the bed will not move as you are performing care. Raising the bed helps you to remember to use good body mechanics. This prevents injury to you and to residents.

Ending Steps

Make resident comfortable.	Make sure sheets are wrinkle-free and lie flat under the resident's body. This helps prevent pressure ulcers. Replace bedding and pillows. Check that the resident's body is in proper alignment. This promotes comfort and health after you leave the room.
Return bed to lowest position. **Remove privacy measures.**	Lowering the bed provides for residents' safety. Remove extra privacy measures added during the procedure. This includes anything you may have draped over and around residents, as well as privacy screens.
Leave call light within resident's reach.	A call light allows residents to communicate with staff as necessary. Making the decision not to respond to a call light is considered neglect.
Wash your hands.	Handwashing is the most important thing you can do to prevent the spread of infection.
Be courteous and respectful at all times.	Say "thank you" before you leave. It is the polite and proper thing to do. Ask residents if they need anything else. Let them know that you are leaving. This promotes respect.
Report any changes in the resident to the nurse. **Document procedure using facility guidelines.**	You will often be the person who spends the most time with a resident, so you are in the best position to note any changes in a resident's condition. Every time you provide care, observe the resident's physical and mental capabilities, as well as the condition of the body. For example, a change in a resident's ability to dress himself may signal a greater problem. After you have finished giving care, document the care using facility guidelines. Do not record care before it is given. If you do not document the care you gave, legally it did not happen.

In addition to the beginning and ending steps listed above, remember to follow infection prevention guidelines. Even if a procedure in this book does not tell you to wear gloves or other PPE, there may be times when it is appropriate.

For example, the procedure for giving a back rub does not include gloves. Gloves are usually not required for a back rub. However, if the resident has open sores on his back, gloves are necessary.

1
The Nursing Assistant in Long-Term Care

Nurses' Aides: Helping Hands During World War II

One of the early times nurses' aides were used in America was during World War II. Various hospitals, along with the American Red Cross, trained nurses' aides in 1941 to help deal with a shortage of nurses due to the war. Employers in the United States expected nurses' aides to volunteer during this time. The country set a goal of training 100,000 nurses' aides to assist nurses with patient care. These aides worked each day without being paid. Imagine being hired today as a nursing assistant and being expected to do the job without pay!

"A professor can never better distinguish himself in his work than by encouraging a clever pupil, for the true discoverers are among them, as comets amongst the stars."

Carl Linnaeus, 1707-1778

"If one advances confidently in the direction of his dreams, and endeavors to live the life which he has imagined, he will meet with a success unexpected in common hours."

Henry David Thoreau, 1817-1862
from *Walden*

1. Define important words in this chapter

accountable: answerable for one's actions.

activities of daily living (ADLs): personal daily care tasks, including bathing, skin, nail, and hair care, walking, eating and drinking, mouth care, dressing, transferring, and toileting.

acute care: 24-hour skilled care for short-term illnesses or injuries; generally given in hospitals and ambulatory surgical centers.

adaptive devices: special equipment that helps a person who is ill or disabled perform ADLs; also called assistive devices.

adult daycare: care given to adults at a facility during daytime work hours.

assisted living: a residence for people who require some help with daily care, but who need less care than a long-term care facility offers.

assistive devices: special equipment that helps a person who is ill or disabled perform ADLs; also called adaptive devices.

care team: the group of people with different kinds of education and experience who provide resident care.

chain of command: the order of authority within a facility.

charge nurse (nurse-in-charge): a nurse responsible for a team of healthcare workers.

chronic: the term for an illness or condition that is long-term or long-lasting.

cite: in a long-term care facility, to find a problem through a survey.

conscientious: guided by a sense of right and wrong; principled.

continuity of care: coordination of care for a resident over time, during which the care team is always exchanging information about the resident and working toward shared goals.

courteous: polite, kind, considerate.

delegation: transferring authority to a person for a specific task.

dementia: the loss of mental abilities, such as thinking, remembering, reasoning, and communicating.

diagnosis: the identification of a disease by its signs and symptoms and from the results of different tests.

empathetic: identifying with and understanding another's feelings.

first impression: a way of classifying or categorizing people at the first meeting.

functional nursing: method of care assigning specific tasks to each team member.

holistic: care that involves the whole person; this includes his or her physical, social, emotional, and spiritual needs.

home health care: care that takes place in a person's home.

hospice care: care for people who have approximately six months or less to live; care is available until the person dies.

inter-generational care: mixing children and the elderly in the same care setting.

Joint Commission: a not-for-profit organization that evaluates and accredits different types of healthcare facilities.

length of stay: the number of days a person stays in a healthcare facility.

liability: a legal term that means a person can be held responsible for harming someone else.

licensed practical nurse (LPN) or licensed vocational nurse (LVN): licensed nurse who has completed one to two years of education; LPN/LVN administers medications, gives treatments, and may supervise daily care of residents.

long-term care: 24-hour care provided for people with ongoing conditions who are generally unable to manage their ADLs.

nursing assistant (NA/CNA): person who performs assigned nursing tasks and gives personal care.

outpatient care: care usually given for less than 24 hours to people who have had treatments, procedures, or surgery.

pet therapy: the practice of bringing pets into a facility or home to provide stimulation and companionship.

policy: a course of action to be followed.

primary nursing: a method of care in which the registered nurse gives much of the daily care to residents.

procedure: a method, or way, of doing something.

professionalism: the act of behaving properly for a certain job.

registered nurse (RN): a licensed nurse who has completed two to four years of education; RNs assess residents, create the care plan, monitor progress, provide skilled nursing care, give treatments, and supervise the care given by nursing assistants and other members of the care team.

rehabilitation: a program of care given by a specialist or a team of specialists to restore or improve function after an illness or injury.

resident: a person living in a long-term care facility.

resident-focused care: method of care in which the resident is the primary focus; residents and their families actively participate in care and their choices are honored by caregivers whenever possible.

sandwich generation: people responsible for the care of both their children and aging relatives.

skilled care: medically-necessary care given by a skilled nurse or therapist.

subacute care: care for an illness or condition given to people who need less care than for an acute (sudden onset, short-term) illness or injury but more than for a chronic (long-term) illness.

team leader: a nurse in charge of a group of residents for one shift of duty.

team nursing: method of care in which a nurse acts as a leader of a group of people giving care.

trustworthy: deserving the trust of others.

2. Describe healthcare settings

Welcome to the rewarding world of caring for others! No work is more appreciated or valued. Your work will make an important difference in the lives of many people.

Nursing assistants have many job opportunities. Where you work will depend on you, your schedule, and the type of resident you prefer. More information on finding a job is in Chapter 28.

Each healthcare setting is unique; however, there are some similar tasks that will be performed in every setting. This textbook will focus on **long-term care** for elderly residents.

Long-term care (LTC) facilities provide 24-hour skilled care for people who are no longer eligible for hospital care, but are unable to be cared for at home. **Skilled care** is medically-necessary care given by a skilled nurse or therapist. This care is available 24 hours a day. It is ordered by a doctor, and involves a treatment plan.

Long-term care assists people with ongoing, chronic medical conditions, and is usually given for an extended period of time. **Chronic** means that the conditions last a long period of time, even a lifetime. Examples of chronic conditions include physical disabilities, heart disease, and recovery from stroke. Other terms for long-term care facilities are:

- Nursing homes
- Nursing facilities
- Skilled nursing facilities
- Extended care facilities

A long-term care facility is the resident's home (Fig. 1-1). This is why we call people in these facilities **residents**. It will be the resident's home

until he or she returns home, moves to another place, or dies. You must always remember that when you knock on the door and walk into a resident's room, it is the very same thing as knocking on the door of your neighbor's home. Always treat residents' rooms with respect.

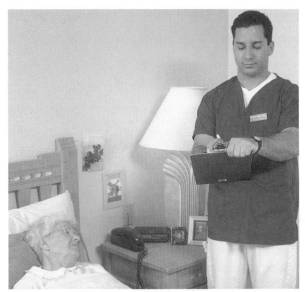

Fig. 1-1. A long-term care facility is the resident's home. Treat their rooms and possessions with respect.

In **assisted living** facilities, residents are generally more independent. Staff are available to provide whatever daily care the resident needs, such as bathing and dressing. Sometimes staff give help with medications. Residents in assisted living do not usually need skilled care.

Many assisted living centers have a stair-step method of handling residents' needs. The stair-step method means that a person is admitted to a facility when he is still fairly independent. As he requires more care, the level of placement within the facility changes. The advantage this provides is that the resident is not moved from facility to facility.

Home health care is care that takes place in a person's home (Fig. 1-2). In some ways, working as a home health aide is similar to working as a nursing assistant. Almost all care in this textbook applies to home health aides. Most of the personal care and basic nursing procedures are the same. Home health aides may also clean the home, shop for groceries, do laundry, and cook. They will work more independently, although a supervisor monitors their work, and they may have more contact with the family. The advantage of home health care is that clients do not have to leave home. They may have lived in their homes for many years, and staying at home is more comforting for most people.

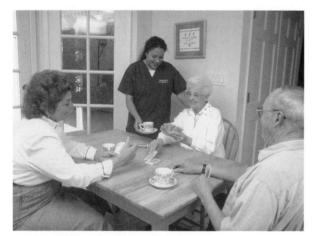

Fig. 1-2. Home care is performed in a person's home.

Adult daycare is given at a facility during daytime working hours. Generally, adult daycare is for people who need some help, but who are not seriously ill or disabled. In the past, aging family members were cared for mostly at home. Today, the **sandwich generation**—the generation caring for children and aging parents at the same time—is often unable to spend enough time at home. If no one can care for an elderly relative at home, or if a person needs a break from caregiving, adult daycare is a good option for busy families.

Some centers have merged adult and child daycare and offer **inter-generational care**. With this type of care, the young and the elderly are able to spend their days together (Fig. 1-3). Many elderly people live far away from close family or do not have family. This kind of care provides "grandparents" or "grandchildren" for those who have none or who live too far away from their own families.

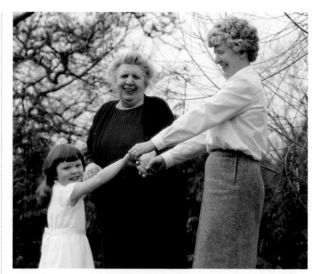

Fig. 1-3. Inter-generational care provides an opportunity for the elderly and the young to spend time together.

Acute care is given in hospitals and ambulatory surgical centers (Fig. 1-4). It is for people who require care for illnesses or injuries. People are also admitted for short stays for surgery. The length of time the person remains will vary depending upon the illness. Acute care is 24-hour skilled care for short-term illnesses or injuries.

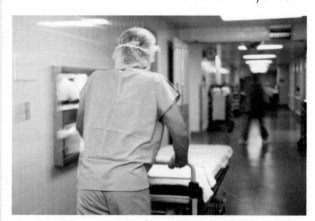

Fig. 1-4. Acute care is performed in hospitals.

Subacute care can be given in a long-term care facility or a hospital. It is used for people who need less care than for an acute illness, but a higher level of care and observation than is given in long-term care. The cost is usually less than hospital care, but more than long-term care. Subacute care will be covered in depth in Chapter 26.

Outpatient care is usually given for less than 24 hours. It is for people who have had treatments or surgery and need short-term skilled care. They are sent home with instructions for further care. Families or friends may play a part in their successful recovery.

Rehabilitation is care given by a specialist or a team of specialists. Physical, occupational, and speech therapists help restore or improve function after an illness or injury. You will learn more about these specialists in Learning Objective 9 of this chapter. Information on rehabilitation is located in Chapter 25.

Hospice care is for people who have approximately six months or less to live. Hospice workers give physical and emotional care and comfort until a person dies, and they also support families during this process. Hospice care can take place in facilities or in homes.

Tip

Pet Therapy

Another addition to adult daycare, inter-generational care, or long-term care is pet therapy. **Pet therapy** provides different kinds of animals to brighten the days of older adults. The Delta Society, founded in 1977 by a physician and a veterinarian, is a national organization dedicated to the therapeutic bond between animals and humans. The group welcomes inquiries from owners interested in volunteering good-natured dogs. You can contact the society by visiting their website, deltasociety.org. Many people love having animals nearby and become attached to them. Allergies or fear of animals must be taken into account when using pet therapy.

Trivia

Early Nursing Schools

The early nursing schools in the 1800s and early 1900s had very strict rules for their students. The classes at that time were made up of women, and they normally lived together in the same building. The schools usually had women who acted as housemothers for the students. Rigid curfews, rules restricting smoking, drinking, and profanity, separation of the sexes, and specific dress codes were strictly enforced. Women were normally not allowed to date or marry, and those who broke the rules suffered severe punishment. The nursing students were expected to work long hours and, in addition to caring for patients, had to wash and wax floors and do chores that today are duties of other employees.

3. Explain Medicare and Medicaid

The Centers for Medicare & Medicaid Services (CMS) is a federal agency within the United States Department of Health and Human Services (Fig. 1-5). CMS runs two national healthcare programs, Medicare and Medicaid. They both help pay for health care and health insurance for millions of Americans. CMS has many other responsibilities as well.

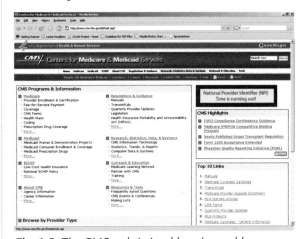

Fig. 1-5. *The CMS website's address is cms.hhs.gov.*

Medicare is a health insurance program for people who are 65 years of age or older. Medicare also covers people younger than 65 who are disabled or ill and cannot work.

Medicare has four parts. Part A helps pay for care in a hospital or skilled nursing facility or for care from a home health agency or hospice. Part B helps pay for doctor services and other medical services and equipment. Part C allows private health insurance companies to provide Medicare benefits. Part D helps pay for medications prescribed for treatment. Medicare will only pay for care it determines to be medically necessary.

Medicaid is a medical assistance program for low-income people. It is funded by both the federal government and each state. Eligibility is determined by income and special circumstances. People must qualify for this program.

Medicare and Medicaid pay long-term care facilities a fixed amount for services. This is based on the resident's needs upon admission.

4. Describe the residents for whom you will care

There are some general statements that can be made about residents in long-term care facilities. However, more important than understanding the entire population is understanding each individual for whom you will care. Make sure you know how to care for residents based on their specific needs, illnesses, and preferences.

According to the National Center for Health Statistics, over 88 percent of long-term care residents in the U.S. are over age 65. Only 11.7 percent are younger than 65. Over 71 percent of residents are female. More than 85 percent are Caucasian (Fig. 1-6). This is a much larger percentage than the U.S. population as a whole. About one-third of residents come from a private residence; almost 64 percent come from a hospital or other facility.

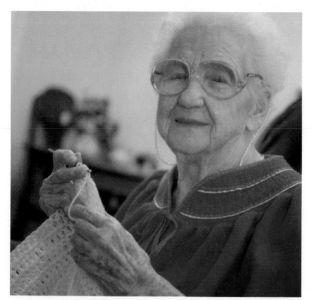

Fig. 1-6. *Caucasian women make up a high percentage of residents in long-term care facilities.*

The **length of stay** is the number of days a person stays in a healthcare facility. The length of stay of over two-thirds of residents in long-term care is six months or longer. These residents need enough help with their activities of daily living to require 24-hour care. Often, they did not have caregivers available to give sufficient care for them to live in the community. The groups with the longest average stay are the developmentally disabled. They are often younger than 65. You will learn more about these groups in Chapter 5.

The other third of residents stay for less than six months. This group generally falls into two categories. The first category is made up of residents admitted for terminal care. They will probably die in the facility. The second category is made up of residents admitted for rehabilitation or temporary illness. They will usually recover and return to the community. As you can imagine, care of these residents may be very different.

Dementia is defined as the loss of mental abilities, such as thinking, remembering, reasoning, and communicating. Various studies place the number of residents with dementia in long-term care facilities between 50 and 90 percent. Dementia and other mental disorders are major causes of admissions to care facilities. Many residents are admitted with other disorders as well. However, the disorders themselves are often not the main reason for admission. It is most often the lack of ability to care for oneself and the lack of a support system that leads people into a facility.

A support system is vital in allowing the elderly to live outside a facility. For every elderly person living in a long-term care facility, at least two with similar disorders and disabilities live in the community.

You may notice the lack of outside support given to your residents. It is one reason you will care for the "whole person" instead of only the illness or disease. Residents have many needs besides bathing, eating, drinking, and toileting. These needs will go unmet if staff do not work to meet them.

5. Describe the nursing assistant's role

A **nursing assistant (NA/CNA)** performs assigned nursing tasks. Most of the tasks deal with helping care for residents. Examples of nursing tasks include taking residents' temperature and blood pressure. A nursing assistant also assists residents with **activities of daily living (ADLs)**, which are personal daily care tasks, such as bathing, skin, nail, and hair care, walking, eating and drinking, mouth care, dressing, transferring, and toileting.

Common nursing assistant tasks include the following:

- Serving trays and feeding residents (Fig. 1-7)

- Helping residents dress and undress

- Bathing residents

- Shampooing hair

- Shaving residents

- Bedmaking

- Tidying residents' living areas

- Measuring vital signs, including temperature, pulse, respiration, blood pressure and observing and reporting pain levels

- Helping residents with toileting needs

- Assisting with mouth care

- Giving back rubs

- Observing and reporting changes in residents' conditions

- Reporting residents' complaints to the nurse

- Helping residents move safely around the facility

- Caring for equipment

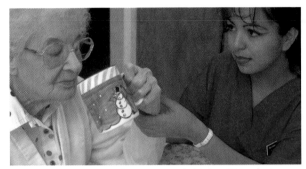

Fig. 1-7. Helping residents eat and drink will be an important part of your job.

Nursing assistants are generally not allowed to give medications. Other tasks that nursing assistants usually do not perform include inserting and removing tubes, giving tube feedings, and changing sterile dressings.

Nursing assistants can have many different titles. Examples include "nurse aide," "patient care attendant," "health care assistant," "patient care technician," and "personal care assistant." This book will use the term "nursing assistant."

6. Discuss professionalism and list examples of professional behavior

Understanding how to be professional is the first step to success in the healthcare field. Professional behavior is vital in the workplace. **Professionalism** has to do with behaving properly on the job. Everything about the way you present yourself to others in a healthcare setting will be closely observed. Dressing appropriately, speaking well, and being dependable and responsible are all part of professionalism. A healthcare facility is a place where professional behavior is expected. Follow these guidelines to behave professionally:

Guidelines: Professional Behavior

G Be neatly dressed and groomed. Keep your uniform and shoes clean.

G Do not discuss personal problems or personal situations with residents. At work, conversation focuses on the resident, not the caregiver.

G Be on time when you are scheduled to work. Call in a timely manner if you are sick or cannot report for duty as scheduled.

G Avoid unnecessary absences. When you are absent, your co-workers have more work to complete.

G Never leave your job early without permission. Report to the nurse in charge when leaving your unit for any reason.

G Do not report to work under the influence of drugs and/or alcohol.

G Keep a positive attitude.

G Do not gossip or speak badly about co-workers or bosses.

G Speak politely to all persons in the facility. Treat all visitors with courtesy and respect.

G Address residents, family members, and visitors in the way they wish to be addressed. Never call someone "honey," "dear," or "sweetie."

G Do not curse or use inappropriate language.

G Keep all resident information confidential.

G Follow all facility policies and procedures.

G Report concerns or problems to your supervisor.

G Meet and maintain all educational requirements.

G Ask questions when you do not understand something.

G Be honest. Document and report carefully and truthfully (Fig. 1-8).

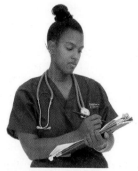

Fig. 1-8. *Writing down what you observe is one of your most important duties.*

G Accept constructive criticism gracefully and learn from it. Constructive criticism is meant to help you improve your performance. An example is, "You need to document care more accurately."

G Do not accept tips or gifts from residents, their families, or other visitors.

G Be loyal to your facility. Be a positive role model.

Behaving professionally will be an ongoing focus of this textbook. Pay attention to this information. Professionalism can earn you the respect of others and help you advance in your job. Not behaving professionally can result in poor performance evaluations, negative relationships with residents and other staff members, and the loss of your job. Always strive to be professional.

7. List qualities that nursing assistants must have

The best nursing assistants have the qualities listed below. As you read through this list, ask yourself whether or not you have these qualities. Nursing assistants should be:

Patient and understanding: Working with ill or disabled people requires patience and understanding. People who are patient remain calm. They are able to put up with difficulties without complaining.

Honest and trustworthy: An honest person tells the truth and can be trusted. Co-workers will depend on honesty in planning care. Employers count on truthful observations and documentation. Residents count on nursing assistants to keep their confidential information private.

Conscientious: Nursing assistants must be conscientious. People who are conscientious are guided by a sense of right and wrong. They always try to do their best. They are alert, observant, accurate, and responsible.

Enthusiastic: People who are enthusiastic have a positive attitude. They are encouraging. They show interest in others, including their situations and problems (Fig. 1-9). Enthusiastic people have a positive influence on others.

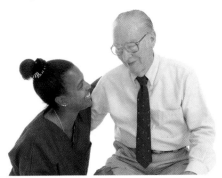

Fig. 1-9. You will be expected to be enthusiastic, cheerful, and positive.

Courteous and **respectful**: Nursing assistants must be kind, polite, and considerate. They should respect others' beliefs, even if they are different from their own.

Empathetic: Empathetic people care about other people's problems. They can think about what it would be like to be ill and dependent on others for help.

Dependable and responsible: Nursing assistants must be at work on time and avoid too many absences. They should always follow policies and procedures. Nursing assistants must be able to be counted on to do their tasks properly.

Humble and open to growth: People who are humble are willing to admit when they have made a mistake. They can accept their limitations. They hold themselves **accountable**. This means that they can admit when they make a mistake and apologize. They can ask others for help when they need it.

Tolerant: Nursing assistants must not judge others. They should keep their opinions to themselves and see people as individuals.

Unprejudiced: Nursing assistants work with different people from many backgrounds. They must give each person quality care regardless of age, gender, sexual orientation, religion, race, ethnicity, or condition.

8. Discuss proper grooming guidelines

Making positive **first impressions** can help you obtain the things you want, such as getting a job. Nursing assistants must pay attention to the way they present themselves to residents, their family members and friends, and to other staff members. Good grooming is essential to making a good first impression. Some important grooming guidelines are listed below:

Guidelines: Grooming

G Keep your uniform clean, neat, and pressed. Make sure your uniform fits you properly.

G Bathe or shower every day. Wear deodorant or anti-perspirant.

G Brush your teeth at least twice a day.

G Avoid using strongly-scented items, such as perfume, cologne, after-shave, body washes, body creams and lotions, hair spray, and fabric softeners.

G Keep your hair neatly tied back and away from your face.

G Keep beards trimmed and neat-looking.

G Apply makeup lightly or use none at all.

G Keep nails short, filed, and clean. As older people have fragile skin, this is very important. Follow facility policy regarding nail polish. It may not be allowed.

G Do not wear artificial nails. Artificial nails harbor bacteria, no matter how well you wash your hands.

G Keep shoes and laces clean. Shoes should be in good condition. They should be comfortable. They should not look worn and old. Change or wash shoelaces when they become soiled.

G Wear as little jewelry as possible. Sharp edges on jewelry can scratch or tear fragile skin. Remove rings and bracelets while working. They collect bacteria and can cause infection. They may also cause problems with wearing gloves. Remove necklaces while working; necklaces may also hide bacteria. Confused residents may pull on necklaces and break them. Wear small earrings that will not snag on things and that confused residents cannot pull on.

You will need to wear a simple, waterproof watch and an identification badge (Fig. 1-10). You will need a watch to take a resident's pulse and respirations and record events. An identification badge identifies you to residents, visitors, and other staff members.

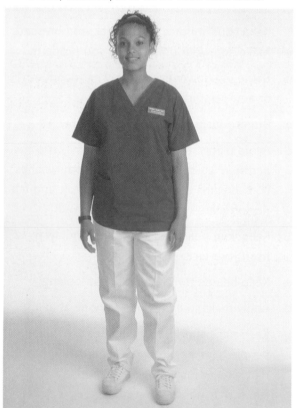

Fig. 1-10. Wearing a clean uniform, a watch, and identification badge are examples of professional behavior.

Tip

Kill the scent!

Residents may have allergies that are worsened by scents. Residents may also be very aware of scents because they do not feel well. Think about how you feel when you are sick. You must always try to meet the needs of residents in every way. That means respecting their individual problems and putting their comfort first. Avoid using heavily-scented items.

9. Define the role of each member of the care team

The **care team** consists of many members who have had different training and experience in order to provide care for each resident (Fig. 1-11). The resident is the most important part—the center—of the care team. Members of the care team include the following:

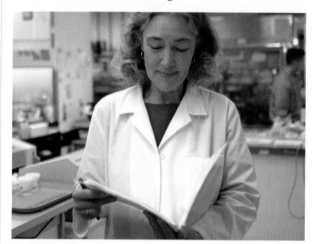

Fig. 1-11. The care team is made up of many different types of professionals.

Resident and Resident's Family: The care team revolves around the resident. Residents make choices about their care. They help plan their care. The resident's family and friends may help with these decisions. They play another important role, too. Family and friends may share vital information about the resident with the care team. This information includes the resident's health and medical record, personal preferences, rituals, and routines.

Nurse: A nurse assesses residents, creates the care plan, monitors progress, and gives treatments. Your immediate supervisor may be a registered nurse (RN), a licensed practical nurse (LPN), or a licensed vocational nurse (LVN). An explanation of the different types of nurses follows in the next three paragraphs.

Registered Nurse (RN): A person who has graduated from a state-licensed nursing program (two to four years of education) and has passed a national examination.

Licensed Practical or Licensed Vocational Nurse (LPN/LVN): A person who has graduated from a state-licensed nursing program (one to two years of education) and has passed a national examination.

Advanced Practice Nurse (APRN): an advanced practice nurse is a registered nurse who has completed training at the graduate level as a certified nurse practitioner (CNP), nurse anesthetist (CRNA), nurse midwife (CNM), or clinical nurse specialist (CNS). There are also other types of advanced practice nurses such as the gerontological nurse practitioner (GNP).

Physician or Doctor [MD (medical doctor) or DO (doctor of osteopathy)]: A doctor diagnoses disease or disability and prescribes treatment. A **diagnosis** is the identification of a disease by its signs and symptoms and/or results from testing. A doctor has graduated from medical school after first receiving a bachelor's degree. Many doctors also take specialized training programs after medical school.

Medical Social Worker (MSW): A medical social worker helps with social needs. For example, an MSW helps residents find compatible roommates. An MSW also helps with support services, such as counseling and financial assistance.

Physical Therapist (PT): A physical therapist gives therapy in the form of heat, cold, massage, ultrasound, electricity, and exercise to muscles, bones, and joints (Fig. 1-12). This is done to improve blood circulation, promote healing, ease pain, and help the resident regain mobility.

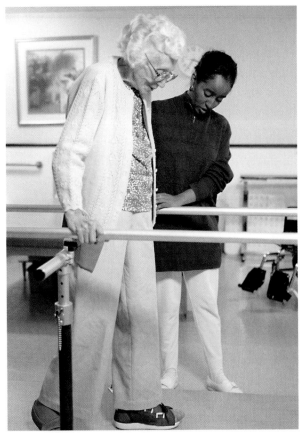

Fig. 1-12. *A physical therapist helps exercise muscles, bones, and joints to improve strength or restore abilities.*

Occupational Therapist (OT): An occupational therapist works with people who need help with activities of daily living (ADLs). An OT evaluates a resident's ability to do these activities, and **assistive** or **adaptive devices** may be ordered to help. These devices help residents perform ADLs. An example is a special spoon that helps a person feed himself (Fig. 1-13).

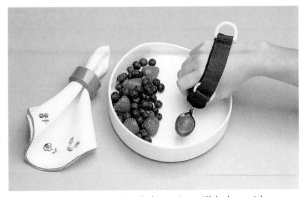

Fig. 1-13. *An occupational therapist will help residents learn to use adaptive devices, such as this special spoon and plate.* (PHOTO COURTESY OF NORTH COAST MEDICAL, INC. 800-821-9319)

Registered Dietitian (RDT): A registered dietitian or nutritionist assesses nutritional status and plans a care program. A dietitian creates diets for residents with special needs. These special diets can improve health and help manage illness.

Speech-Language Pathologist (SLP): A speech-language pathologist or speech therapist teaches exercises to help the resident improve or overcome speech problems. An SLP also evaluates a person's ability to swallow food and drink.

Activities Director: The activities director plans activities, such as bingo or special performances, to help residents socialize and stay physically and mentally active.

Nursing Assistant or Certified Nursing Assistant (NA or CNA): The nursing assistant does assigned tasks, such as taking a resident's temperature. NAs also give personal care, such as bathing residents, brushing their teeth, and assisting with toileting. Nursing assistants are some of the most important team members because they have the most direct contact with residents. If a resident's health changes from day to day, they will often be the first ones to notice this change. Nursing assistants must report any changes in a resident's condition to the nurse promptly. The federal government requires that nursing assistants have at least 75 hours of training. Some states require more than 75 hours of training.

Nursing assistant may be abbreviated as "NA," which usually means the person has completed a state-accredited nursing assistant training program. A certified nursing assistant (CNA) generally has advanced further by passing the state test for certification. You will learn more about training requirements in Chapter 2.

10. Discuss the facility chain of command

The **chain of command** describes the line of authority in the facility. For example, the nurse

will usually be the nursing assistant's immediate supervisor. If a nursing assistant has a problem with another department, he or she will report this to the proper person. This is usually an immediate supervisor or the **charge nurse**, who is a nurse responsible for a team of healthcare workers. The nursing assistant would not go directly to the department to tell them of the problem. That would not be following the chain of command (Fig. 1-14).

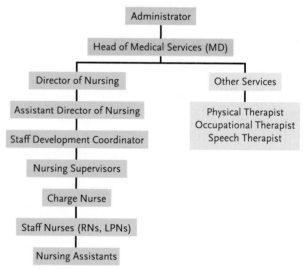

Fig. 1-14. *The chain of command describes the line of authority in a facility and helps ensure that the resident receives proper care.*

The chain of command also helps to protect staff from **liability**. Liability is a legal term. It means a person can be held responsible for harming someone else. Consider this example: A nursing assistant gives care to a resident and he is injured. If the care was assigned and was done according to policy and procedure, the nursing assistant may not be liable, or responsible, for hurting the resident. However, if a nursing assistant performs a task that is not assigned to her or is not within her scope of practice, and it harms a resident, she could be held responsible. That is why it is important to follow instructions and the chain of command. Doing this helps lessen the risk of liability. When handling any problem, speak with your supervisor first.

11. Explain "The Five Rights of Delegation"

When planning care, nurses have to decide which tasks to delegate to others. This includes nursing assistants. **Delegation** means transferring authority to a person for a specific task. Licensed nurses are accountable for care, including all delegated tasks. The National Council of State Boards of Nursing has identified "The Five Rights of Delegation." This can be used as a mental checklist to help nurses in the decision-making process.

"The Five Rights of Delegation" are the "Right Task," "Right Circumstance," "Right Person," "Right Direction/Communication," and "Right Supervision/Evaluation." Before delegating tasks, nurses consider these questions:

- Is there a match between the resident's needs and the nursing assistant's skills, abilities, and experience?

- What is the level of resident stability?

- Is the nursing assistant the right person to do the job?

- Can the nurse give appropriate direction and communication?

- Is the nurse available to give the supervision, support, and help that the nursing assistant needs?

There are questions you may want to consider before accepting a task:

- Do I have all the information I need to do this job? Are there questions I should ask?

- Do I believe that I can do this task? Do I have the necessary skills?

- Do I have the needed supplies, equipment, and other support?

- Do I know who my supervisor is, and how to reach him/her?

- Have I told my supervisor of my special needs for help and support?

- Do we both understand who is doing what?

Never be afraid to ask for help. Always ask if you need more information or if you are unsure about something. If you feel that you do not have the skills for a task, talk to the nurse.

12. Describe four methods of nursing care

The nursing profession takes a holistic view of resident care. The word "holistic" comes from a Greek word meaning "whole." **Holistic** means considering a whole system, such as a whole person, and not dividing the system up into parts. Holistic care is caring for the whole person. This includes his or her physical needs, as well as other needs, such as social, emotional, intellectual, and spiritual (Fig. 1-15). Meeting these needs helps improve residents' quality of life. You will learn more about these needs in Chapter 5.

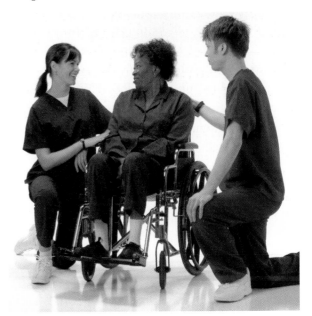

Fig. 1-15. *Caring for residents holistically means considering their emotional needs as well as their physical needs.*

Over the years, the nursing profession has seen many changes. Many types of nursing care have been used at facilities. Each facility chooses the type that provides the best care for their residents.

Resident-Focused Care: This style of nursing care focuses on the resident and his or her family. It is based upon a partnership between the residents, their families and their caregivers. Residents and families are active participants in care. Choices made by residents and their families are honored by caregivers whenever possible. Families are encouraged to participate in the actual care. Healthcare providers and caregivers share useful and accurate information with residents and families.

Team Nursing: A registered nurse has the role of the **team leader** in this method. Assignments are made, care is given, and the team members report to the team leader throughout the day. The resident's care is managed efficiently and cooperatively by using this team approach to care.

Primary Nursing: With this method, a registered nurse gives much of the daily care to residents. This type of care allows for a closer relationship between the nurse and the residents. Consistency and continuity of care are positive results of this method. **Continuity of care** is coordination of care for a resident over time. The nursing team exchanges information about the resident throughout the day, while working toward shared goals.

Functional Nursing: Staff provide care to large numbers of residents during each shift using this method. Each member of the care team is given one or more specific tasks to complete for a large number of residents. For example, one team member is assigned to measure vital signs on all residents in the unit. Another completes all of the daily weights. One nurse administers medications, while another gives treatments. This type of care is not as organized as other methods. Staff may not have enough time to accurately observe each resident, and changes in a resident's condition may be overlooked.

13. Explain policy and procedure manuals

All facilities have manuals outlining policies and procedures. A **policy** is a course of action to be taken every time a certain situation occurs. The policy manual has information about every facility policy. For example, one basic policy is that the chain of command must always be followed.

A **procedure** is a specific method, or way, of doing something. The procedure manual has information on the exact way to complete every procedure. For example, there will be a procedure for giving a resident a bed bath.

Everyone needs a reminder about how to perform a task from time to time. The procedure manual serves as a guide if you want to review the steps in a procedure. Do not hesitate to look at the procedure manual. Nursing assistants who ask questions when they are unsure provide safer resident care. Acting confident when you are unsure of how to perform a procedure can be dangerous. Always ask if you have questions.

The policy and procedure manuals are usually kept together. Know where these manuals are so that you may review them when necessary.

14. Describe the long-term care survey process

Inspections are done to make sure long-term care facilities (and home health agencies) are following state and federal regulations. Inspections are done periodically by the state agency that licenses facilities. These inspections are called surveys. They may be done more often if a facility has been cited for problems. To **cite** means to find a problem through a survey. Inspections may be done less often if the facility has a good record. Inspection teams include a variety of trained healthcare professionals.

Surveyors study how well the staff cares for its residents. They focus on how residents' nutritional, physical, social, emotional, and spiritual needs are being met. They interview residents and families and observe the staff's interactions with residents and the care given. They review resident charts and observe meals. Surveys are one reason the "paperwork" part of a nursing assistant's job is so important.

If a facility is cited for not following a federal regulation, surveyors use special tags to note these problems. When surveyors are in your facility, try not to be nervous. Give the same great care you do every day. Answer any questions to the best of your ability. If you do not know the answer, be honest. Never guess. Tell the surveyor that you do not know the answer, but will find out as quickly as possible. Then do just that.

The **Joint Commission**, formerly the Joint Commission on Accreditation of Healthcare Organizations (JCAHO), is an independent, not-for-profit organization whose standards focus on improving the quality and safety of care provided by healthcare facilities. The Joint Commission makes sure each facility is following the standards of care by inspecting and evaluating different types of healthcare facilities. The Joint Commission's surveys are not associated with state inspections.

Facilities join the Joint Commission on a voluntary basis; some do not participate in this process. In order to receive the Joint Commission's approval, facilities must pass evaluations at least every three years. A facility may be visited more often if problems are found.

Chapter Review

1. Describe long-term care (LO 2).

2. Whom does Medicare insurance cover (LO 3)?

3. Who makes up the majority of residents in long-term care facilities—men or women (LO 4)?

4. List ten common nursing assistant tasks (LO 5).

5. What are three tasks that nursing assistants do not usually perform (LO 5)?

6. List ten ways a nursing assistant can show professional behavior (LO 6).

7. List each of the ten qualities in Learning Objective 7. For each quality, write one example of a way that a nursing assistant can demonstrate that quality (LO 7).

8. Describe ten grooming guidelines for nursing assistants (LO 8).

9. Who is the most important part of the care team (LO 9)?

10. Choose four members of the care team and describe the roles they play (LO 9).

11. Define the chain of command (LO 10).

12. List the "Five Rights of Delegation" (LO 11).

13. Give a brief description of the four methods of nursing care (LO 12).

14. What is a policy? What is a procedure (LO 13)?

15. When surveyors visit a facility, what do they study and observe (LO 14)?

16. When a surveyor asks a nursing assistant a question she does not know the answer to, how should she respond (LO 14)?

2
Ethical and Legal Issues

The First Code of Ethics

An English physician named Thomas Percival wrote a code of ethics called "Percival's Medical Ethics" in 1803. Here is a sample from that first code of ethics: "A physician ought not to abandon a patient because the case is deemed incurable, for his attendance may continue to be highly useful to the patient, and comforting to the relatives around him . . ." In 1847, Percival's Medical Ethics was used to help develop the American Medical Association's first code of ethics. The American Medical Association Principles is still the code of ethics that physicians use today.

"It's a funny thing about life, if you refuse to accept anything but the best, you very often get it."

W. Somerset Maugham, 1874-1965

"Wherever there is a human being, I see God-given rights inherent in that being, whatever may be the sex or complexion."

William Lloyd Garrison, 1805-1879

1. Define important words in this chapter

abuse: causing physical, mental, emotional, or financial pain or injury to someone.

active neglect: purposely harming a person physically, mentally, or emotionally by failing to provide needed care.

advance directives: legal documents that allow people to decide what kind of medical care they wish to have if they are unable to make those decisions themselves.

assault: the act of threatening to touch a person without his or her consent.

battery: touching a person without his or her consent.

civil law: private law; law between individuals.

criminal law: public law; related to committing a crime against the community.

DNR (do-not-resuscitate): an order that tells medical professionals not to perform CPR.

domestic violence: physical, sexual, or emotional abuse by spouses, intimate partners, or family members.

durable power of attorney for health care: a signed and dated legal document that appoints someone to make the medical decisions for a person in the event he or she becomes unable to do so.

ethics: the knowledge of right and wrong; standards of conduct.

etiquette: the code of proper behavior and courtesy in a certain setting.

false imprisonment: the unlawful restraint of someone which affects the person's freedom of movement; includes both the threat of being physically restrained and actually being physically restrained.

financial abuse: the act of stealing, taking advantage of, or improperly using the money, property, or other assets of another.

HIPAA (Health Insurance Portability and Accountability Act): a federal law that sets standards for protecting the privacy of patients' health information.

invasion of privacy: a violation of the right to be left alone and the right to control personal information.

involuntary seclusion: separating or confining a person from others against the person's will.

laws: rules set by the government to help protect the public.

living will: a document that states the medical care a person wants, or does not want, in case he or she becomes unable to make those decisions.

malpractice: a negligent or improper act by a professional that results in damage or injury to a person.

mandated reporters: people who are required to report suspected or observed abuse or neglect due to their regular contact with vulnerable populations, such as the elderly in long-term care facilities.

misappropriation: the act of taking what belongs to someone else and using it illegally for one's own gain.

NATCEP (Nurse Aide Training and Competency Evaluation Program): part of OBRA that sets minimum requirements for nursing assistants for training and testing.

negligence: actions, or a failure to act or give proper care, that result in injury to a person.

OBRA (Omnibus Budget Reconciliation Act): federal law that includes minimum standards for nursing assistant training, staffing requirements, resident assessment instructions, and information on rights for residents.

ombudsman: person assigned by law as the legal advocate for residents.

passive neglect: unintentionally harming a person physically, mentally, or emotionally by failing to provide needed care.

physical abuse: intentional or unintentional treatment that causes harm or injury to a person's body.

protected health information (PHI): information that can be used to identify a person and relates to the patient's past, present, or future physical or mental condition, including any health care the patient has had, or payment for that health care.

psychological abuse: any behavior that causes a person to feel threatened, fearful, intimidated, or humiliated in any way.

Residents' Council: a group of residents who meet regularly to discuss issues related to the long-term care facility.

Residents' Rights: rights identified in OBRA that relate to how residents must be treated while living in a long-term care facility; they provide an ethical code of conduct for healthcare workers.

scope of practice: defines the tasks that healthcare providers are legally permitted to perform as allowed by state or federal law.

sexual abuse: forcing a person to perform or participate in sexual acts against his or her will.

sexual harassment: any unwelcome sexual advance or behavior that creates an intimidating, hostile or offensive working environment.

substance abuse: the use of legal or illegal drugs, cigarettes, or alcohol in a way that is harmful to the abuser or to others.

verbal abuse: the use of language—spoken or written—that threatens, embarrasses, or insults a person.

workplace violence: verbal, physical, or sexual abuse of staff by residents, other staff members, or visitors.

2. Define the terms "law," "ethics," and "etiquette"

There are many legal and ethical terms that relate to resident care. **Ethics** are the knowledge of what is right and wrong; they help guide conduct. Ethics help us make decisions at home, in the workplace, or in the community. In healthcare, ethics guide the people giving care. For example, keeping a resident's information confidential is ethical behavior. It is also the law.

Laws are rules set by the government to help protect the public. In healthcare, laws protect those receiving care (Fig. 2-1). For example, there is a law against stealing a resident's belongings.

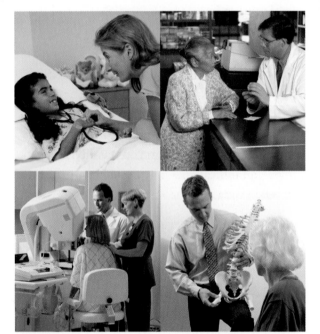

Fig. 2-1. *All healthcare providers must behave ethically and follow the law.*

Laws can be civil or criminal. **Criminal laws** are written to protect society from people or organizations that try to do them harm. This type of law protects the public. It is also called "public law." **Civil law** refers to disputes between individuals. Problems with landlords, conflicts with neighbors, and divorce issues are examples of areas covered by civil law. Civil law is sometimes referred to as "private law."

Criminal law includes these offenses (crimes):

- A misdemeanor is any crime that is not a felony. It is not as serious an offense as a felony. Disturbing the peace is an example of a misdemeanor. Punishment may include community service time, a fine, and/or a short prison term.

- A felony is a more serious crime than a misdemeanor. Murder and bribery are examples of felonies. Punishment may include a longer prison term, such as life without parole, or even a death sentence.

Etiquette is the code of proper behavior and courtesy in a certain setting. For example, identify yourself when you answer the phone at your facility. Ask, "How may I help you?" This is proper telephone etiquette.

3. Discuss examples of ethical and professional behavior

A nursing assistant's ethics play an important part in his or her success as a care team member. Professional and ethical behavior is vital to the safety and well-being of the residents. Below are guidelines for behavior that nursing assistants must follow:

Guidelines: Legal and Ethical Behavior

G Keep all resident information confidential (private). This is one of the Residents' Rights covered later in this chapter. All team members must keep resident information confidential. You can only discuss residents with specific members of the care team.

G Keep staff information confidential. Do not share private information about your coworkers at home or anywhere else.

G Be honest at all times. Communicate honestly and clearly with members of the care team. Be honest when documenting resident care.

Be truthful when reporting the hours you have worked. Do not take items that do not belong to you.

G   Be trustworthy. Trusting others is important in facilities. Residents must be able to trust staff members. Employers must be able to trust their employees. Employees need to trust their supervisors. One way employees can show that they are trustworthy is to be at work on time each day. When an employee often fails to show up for work, the boss cannot trust or count on that employee. Employers also trust that employees will come to them if they have a problem. This is following the chain of command.

G   Do not accept tips or gifts from residents or their family members or friends (Fig. 2-2).

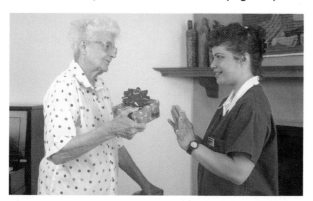

Fig. 2-2. Nursing assistants should not accept money or gifts because it is unprofessional and can lead to conflict.

G   Report abuse or suspected abuse of residents. You will learn more about abuse in Learning Objective 7 of this chapter.

G   Do not report to work under the influence of alcohol or drugs.

G   Follow all facility policies, rules, and procedures. Document care you give accurately and promptly.

G   Do your assigned tasks. If you make a mistake, report it promptly to the nurse. This can help minimize damage and prevent any further problems.

G   Be positive and professional. Residents deserve caregivers who will try to make their days as pleasant as possible. A person who is cheerful and encouraging is someone others like to be around.

G   Be tactful. Tact is the ability to understand what is proper and appropriate when dealing with others. It is the ability to speak and act without offending others.

G   Treat all residents with respect, and be empathetic. Respect means allowing others to believe or act as they wish to do. Empathy means being able to share in and understand the feelings and troubles of others. A caring person is empathetic with a person who is ill. A caring person also respects an ill person's actions or beliefs about the illness, despite her own feelings.

G   Be patient. Nursing assistants have to deal with residents' troubles and pain without being frustrated. Activities of daily living (ADLs), such as eating, dressing, and toileting, may take older people much longer and use up much of their energy, leaving them tired (Fig. 2-3). Residents should be allowed to do tasks at their own pace. The more patient you are, the better care you will provide.

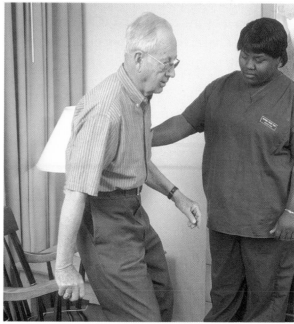

Fig. 2-3. Older adults may need extra time with ADLs. Be patient and allow them to do tasks at their own pace.

Tip

Gifts and Tips

Accepting gifts or tips is not allowed in the health-care field. It is unprofessional and can lead to conflict. Nursing assistants and other staff receive payment from the facility for the work they do. If a resident, family member, or visitor offers to tip you or tries to give you a gift, politely refuse. Explain that it would not be ethical for you to accept it and that it is against the facility's policies.

4. Describe a nursing assistant code of ethics

Many facilities have adopted a formal code of ethics. This helps their employees deal with issues of right and wrong. Codes of ethics differ, but all revolve around the idea that a resident is a valuable person who deserves ethical care. A sample code of ethics for nursing assistants is shown below:

1. I will strive to provide and maintain the highest quality of care for my residents. I will fully recognize and follow all of the Residents' Rights.

2. I will communicate well, serve on committees, and read all material as provided and required by my employer. I will attend educational in-services, and join organizations relevant to nursing assistant care.

3. I will show a positive attitude toward my residents, their family members, staff, and other visitors.

4. I will always provide privacy for my residents. I will maintain confidentiality of resident, staff, and visitor information.

5. I will be trustworthy and honest in all dealings with residents, staff, and visitors.

6. I will strive to preserve resident safety. I will report mistakes I make, along with anything that I deem dangerous, to the right person(s).

7. I will have empathy for my residents, other staff, and all visitors, giving support and encouragement when needed.

8. I will respect all people, without regard to age, gender, ethnicity, religion, economic situation, sexual orientation, or diagnosis.

9. I will never abuse my residents in any way. I will always report any suspected abuse to the proper person immediately.

10. I will strive to have the utmost patience with all people at my facility.

Tip

Never call yourself a nurse.

Nursing assistants must *never* identify themselves as nurses. Nurses have had more education and training than nursing assistants. Nurses have different responsibilities than nursing assistants do. Calling yourself a nurse could result in injury to yourself or others, a lawsuit, and/or being fired from your job. So never use the term "nurse" lightly; always identify yourself as a nursing assistant.

5. Explain the Omnibus Budget Reconciliation Act (OBRA)

The Omnibus Budget Reconciliation Act (OBRA) was passed in 1987. It has been updated many times since then. OBRA was written in response to reports of poor care and abuse in long-term care facilities. Congress decided to set minimum standards of care. This included standardizing training of nursing assistants.

OBRA requires that the **Nurse Aide Training and Competency Evaluation Program (NATCEP)** set minimum requirements for nursing assistants. Nursing assistants must complete at least 75 hours of training. However, programs may exceed these minimums. Many states require 80 to 150 program hours in theory and clinical skills. These skills include basic nursing skills, personal care skills, restorative skills, and training for mental health and social service needs, Residents' Rights, and safety and emergency care.

Nursing assistants must also pass a competency evaluation (testing program) before they can be employed. The exam consists of both written and demonstrated nursing skills. Nursing assistants must also attend regular in-service education classes (Fig. 2-4).

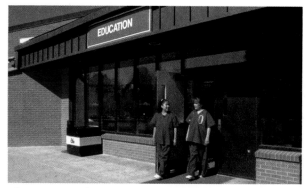

Fig. 2-4. *Completing in-service education successfully is an OBRA requirement for nursing assistants.*

OBRA also requires that states keep a current list of nursing assistants in a state registry. In addition, OBRA identifies standards that instructors must meet in order to train nursing assistants. OBRA sets guidelines for minimum staff requirements and specifies services that long-term care facilities must provide.

Another important part of OBRA is the resident assessment requirements. OBRA requires complete assessments on every resident. The assessment forms are the same for every facility. The MDS (Minimum Data Set) is a resident assessment system that was developed in 1990. It is revised periodically. The MDS is a detailed form with guidelines for assessing residents. You will learn more about the MDS in Chapter 3.

OBRA also identifies important rights for residents in long-term care facilities. You will learn about these rights in Learning Objective 6.

OBRA regulations are important to nursing assistant practice because they do these things:

- Give recognition through certification and registration

- Help define the nursing assistant's **scope of practice**, which specifies the tasks that nursing assistants are legally permitted to perform as allowed by state or federal law

- Provide better uniformity of care

- Promote educational standards

Tip

What is the State Board of Nursing?

In your state, this agency might have a different name. However, the responsibilities will be similar. The State Board of Nursing is in charge of licensing all nurses and testing and certification of nursing assistants. This agency may also handle issues and problems with nurses and nursing assistants.

Tip

Reciprocity

When you have completed an approved nursing assistant course, you may be eligible for nursing assistant certification. When you move to another state, your certification may transfer to that state. This is called "reciprocity." Before moving to another state, contact the agency there that handles nursing assistant issues and find out if you qualify for reciprocity. If needed, gather important paperwork from your original state before you leave. Obtaining a new certificate in your new state is your responsibility and will be necessary before you can begin working there.

6. Explain Residents' Rights

Residents' Rights specify how residents must be treated while living in a facility. They provide an ethical code of conduct for healthcare workers. Facilities give residents a list of these rights and review each right with them. Be familiar with these legal rights. Residents' Rights are very detailed, and they include the following:

Quality of life: Residents have the right to the best care available. Dignity, choice, and independence are important parts of quality of life.

Services and activities to maintain a high level of wellness: Residents must receive the correct care. Facilities are required to develop a care plan that helps determine residents' daily activities. Residents' care must keep them as healthy as possible. Their health should not decline as a direct result of the facility's care.

The right to be fully informed about rights and services: Residents must be told what services are offered and what the fee is for each service. Residents must be given a copy of their legal rights, along with the facility's rules and regulations. These rights must be in a language that each resident can understand. Residents must be given the names and phone numbers of state agencies related to quality of care, such as the ombudsman. Survey results must be shared with residents if they request to see them. Residents have the right to be notified about any change of room or roommate. Residents have the right to communicate with someone who speaks their language. They have the right to assistance for any sensory impairment, such as hearing loss.

The right to participate in their own care: Residents have the right to participate in planning their treatment, care, and discharge (Fig. 2-5). They have the right to change care providers at any time. Residents have the right to refuse medication, treatment, care, and restraints. They have the right to be told of changes in their condition. They have the right to review their medical record.

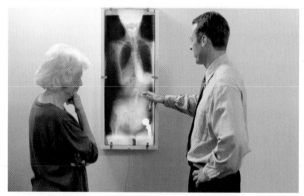

Fig. 2-5. *Residents have the right to be informed about their care and to make decisions about the kind of care they want.*

The right to make independent choices: Residents can make choices about their doctors, care, and treatments. They can make personal decisions, such as what to wear and how to spend their time. They can join in community activities, both inside and outside the care facility.

They have the right to act within a Residents' Council.

A **Residents' Council** is a group of residents who meet regularly to discuss issues related to the long-term care facility. This Council gives residents a voice in facility operations. Topics of discussion may include facility policies, decisions regarding activities, concerns, and problems. The Residents' Council offers residents a chance to provide suggestions on improving the quality of care. Council executives are elected by residents. Family members are invited to attend meetings with or on behalf of residents. Staff may participate in this process when invited by Council members.

The right to privacy and confidentiality: Residents have the right to speak privately with anyone, the right to privacy during care, and the right to confidentiality regarding every aspect of their lives. They have the right to send mail and receive mail that is unopened (Fig. 2-6). Their medical and personal information cannot be shared with anyone but the care team. You will learn more about confidentiality in Learning Objective 11 of this chapter.

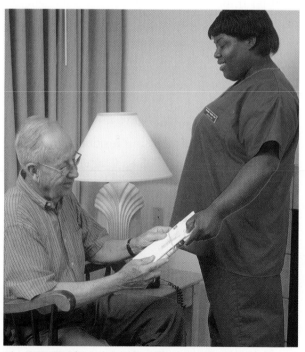

Fig. 2-6. *Residents have the right to privacy, which includes being able to receive unopened mail.*

The right to dignity, respect and freedom: Residents must be respected and treated with dignity by caregivers. Residents cannot be abused, mistreated, or neglected in any way.

The right to security of possessions: Residents' personal possessions must be safe at all times. They cannot be taken or used by anyone without a resident's permission. Residents have the right to file a complaint with the state agency for misappropriation of property. **Misappropriation** is taking what belongs to someone else and using it illegally for one's own gain. Residents have the right to control their finances or to choose someone else to do it for them. They have the right to not be charged for any care covered by Medicaid or Medicare.

Rights during transfers and discharges: Residents have the right to be informed of and to consent to any location changes. Residents can be moved from the facility if their safety is at risk, if their health has improved, if the move is needed to protect others at the facility, or if payment for care is not received by the facility. Residents also have the right to stay in a facility unless a transfer or discharge is needed.

The right to complain: Residents have the right to complain without any fear for their safety or care. They also have the right to a quick response to their concerns.

The right to visits: Residents have the right to visits from doctors, family members, friends, ombudsmen, clergy members, legal representatives, or any other person (Fig. 2-7).

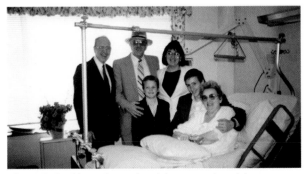

Fig. 2-7. Residents have the right to receive visitors at any reasonable hour.

Rights with regard to social services: The facility must provide residents with access to social services. This includes counseling, assistance in solving problems with others (mediation), and help contacting legal and financial professionals.

Throughout this book you will see special boxes that will teach you how to promote Residents' Rights. Pay close attention to this information. You must obey legal and ethical workplace guidelines.

7. Explain types of abuse and neglect

Preventing abuse and neglect is a very important part of Residents' Rights. In order to do this, it helps if you understand more about the different types of abuse and neglect. **Abuse** means causing physical, mental, emotional, or financial pain or injury to someone. There are many different types of abuse, including the following:

Physical abuse is intentional or unintentional treatment that causes harm to a person's body. Physical abuse includes hitting, kicking, cutting, burning, pushing, or touching a resident in any way that causes pain or injury. It also includes rough handling of a person. Pushing a resident to move faster is one example of physical abuse. Hitting or pinching a resident is another example. Holding or restraining a resident is also considered abuse.

Psychological abuse is any behavior that causes a person to feel threatened, fearful, intimidated, or humiliated in any way. It also includes verbal abuse. **Verbal abuse** involves the use of language—spoken or written—that threatens, embarrasses, or insults a person. Threatening to harm a resident if he tells another caregiver about a problem is one example of psychological abuse. Sharing private or potentially embarrassing issues among residents is another example of psychological abuse.

Sexual abuse is forcing a person to perform or participate in sexual acts. Any kind of sexual behavior that causes a person to be fearful and feel threatened sexually is sexual abuse. For example, showing sexually explicit magazines to residents is sexual abuse. Rubbing against a resident inappropriately during personal care is also sexual abuse.

Financial abuse is the act of stealing, taking advantage of, or improperly using the money, property, or other assets of another person. For example, offering to give a resident "special" care if the resident pays the nursing assistant for it is financial abuse. Stealing money from a resident is also considered financial abuse.

Assault is threatening to touch a person without his or her consent. The person feels fearful that he or she will be harmed. Telling a resident that she will be slapped if she does not stop yelling is an example.

Battery means a person is actually touched without his or her consent. An example is a nursing assistant hitting or pushing a resident. This is also considered physical abuse. Performing a procedure on a resident who has refused the procedure is also considered battery.

Domestic violence is abuse by spouses, intimate partners, or family members. It can be physical, sexual, or emotional. The victim can be a woman or man of any age or a child.

Workplace violence is abuse of staff by other staff members, residents, or visitors. It can be verbal, physical, or sexual. One staff member hitting another staff member is an example of workplace violence. Another example is a resident who insults a nursing assistant's culture. Workplace violence also includes improper touching and discussion about sexual subjects.

False imprisonment is the unlawful restraint of someone which affects the person's freedom of movement. Both the threat of being physically restrained and actually being physically restrained are false imprisonment. Not allowing a resident to leave the building is also considered false imprisonment. This does not include some

people with dementia, who may be confined for their safety.

Involuntary seclusion is separating a person from others against the person's will. A resident who is made to stay in her room with the door closed during the dinner hour is a victim of involuntary seclusion.

Sexual harassment is any unwelcome sexual advance or behavior that creates an intimidating, hostile or offensive working environment. Requests for sexual favors, unwanted touching, and other acts of a sexual nature are examples of sexual harassment. A supervisor telling a team member that if she has sex with him, she will get the work schedule she wants is an example of sexual harassment.

Substance abuse is the use of legal or illegal drugs, cigarettes, or alcohol in a way that harms oneself or others. Substances can be legal, or even prescribed, and still be abused. For example, alcohol and cigarettes are legal for adults, but are often abused. Over-the-counter medications can be addictive and harmful (Fig. 2-8). Even paint or glue may be abused. Information on signs of substance abuse is in Chapter 22.

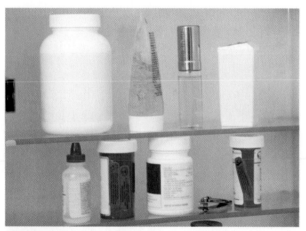

Fig. 2-8. Both prescription and non-prescription drugs can be abused.

Neglect can be divided into two categories: active neglect and passive neglect. **Active neglect** means purposely harming a person physically, mentally, or emotionally by failing to provide needed care. Examples include deliberately leaving a bedridden resident alone for lengthy periods, ignoring a resident's call light, or willfully denying the resident food, medication, dentures, or eyeglasses. **Passive neglect** is unintentionally harming a person physically, mentally, or emotionally by failing to provide needed care. The caregiver may not know how to properly care for the resident, or may not understand the resident's needs. An example of passive neglect is forgetting to bring water to a resident who has a doctor's order to drink extra fluids.

Negligence is actions, or a failure to act or give proper care, that result in injury to a person. A nursing assistant who forgets to lock the bed wheels before transferring a resident to a chair is being negligent. The bed can roll backward and cause the resident to fall and injure herself. **Malpractice** occurs when a negligent or improper act by a doctor, nurse, or other professional results in damage or injury to a person.

If you see or suspect that a resident is being abused in any way, you are legally required to report it. Report abuse immediately to your supervisor. Document any complaints of abuse reported to you and anything you witness yourself. If action is not taken, keep reporting up the chain of command. Do this until action is taken. If no appropriate action is taken at the facility, call the state abuse hotline. If no abuse hotline exists, contact the proper state agency. You can report abuse in a way that protects you and does not identify you. These agencies are required to promptly investigate reports of abuse.

If residents want to make a complaint of abuse themselves, you must assist in every possible way. This includes informing them of the process and their rights.

Never retaliate against a resident making a complaint of abuse. If you witness another team member retaliating against a resident who made a complaint, you must report it. Follow the chain of command. All care team members are responsible for residents' safety.

Residents' Rights

They are all your residents.

All of the residents in your area or unit are your residents. Even though you may be assigned a certain number of residents, you must still respond to any resident in need. Never say, "He/she is not my resident."

8. Recognize signs and symptoms of abuse and neglect

Abuse can be suspected when staff observe certain signs and symptoms. All care team members must look for these signs and report them. Many of the signs of abuse are listed below.

Observing and Reporting: Abuse and Neglect

Signs of physical abuse include:

- O/R Unexplained broken bones
- O/R Unexplained bruising
- O/R Similar injuries that occur over and over, such as an injury shaped like a belt buckle
- O/R Burns of unusual shape and in unusual locations; cigarette burns
- O/R Bite marks or scratches
- O/R Unexplained weight loss
- O/R Dehydration
- O/R Dry, cracked, torn or bleeding skin
- O/R Missing hair
- O/R Broken or missing teeth
- O/R Blood in underwear
- O/R Bruising in the genital area

Signs of psychological abuse include:

- O/R Depression or withdrawal (Fig. 2-9)
- O/R Mood swings
- O/R Fear and anxiety, especially when a certain caregiver is present

○/R Lack of appetite

○/R Fear of being left alone

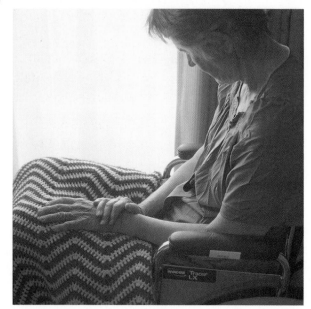

Fig. 2-9. *Withdrawal and depression are important signs to report.*

Signs of neglect include:

○/R Sores on the body

○/R Weight loss, poor appetite

○/R Dehydration

○/R Frequent complaints of hunger or thirst

○/R Strong smell of urine

○/R Unclean body

○/R Dirty, matted, or unstyled hair

○/R Ragged or dirty fingernails

○/R Soiled clothes or bed linens or incontinence briefs not being changed

○/R Ripped or torn clothing

○/R Damaged or poorly-fitting hearing aids, glasses, or dentures

○/R Unanswered call lights

Other signs of abuse include:

○/R Missing doctor's appointments

○/R Changing doctors frequently

○/R Wearing makeup or sunglasses to hide injuries

○/R Family concern that abuse is occurring

○/R Person not taking his medication

○/R Caregiver not allowing anyone to be alone with the resident

Remember that nursing assistants are legally required to report abuse or suspected abuse. Nursing assistants are considered "mandated reporters." **Mandated reporters** are people who are required to report suspected or observed abuse or neglect because they have regular contact with vulnerable populations, such as the elderly in long-term care facilities.

9. Describe the steps taken if a nursing assistant is suspected of abuse

When a report of abuse by a nursing assistant is made, the NA is usually suspended immediately. The NATCEP (Nurse Aide Training and Competency Evaluation Program) is notified, as well as the facility administrator. Adult Protective Services (APS) may be notified. A full, confidential investigation is completed. The facility will protect the resident and the person who reported the abuse from retaliation. If the investigation does not prove the claim of abuse, the NA returns to work. If the investigation shows that there might be truth to the claim, specific actions are taken.

The NATCEP outlines steps that must be followed. These steps include investigation, notification, a hearing, decision of the hearing, and the appeals process. If the findings show that abuse did occur, the nursing assistant is placed on the abuse registry, in addition to other possible legal penalties. The abuse registry is shared with other states. Employers check this registry before hiring nursing assistants.

10. Discuss the ombudsman's role

The word "ombudsman" originally came from a Scandinavian word. In parts of Scandinavia, an ombudsman is a government official who investigates citizens' complaints. In long-term care facilities in the U.S., an **ombudsman** is the legal advocate for residents. The ombudsman visits the facility and listens to residents. He or she decides what course of action to take if there is a problem. An ombudsman can help settle disputes and resolve conflicts. He or she provides an ongoing presence in nursing homes to monitor care and conditions (Fig. 2-10).

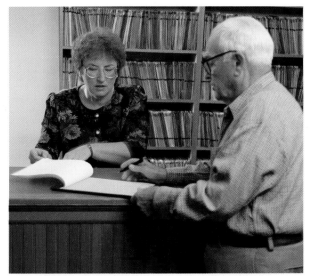

Fig. 2-10. An ombudsman is a legal advocate for residents who visits the facility and listens to residents. He or she also works with other agencies to resolve complaints.

An ombudsman typically performs these duties:

- Advocates for Residents' Rights and quality care

- Educates consumers and care providers

- Investigates and resolves complaints; works with investigators from the police, Adult Protective Services, and health departments

- Appears in court and/or in legal hearings

- Gives information to the public

In some states, a group of specially-selected people may also investigate reports of abuse that occur in healthcare facilities.

There are also state agencies that can assist people with concerns about a facility. Know the name of your state's department that handles facility complaints. Some examples of departments that a resident or his family can contact are the State Department of Health and the State Department of Health and Human Services.

For more information about the ombudsman program, contact the department in your state that handles elder care or your legal aid society.

11. Explain HIPAA and related terms

One of the most important parts of a nursing assistant's job is to keep resident information confidential. Staff will learn residents' health information from the residents themselves, their families, and from their medical records. They may also learn personal information about a resident's finances or relationships. This information cannot be shared with anyone except other care team members.

The Health Insurance Portability and Accountability Act (HIPAA) was passed in 1996. It has been revised a few times since then. This law sets standards for protecting the privacy of patients' health information. It identifies certain **protected health information (PHI)** that must remain confidential. It was also passed to facilitate the transfer of PHI for payment and research needs.

PHI is information that can be used to identify a person and relates to the patient's past, present, or future physical or mental condition; any health care that patient has had; or payment for that health care. PHI includes the patient's name, address, telephone number, medical record, social security number, e-mail address, and other information. This information must remain secure at all times, both inside and outside of the facility. All healthcare organizations must take special steps to protect health information. Only people who must have information for care or to process records can have access to this information (Fig. 2-11).

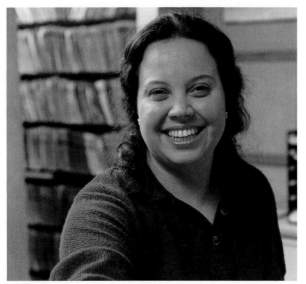

Fig. 2-11. *HIPAA requires that special care be taken to keep medical records confidential. Only people who give care or process records should have access to this information.*

The Health Information Technology for Economic and Clinical Health (HITECH) Act became law at the end of 2009. It was enacted as a part of the American Recovery and Reinvestment Act of 2009. HITECH was created to expand the protection and security of consumers' electronic health records (EHR). HITECH increases civil and criminal penalties for sharing or accessing PHI and expands the ability to enforce these penalties. HITECH also offers incentives to providers and organizations to adopt the use of EHR.

HIPAA applies to all healthcare providers, including doctors, nurses, nursing assistants, and other care team members. Nursing assistants must never share any protected information with anyone who is not directly involved in the resident's care. For example, if a friend asks you about a resident's condition, the correct response is "I cannot share that information. It is confidential." Only people who have a legal reason to know about the resident, such as members of the care team, can share health information. Staff can keep information confidential in these ways:

- Do not give health information on the tele-
phone unless you know you are speaking with an approved staff member.

- Do not give any personal information to any visitors, no matter who they are.

- Never share a medical record with anyone other than a staff member directly involved in the resident's care.

- Do not discuss residents in any public area, such as the dining room/cafeteria, a restaurant, store, or waiting room (Fig. 2-12). Use private areas at the facility to give reports.

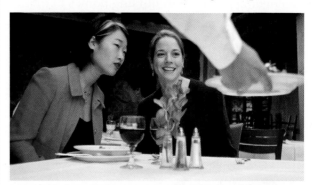

Fig. 2-12. *Do not discuss any information about residents in public places, such as grocery stores or restaurants. Only discuss residents' information with the care team.*

- Do not bring your family or friends to the facility to meet residents.

- Double-check fax numbers before faxing information. Use a cover sheet with a confidentiality statement.

- Return charts to their proper place after use. Hand charts directly to team members if transferring a resident to another unit or for a test.

- Dispose of personal notes regarding resident care (for example, notes taken during care reports) prior to leaving work for the day. They may need to be shredded or put in a special area. Follow facility policy.

- When finished with any computer work, logout and/or exit the web browser. Do not share your personal passwords with others.

- Do not include private information in

e-mails. You do not know who has access to your messages.

- Do not share resident information on any social networking site, such as Facebook or Twitter.

- Do not take photos of residents and share them, including via cell phones, e-mail, social networking sites, or other websites.

- Give any documents you find with a resident's information to the nurse.

There can be serious penalties if you do not protect confidentiality and follow HIPAA guidelines. Team members may have to pay a fine and can even be sentenced to prison. All healthcare workers must follow HIPAA regulations.

Invasion of privacy is a legal term. It means violating a person's right to be left alone or exposing information about that person without his or her consent. This includes releasing private facts, such as a medical record or even a photograph, without the person's consent. For example, invasion of privacy could be charged if a caregiver released medical information about a resident to a newspaper. Discussing a resident's care or personal affairs with anyone other than your supervisor or another member of the care team could be considered an invasion of privacy, which violates civil law.

12. Discuss the Patient Self-Determination Act (PSDA) and advance directives

The Patient Self-Determination Act (PSDA) is a federal law originally passed in 1990 as an amendment to OBRA. The PSDA requires all healthcare agencies receiving Medicare and Medicaid money to give adults, during admission or enrollment, information about their rights relating to advance directives. **Advance directives** are legal documents that allow people to decide what kind of medical care they wish to

have if they are unable to make those decisions themselves. An advance directive can also designate someone else to make medical decisions for a person if that person is disabled. Rules on how to execute these documents vary from state to state.

Living wills and a durable power of attorney for health care are examples of advance directives. A **living will** states the medical care a person wants, or does not want, in case he or she becomes unable to make those decisions. For example, a person may specify that certain measures are to be taken or withheld if he is in a coma. It is called a "living will" because it takes effect while the person is still alive. It may also be called a "directive to physicians," "health care declaration," or "medical directive."

A **durable power of attorney for health care** is a signed and dated legal document that appoints someone to make the medical decisions for a person in the event he or she becomes unable to do so. This can include instructions about medical treatment the person wants to avoid. Because the term "power of attorney" indicates legal issues, people may think this means that someone can take control of a person's money, property, etc. This document, however, deals only with medical issues.

A **do-not-resuscitate (DNR)** order is another way to honor wishes about health care. A DNR order tells medical professionals not to perform CPR (cardiopulmonary resuscitation). CPR refers to medical procedures used when the heart and lungs have stopped working. You will learn more about CPR in Chapter 8. A DNR order means that providers will not attempt to give emergency CPR if breathing and the heartbeat stops. Generally these orders are used by people who are in the final stages of a terminal illness or who have a very serious condition.

Types of advance directives may be used together, or a person may elect to use one or none at all. Having an advance directive is not legally required. However, it is a good way to make sure a person's wishes regarding medical care are known. An advance directive can be changed or canceled at any time, either in writing, or verbally, or both.

According to the Patient Self-Determination Act, rights relating to advance directives that must be given upon admission include the following:

- The right to participate in and direct health-care decisions

- The right to accept or refuse treatment

- The right to prepare an advance directive

- Information on policies that govern these rights

The PSDA requires that facilities give new residents the facility's policies on handling advance directives. Each facility must ask residents what advance directives they have and obtain copies of these documents. In addition, facilities must offer education to the staff about advance directives. The act prohibits discriminating against a patient who does not have an advance directive.

Tip

Wills and Living Wills

A living will is different from a will. A living will is a type of advance directive that states the medical care a person wants, or does not want, in case he or she becomes unable to make those decisions. A will is a legal document that details how a person wants his possessions to be disposed of after his death. If a resident tells you that he or she wants to prepare a will, notify the nurse. Many facilities have a rule that staff should not witness a will, even if a resident asks you to do so. Know your facility's policy about witnessing any legal documents.

Chapter Review

1. What are ethics (LO 2)?

2. Give one example of a law that must be followed (LO 2).

3. List five ways that a nursing assistant can be-

have ethically. Give an example of each that is not listed in the textbook (LO 3).

4. Describe five points of a typical nursing assistant code of ethics (LO 4).

5. Explain what OBRA covers (LO 5).

6. What is the minimum number of hours of training that a nursing assistant must complete (LO 5)?

7. What are ten different Residents' Rights (LO 6)?

8. Why do you think Residents' Rights are so important (LO 6)?

9. List eight different kinds of abuse and give one example of each (LO 7).

10. What are active neglect and passive neglect (LO 7)?

11. Give an example of negligence (LO 7).

12. What is a nursing assistant's responsibility if she sees or suspects abuse (LO 7)?

13. List 20 signs of abuse and/or neglect (LO 8).

14. What generally happens to a nursing assistant after a report of abuse has been made about him or her (LO 9)?

15. Describe some of the typical duties of an ombudsman (LO 10).

16. With whom may a nursing assistant share a resident's health information (LO 11)?

17. What does HIPAA protect (LO 11)?

18. List four examples of PHI (LO 11).

19. To which members of the care team does HIPAA apply (LO 11)?

20. What are advance directives (LO 12)?

21. List four rights related to advance directives that the PSDA requires be given to new residents (LO 12).

3
Communication Skills

Hippocrates: The "Father of Medicine"

Hippocrates was a Greek physician who lived around the year 400 B.C. Known as the "Father of Medicine," Hippocrates formed some of the earliest medical words in his writings. The Hippocratic Oath, a code of ethics, is named after him. Many new doctors continue to take this oath today.

In approximately 100 A.D. the early Romans developed the basis for the medical language of today. The Romans started keeping records of new words they developed from all of their experiences with wounded soldiers in the battlefield. This impressive recordkeeping by the Romans, along with the prior work of Hippocrates, laid the groundwork for Greek and Latin to become the two primary languages of medicine.

"Old age, especially an honored old age, has so great authority, that this is of more value than all the pleasures of youth."
Marcus Tullius Cicero, 106-43 B.C.

"Never promise more than you can perform."
Publilius Syrus, 100 B.C.

1. Define important words in this chapter

active listening: a way of communicating that involves giving a person your full attention while he is speaking and encouraging him to give information and clarify ideas; includes nonverbal communication.

barrier: a block or an obstacle.

body language: all of the conscious or unconscious messages your body sends as you communicate, such as facial expressions, shrugging your shoulders, and wringing your hands.

care conference: a meeting to share and gather information about residents in order to develop a care plan.

care plan: a written plan for each resident created by the nurse; outlines the steps taken by the staff to help the resident reach his or her goals.

charting: the act of noting care and observations; documenting.

code: in health care, an emergent medical situation in which specially-trained responders provide resuscitative measures to a person.

code status: formally written status of the type and scope of care that should be provided in the event of a cardiac arrest, other catastrophic failure, or terminal illness; terms and acronyms are used to identify the care desired by the person, such as "DNR" (do not resuscitate) and "no code."

critical thinking: the process of reasoning and analyzing in order to solve problems; for the nursing assistant, critical thinking means making good observations and promptly reporting all potential problems.

culture: a set of learned beliefs, values, traditions, and behaviors shared by a social, ethnic, or age group.

edema: swelling in body tissues caused by excess fluid.

incident: an accident, problem, or unexpected event during the course of care.

incident report: a report documenting an incident and the response to the incident; also known as an occurrence report or event report.

medical chart: written legal record of all medical care a patient, resident, or client receives.

Minimum Data Set (MDS): a detailed form with guidelines for assessing residents in long-term care facilities; also details what to do if resident problems are identified.

nonverbal communication: communication without using words, such as making gestures and facial expressions.

nursing process: an organized method used by nurses to determine residents' needs, plan the appropriate care to meet those needs, and evaluate how well the plan of care is working; five steps are assessment, diagnosis, planning, implementation, and evaluation.

objective information: factual information collected using the senses of sight, hearing, smell, and touch; also called signs.

orientation: a person's awareness of person, place, and time.

prefix: a word part added to the beginning of a root to create a new meaning.

prioritize: to place things in order of importance.

root: the main part of a word that gives it meaning.

rounds: physical movement of staff from room to room to discuss each resident and his or her care plan.

sentinel event: an unexpected occurrence involving death or serious physical or psychological injury.

subjective information: information collected from residents, their family members and friends; information may or may not be true, but is what the person reported; also called symptoms.

suffix: a word part added to the end of a root or a prefix to create a new meaning.

verbal communication: communication involving the use of spoken or written words or sounds.

vital signs: measurements—temperature, pulse, respirations, blood pressure, pain level—that monitor the functioning of the vital organs of the body.

2. Explain types of communication

Communication is the exchange of information with others. It is a process of sending and receiving messages. People communicate with signs and symbols, such as words, drawings, and pictures; they also communicate with behavior.

People have different roles during communication. A person can be the "sender" or the "receiver." The person who communicates first is the "sender," sending a message. The person who receives the message is called the "receiver." Receiver and sender switch roles as they communicate. The third step is giving feedback. The receiver repeats the message or responds to it to let the sender know the message was received and understood. All three steps must occur before the process is complete. During a conversation, this process occurs over and over (Fig. 3-1).

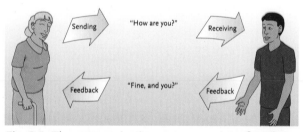

Fig. 3-1. The communication process consists of sending a message, receiving the message, and giving feedback.

Communicating verbally means using words. Speaking and writing are two ways of communicating verbally. Oral reports are an example of **verbal communication**. You will learn more about these reports in Learning Objective 18. Verbal communication also includes the way in which words are spoken or written. How the voice sounds when a person speaks says as much as the words he uses. For example, if a nursing assistant sounds irritated when saying, "Let me know if you need anything else," the resident may feel that the nursing assistant does not want to be bothered. The resident may not want to communicate a need because he fears it will make the nursing assistant angry. The words a person chooses send a message as well. Always use a pleasant tone of voice with residents, and carefully consider your choice of words before speaking.

When writing information, be clear and direct. Check to see if you are using the right words so that you will be understood. Also make sure to write clearly so that others can read your information correctly.

Nonverbal communication is communicating without using words. **Body language** is a form of nonverbal communication. Body language has to do with all of the conscious or unconscious messages your body sends as you communicate. It includes posture, body movements, facial expressions, and gestures (Fig. 3-2). Body language can add positive or negative messages during communication. For example, if you smile and tell a resident, "I'll be glad to help you find your glasses, Mrs. Martinez," it communicates that you are willing to help. However, if you roll your eyes while responding, it sends a message that you are annoyed by the request.

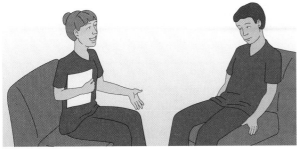

Fig. 3-2. Just as with speaking, body language sends messages. Which of these people seems more interested in their conversation—the person slouching in his chair on the right or the person sitting up straight and smiling on the left?

Touch is another important part of nonverbal communication. Some people are more comfortable with being touched than others. Some find it comforting, while others may be offended by it. Nursing assistants have to touch residents during care. However, if a resident is not comfortable being touched, limit touch as much as possible. Always ask permission before touching a resident.

Examples of positive nonverbal communication include the following:

- Smiling in a friendly manner
- Leaning forward to listen
- Nodding while a person is speaking
- With permission, putting your hand over a resident's hand while listening to her

Examples of negative nonverbal communication include the following:

- Rolling your eyes
- Crossing your arms in front of you
- Tapping your foot
- Pointing at someone while speaking

As you read the examples of body language, think about how each would make you feel. If a resident seems offended by your behavior, think about what you might be communicating with your body. Make positive changes in your body language. It will improve the way you relate to other people.

To communicate properly, do the following:

- Use appropriate words. Make sure residents are able to understand what you say. Use proper words and terms with care team members.
- Be aware of your body language.
- Use an acceptable tone of voice. Communicate caring and concern.
- Wait for responses. Let pauses happen. Do not interrupt or try to finish the person's sentences.
- Practice active listening. **Active listening** involves giving residents your full attention

while they are speaking. Maintain good eye contact. Use phrases that encourage them to keep speaking and to clarify their communication. Examples are "Yes," "Hmm," "I see," and "I understand." "Go on" is another example. Repeat the resident's message to show you have been listening closely. Active listening also includes nonverbal communication, such as nodding and smiling. Show residents you are really interested in what they have to say.

- Use facts when communicating. A fact is something that is definitely true. An opinion is something believed to be true, but not proven to be true. For example, "Ms. Simpson weighs 155 pounds" is a fact. "Ms. Simpson looks thinner" is an opinion. It might be true, but cannot be backed up with evidence. If you give an opinion to the care team, make it clear that what you are saying is an opinion, not a fact. Both facts and opinions are valuable to the care team. However, using mostly facts will help you communicate more effectively.

3. Explain barriers to communication

Some residents will have trouble understanding or using verbal (spoken or written) communication. This is due to a barrier that prevents proper communication. A **barrier** is a block or an obstacle. For example, a resident who is hearing-impaired may not understand you when you are explaining a care procedure.

These are some barriers and ways to avoid them (Fig. 3-3):

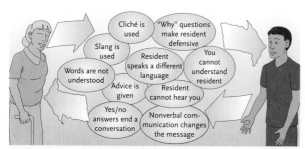

Fig. 3-3. *Barriers to communication.*

Resident does not hear you, does not hear correctly, or does not understand. Stand directly facing the resident. Speak slowly. Make sure each word is spoken clearly. Do not shout, whisper or mumble. Speak in a low, pleasant voice. Use a professional tone of voice. If the resident wears a hearing aid, check to see that it is on and works properly.

Resident is difficult to understand. Be patient. Take the time to listen. Ask the resident to repeat or explain. State the message in your own words to make sure you have understood. If the resident becomes frustrated, take a break and try again in a few minutes or find someone else to listen with you.

NA, resident, or others use words that are not understood. Do not use medical terminology with residents or their families. Use simple, everyday words. Do not pretend to understand what a word means. Ask what a word means if you are not sure.

NA uses slang or profanity. Avoid slang; it can confuse the message. It may not be understood and is unprofessional. Never use profanity, even if the resident does.

NA uses clichés. Clichés are phrases that are used repeatedly and do not really mean anything. For example, "Everything will be okay" is a cliché. Instead of using a cliché, listen to what your resident is really saying. Respond with a meaningful and thoughtful message. For example, if a resident is afraid of having a bath, say, "I understand that it seems scary to you. What can I do to make you feel more at ease?" Do not say, "Oh, it'll be over before you know it."

NA responds with "why." Try not to ask "why" when a resident speaks. "Why" questions make people feel defensive. For example, a resident may say she does not want to participate in an activity. If you ask, "Why not?" you may get an angry response. Instead, ask, "Are you too tired to do this? Is there something else you want to do?" The resident may then be willing to discuss the issue.

NA gives advice. Do not offer your opinion or give advice. Residents and family members should make decisions on their own or with help from doctors. Giving medical advice is not within your scope of practice. It could be dangerous. People with more education, such as doctors, can give medical advice.

NA asks questions that only require yes/no answers. Ask open-ended questions that need more than a "yes" or "no" answer. Yes and no answers end conversation. For example, if you want to know what a resident likes to eat, do not ask "Do you like meatloaf?" Instead, try "What are some of your favorite foods?"

Resident speaks a different language. If a resident speaks a different language than you do, speak slowly and clearly. Keep your messages short and simple. Be alert for words the resident understands. Also be alert for signs that the resident is only pretending to understand you. You may need to use pictures and gestures to communicate. Ask the resident's family, friends, or other staff members who speak the resident's language for help. Be patient and calm.

NA or resident uses nonverbal communication. Nonverbal communication can change the message. Be aware of your body language and gestures. Look for nonverbal messages from residents and clarify them. For example "Ms. Gold, you say you're doing well but you seem to be in pain. Is that true? Can I help in any way?"

4. List ways that cultures impact communication

The world is full of many different cultures. A **culture** is a set of learned beliefs, values and behaviors shared by a social, ethnic, or age group. Cultures communicate in many different ways.

The use of eye contact varies from culture to culture. One culture may believe a person should look another person in the eye when speaking. That culture may think it is a sign of honesty or respect. Another culture may find this rude or aggressive. People may view looking someone in the eye as disrespectful. Learn about your residents' behaviors and preferences. If a resident is sensitive to eye contact, try to limit it as much as possible.

As you learned earlier, touch is another important way to communicate. Touch practices differ from one culture to another (Fig. 3-4). Preferences regarding touch may also just be a part of a person's personality. You will need to touch residents during daily care. However, if a resident is uncomfortable with touch, respect this.

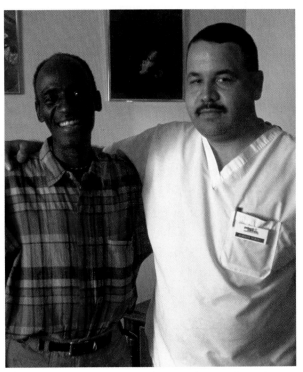

Fig. 3-4. *How a person perceives touch may depend on his background.*

Examples of acceptable touch include the following:

- Giving residents respectful personal care, such as bathing, dressing, feeding, and shaving

- Hugging, if the resident permits or asks for it

- Holding a resident's hand when she asks you to

Examples of unacceptable touch include the following:

- Sitting on a resident's lap or asking a resident to sit on your lap
- Kissing a resident
- Hugging a resident who pulls away from you
- Inappropriately touching or rubbing against a resident or staff member

Language barriers can be a problem when communicating. A resident's first language may be different than yours. One way to deal with this is to use an interpreter. An interpreter is a person who speaks the resident's language and can translate words from another language to explain the message. A slight change in pronunciation can change the meaning of words. An interpreter will make sure that residents can fully understand the information you are giving them. Picture cards and flash cards can also assist with communication.

You can also try to learn a few words or phrases in a resident's native language. An interpreter can help with that. A resident's family and friends may also be able to help. Hearing a few words in residents' native languages may be comforting to them. Do not speak with other staff in a different language in front of residents.

5. Identify the people you will communicate with in a facility

There are many people you will communicate with on a daily basis while in a facility. Some of these people are listed below.

Doctors, Nurses, Supervisors, Managers, and Other Staff Members

As you learned in Chapter 1, there are different care team members. Nursing assistants will communicate with the care team both verbally and nonverbally. Charting information and using the telephone and call systems are other ways you will communicate. You may use a computer and be involved in care planning. More

information on each of these methods is listed later in the chapter. Be familiar with them, as they promote better communication with the care team.

Other Departments

Nursing assistants will communicate with other departments, such as the dietary department. This may happen in person or over the phone. A good relationship with other departments in a facility is very important. It helps deliver excellent, organized care. Be positive in your dealings with other departments. Keep communication open and friendly. If you experience a problem with another department, report it to the nurse.

Residents

The most important communication with residents happens each time you greet them. At that time, you will introduce yourself and identify the resident. You will explain the procedure you are going to be doing and encourage the resident's participation. You will do this for every resident each time you provide care. Facilities may use name bands or photos to help identify residents. Identifying residents before you perform care is a vital part of promoting safety in the workplace. Explaining care before you give it is an important part of communication. It's also part of Residents' Rights.

Families and Visitors

The care team should try to have a good, open relationship with residents' families and friends. One way to do this is to always respond immediately when a resident calls for help. This lets family and friends know that you are taking proper care of their loved ones. Responding immediately to requests also helps prevent injury. Families are a rich source of information regarding residents' likes, dislikes, and histories (Fig. 3-5). Ask them about residents' preferences and experiences. You will learn more and be able to provide better care.

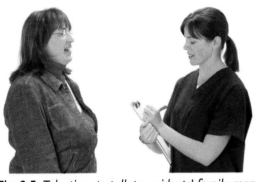

Fig. 3-5. *Take time to talk to residents' family members about residents' preferences, routines, and histories.*

The Community

Staff may receive calls from doctors' offices or clinics. Staff from these offices may visit the facility. Refer any questions to your supervisor. Keep all resident and staff information confidential unless you have been instructed otherwise.

6. Understand basic medical terminology and abbreviations

In order to communicate well with care team members, you will need to learn medical language. You will use medical terms for specific conditions. For example, **edema** is swelling in body tissues caused by excess fluid.

Medical terms are made up of these word parts: roots, prefixes, and suffixes. A **root** is the main part of the word that gives it meaning. For example, the root "scope" means an instrument to look inside. The prefix "oto" means ear. An otoscope is an instrument used to examine the ear.

A **prefix** comes at the front of the word. It works with a word root to make a new term. For example, the prefix "brady" means slow. The root "cardia" means heart. "Bradycardia" means slow heart rate or pulse.

A **suffix** is found at the end of a word. A suffix by itself does not form a full word. When you add a prefix or a root, the suffix turns it into a working medical term. For example, the suffix "meter" means measuring instrument. The prefix "thermo" means heat. A thermometer is

an instrument that measures body temperature. One of the most common suffixes is "-logy," which means the study of something. You will mostly see it when it refers to a medical specialty, such as cardiology. Cardiology is the study of the heart.

Very soon you will be able to look at word parts and recognize them immediately. Your instructor has more examples of roots, prefixes, and suffixes for you to review.

When speaking with residents and their families, use simple, non-medical terms. When you speak with the care team, medical terms will help you give more complete information.

Abbreviations are another way to communicate more efficiently. For example, the abbreviation "p.r.n." means "when necessary." "Stat" means "immediately." "BP" or "B/P" means blood pressure. Learn the standard medical abbreviations your facility uses. Use them to report information concisely and accurately. You may need to know these abbreviations to read assignments, care plans, or medical charts. A brief list of abbreviations is below. A more comprehensive list is found at the end of this textbook, but it is not a complete list. Check with your facility to see if there are others you must know.

ADLs	activities of daily living
amb	ambulatory
BID, b.i.d.	two times a day
BM	bowel movement
BP, B/P	blood pressure
$\bar{c}$	with
c/o	complains of
DNR	do not resuscitate
Dx, dx	diagnosis
h, hr	hour
H_2O	water
I&O	intake and output
inc	incontinent

isol	isolation
IV	intravenous (within vein)
meds	medications
min	minute
mL	milliliter
NKA	no known allergies
NPO	nothing by mouth
PPE	personal protective equipment
p.r.n., prn	when necessary
q2h, q3h, etc.	every 2 hours, every 3 hours, and so on
q.h., qh	every hour
$\bar{s}$	without
stat	immediately
T, temp	temperature
TID, t.i.d.	three times a day
TPR	temperature, pulse, and respiration
v.s., VS	vital signs
w/c, W/C	wheelchair

Residents' Rights

Showing off is rude.

Do not use medical terminology when speaking to residents or their families or friends. This may prevent them from understanding a procedure or important information. They may not tell you that they do not understand or they may not want to appear as if they do not know something. When talking with residents, speak in simple, everyday language.

7. Explain how to convert regular time to military time

Facilities may use the 24-hour clock, or military time, to document information (Fig. 3-6). Regular time uses numbers 1 through 12 to show each of the 24 hours in a day. In military time, the hours are numbered from 00 to 23. Using this system, midnight is expressed as 00, 1 a.m. is 01, 1 p.m. is 13, and so on.

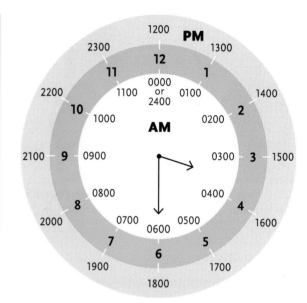

Fig. 3-6. *Divisions in the 24-hour clock.*

Both regular and military time list minutes and seconds the same way. The minutes and seconds do not change when converting from regular to military time. Regular time uses a.m. and p.m. to show what time of day it is. These are not used in military time, since specific numbers show each hour of the day.

To change the regular hours between 1:00 p.m. to 11:59 p.m. to military time, add 12 to the regular time. For example, to change 4:00 p.m. to military time, add 4 + 12. The time is expressed as 1600 hours. To change 1:42 p.m. to military time, add 1 + 12. The minutes do not change. The time is expressed as 1342 hours.

Midnight is the only time that differs. Midnight is often written as 0000. However, some places use 2400 to express midnight. This follows the rule of adding 12 to the regular time. Follow your facility's policy on this.

To change from military time to regular time, subtract 12 from the hours. Again, the minutes do not change. For example, to change 1600 hours to standard time, subtract 16 - 12. The time is expressed as 4:00 p.m. To change 2210 hours to standard time, subtract 22 - 12. The result is 10:10 p.m.

Examples of the way the numbers are written follow:

Regular to Military
3:00 p.m. = 1500 (fifteen-hundred hours)

Military to Regular
1115 = 11:15 a.m.

8. Describe a standard resident chart

The **medical chart**, or medical record, is the legal record of a resident's care. What is written in the chart is considered in court to be what actually happened. This chart is saved as long as the law dictates that it be kept. It is saved in case other care providers need to refer to the chart. A provider may need medical history or information about an advance directive. Lawyers or judges may also request to see a chart if there is a legal need. The information found in the medical chart includes the following:

- Admission forms
- Resident's history and results of physical examinations
- Care plans
- Doctors' orders
- Doctors' progress notes
- Nursing assessments
- Nurses' notes
- Notes from physical therapists, occupational therapists and other specialists
- Flow sheets
- Graphic record
- Intake and output record
- Consent forms
- Lab and test results
- Surgery reports
- Advance directives

Your responsibility with the resident's chart is to gather information and report it to the nurse. You will write down your observations and care. This is called **charting**. You may also use a computer to record this information. You will read more about documentation in the next Learning Objective.

Some facilities allow nursing assistants to chart in a medical record. Others limit nursing assistants' charting to certain forms. Follow your facility's policies. Remember, all of the information you see or add to a chart is confidential.

9. Explain guidelines for documentation

Nursing assistants chart, or document, all resident care that they provide. They also document their observations. It is very important to document accurately (Fig. 3-7). Documentation provides an up-to-date record of each resident's status and care. As you learned before, the medical chart is a legal document. Documentation is a legal record of all resident care. Documentation is also important for planning residents' care. General documentation guidelines are listed below.

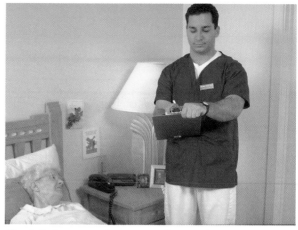

Fig. 3-7. Documenting accurately provides important information about residents to the care team.

Guidelines: Accurate Documentation

- **G** Keep all information in the chart confidential.
- **G** Document immediately after care is given. Record your notes carefully. Never record any care before it is done.
- **G** Use black ink when documenting. Write neatly.
- **G** Sign each note you make in the chart. Sign your name and title. Some states require you to list your full name; others require your first initial and last name. Write it the way your state requires. For example, Max Johnson, NA (or CNA) or M. Johnson, NA. Use the correct date and time.
- **G** Use only facts, not opinions, when documenting. Write exactly what the person has said, or what you see, hear, smell, or touch. The words "seems," "appears to be," or "looks like" are not used in charting. For example, "The resident doesn't seem to like her family" is an opinion. "The resident yelled at her relatives and asked them to leave" is a fact.
- **G** If you make a mistake, draw one line through it. Write the correct information. Write your initials and the date (Fig. 3-8). Do not erase what you have written. Do not use correction fluid. Documentation done on a computer is time-stamped; it can only be changed by entering another notation.

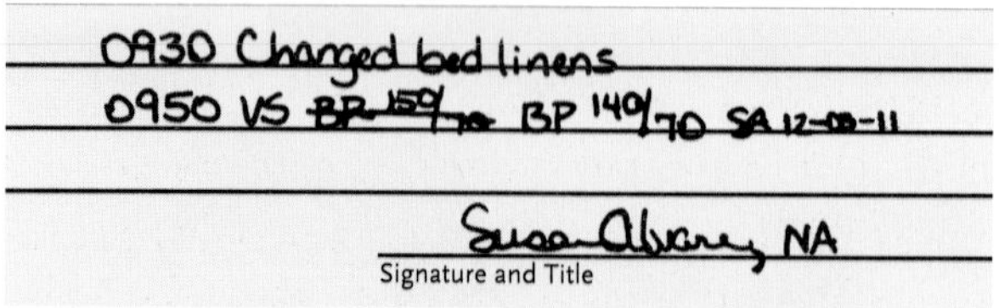

Fig. 3-8. One example of how to correct a mistake.

- **G** Use only your facility's accepted abbreviations and terms. A sample list of abbreviations is at the back of this book.
- **G** Use comparisons to describe size instead of words like "large," "medium," or "small." For example, "There is a spot of blood on her bandage the size of a dime."

All facilities will have policies and procedures for documenting. Follow them. Some facilities will require documentation on a "check-off" sheet. This is also called an ADL (activities of daily living) or flow sheet (Fig. 3-9). You will learn more about ADLs in Chapter 12.

ADL FLOW RECORD

SELF-PERFORMANCE Code 4, 3, 2, 1, 0
4 - Total Dependence
3 - Extensive Assistance - patient/resident involved but staff performed weight bearing assistance
2 - Limited Assistance - some physical help provided
1 - Supervision - oversight, encouragement or cueing
0 - Independent - no help or oversight

SUPPORT
3 = 2 person assist
2 = 1 person assist
1 = Set-up only
0 = No help required
Did not occur (can not be coded for bed mobility)

Record Self Performance in Top of Box
Record Support Provided in Lower Box

MONTH: ______ YEAR: ______

	Day	1	2	3	4	5	6	7	8	9	10	11	12	13	14	15
BED MOBILITY — How a resident moves to and from a lying position, turns side to side, and positions body while in bed.	11-7															
	7-3															
	3-11															
EATING — How a resident eats/drinks regardless of skill (includes G-tube and TPN).	11-7															
	7-3															
	3-11															
TRANSFERS — How resident moves to and from bed, chair, wheelchair, standing.	11-7															
	7-3															
	3-11															
TOILET USE — How resident uses the toilet room/commode/bedpan/urinal.	11-7															
	7-3															
	3-11															
DRESSING — How resident dresses self (street clothes)	11-7															
	7-3															
	3-11															
FLUIDS — Number of times resident offered fluids	11-7															
	7-3															
	3-11															

NAME–Last | First | Middle | Attending Physician | Record No. | Room/Bed

Form 3140HH © 2001 Briggs, Des Moines, IA 50306 PRINTED IN U.S.A.
DON'T BREAK THE LAW MAKE THE CALL 1-800-247-2343 www.BriggsCorp.com

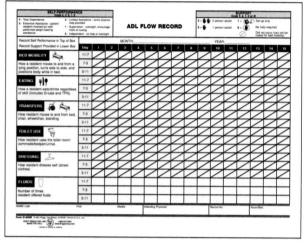

Fig. 3-9. Some facilities use ADL or flow sheets. (REPRINTED WITH PERMISSION OF BRIGGS CORPORATION, 800-247-2343, WWW.BRIGGSCORP.COM)

> **Tip**
>
> **Little Letters, Big Meanings**
>
> Have you ever wondered what the following little abbreviations mean?
>
> **et al.** (Latin *et alia*): means "and other things." Only "al" has a period at the end.
>
> **i.e.** (Latin *id est*): means "that is." Both letters have a period.
>
> **e.g.** (Latin *exempli gratia*): means "for example." Both letters have a period.

10. Describe the use of computers in documentation

Some care facilities require that computers be used to document information. Computers can easily store information that can be retrieved when it is needed. This is usually faster and more legible than writing by hand.

In some facilities, a computer is in every resident's room. Staff input information each time they enter and leave the room. In other facilities, a computer is moved from room to room. Documenting using computers replaces time-consuming paper charting, although some paperwork may still need to be done.

Facilities will train staff on computer use. Nursing assistants must follow the rules for computerized charting. These are some general rules for computer use:

- Do not share your personal password or log-in ID with anyone.
- Do not access personal e-mail accounts at work.
- Do not view inappropriate websites from work.
- Log off and/or exit the web browser when you are done with charting or using the computer.
- HIPAA privacy guidelines apply to computer use. Be careful about who can see private or protected health information (PHI) on the computer screen.

11. Explain the Minimum Data Set (MDS)

The **Minimum Data Set (MDS)** manual is an assessment tool developed by the federal government. It gives long-term care facilities a structured, standardized approach to care. The original edition was produced in 1990. The manual is revised periodically.

The MDS is a detailed form with guidelines for assessing residents. It also explains what to do if resident problems are identified. The manual provides examples and definitions for nurses to help them complete the assessments accurately (Fig. 3-10).

Nurses must complete the MDS for each resident within 14 days of admission and again each year. In addition, the MDS for each resident must be reviewed every three months. A new MDS is done when there is any major change in a resident's condition.

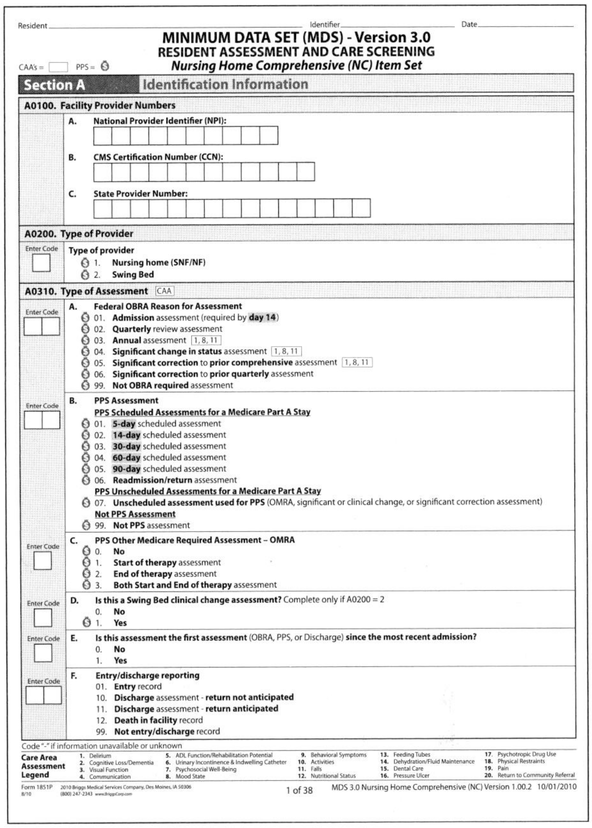
Resident ______ Identifier ______ Date ______

MINIMUM DATA SET (MDS) - Version 3.0
RESIDENT ASSESSMENT AND CARE SCREENING
Nursing Home Comprehensive (NC) Item Set

CAA's = ☐ PPS =

Section A — Identification Information

A0100. Facility Provider Numbers
A. **National Provider Identifier (NPI):**
B. **CMS Certification Number (CCN):**
C. **State Provider Number:**

A0200. Type of Provider
Enter Code
Type of provider
1. **Nursing home (SNF/NF)**
2. **Swing Bed**

A0310. Type of Assessment CAA
Enter Code
A. **Federal OBRA Reason for Assessment**
01. **Admission** assessment (required by **day 14**)
02. **Quarterly** review assessment
03. **Annual** assessment 1, 8, 11
04. **Significant change in status** assessment 1, 8, 11
05. **Significant correction** to **prior comprehensive** assessment 1, 8, 11
06. **Significant correction** to **prior quarterly** assessment
99. **Not OBRA required** assessment

Enter Code
B. **PPS Assessment**
PPS Scheduled Assessments for a Medicare Part A Stay
01. **5-day** scheduled assessment
02. **14-day** scheduled assessment
03. **30-day** scheduled assessment
04. **60-day** scheduled assessment
05. **90-day** scheduled assessment
06. **Readmission/return** assessment
PPS Unscheduled Assessments for a Medicare Part A Stay
07. **Unscheduled assessment used for PPS** (OMRA, significant or clinical change, or significant correction assessment)
Not PPS Assessment
99. **Not PPS** assessment

Enter Code
C. **PPS Other Medicare Required Assessment – OMRA**
0. **No**
1. **Start of therapy** assessment
2. **End of therapy** assessment
3. **Both Start and End of therapy** assessment

Enter Code
D. **Is this a Swing Bed clinical change assessment?** Complete only if A0200 = 2
0. **No**
1. **Yes**

Enter Code
E. **Is this assessment the first assessment** (OBRA, PPS, or Discharge) **since the most recent admission?**
0. **No**
1. **Yes**

Enter Code
F. **Entry/discharge reporting**
01. **Entry** record
10. **Discharge** assessment - **return not anticipated**
11. **Discharge** assessment - **return anticipated**
12. **Death in facility** record
99. **Not entry/discharge** record

Code "-" if information unavailable or unknown

Care Area Assessment Legend
1. Delirium 2. Cognitive Loss/Dementia 3. Visual Function 4. Communication 5. ADL Function/Rehabilitation Potential 6. Urinary Incontinence & Indwelling Catheter 7. Psychosocial Well-Being 8. Mood State 9. Behavioral Symptoms 10. Activities 11. Falls 12. Nutritional Status 13. Feeding Tubes 14. Dehydration/Fluid Maintenance 15. Dental Care 16. Pressure Ulcer 17. Psychotropic Drug Use 18. Physical Restraints 19. Pain 20. Return to Community Referral

Form 1851P 8/10 2010 Briggs Medical Services Company, Des Moines, IA 50306 (800) 247-2343 www.BriggsCorp.com
1 of 38
MDS 3.0 Nursing Home Comprehensive (NC) Version 1.00.2 10/01/2010

Fig. 3-10. *A sample MDS form.* (REPRINTED WITH PERMISSION OF THE BRIGGS CORPORATION, 800-247-2343, WWW.BRIGGSCORP.COM)

The MDS helps the care team identify problems with a resident's health. Always report changes you notice to the nurse. The reporting you do on changes in your residents may trigger a needed assessment. Changes may be a sign of a problem or illness. By reporting them right away, a new MDS assessment can be done, if needed.

12. Describe how to observe and report accurately

Nursing assistants spend more time with residents than any other care team member. Because of this, they may observe more changes in residents than other team members. Reporting these observations accurately and in a timely manner is very important. They are vital to the care plan.

A **care plan** is a written plan developed by the nurse, using data collected from the resident, his or her family, and care team members. It outlines the steps and tasks that the care team must perform to help the resident achieve his or her goals (Fig. 3-11). The care plan must be followed very carefully.

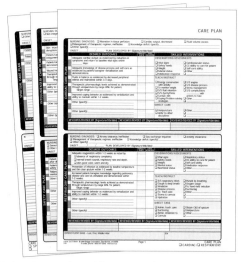

Fig. 3-11. *A sample resident care plan.* (REPRINTED WITH PERMISSION OF BRIGGS CORPORATION, 800-247-2343, WWW.BRIGGSCORP.COM)

In order to plan care, nurses collect information from staff. Nursing assistants will report signs and symptoms that they observe. This information will be either objective or subjective.

Objective information is information based on what you see, hear, touch, or smell; it is collected using four of the five senses: sight, hearing, smell, and touch. It is also called "signs." **Subjective information** is information collected from something that residents or their families reported to you, and it may or may not be accurate. It is also called "symptoms." Subjective information is something you cannot or did not observe. This is information the "subject" is telling you, so it is an opinion. Objective information may confirm subjective information.

An example of objective information is "Mr. Hartman is rubbing his temples and holding his head." A subjective report might be, "Mr. Hartman says he has a headache." Both objective and subjective reports are valuable.

Your observations can alert staff to possible problems. To report accurately, observe accurately. Use medical terminology when making and recording observations.

To use the four senses to gather information (Fig. 3-12), do the following:

Sight: Look for changes in appearance, such as redness, swelling, rashes, discharge, and changes in the eyes or ears or ability to move.

Hearing: Listen to what the resident tells you. Make sure he is making sense. Check to see if his breathing is normal. Note if he coughing, moaning, or gasping. Report if he is showing emotions such as anger or sadness.

Smell: Check for odors coming from the resident's body or mouth. Odors can indicate an infection, a need for bathing, or poor mouth care.

Touch: Note if the skin seems hot or cold. Check to see if it is dry or moist.

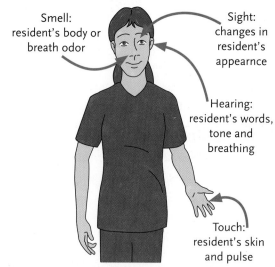

Fig. 3-12. *Reporting what you observe means using four of your senses.*

Other ways for you to observe residents accurately include the following:

- Note any change in orientation. **Orientation** is a person's awareness of person, place, and time. Does the resident know who he is, who you are, where he is, and what year it is?

- Check to see if the resident's vital signs are normal or abnormal. **Vital signs** are the measurements—temperature, pulse, respirations, blood pressure, pain level—that monitor the function of the vital organs of the body. (Vital signs will be covered in depth in Chapter 13.)

- Report any change in ability. Has there been a change in the resident's ability to move any part of her body? Can the resident perform all of the regular daily activities that she could yesterday? Can the resident see, hear, smell, touch, and taste the same today?

- Report other important changes, such as changes in weight or overall appetite, changes in ability to urinate or have a bowel movement, and changes in mood.

Accurate documentation and prompt reporting are important to residents' well-being. How do you determine what to report immediately to the nurse and which signs and symptoms can wait until later? This involves critical thinking. Nursing assistants do not try to solve problems or make decisions about residents' health. This is the nurse's role. For the nursing assistant, **critical thinking** is making good observations and promptly reporting all potential problems.

Signs and symptoms that should be reported will be discussed in this book. In addition, anything that endangers residents should be reported immediately, including the following:

- Wheezing
- Difficulty breathing
- Chest pain or pressure
- Pain in calf of leg
- Blurred vision
- Slurred speech
- Vomiting
- Sudden limp or change in ability to walk
- Numbness or loss of feeling in one side of the body or in arms or legs
- Abdominal pain
- Change in vital signs

- Headache
- Resident fall

A resident's condition will need to be checked closely. Sometimes a nurse will ask you to report every change, no matter what the change is. If this is the case, you will report each change to the nurse as it happens.

13. Explain the nursing process

To communicate with other care team members, nurses use the **nursing process**. This is an organized method used by nurses to determine residents' needs, plan the appropriate care to meet those needs, and evaluate how well the plan of care is working. The process has five steps:

- Assessment: getting information from many sources, such as medical history and a physical assessment, and reviewing it; the purpose is to identify actual or potential problems

- Diagnosis: the identification of health problems after looking at all the resident's needs; completed to create a care plan

- Planning: in agreement with the resident, goals are set and a care plan is created to meet the resident's needs

- Implementation: putting the care plan into action; giving care

- Evaluation: a careful examination to see if goals were met or progress was achieved; if progress is slow or if the problem worsened, the care plan must be changed

This process constantly changes as new information is collected. Good communication between all team members and the resident is vital. It helps ensure the success of this process. The nursing assistant's accurate observations and reports are an important part of helping to meet the resident's care needs.

14. Discuss the nursing assistant's role in care planning and at care conferences

Nursing assistants have an important role in care planning. Care plans are prepared from the observations of staff caring for the resident. At care planning meetings, do not be afraid to share your observations. If you are unsure about what information to share, talk to the nurse before the meeting.

Care plans may be written at a special care conference. The **care conference** is a meeting to share and gather information (Fig. 3-13). This is done in order to develop care plans for residents. Care team members may attend. Each team member may share important information used to create or add to the care plan. Residents and their families and friends may also attend the care conference. Members of the community, such as ombudsmen, share helpful information too. Care plans are usually kept at the nurse's station or by the resident's room.

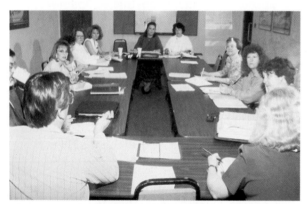

Fig. 3-13. *A care conference is a meeting to share information and to develop a resident's care plan.*

Remember that HIPAA privacy guidelines apply to care plans. Do not share a resident's information with anyone not directly involved with the resident's care.

15. Describe incident reporting and recording

Incident reports are vital to the safety of the staff and residents. An **incident** is an accident,

problem, or unexpected event during the course of care. It is something that is not part of the normal routine. A mistake in care, such as feeding the resident from the wrong meal tray, is an incident. A resident fall or injury is also an incident. Accusations by residents against staff and employee injuries are other types of incidents.

A **sentinel event** is an unexpected occurrence involving death or serious physical or psychological injury. Events are called "sentinel" because they signal the need for an immediate investigation and response. An example of this type of event is a resident falling out of bed and breaking a hip or a medication error that results in a resident's death.

An **incident**, occurrence, or event **report** is a report documenting the incident and the response to it. After the incident occurs, this report must be completed as soon as possible. This is so you do not forget important details. The information in an incident report is confidential. Give the report to the charge nurse (Fig. 3-14).

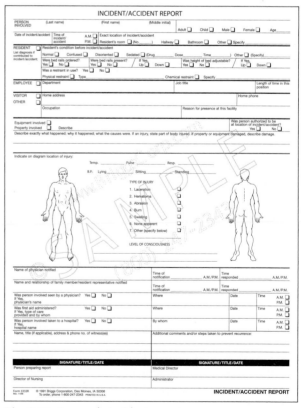

Fig. 3-14. *A sample incident report.* (REPRINTED WITH PERMISSION OF BRIGGS CORPORATION, 800-247-2343)

Always complete an incident report if you are injured in any way, no matter how slightly, while on the job. This protects you and identifies that the injury occurred at work. Nurses may sign and add information to an incident report. The nurse will complete these reports for any accident or injury to residents or visitors. You may be asked to add information regarding residents or visitors.

Include exactly what you saw. State the time and the condition of the resident or visitor. Describe the person's reaction to the incident. State the facts. Do not give your opinion.

Tip

Incident Reports

Do not let anyone try to talk you out of filling out an incident report. It is important to have these reports on file. Complete it the same day the incident occurs, as soon as possible.

16. Explain proper telephone etiquette

When you use the telephone during your shift, you are representing your facility to the community. You must follow rules for proper telephone etiquette. These include the following:

- When greeting a caller, cheerfully say, "Good morning," "Good afternoon," or "Good evening."

- Identify your facility: "Evergreen Facility."

- Identify yourself and your position: "Carol Scott, Nursing Assistant."

- Listen closely to the caller's request. Write down messages. Ask for correct spelling of names. In emergencies, take action immediately.

- Get a telephone number, if needed.

- Say "Thank you," and "Goodbye."

General rules for telephone use include the following:

- Do not give out any information about staff or residents over the phone. For example, if someone calls and asks, "Does Susie Hawkins work there?" respond with, "Please hold and I will get my supervisor to help you." Most facilities have this policy due to the increase in domestic violence and other problems, like stalking. Creditors may also call looking for people who owe them money. People may call to ask about a resident's condition. Remember that all resident and staff information is confidential. It must not be given over the telephone. Refer this type of phone call to a supervisor.

- You may place a caller on hold if you need to get someone to take the call. Ask the caller if she can hold first. Ask for help and training on this if you need it.

- You may have to transfer a call. If you do not know how to transfer, ask for training on this.

- Follow your facility's policy on personal phone calls.

- Follow your facility's policy on cell phone use. Cell phones may not be allowed at work.

17. Describe the resident call system

Residents signal staff that they need them by using the facility call system. Other terms for this system are "signal light," or "call light." This system allows residents to call for help when needed. Think of this system as a resident's lifeline. A lifeline is something that connects a person to help when it is needed; it can literally save someone's life. Always respond to call lights promptly. Do not ignore call lights. Doing so can be considered abuse and/or neglect. Answer all call lights, even for people who are not your assigned residents. Always leave the call light within the resident's reach before leaving his room (Fig. 3-15).

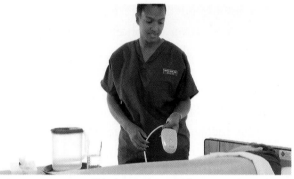

Fig. 3-15. Keep call lights within residents' reach so they can call you when needed.

18. Describe the nursing assistant's role in change-of-shift reports and "rounds"

There are two types of shift reports: start-of-shift report and end-of-shift report. Nursing assistants usually are asked to be at the start-of-shift reports. Nurses are present for both types of reports. The care team gathers to discuss and plan residents' care for a shift. Shifts vary by facility; they are usually 8, 10, or 12 hours in length.

Guidelines: Shift Reports

For start-of-shift reports

G Arrive on time.

G Each staff member is given his or her assignment for the shift. This assignment lists residents for whom every staff member will be responsible during that shift. However, every resident is "your" resident. You must respond to any resident who needs your help. Listen for important information about all of the residents in your area.

G The staff listens to a nurse from the prior shift who reports on the care of each resident. Examples of information passed to the next shift are falls that occurred, appetite problems, difficulties with urination, complaints of pain, or changes in the ability to move. Listen carefully to this information.

G The nurses give special instructions to the other staff members who will be providing resident care. Ask any questions you have about your residents. Special information shared during a report may include new admissions and transfers or discharges from the facility.

For end-of-shift reports

G Report to the nurses before the end-of-shift report. This gives nurses important information you gathered about residents during your shift. Examples are changes in pulse or temperature and skin changes that could signal the start of a pressure ulcer. Nurses will share this information with the staff for the next shift.

Some facilities use a method of reporting called "**rounds**." Staff members move from room to room and discuss each resident and the care plan. You may be involved in rounds at your facility. If you are, listen closely. Take notes (Fig. 3-16). Offer valuable information gathered about residents to staff. Sometimes this method makes residents feel better cared for. Residents may be reassured by the fact that many people can help them when needed.

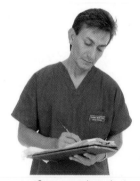

Fig. 3-16. Take notes if you need to during rounds so that you can remember resident information. Remember that HIPAA rules apply when gathering information and reporting.

The Hand-Off Transfer Process

A hand-off is the transfer of a resident and all of the care responsibilities for that resident to another caregiver or team of caregivers. A hand-off also involves the acceptance of that resident by the receiving caregiver or receiving team. The goal is an effective transfer of the resident's care and the thorough transmission of resident information. Thus, the new caregivers can provide safe, thorough, and effective care. The hand-off process involves "senders" and "receivers." Senders are caregivers transferring care of the resident, and receivers are caregivers accepting the care of the resident. The Joint Commission is focusing on improvement of the hand-off process in facilities in order to provide safer, quality care.

19. List the information found on an assignment sheet

An assignment sheet lists residents and all of the tasks that you must do for them. Certain tasks are done daily. These daily tasks are called activities of daily living (ADLs). Range of motion (ROM) exercises may be listed on the sheet. These are exercises done to bring joints through a full range of movement. A resident's **code status** tells the staff the type and scope of care that should be provided in the event of a cardiac arrest, other catastrophic failure, or terminal illness. In health care, a "**code**" is an emergent medical situation in which specially-trained responders provide resuscitative measures to a person. Assignment sheets contain the following information:

- Names and room numbers of residents

- The medical diagnosis of each resident

- Code status

- Activity level

- Range of motion (ROM) exercises

- Bathing information

- Diet orders

- Fluid orders

- Bowel and bladder information

- How often to measure vital signs

- Treatments to be performed

- Special tests and other procedures to be performed

Tip

Show up!

Assignments are based on the number of residents and the number of staff members available on that shift. It is important to work every day you are scheduled. Missing a day can put residents in danger. It can also put staff at risk of injury due to having too many residents to care for.

If you are sick, call your supervisor to discuss taking a day off, as you could transmit your illness to others. Illnesses can be more serious in elderly people.

If you must be absent, call your facility early to tell them. Your supervisor can then promptly begin the process of finding a staff member to replace you.

20. Discuss how to organize your work and manage time

Following report, you will begin your day of caring for residents. Staff members will have duties to complete at certain times of the day. In order to complete your assignments each day, you must learn to organize your work. Here is an example of how you might organize a work day:

After you receive your assignment, make rounds on all of your residents. Check to see if any residents require immediate help or care. If residents have their call lights within reach and do not need immediate help, write down anything important on your assignment sheet. Write down any needed reminders on a notepad. For example, list special tests a resident needs. Ask the nurse if there are any special orders that may not have been added yet to the resident's care plan. When you feel you have all of the needed information, decide which resident you will care for first.

Here are some other basic tips for organization and time management:

Plan ahead. Take the time to list everything you have to do, including special tasks. Check to see if you have all the supplies needed for a procedure. This will get you focused.

Prioritize. Identify the most important things to get done. Do these first.

Make a schedule. Write out the hours of the day and fill in when you will do what. This will help you be realistic.

Combine activities. Can you visit with residents while providing care? Work more efficiently when you can.

Get help. It is not reasonable for you to try to do everything. Sometimes you will need help to ensure a resident's safety. Do not be afraid to ask for help. If you cannot complete an assignment for any reason, notify the nurse.

Each facility will have its own schedule of events and care. Duties at the beginning of a shift include setting up residents for mealtime, bathing residents, and measuring residents' vital signs.

These are only a few of the duties you may have on a given day. Many things can happen to affect the work day. Adapt quickly to changing situations. A new admission, a staff member going home, or a resident transferring to a hospital are some things that may happen to change your day. Make sure each resident has the call light within reach and is safe before you leave them to do anything else.

Tip

Organizing Your Work

It is important to prioritize and organize your work every day. Do you use sticky notes to remind yourself to do things at home? Many nursing assistants use a similar method at work. A small notebook can make the difference between feeling organized and being overwhelmed.

Chapter Review

1. What is the difference between verbal and nonverbal communication (LO 2)?

2. Write one example each of positive and negative nonverbal communication not listed in the textbook (LO 2).

3. Why should "yes" or "no" questions be avoided (LO 3)?

4. A resident tells a nursing assistant that he is scared of a medical test that is going to be performed. Instead of using a cliché, such as "Oh, everything will be fine," what could the nursing assistant say (LO 3)?

5. What does the word "culture" mean (LO 4)?

6. What can help overcome a language barrier with a resident (LO 4)?

7. What does a nursing assistant do each time he or she greets a resident (LO 5)?

8. Should nursing assistants use medical terms when speaking with residents (LO 6)?

9. Define "prefix," "root," and "suffix" (LO 6).

10. Convert 8:33 p.m. to military time (LO 7).

11. Convert 11:10 a.m. to military time (LO 7).

12. List eight items found on a resident's chart (LO 8).

13. With whom can a nursing assistant's observations about residents be shared (LO 8)?

14. When should care be documented (LO 9)?

15. Why is documentation so important (LO 9)?

16. Do HIPAA guidelines apply to computer use (LO 10)?

17. What is the MDS manual? How does a nursing assistant's reporting impact it (LO 11)?

18. List the four senses that are used in accurate observing and reporting (LO 12).

19. What does critical thinking mean for the nursing assistant (LO 12)?

For each of the following five statements, decide whether it is an objective sign or subjective symptom observation. Write "S" for subjective or "O" for objective (LO 12).

20. Resident says she has a sore throat. ___

21. Resident has dark red urine. ___

22. Resident states, "I have a hard time catching my breath." ___

23. Resident is running a fever. ___

24. Resident has blisters on her feet. ___

25. List the five steps in the nursing process (LO 13).

26. How does a nursing assistant contribute to care planning (LO 14)?

27. What is an incident (LO 15)?

28. When should an incident report be completed (LO 15)?

29. Give an example of a proper greeting when answering the phone (LO 16).

30. Why is a call light a resident's lifeline (LO 17)?

31. Describe the nursing assistant's role in rounds at a facility (LO 18).

32. List seven items found on an assignment sheet (LO 19).

33. Give an example of how to combine activities to manage time better (LO 20).

34. What does "prioritize" mean (LO 20)?

4

Communication Challenges

The Navajo Code Talkers

During World War II, the Japanese were able to break almost any American military code. So in 1942, a young Navajo man approached top-ranking U.S. military staff with an idea of how to use the Navajo language as a code. He believed the code would help communicate military messages securely. Many Native Americans, including some teenagers, became Marines and went to work as "Code Talkers." They used a form of the Navajo language to send top-secret messages during the war. In 1943, there were about 200 Navajo Code Talkers, and ultimately, around 400 Code Talkers were sent to the Pacific to serve in World War II. The code was never broken. The Navajo Code Talk remained classified information until 1968. The Navajo Code Talkers played a vital role in the victory of the United States in World War II. Some of the original Navajo Code Talkers were awarded Congressional Gold Medals in 2001.

"A wise old owl sat on an oak,
The more he saw the less he spoke;
The less he spoke the more he heard;
Why aren't we like that wise old bird?"

Edward Hersey Richards, 1874-1957
from *Wise Old Owl*

"The important thing is to not stop questioning."

Albert Einstein, 1879-1955

1. Define important words in this chapter

airway: the natural passageway for air to enter into the lungs.

anxiety: uneasiness, often about a situation or condition.

artificial airway: any plastic, metal, or rubber device inserted into the respiratory tract for the purpose of maintaining an airway and facilitating ventilation.

coma: state of unconsciousness in which a person is unable to respond to any change in the environment, including pain.

combative: violent or hostile.

confusion: the inability to think clearly and logically.

defense mechanisms: unconscious behaviors used to release tension and/or help a person cope with stress.

depression: an illness that causes social withdrawal, lack of energy, and loss of interest in activities, as well as other symptoms.

disorientation: confusion about person, place, or time; may be permanent or temporary.

impairment: a partial or complete loss of function or ability.

masturbation: to touch or rub sexual organs in order to give oneself or another person sexual pleasure.

tracheostomy: a surgically-created opening through the neck into the trachea.

ventilation: in medicine, the exchange of air between the lungs and the environment.

2. Identify communication guidelines for visual impairment

Some residents you care for will be visually impaired. An **impairment** is a partial or complete loss of function or ability. Several diseases can cause visual impairment or blindness. Diabetes and glaucoma are two examples. You will learn more about these diseases in Chapters 22 and 23. A visual impairment is also something that can exist at birth. People of all ages can be visually impaired. It can affect one or both eyes.

Guidelines: Visual Impairment

G Announce yourself and greet the resident when you first enter the room. Do not touch him before you have identified yourself. Tell him why you are there.

G Look at the resident the entire time you are speaking with him.

G Make sure there is proper lighting in the room.

G Tell the resident about the care you are going to perform. Keep talking to him during care.

G Do not shout.

G Use the face of an imaginary clock to explain the position of objects (Fig 4-1). If you are taking the resident to a new area, orient him to the room. For example, say "There is a table with four chairs around it at 3 o'clock. There is a sofa at 7 o'clock." Do not use words such as "see," "look," and "watch."

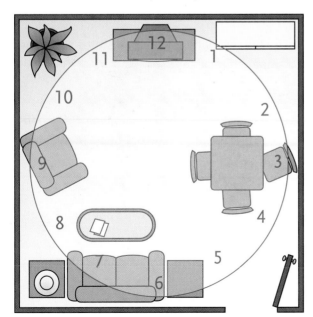

Fig. 4-1. The face of a clock can explain the position of objects.

G Make sure the resident has his glasses on, if he wears them. Check to see that they are clean, fit properly, and are in good condition (Fig. 4-2). If they are damaged or do not fit properly, report this to the nurse.

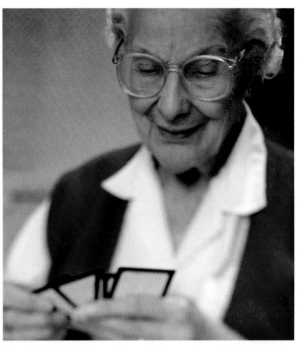

Fig. 4-2. Glasses must be on the person and should be clean, fit properly, and be in good condition.

G Do not move personal items or furniture without the resident's permission. If he agrees, tell him the new location of the items.

G Put everything back where you found it.

G Read menus to the resident.

G Encourage the resident to use his other senses, such as smell, touch, and hearing.

G Announce when you are going to leave the area.

G Do not play with or distract guide dogs, if residents use them.

G There are many helpful items for people with visual impairments. Books on tape or CD, large-print books and newspapers, and large clocks are examples. Offer them when available.

G Be empathetic. Try to imagine what it feels like to not be able to see or see well.

3. Identify communication guidelines for hearing impairment

Residents may have different kinds of hearing losses. Having a partial hearing loss in one ear is one example. Being completely unable to hear at all is another example. Hearing may also be temporarily impaired due to the noise level in the room.

Most hearing loss occurs gradually. The person will, over time, notice changes. The following list shows some symptoms of hearing loss. If you notice any of these, report them to the nurse.

Observing and Reporting: Hearing Loss

O/R Trouble hearing high-pitched noises

O/R Trouble hearing soft consonants, such as "s" and "t"

O/R Trouble hearing what is said in a setting that has background noise

O/R Not understanding the meaning of words

O/R Being unable to hear people when they are not in the same room

O/R Favoring one ear over the other one

O/R Avoiding movies or special events due to not being able to understand the dialogue

O/R Resident complains of ringing in the ears

O/R Resident complains of pain in one or both ears

Guidelines: Hearing Impairment

G Get the resident's attention before speaking. Do not approach her from behind, as she may not hear you come in. Walk in front of her if possible.

G Stand or sit so that the resident can see your face. Make sure there is proper lighting in the room. The light should be on your face, rather than the resident's (Fig. 4-3).

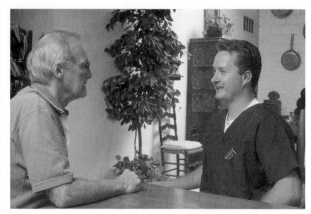

Fig. 4-3. *Speak face-to-face in good light.*

G Look directly at the resident while speaking. A hearing-impaired resident may read lips.

G If the resident uses a hearing aid, make sure it is turned on (Fig. 4-4). More information on hearing aids is in Chapter 22.

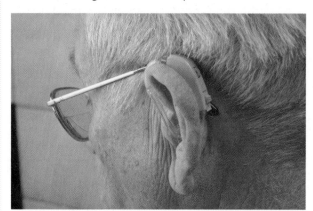

Fig. 4-4. *Make sure hearing aids are turned on.*

G Be familiar with any hand gestures a hearing-impaired resident uses.

G Turn off TV or radios.

G Speak clearly in a low tone of voice. Do not shout. If the person favors one ear, speak to that side.

G Lower the pitch of your voice.

G Do not chew gum or cover your mouth with your hand while speaking.

G Do not exaggerate pronunciation of words.

G Use simple words and short sentences.

G Use pen and paper or picture cards when needed.

4. Explain defense mechanisms as methods of coping with stress

Communicating with residents under stress requires empathy and sensitivity. Words must be carefully chosen so that you do not increase the person's stress level. Residents who are stressed may use defense mechanisms. **Defense mechanisms** are unconscious behaviors used to release tension and/or help a person cope with stress. They help to block uncomfortable or unpleasant feelings which may cause anxiety.

Defense mechanisms prevent the person from facing the real reason a situation has occurred. Overuse of these mechanisms keeps a person from understanding his or her emotional issues and actions.

Defense mechanisms include the following:

Denial: Blocking reality; rejecting the thought or feeling—for example, a resident refuses to believe his diagnosis of cancer.

Displacement: Transferring a strong feeling to a less threatening object—for example, a resident who is mad at her aunt yells at the nursing staff.

Projection: Seeing feelings in others that are actually one's own—for example, a staff member says that a resident does not like her.

Rationalization: Making excuses to justify something—for example, an elderly man fails a driving test and says the test was "unfair."

Repression: Blocking painful events or feelings from the mind—for example, a woman cannot recall abuse she suffered as a child.

Regression: Going back to behavior from the past for comfort—for example, a resident who is stressed starts to rock back and forth.

5. List communication guidelines for anxiety or fear

Anxiety is uneasiness, often about a situation or condition. Feeling anxious is not the same as feeling afraid. Anxiety is a vague emotional state. The unpleasant feelings are coming from the anticipation of something bad that could happen or a future danger. The danger is not happening in the present time. With fear, one is dealing with the present. Fear is a reaction to an actual danger. The resident who is fearful is dealing with a threat of some kind.

There are physical symptoms of anxiety. They include nausea, shaking, sweating, chest pain, and rapid heartbeat. The goal of communicating with an anxious person is to reduce the anxiety and stress levels.

Guidelines: Anxiety or Fear

G   Greet the resident when you first enter the room. Do not touch him before you have identified yourself. Use touch only if it does not upset him.

G   Speak softly. Reduce the noise level.

G   Speak slowly and calmly.

G   Listen to the resident. Be patient. Ask gentle questions to try to identify the cause of the anxiety or fear.

G   Be empathetic. Be calm and reassuring.

G   Avoid demanding behavior.

G   Reassure the resident that he is safe.

More information on anxiety and related disorders is in Chapter 22.

6. Discuss communication guidelines for depression

Depression is a mental illness that causes withdrawal, lack of energy, and loss of interest in activities, as well as other symptoms. It can be managed or even cured. There are many different types and degrees of depression, and you will learn more about these in Chapter 22.

Residents who have recently moved into a facility may be depressed. They have had many changes and personal losses in their lives. Examples of losses include the loss of spouse, family, and friends. Other losses are the loss of health, independence, mobility, and the ability to care for oneself. A chemical imbalance may also cause depression.

Residents may have moved out of their home and into a facility full of strangers. Residents may not have family near, or close family may not choose to visit them. They will probably have to share a room with someone, possibly for the first time in their lives. One of these factors can be enough to make a person depressed. However, residents may have to deal with all of these problems at once. It is not surprising that some become depressed.

Depression is not something people can overcome by choosing to be well. It is an illness like any other illness. Your role is to be supportive and compassionate. Try to make each day as pleasant an experience as possible for residents.

Guidelines: Depression

G   Be pleasant, respectful, and supportive.

G   Use touch if it helps comfort the resident.

G   Sit down and listen carefully. Lean forward and keep good eye contact. This body language helps show you are interested (Fig. 4-5).

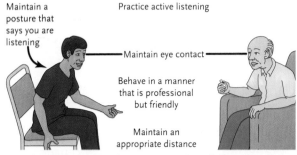

Maintain a posture that says you are listening

Practice active listening

Maintain eye contact

Behave in a manner that is professional but friendly

Maintain an appropriate distance

Fig. 4-5. Practice good communication skills with residents who are depressed.

G   Think before you speak. Try to empathize with the resident's feelings and situation.

G   Use a normal tone of voice when speaking. Use simple, clear statements. Do not talk to adults as if they were children.

G   Talk about feelings if the resident wishes.

G   Encourage social interaction.

Report a resident's depression to the nurse immediately. A list of signs of depression to report is in Chapter 22.

7. Identify communication guidelines for anger

Anger is a natural human emotion. You may see residents, their families and friends, and staff members express anger. Anger has many causes. Residents may feel angry due to illness, fear, pain, grief, loneliness, or a loss of independence. Even minor things, such as a change in the dinner menu, can trigger anger. Anger may also just be a part of someone's personality.

Some people express anger by yelling, throwing things, being sarcastic, pacing, and by exhibiting threatening behavior. Narrowed eyes, clenched fists, and raised fists are other signs of anger. Anger can also be expressed by withdrawing, being silent, or sulking. Anger can be difficult to handle. Always report angry behavior to the nurse at the first sign of it.

If a resident's anger makes it so that he or she requires more time from staff, a care conference may be scheduled. Care plans can be developed to reduce the behavior. Your input at a care conference is valuable. Offer ideas to help identify the cause of the anger and thoughts about how to stop it.

Guidelines: Angry Behavior

G   Be pleasant and supportive. Let the resident know you are there for him and that you are available to help.

G   Try to find out what caused the resident's anger. Listen closely as he speaks. Note the exact words the resident uses. Being silent may help him explain.

G   Watch the resident's body language.

G   Think before you speak. Empathize with the resident. Try to understand what he is feeling.

G   Do not argue with an angry resident. Stay calm. Speak in a normal tone of voice. Consider your responses carefully.

G   Treat the resident with dignity and respect.

G   Answer call lights promptly.

G   If the resident's anger increases, get the nurse immediately. Stay at a safe distance if the resident becomes violent.

G   Try to involve the resident in activities, such as taking a walk or listening to music.

8. Identify communication guidelines for combative behavior

When anger increases, a person may become combative. **Combative** means violent or hostile. Such behavior includes hitting, shoving, kicking, throwing things, and insulting others.

Combative behavior may be due to a disease affecting the brain. It may be due to a worsening of anger or frustration. Medication or changes in health may cause a resident to become combative. Combativeness may be linked to behaviors seen, expected, accepted, or practiced in a person's childhood. In general, combative behavior is not a reaction to you. Try not to take it personally.

Even though it is probably not personal, a combative resident is a threat to you, other staff, other residents, and visitors. Your responsibility is to keep everyone safe. If you see a resident becoming combative, call for the nurse right away. Combative behavior requires special techniques.

Guidelines: Combative Behavior

G   Call for the nurse immediately or get someone to call her. Use the call light if you need to contact someone. Try not to leave the resident alone.

G   Keep yourself and other people at a safe distance from the resident. If a resident tries to hit you, or does hit you, never hit back (Fig. 4-6).

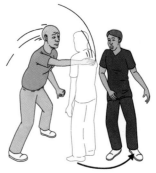

Fig. 4-6. *If a resident tries to hit you, step out of the way if you can. Never hit back even if a resident strikes you.*

G   Stay calm. Do not appear threatening to the resident.

G   Be reassuring. Try to find out what triggered the behavior.

G   Do not respond to insults.

G   Follow the direction of the nurses.

G   Report facts you know.

G   When anger passes, sit with the resident for awhile to provide comfort.

9. Identify communication guidelines for inappropriate sexual behavior

Older adults, like all humans, are sexual beings. Residents have the right to choose how they express their sexuality. They have the right to make choices about sex. There is a variety of sexual behavior in all age groups. This is also true of residents.

However, sometimes residents will show inappropriate sexual behavior. This behavior does not seem normal or makes you or others uncomfortable. It includes sexual advances or comments. Inappropriate behavior also includes things like residents removing clothing in public places, such as the dining room or hallway.

This behavior can be due to illness, dementia, confusion, or medication (Fig. 4-7). Changes in the brain may make a person unable to tell the difference between proper and improper behavior. Use the following guidelines to help deal with inappropriate sexual behavior.

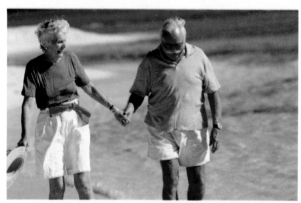

Fig. 4-7. *Older adults are sexual beings and have the right to make choices about sex. However, illness, dementia, confusion, and medication may cause inappropriate sexual behavior, which is something that must be reported to the nurse.*

Guidelines: Inappropriate Sexual Behavior

G   If you encounter an embarrassing situation, do not overreact. Be professional. Remain calm and try to distract the person. If this does not work, gently direct the resident to a private area. Tell the nurse.

G   Listen to the resident if he or she wants to talk.

G   Do not judge the behavior.

G   Sometimes a confused resident will show inappropriate behavior that is due to having a rash, or clothes that are too tight, too hot, or too scratchy. The resident might just need to go to the bathroom. Watch for these problems.

G   Always report all inappropriate behavior to the nurse.

It is important to remember that there is also normal, appropriate sexual behavior. All human beings need love and affection. Residents are sexual beings and can express their sexual needs. They have the right to engage in mutually-agreed-upon sexual relationships. Residents also have the right to masturbate. **Masturbation** means to touch or rub sexual organs in order to give oneself or another person sexual pleasure. Masturbation is a normal expression of satisfying sexual needs in all persons, including the elderly. If you witness consenting adults in a sexual situation, provide privacy and leave the area. See Chapter 5 for more information on sexual needs.

10. Identify communication guidelines for disorientation and confusion

Disorientation is confusion about person, place, or time. This condition may be permanent due to an injury or disorder in the brain. It can also be temporary due to dehydration, constipation, hypoxia (lack of oxygen to the brain), or medication. Orientation was first discussed as a way to observe residents accurately in Chapter 3. When a resident is oriented, it means he can identify who he is and who you are (person), the city, state, and facility he is in (place), and the correct time (time of day, year, season, e.g. spring). A resident who is disoriented may not be able to express one or more of these things.

Confusion is the inability to think clearly and logically. A confused person has trouble focusing his attention and may feel disoriented. A confused resident may not remember to finish his meal or may not be able to locate his room. Confusion interferes with the ability to make decisions and may change a person's personality. When a resident is confused, he may not be able to identify his name, the date, other people, or where he is. Confusion can be a temporary or permanent state.

Confusion is often due to a physical problem, such as a stroke. You will learn more about strokes, also called cerebrovascular accidents (CVA), in Chapter 22. Confusion can also be caused by:

- Urinary tract infection
- Low blood sugar
- Head trauma or head injury
- Dehydration
- Nutritional problems
- Fever
- Sudden drop in body temperature
- Lack of oxygen
- Medications
- Infections
- Brain tumor
- Illness
- Loss of sleep
- Seizures
- Constipation
- Not using a hearing aid when it is necessary

Guidelines: Disorientation or Confusion

G   Do not leave a confused resident alone.

G   Stay calm. Provide a quiet environment.

G   Speak in a lower tone of voice. Speak clearly and slowly.

G   Introduce yourself each time you see the resident. Remind the resident of his or her location, name, and the date. A calendar can help with this (Fig. 4-8).

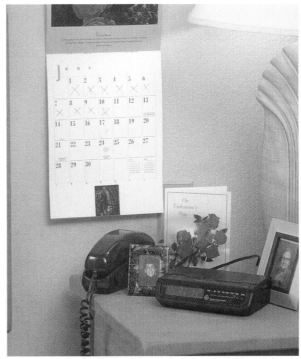

Fig. 4-8. *Personal photos and a calendar can help remind a resident who he is and what the date is.*

G   Repeat directions if needed. Use short, simple sentences. Break tasks into steps.

G   Be patient with the resident. Do not rush her.

G   Listen to the resident closely. Observe how the resident is communicating. Watch his body language. Do not focus on the words alone.

G   Tell the resident about plans for the day. Keep a routine.

G   Encourage the use of eyeglasses and hearing aids. Make sure they are clean and are not damaged.

G   Tell the resident when you are leaving the area. Repeat if needed.

G   Report observations to the nurse.

11. Identify communication guidelines for the comatose resident

You may be assigned to care for a resident who is comatose. A **coma** is a state of unconsciousness. A person in a coma cannot respond to any change in the environment, including pain. It usually occurs due to an illness, such as meningitis, a condition, such as a drug overdose, or an injury, such as a motor vehicle accident. A comatose resident deserves your respect in the same way that an alert resident does.

Guidelines: Comatose Resident

G Introduce yourself when entering the resident's room.

G Explain each procedure you will be performing. List the steps you will take.

G Do not hold personal discussions while caring for a comatose resident.

G Announce when you are going to leave the room.

Related Terms

A **coma** is a state of unconsciousness in which a person is unable to be aroused, even by powerful stimulation. The person does not respond to pain, does not open his or her eyes, and does not speak.

A person in a coma can transition to a **persistent vegetative state (PVS)**, which means the person may have some level of consciousness. He may open his eyes and have some facial movements, but these are mostly physical reactions and not a response to external stimuli.

A **minimally conscious state (MCS)** is different than a coma or vegetative state. The person exhibits some cognitive behavior and shows sporadic signs of consciousness, such as crying or laughing appropriately.

Residents' Rights

Unconscious Residents

Even when people are unconscious, they still may be able to hear what is going on around them. Unconscious people have been known to regain consciousness and relate many of the things they heard while they were unconscious. Limit your discussions to appropriate subjects. Speak respectfully, and explain what you are doing. Do not talk about anything personal while giving care. Speak to unconscious residents as you would to any resident.

12. Identify communication guidelines for functional barriers

Residents may have a functional problem that interferes with their ability to speak. Some causes of these problems are difficulty breathing, physical problems with the mouth or lips, or an artificial airway.

When a resident has trouble breathing, never push him or her to speak. It can make breathing more difficult. Allow plenty of pauses between words and sentences.

Physical problems of the lips, mouth, and tongue can make speech difficult. They include the following:

• Lip, mouth or tongue sores of any kind

• Dental problems of any kind, including missing teeth, mouth pain, and dental work

• Poorly-fitting dentures (artificial teeth)

• Birth defects like cleft palate

• Paralysis of one side of the mouth due to stroke

An **airway** is the passageway for air to move into and out of the lungs. An **artificial airway** is any plastic, metal, or rubber device inserted into the respiratory tract for the purpose of maintaining an airway and facilitating ventilation. **Ventilation** is the exchange of air between the lungs and the environment. An artificial airway is needed when the airway is obstructed due to illness, injury, secretions, or inhaling fluid into the lungs. Sometimes it is needed when a person has surgery. Some residents who are unconscious will need an artificial airway.

A **tracheostomy** is a common type of artificial airway seen in long-term care. An opening is made in the neck, either surgically or percutaneously (through the skin, usually in an emergency), into the trachea (windpipe) so that the air can reach the person's lungs. This procedure can be temporary or permanent. Tracheostomies may be used while a person is recovering from an acute illness. A person with cancer of the head or neck area may also require a tracheostomy. In addition, they may be used when a person needs a ventilator. While a tracheostomy is in place, the person may be unable to speak. More information on artificial airways is in Chapter 26.

Guidelines: Functional Barriers

G　Give the resident plenty of time to speak. Be patient.

G　Ask the resident to write down anything you do not understand.

G　Do not tire the person. Use a communication board or picture cards if the resident becomes tired. (You will learn more about these in Chapter 22.)

G　Do not remove a resident's oxygen for any reason. Only nurses remove oxygen.

G　Report mouth sores, poorly-fitting dentures, or complaints of mouth pain to the nurse.

G　Use other methods of communication if the person cannot speak. Try writing notes, drawing pictures, and using communication boards (Fig. 4-9). Watch for hand and eye signals. For example, you can use one blink for "yes" and two blinks for "no."

G　Be reassuring and calm. Be empathetic. It can be frightening and uncomfortable to have an artificial airway. Some residents may choke or gag. Imagine how it might feel to have a tube in your nose, mouth, or throat.

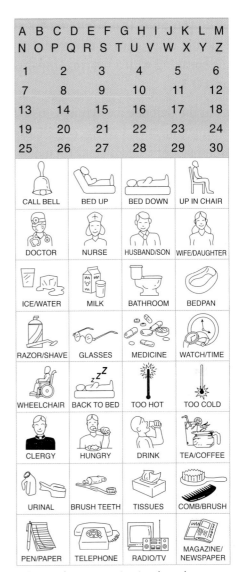

Fig. 4-9. A sample communication board.

Chapter Review

1.　What should the nursing assistant do first when dealing with a resident with a visual impairment (LO 2)?

2.　How can a nursing assistant explain the position of objects to a visually-impaired resident (LO 2)?

3.　When speaking with a hearing-impaired resident, whose face should the light be on, the nursing assistant's or the resident's (LO 3)?

4. Why do you think that a nursing assistant should not chew gum or cover her mouth while speaking with a hearing-impaired resident (LO 3)?

5. Look at the defense mechanisms listed in Learning Objective 4. Write one example of how a resident could display each defense mechanism listed (denial, displacement, projection, rationalization, repression, regression) (LO 4).

6. What is the difference between anxiety and fear (LO 5)?

7. List four losses that could cause residents to be depressed (LO 6).

8. Can a person who is depressed simply choose to be well (LO 6)?

9. List five possible causes of anger (LO 7).

10. If a resident hits a nursing assistant first, is it okay for the nursing assistant to strike back (LO 8)?

11. What can cause inappropriate sexual behavior (LO 9)?

12. What are reasons a resident might exhibit what appears to be inappropriate behavior (LO 9)?

13. Define "disorientation" and "confusion" (LO 10).

14. Are disorientation and confusion always permanent states (LO 10)?

15. Why should a nursing assistant explain procedures and introduce herself to an unconscious resident (LO 11)?

16. What are other possible methods of communication if a person cannot speak (LO 12)?

17. List three physical problems of the lips, mouth, and tongue that make speech difficult (LO 12).

18. What is an artificial airway (LO 12)?

5 Diversity and Human Needs and Development

The Black Death: The Plague That Didn't Discriminate

In the 14th century, the bubonic plague, also known as the "Black Death," first reared its ugly head. The name Black Death came from the black areas on the skin commonly seen in plague patients. It is thought to have developed in the Far East. This plague moved across Asia and into North Africa, slipping into Europe by way of Italy. Italian merchants at the time traveled to Asia searching for beautiful wares to sell. When they set sail for home, they carried the specter of the Black Death with them to Italy without realizing it. The plague spread from Italy across Europe to England. An estimated 60 million people died of the plague from 1340 to 1350. The plague killed people from many cultures and ethnic groups. Disease strikes everyone from every age group. It truly does not discriminate.

"The great law of culture is: Let each become all that he was created capable of being."

Thomas Carlyle, 1795-1881

"Religion is a great force—the only real motive force in the world: but what you fellows don't understand is that you must get at a man through his own religion and not through yours."

George Bernard Shaw, 1856-1950

1. Define important words in this chapter

ageism: stereotyping of, prejudice toward, and/or discrimination against the elderly.

agnostic: a person who claims that he does not know or cannot know if God exists.

atheist: a person who claims that there is no God.

Buddhism: a religion that follows the teachings of Buddha.

Christianity: a religion that follows the teachings of Jesus Christ.

cultural diversity: the variety of people living and working together in the world.

developmental disability: a chronic condition that restricts physical and/or mental abilities.

health: state of physical, mental, and social well-being.

Hinduism: a religion that believes in the unity of everything and that all are a part of God.

Islam: a religion that follows the prophet Muhammad and the Five Pillars of Islam.

Judaism: a religion that follows the teachings of God as given to Moses in laws and commandments.

mores: the accepted traditional customs of a particular social group.

need: something necessary or required.

psychosocial needs: needs which involve social interaction, emotions, intellect, and spirituality.

puberty: the period at which a person develops secondary sex characteristics.

religion: a set of beliefs and practices followed by a group of people.

spirituality: of or relating to the concerns of the spirit, the sacred, or the soul.

stereotype: a biased generalization about a group that is usually based on opinions and distorted ideas.

transcultural nursing: the study of various cultures with the goal of providing care specific to each culture.

wellness: successfully balancing things that happen in everyday life; includes five different types: physical, social, emotional, intellectual, and spiritual.

2. Explain health and wellness

The World Health Organization has defined the word **health** as "a state of complete physical, mental, and social well-being, and not merely the absence of disease or infirmity." This view of health looks at the whole person. It also takes the focus off disease and redirects it to healthy attitudes and lifestyles. In recent years, we have seen much information on health, wellness, and healthy living.

Wellness has to do with successfully balancing things that happen in our everyday lives. There are five types of wellness: physical, social, emotional, intellectual, and spiritual. Physical wellness includes things like being able to complete everyday tasks. Social wellness has to do with relating to other people. Emotional wellness covers managing stress and expressing feelings. Intellectual wellness deals with growing and learning throughout the life span. Spiritual wellness includes religious beliefs, ethics, values, and mores. **Mores** are the accepted traditional customs of a particular social group.

3. Explain the importance of holistic health care

You first learned about holistic health care in Chapter 1. Care team members should view resident care in a holistic way. Holistic health care involves considering the whole person, which includes his physical and psychosocial needs (Fig. 5-1). **Psychosocial needs** include social contact, emotions, thought, and spirituality. A simple example of holistic health care is taking time to

talk with residents while helping them bathe. You are meeting a physical need with the bath and meeting the psychosocial need for interaction with others at the same time. You will learn more about these needs in Learning Objective 4.

Health care is formed around the thought that harmony or balance in one's life promotes good health. If the balance is disturbed, illness can result. Holistic health care supports the harmony, which can improve a resident's chances of living a better life.

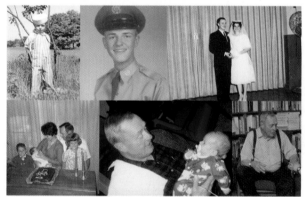

Fig. 5-1. *Remember that residents are people, not just lists of illnesses and disabilities. They have many needs, like you. Many have had rich lives with wonderful experiences. Take time to care for your residents as whole people.*

4. Identify basic human needs and discuss Maslow's "Hierarchy of Needs"

All human beings have the same basic physical needs. A **need** is something necessary for a person to survive and grow. Physical needs include:

- Food and water

- Protection and shelter

- Activity

- Sleep and rest

- Safety

- Comfort, especially freedom from pain

Human beings also have psychosocial needs. Although they are not as easy to define as physical needs, psychosocial needs include:

- Love and affection

- Acceptance by others

- Security

- Self-reliance and independence in daily living

- Contact with others

- Success and self-esteem

Abraham Maslow was a psychologist who researched human behavior. He developed a model to show how physical and psychosocial needs are arranged in order of importance. He believed that physical needs must be met before psychosocial needs can be met. His theory is called Maslow's "Hierarchy of Needs" (Fig. 5-2).

The needs at the bottom of the pyramid are physical needs. They are the ones that must be met to survive. For example, a person can live only a few days without water. Nursing assistants (NAs) can help residents meet these needs by encouraging them to eat and drink. NAs can provide a quiet place for residents to rest. They can also help residents with toileting whenever they need it.

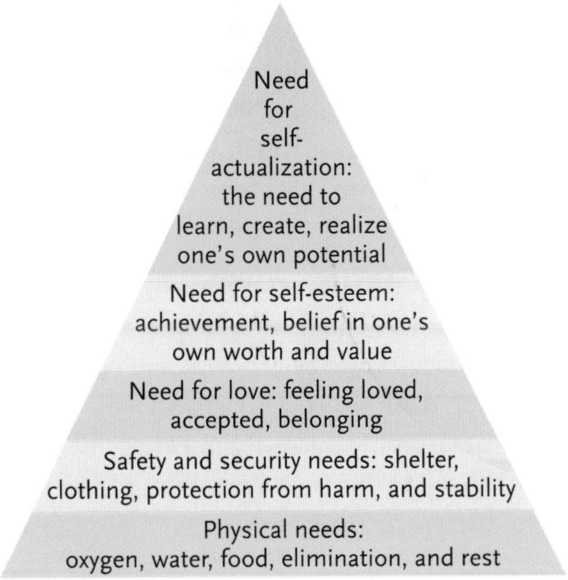

Need
for
self-
actualization:
the need to
learn, create, realize
one's own potential

Need for self-esteem:
achievement, belief in one's
own worth and value

Need for love: feeling loved,
accepted, belonging

Safety and security needs: shelter,
clothing, protection from harm, and stability

Physical needs:
oxygen, water, food, elimination, and rest

Fig. 5-2. An illustration of Maslow's Hierarchy of Needs.

The second level is safety and security needs. These include shelter, clothing, protection from

harm, and stability. For example, moving a person from her home into a facility can cause anxiety. Because it is not yet a stable environment, new residents may find it hard to adapt. It may take time for them to feel comfortable in their new home. Nursing assistants can help residents by being compassionate and empathetic. They can listen to residents when they want to talk. NAs can reassure residents that they are receiving quality care.

The third level is love, acceptance, and belonging. When residents move into a facility, they may be separated from their loved ones. Living in a new place with strangers can be very lonely. This is especially true if loved ones do not visit as often as before. Residents need to feel as if they belong in their new home. NAs can help by welcoming them and making them feel listened to and cared for. NAs can encourage residents to interact with other residents and staff.

The fourth level is the need for self-esteem. Residents may feel less of a sense of self-worth as they become dependent on others. They will need help with tasks they have performed alone all their lives. NAs can help by encouraging residents to be as independent as possible. You will learn more about doing this throughout this textbook. The more residents can care for themselves, the better they will feel about themselves. NAs should praise successes, no matter how small. This maintains dignity and self-esteem.

According to Maslow's theory, self-actualization is the highest need a person can achieve. A person must reach his or her highest potential to become self-actualized. People rarely reach this level in every single part of their lives. Residents will each be at different stages in this process. Some residents will be content with the level they have reached in life. They may spend their days quietly watching television or reading. Other residents will still be striving to do more. For example, a resident might help other residents read mail or write letters, or volunteer to oversee special activities.

Ensure easy access to food and drink.

Helping residents meet their basic needs, such as eating and drinking, is part of honoring their legal rights. When food is delivered to residents' rooms, trays must be set up in a timely manner. Their trays must be prepared so they can eat as easily as possible. Not bothering to open a milk carton or to cut up food when needed can prevent a resident from maintaining a healthy diet. This can be considered neglectful or abusive behavior. Be attentive to your residents, and help them meet their needs.

5. Identify ways to accommodate cultural differences

As you learned in Chapter 3, "culture" refers to a set of learned beliefs, values, and behaviors. The world is full of many different groups of people. Each group has its unique way of looking at the world. You will have the opportunity to take care of people from many cultures. Having an understanding of cultures will help you give better care to your residents. Your own culture greatly influences you in many ways.

Cultural diversity has to do with the wide variety of people throughout the world. Each culture may have different customs, traditions, religions, behaviors, and lifestyles. Culture and background often have an impact on how a person behaves while ill. **Transcultural nursing** is the study of various cultures with the goal of providing care specific to each culture. Understanding other cultures will help you provide better care. Be sensitive to and respect people who are different from you. Respect and value each person as an individual. It is important to respond to new ideas with acceptance, not prejudice.

There are so many cultures that they cannot all be listed here. There are thousands of different groups in the United States alone (Fig. 5-3). Some examples are Japanese-Americans, Native Americans, and Latinos. The U.S. also has people from many different regions. Each region has its own culture and traditions. For example,

the rural U.S. is much different from the urban U.S. The culture of the Northeast is not the same as the culture of the South.

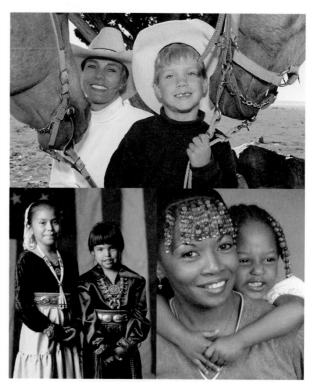

Fig. 5-3. *There are many different cultures in the U.S.*

As you learned earlier, culture can affect ideas about touch or eye contact. It can affect the language people use and the need for an interpreter. Culture also influences food choices. For example, some Korean people eat *kimchi*, which is a type of spicy cabbage. Some Mexican people eat *queso fresco*, which is a type of cheese. You will learn more about food choices in Chapter 14.

Culture also influences the way people seek health care or discuss health issues. Some people will be very comfortable with and open about discussing their health. Others will feel shy and be embarrassed by this. Nursing assistants must be sensitive to differences in how residents feel about discussing their health.

A good nursing assistant becomes familiar with residents' cultures. People may be happy to talk about their backgrounds and educate others about their cultures. Ask residents, their families and friends about special customs or traditions. When nursing assistants are sensitive to cultural differences, residents benefit.

Do not make fun of or disrespect any culture, behavior or belief. When people accept and do not judge others' beliefs or way of life, they can learn new ideas and create lasting relationships. Residents will feel comfortable with you and will look forward to seeing you each day.

Rights with Language

Residents have the right to communicate with someone who speaks their language. They must understand all documents before signing them. They also must understand all care before it is performed. Sometimes a change in pronunciation will change the meaning of what is said. Tell the nurse if you feel you need an interpreter to make sure your meaning is clear.

6. Discuss the role of the family in health care

Families play an important part in most people's lives. The concept of "family" is always changing. Often the support people give each other defines the family more than the particular people involved. There are many different kinds of families (Fig. 5-4):

- Nuclear families (a father and a mother and one or more children)

- Single-parent families (one parent and one or more children)

- Unmarried couples of the same sex or opposite sex, with or without children

- Extended families (parents, children, grandparents, aunts, uncles, cousins, other relatives, and even friends)

- Blended families (divorced or widowed parents who have remarried and have children from previous relationships and/or the current marriage)

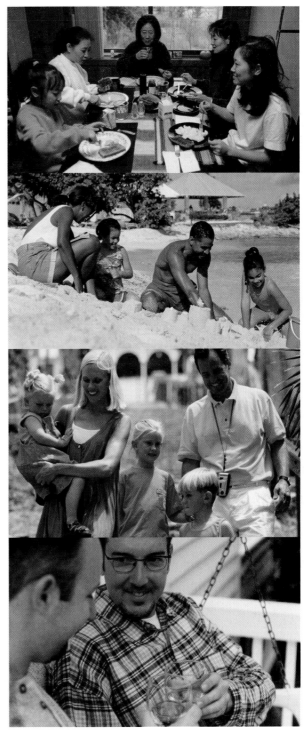

Fig. 5-4. *Families come in all shapes and sizes.*

Treat all kinds of families with respect. Do not judge families, even if they are different from your own idea of what a family is. No family is a "right" or "wrong" kind of family. However, staff may need to be alert if there are concerns about a resident's safety around one or more family members.

Families have an important role in residents' health care. They may provide some of their loved one's care. Friends may also help with their care. They help in many other ways:

- Helping to make care decisions

- Relating routines and preferences to care team members

- Connecting residents to what is going on outside of the facility

- Reading mail

- Helping to prepare menus

- Taking residents on walks

- Going with residents to activities or outside functions

- Bathing or helping with other personal care

- Washing clothing at home

- Shopping for special items, gifts, or cards

- Helping to prepare cards, letters, and gifts

When families visit, do all you can to help residents prepare. Assist them to dress, apply makeup, buy gifts, or anything else they ask. Help them find a private place for the visit, if needed. Pay attention to the needs of the resident and family during the visit. Report questions from the family promptly to the nurse.

7. Explain how to meet emotional needs of residents and their families

Nursing assistants may be of great help to residents and their families and friends. Because NAs are the primary caregivers, they play an important role in the comfort and well-being of residents.

Nursing assistants may be the people residents or their family members turn to when they feel fear, anger, or stress. They may go to NAs during an emotional crisis. For example, if a resident's friend dies, he may come to you needing comfort. If a resident dies, his family may seek you out for comfort or to talk.

When residents come to you with problems or needs, listen closely to what they say. Do not interrupt. Sometimes being quiet while someone talks is enough. Offer support and encouragement. Show that you care. Do not respond with cliches, such as, "You will be fine." You do not know that for a fact. You can ask questions, such as, "How can I help?"

Respond to worry or fear with a meaningful message. Answer any questions asked, if it is within your scope of practice. If any questions have to do with medical issues or advice, report them to the nurse.

Residents sometimes feel that nursing assistants are a part of their family. However, it is important for NAs to maintain professional boundaries. Understanding the limits of professional relationships with residents means behaving in an ethical and responsible way. Residents who are ill and lonely may feel that they need more from staff than what is appropriate. Staff who are overworked, have poor relationships at home, or who are prone to substance abuse may be at risk for inappropriate relationships with residents. It is important to be aware of these factors. If you are unsure about how to maintain a proper emotional distance from residents, always ask a supervisor for help.

NAs should be available for family members or friends of residents, too. Spend as much time with them as possible. Families often seek out nursing assistants because they see them more than other staff. Take time to listen to them when they want to talk (Fig. 5-5). Be reassuring. Families may ask questions regarding residents' care. They may want to know when a resident is bathed or when meals are offered. Answer these types of questions. However, when families ask questions regarding a resident's diagnosis, treatments, and therapies, refer them to the nurse.

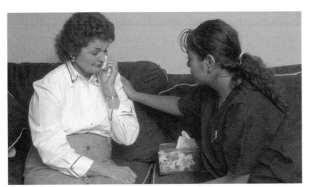

Fig. 5-5. Sometimes listening to a resident's family member is the best way to provide emotional support.

NAs can provide comfort and compassion to residents' families and friends just by being available. When families get sad or upset for any reason, stay with them and seek other help as needed.

8. Explain ways to help residents with their spiritual needs

People have different spiritual needs. Nursing assistants can help residents meet these needs. Residents may feel strongly about their spiritual beliefs. This can help them cope with problems they face. Remember that spirituality is a sensitive area.

Residents may have varying beliefs in God ranging from very strong to no belief. Residents may consider themselves spiritual, but may not believe in God or a higher power. The important thing to remember is to respect all residents' beliefs, whatever they are. Do not make judgments about residents' spiritual beliefs or try to push your own beliefs on residents.

It may help if you know a little about some of the different **religions** and religious practices you may encounter. It is important to know that even if a resident belongs to a religious group, he may not believe or practice everything that religion teaches. There is a variety of faiths and non-faiths. Within each of these, there are many different beliefs. Your job is to accommodate religious practices and requests when possible. Common religions, listed alphabetically, follow:

Buddhism: Buddhism evolved from Siddhartha Gautama, who reached enlightenment and took the title of "Buddha." Buddhists believe that morality, meditation, and wisdom are the path to enlightenment. They believe in reincarnation and that people must travel through birth, life, and death. After these travels, a person can reach Nirvana. Nirvana is the state of peace and happiness and freedom from worry and pain. It is the highest spiritual plane one person can attain. There are many Buddhist texts. The Tipitaka or Pali Canon is the standard scripture collection. The Dalai Lama is considered to be the highest spiritual leader.

Christianity: Christians believe that Jesus Christ was the son of God and that he died so that their sins would be forgiven. Christians believe in heaven and that those who repent their sins before God will be able to go to heaven. There are different branches of the Christian church, such as Catholic or Protestant. There are many subgroups, such as Baptists, Episcopalians, Evangelicals, Lutherans, Methodists, Mormons, and Presbyterians. Christians may be baptized and take communion as a symbol of Christ's sacrifice. The Christian Bible is the sacred text and is divided into two parts: the Old Testament and the New Testament. Religious leaders may be called priests, preachers, pastors, ministers, or deacons.

Hinduism: Hindus believe in the unity of everything, called "Brahman." The purpose of life is to realize that all are part of God. People move through birth, life, death, and rebirth. How a person moves toward enlightenment is determined by karma. Karma is the result of actions in past lives, and actions in this life can determine one's destiny in future lives. Good thoughts and deeds can cause one to be reborn at a higher level, but bad thoughts and deeds may cause a person to be born at a lower level. The Vedas are the primary texts of Hinduism. Holy men are called Sadhus.

Islam: Muslims are followers of the prophet Muhammad [Mohammed]. Muslims worship God; the Arabic term for God is "Allah." The Five Pillars of Islam include reciting the profession of faith, ritual prayer five times daily at certain times of the day, fasting during the month called "Ramadan," charitable donations to the poor and needy, and pilgrimage to Mecca. Mecca is the Muslim holy city. Muslims worship at mosques and follow specific religious practices related to food and drink. For example, Muslims usually do not eat pork or drink alcohol. The sacred text of Islam is the Qur'an [Koran]. The Qur'an is believed to be the literal word of God as revealed to Muhammad. Titles of Islamic religious leaders include ayatollah, caliph, imam, mufti, and mullah.

Judaism: Judaism is the religion of the Jewish people. It is divided into Reform, Conservative, and Orthodox movements. Jewish people believe there is one God. They believe God is merciful and that they should follow God's laws. Jewish people believe that God gave them laws and commandments through Moses in the form of the Torah. Jewish services are held on Friday evenings and sometimes on Saturdays in synagogues or temples. The Sabbath day, called "Shabbat," is a special day of rest. Jewish people may not do certain things on the Sabbath. This lasts from Friday sundown to Saturday sundown. Religious leaders are called rabbis.

Spirituality refers to concerns of the spirit, the sacred, or the soul. Some consider themselves to be spiritual, but not religious. Others believe that their spiritual self is the same as their religious self. Spirituality centers around thoughts of a spiritual aspect of life and nature beyond worldly things. It may be associated with inner peace and well-being. It may refer to a person's beliefs about the overall meaning or purpose of life.

Many Native American tribes follow spiritual traditions. Their belief systems often include the idea that everything—people, animals, oceans, trees, and other things—has a spirit. The importance of community and a love of the environment can play an important part in the lives of Native Americans. Traditions generally include special ceremonies and rituals.

As mentioned earlier, some people may not believe in God or a higher power at all. They may identify themselves as **agnostic**. Agnostics claim that they do not know or cannot know if God exists. They do not deny that God might exist, but they feel there is no true knowledge of God's existence.

Atheists are people who claim that there is no God. This is different from what agnostics believe. Atheists actively deny the existence of any deity (higher power). For many atheists, this belief is as strongly held as any religious belief.

Here are some ways you can help residents meet their spiritual needs:

- Honor dietary restrictions. Dietary restrictions are rules about what and when followers can eat. For example, Muslims may not eat shellfish. Catholics may not eat meat on Fridays during Lent. Orthodox and Conservative Jewish people may eat only kosher foods and may not eat pork. Do not judge any dietary restrictions. Report fasting requests to the nurse.

- Report requests to see clergy to the nurse promptly. Give privacy for clergy visits (Fig. 5-6).

- Respect all religious items. Handle religious items carefully. When asked, help residents apply religious articles of clothing.

- Allow time and privacy for prayer. If you are asked to do so, read religious materials aloud.

- Residents have the right to attend religious services if they choose to do so. Make sure residents who want to go to these services are ready on time and are helped to the proper site.

- Report to the nurse or social worker if a resident needs help finding spiritual resources.

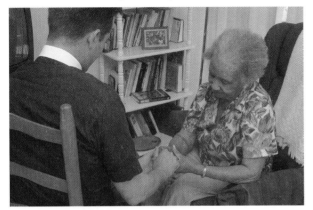

Fig. 5-6. *Be welcoming and give privacy when residents receive a visit from a spiritual leader.*

Residents' spiritual or religious beliefs or non-beliefs may be different from yours. Do not try to change someone's religion or tell a resident that his belief or religion is wrong. Do not express judgments or say anything negative about a religious group. Never insist that a resident join in a religious activity, and never interfere with a religious practice.

Spiritual needs are different for each person. Respect residents' religions or beliefs. Listen carefully when they want to talk about them. When you respect and provide support for each resident's spiritual concerns, you are helping to meet their needs.

9. Identify ways to accommodate sexual needs

Humans are sexual beings, and they continue to have sexual needs throughout their lives. Sexuality is not just about having sex. Sex and sexuality have been defined in this way: sex is something a person does, while sexuality is something a person is. Sexual orientation is a person's preference for one gender or the other. Sexual orientation or identity plays a big part in human sexuality.

Terms defining sexual identity include:

- Heterosexual: A person whose sexual preference is for people of the opposite sex; also known as "straight."

- Homosexual: A person whose sexual preference is for people of the same sex; terms "gay" and "lesbian" are usually preferred.

- Gay: 1. A person whose sexual preference is for people of the same sex. 2. A man whose sexual preference is for men.

- Lesbian: A woman whose sexual preference is for women.

- Bisexual: A person whose sexual preference is for people of both sexes.

- Transsexual: 1. One who wishes to be accepted by society as a member of the opposite sex. 2. One who has undergone a sex change operation.

- Transgender: A person whose gender identity conflicts with his or her birth sex (sex assigned at birth due to anatomy).

- Transitioning: The process of changing genders.

A common myth is that elderly people no longer have sexual needs or desires. That is not true. Sexual urges do not end due to age or admission to a care facility. Many things can affect residents' sexual needs. Illness and disability can affect sexual desires, needs, and abilities. However, do not assume you know what impact a disability has had on sexuality. A disability may limit the ability to meet sexual needs, but not lessen sexual desire. Many people in wheelchairs can have sexual and intimate relationships.

Living environments may also affect sexuality. In care facilities, a lack of privacy and no available partner are often reasons for a lack of sexual expression. Be sensitive to privacy needs.

Sexuality is a very important part of every human being. And in every age group, there is a variety of sexual expression and behavior. Do not judge any sexual behavior you see (Fig. 5-7). An attitude that any expression of sexuality by the elderly is either "disgusting" or "cute" is inappropriate. It deprives residents of their right to dignity and respect.

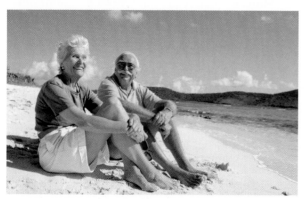

Fig. 5-7. *Elderly people continue to have sexual needs and desires. Do not judge any sexual behavior you see.*

Here are ways you can help residents with their sexual needs:

• Always knock and wait for permission to enter before going into residents' rooms. Honor "Do Not Disturb" signs if your facility uses them.

• If you encounter any sexual situation between consenting adults, provide privacy and leave the room. Do not discuss what you saw with other staff members. Consenting adults are allowed to have sexual relationships. Residents may also masturbate, which means to rub or touch sexual organs to give oneself pleasure.

• Do not judge sexual choices or residents' sexual orientation. Do not judge the sexual orientation of residents' family members or friends.

• If you ever see a resident being sexually abused, remove the resident from the situation immediately. Make sure he or she is taken to a safe place, then report this to the nurse. Never delay in reporting sexual abuse.

If a sexual situation is disturbing or inappropriate, ask a nurse for help. Tips on dealing with sexually-inappropriate behavior are in Chapter 4.

More information on sexual needs of the elderly is in Chapter 17.

10. Describe the stages of human growth and development

Human growth and development is an ongoing and complex process. Growth refers to the physical changes that can be measured. Development means the emotional, social, and physical changes that occur. Each person's growth and development will differ. One child may walk at nine months old, while another will not walk until over a year old.

Many things affect growth and development. These include the parents' involvement, the child's surroundings, nutrition, exercise, medical care, and overall lifestyle.

There are different types of development. Cognitive development focuses on how children think and learn. Language development focuses on gaining language skills. Moral development deals with forming a sense of right and wrong. Motor development is gaining an ability to do things like grasp things, use scissors, and draw. Physical development deals with the changes that happen to the body during growth. Sexual development has to do with the reproductive changes that occur when people reach puberty. Social development is the process of learning to relate to other people.

Infants (Birth to 12 months)

Babies grow quickly during the first year. Infants tend to triple birth weight in the first year of life. Physical development in infancy moves from the head down (Fig. 5-8). For example, infants gain control over the neck muscles before the muscles in their shoulders. Infants learn to grasp, lift their heads, and crawl. They may be able to pick things up toward the end of the first year. Infants are totally dependent on others for care. Touch is important as a communication tool. Touch helps babies grow and thrive.

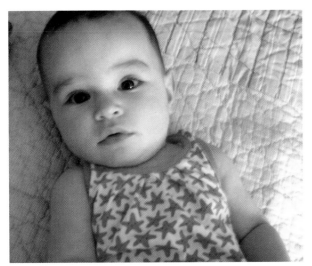

Fig. 5-8. An infant's physical development moves from the head down.

Toddler (Ages 1 to 3)

Toddlers grow fast between the ages of one and three. Most toddlers can move about quickly, and run and jump. During the toddler years, speech improves. Toddlers gain coordination of their limbs and learn to control their bladders and bowels (Fig. 5-9). It is important to protect toddlers as they explore their world, for they often take risks. They do not understand what kinds of things can harm them. Parents begin to teach them language, the difference between right and wrong, and accepted behavior.

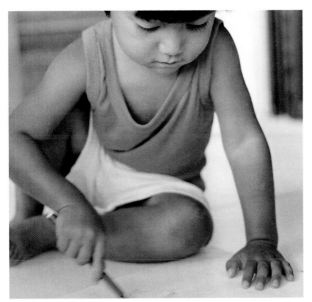

Fig. 5-9. Toddlers gain coordination of their limbs.

Pre-School (Ages 3 to 6)

Pre-school-age children become more independent and have social relationships. They play better with other children, and they can play in groups (Fig. 5-10). Their language abilities improve. Pre-schoolers learn to care for themselves. They become more physically coordinated, and their sense of imagination develops. Playing dress-up in parents' clothing is common.

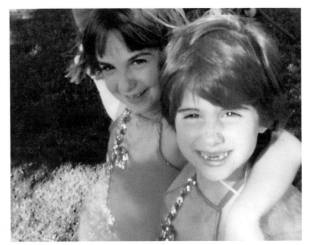

Fig. 5-10. Children in pre-school years develop social relationships.

School-Age (Ages 6 to 12)

School-age children's development centers on cognitive and social development. Entering school is a big adjustment for children and their families. Children learn to get along with each other. They begin to develop a conscience, morals, and self-esteem. During this time, boys develop more muscle, but girls may be larger than boys. The period between nine and twelve is called "pre-adolescence." Hormonal changes occur. There is a growing interest in the opposite sex. Girls may reach puberty in the later years of this stage. During **puberty**, a person develops secondary sex characteristics. In females, secondary sex characteristics include growth of body hair and development of breasts and hips. In males, they include growth of body hair, growth of the testes and the penis, broadening of the shoulders, and a lower voice.

Adolescence (Ages 12 to 18)

During adolescence, genders become sexually mature. Boys tend to reach puberty. If girls did not reach puberty during the prior stage, it will start here. Adolescents may have a hard time adapting to changes caused by puberty (Fig. 5-11). This group becomes more independent. They must make important decisions, mostly by themselves, each day. Moral values that the child has learned play a part in these decisions. Adolescents can sometimes become stubborn and difficult for their parents to handle. They may have mood swings. They are concerned with acceptance from others.

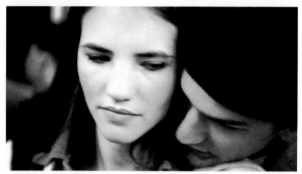

Fig. 5-11. Adolescence is a time of adapting to change.

Young Adulthood (Ages 18 to 40)

Growth has usually been completed by this time. However, boys can continue to grow up to the age of 25. During this stage, people make decisions about whether to continue their education or join the work force. They may meet a life partner. Many couples marry (Fig. 5-12). Some people decide to have children during this time.

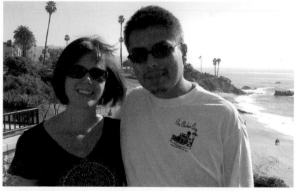

Fig. 5-12. Young adulthood often involves finding long-term mates.

Middle Adulthood (Ages 40 to 65)

During middle adulthood, people usually become more comfortable and stable. Their children may have left home to go to college or to live on their own. This can be a very happy time for people (Fig. 5-13). They may find there is more time and money to spend on themselves. Couples may take trips and spend more time together. A person may decide to begin a second career.

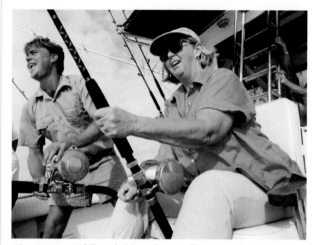

Fig. 5-13. Middle adulthood can offer more free time to take trips and pursue hobbies.

Some people may find themselves in a "mid-life crisis" during this stage. This is a period of unrest due to a desire for change and fulfillment of unmet goals. It has to do with the reality of getting older. A mid-life crisis can occur in both men and women. People may change the way they dress, act, or behave during this time.

Late Adulthood (65 years and older)

People in late adulthood may see many changes. They may retire from jobs. Medical care may be needed for problems that develop during this time. People may have to cope with a loved one's illness or death. Staying connected to others is vital to staying healthy and mentally alert (Fig. 5-14). Hobbies and volunteering can help the person stay connected. It is important to encourage people in this stage to stay as active and involved as possible.

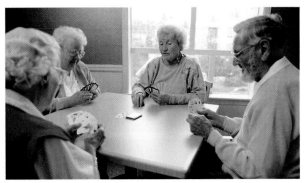

Fig. 5-14. *In late adulthood, it is important to stay connected with others to help remain healthy and active.*

Figure 5-15 outlines the developmental tasks that are required throughout all of the stages of life.

11. Discuss stereotypes of the elderly

It is common for people to have false beliefs about the elderly. A **stereotype** is a biased generalization about a group. These generalizations are usually based on opinions and distorted ideas and often come from television or the movies. These unfair ideas create prejudices against the elderly. Stereotyping of, prejudice toward, and/or discrimination against the elderly is called **ageism**. Common stereotypes of the elderly include the following:

- They cannot remember things.
- They are totally dependent on others.

Infant (Birth to 12 months)	Toddler (Ages 1 to 3)	Pre-School (Ages 3 to 6)	School-Age (Ages 6 to 12)
• Rapid physical growth • Physical development moves from the head down • Learns to lift head and grasp • Begins to crawl and climb • Picks up objects • Smiles, cries, coos, babbles, and laughs	• Learns to walk, run, and jump • Speech improves • Gains coordination of limbs • Learns to control bladder and bowels	• Becomes more independent • Has social relationships • Language ability improves • Learns to care for self • Becomes more physically coordinated	• Learns to get along with other children • Begins to develop a conscience, morals, and self-esteem • During "pre-adolescence" hormonal changes occur • Growing interest in the opposite sex • Girls may reach puberty in the later years of this stage—body hair grows, menstruation and ovulation begin, and breasts and hips develop

Adolescence (Ages 12 to 18)	Young Adulthood (Ages 18 to 40)	Middle Adulthood (Ages 40 to 65)	Late Adulthood (65 years and older)
• Boys reach puberty—body hair grows; the testes and the penis grow; sperm is produced; shoulders broaden; and voice lowers • Girls reach puberty if they have not before • May have a difficult time adapting to changes caused by puberty • Becomes more independent • Makes important decisions • Can become stubborn • Has mood swings • Concerned with acceptance from others	• Growth has usually been completed • Makes decisions about education or careers • May select a mate • May marry • May have children	• Becomes more comfortable and stable • Some changes of aging appear • Children may have left home • May travel more	• Retires from jobs • Changes of aging more apparent • May require medical care for problems • Mobility can become limited • Copes with illness and/or death of loved ones and friends

Fig. 5-15. *The stages of growth and development.*

- They do not have an active sex life.
- They do not like to leave home.
- They are grumpy or grouchy.
- They cannot manage their money.
- They are less intelligent than younger people.
- They have no friends.
- They have no interests.

These ideas are not true of most elderly people. Research has shown that most older people are active and have many interests (Fig. 5-16). They exercise, continue to learn, work, manage their finances, and have intimate relationships. They are relatively independent.

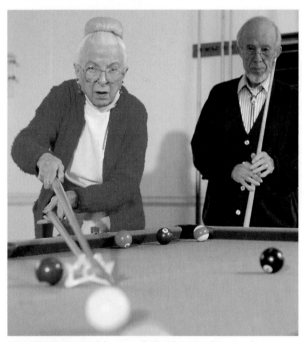

Fig. 5-16. Most older people lead active lives.

Aging is a normal process. There are many emotional and physical changes that occur as people age. These normal changes of aging do not mean that people will always become ill or dependent. You must be able to tell the difference between what is true and what is not true about the aging process. This will help you provide better care for your residents.

12. Discuss developmental disabilities

Developmental disabilities are present at birth or emerge during childhood. A **developmental disability** is a chronic condition; it will exist throughout a person's life. Developmental disabilities restrict physical and/or mental ability. These disabilities prevent a child from developing at a "normal" rate. These disabilities include cerebral palsy, autism, visual or hearing impairment, and an intellectual disability.

Developmental disabilities cause problems with language, mobility, and learning. They also cause difficulty with self-care and the things people do every day. For example, a person may struggle with eating, bathing, walking, or speaking. A brief description of some developmental disabilities follows:

Intellectual Disability: The most common developmental disability is intellectual disability (formerly called "mental retardation"). It causes below-average mental functioning. People have difficulty in learning and problems with social skills. People with an intellectual disability develop at a below-average rate. There are different degrees of this disability.

An intellectual disability is not a disease or mental illness. One method used to identify this disability is the testing of intelligence (IQ). People with an intellectual disability need some support in their day-to-day lives. They may need help with ADLs, such as bathing, eating, moving, and positioning. These individuals may be able to work and live independently, depending upon the severity of the disability.

There are other terms used for an intellectual disability. Examples include "special," "challenged," and "developmentally delayed." Respect each person's wishes on how to refer to this disability.

Cerebral Palsy (CP): Cerebral palsy is a developmental disability that affects movement and balance. It can also cause intellectual disabilities. A person with cerebral palsy suffered brain damage while in the uterus or during birth. This damage can be caused by birth trauma, infection, or a head injury. The part of the brain that was damaged controls muscle tone. People with CP may lack control of their head and have trouble using their arms and hands. They can have poor balance or posture. They may be stiff or limp. CP can cause problems with speech and may affect intelligence.

CP generally does not worsen as the person gets older. Cerebral palsy includes four types: ataxic, athetoid, spastic, and mixed. Most people with CP have spastic cerebral palsy. This means they might move awkwardly and have stiff muscles.

Signs and symptoms of CP can be different for each person. Some people have very mild symptoms. Others are much more severe. Some people with CP also have other disorders, such as hearing or visual impairment or a seizure disorder.

Autism: Autism is a group of developmental disabilities called "ASDs" or "Autism Spectrum Disorders." They are also called "Pervasive Developmental Disorders (PDD)." Asperger syndrome is considered a milder form of this disorder. Autism starts prior to age three and continues through the person's lifetime. It is seen more often in boys. People with autism disorders have trouble with speech, language, and communication. They may have problems relating to other people socially. Autistic people may do specific actions over and over again, such as rocking back and forth.

Guidelines: Developmental Disabilities

G Treat adult residents as adults, regardless of their intellectual abilities.

G Praise and encourage them often, especially for positive behavior.

G Help teach ADLs by dividing tasks into small steps.

G Repeat words to make sure they understand.

G Talk to residents, even if they cannot speak.

G Help residents with cerebral palsy move slowly. They may take longer to adjust their body position.

G Promote independence while ensuring safety. Assist with safe activities and motor functions that are difficult.

G Encourage social interaction.

G Always be patient.

Visual and hearing impairments are also considered developmental disabilities. You learned about these impairments in Chapter 4. A person with a visual or hearing impairment may need a little or a lot of outside support throughout their lives. Having one of these impairments may affect a person's ability to drive, work and communicate. See Chapters 4 and 22 for guidelines for these impairments.

Chapter Review

1. What do the terms "health" and "wellness" mean (LO 2)?

2. Define "holistic care" and describe what it involves (LO 3).

3. What are psychosocial needs (LO 3)?

4. The needs listed at the bottom of Maslow's "Hierarchy of Needs" are physical needs. Identify the physical needs (LO 4).

5. List one example of how a nursing assistant can help with each of the following needs: physical needs, safety and security needs, need for love, need for self-esteem (LO 4).

6. What is cultural diversity (LO 5)?

7. List three things that culture affects (LO 5).

8. List five ways families and friends help with a resident's care (LO 6).

9. Name three ways nursing assistants can respond to the emotional needs of residents and their families (LO 7).

10. Describe five ways nursing assistants can help residents meet their spiritual needs (LO 8).

11. If a nursing assistant encounters a sexual situation between two consenting residents, what should she do (LO 9)?

12. What should a nursing assistant do if she sees a resident being sexually abused (LO 9)?

13. Name one thing that occurs in each stage of human development (LO 10).

14. What is a stereotype (LO 11)?

15. Why should stereotyping be avoided (LO 11)?

16. List three facts about developmental disabilities (LO 12).

17. Why do you think it is important for nursing assistants to treat developmentally disabled residents as adults, regardless of their behavior (LO 12)?

6 Infection Prevention

Semmelweis and Childbed Fever: It was handwashing, plain and simple!

Ignaz Semmelweis (1818-1865) was a Hungarian doctor who practiced and taught medicine in Vienna, Austria during the mid-1800s. He noted that the death rate from childbed fever on a certain maternity ward was higher than on a similar ward at the same facility. The only difference he could find was that doctors and medical students came to the ward where the death rate was higher right after dissecting corpses in the autopsy rooms. The second ward, where the midwives worked, had a much lower death rate. The midwives did not go into the autopsy rooms.

Semmelweis asked the doctors and the medical students to first wash their hands and then soak them in a special solution before and after examining the maternity patients. After this process was initiated, the death rate from childbed fever dropped dramatically. Semmelweis eventually wrote a book on his discovery.

"Cleanliness is a great virtue..."
Charles B. Fairbanks, 1827-1859

"The sick are the greatest danger to the healthy; it is not from the strongest that harm comes to the strong, but from the weakest."
Friedrich Wilhelm Nietzsche, 1844-1900

1. Define important words in this chapter

antimicrobial: an agent that destroys, resists, or prevents the development of pathogens.

autoclave: an appliance used to sterilize medical instruments or other objects by using steam under pressure.

bloodborne pathogens: microorganisms found in human blood that can cause infection and disease.

Bloodborne Pathogen Standard: federal law requiring that healthcare facilities protect employees from bloodborne health hazards.

body fluids: tears, saliva, sputum (mucus coughed up), urine, feces, semen, vaginal secretions, pus or other wound drainage, and vomit.

carrier: person who carries a pathogen usually without signs or symptoms of disease, but who can still spread the disease.

catheter: tube inserted through the skin or into a body opening that is used to add or drain fluid.

C. difficile (C. diff, clostridium difficile): a bacterial illness that can cause diarrhea and colitis; spread by spores in feces that are difficult to kill.

Centers for Disease Control and Prevention (CDC): federal government agency responsible for improving the overall health and safety of the people of the United States.

clean: a condition in which an object has not been contaminated with pathogens.

communicable disease: an infectious disease transmissible by direct contact or by indirect contact.

contagious disease: a type of communicable disease that spreads quickly from person to person.

contaminated: soiled, unclean; having disease-causing organisms or infectious material on it.

cross-infection: the physical movement or transfer of harmful bacteria from one person, object, or place to another, or from one part of the body to another.

dehydration: an excessive loss of water from the body; a condition that occurs when fluid loss is greater than fluid intake.

direct contact: way to transmit pathogens through touching the infected person or his or her secretions.

direct spread: method of transmission of disease from one person to another.

dirty: a condition in which an object has been contaminated with pathogens.

disinfection: a measure used to decrease the spread of pathogens and disease by destroying pathogens.

doff: to remove.

don: to put on.

drainage: flow of fluids from a wound or cavity.

exposure control plan: plan that outlines specific work practices to prevent exposure to infectious material and identifies step-by-step procedures to follow when exposures do occur.

exposure incident: specific eye, mouth, other mucous membrane, non-intact skin, or parenteral contact with blood or other potentially infectious materials that results from the performance of an employee's duties.

fomite: an object that is contaminated with a pathogen and can spread the pathogen to another person.

hand hygiene: washing hands with either plain or antiseptic soap and water or using alcohol-based hand rubs.

hand rubs: an alcohol-containing preparation designed for application to the hands for reducing the number of microorganisms on the hands.

healthcare-associated infection (HAI): an infection associated with healthcare delivery in any setting (e.g., hospitals, long-term care facilities, ambulatory settings, or home care).

hepatitis: inflammation of the liver caused by certain viruses and other factors, such as alcohol abuse, some medications, and trauma.

immunity: resistance to infection by a specific pathogen.

incubation period: the period of time between the time a pathogen enters the body and the time it causes visible signs and symptoms of disease.

indirect contact: a way to transmit pathogens by touching something contaminated by the infected person.

indirect spread: method of transmission of disease from an object, insect, or animal to a person.

infection: the state resulting from pathogens invading and growing within the human body.

infection prevention: set of methods used to control and prevent the spread of disease; formerly known as "infection control."

infectious disease: any disease caused by growth of a pathogen.

isolate: to keep something separate, or by itself.

localized infection: infection limited to a specific part of the body; has local symptoms.

malnutrition: a serious condition in which a person is not getting proper nutrition.

medical asepsis: refers to practices used to reduce and control the spread of microorganisms, such as handwashing.

microbe: a tiny living thing visible only by microscope; also called a microorganism.

microorganism (MO): a tiny living thing not visible to the eye without a microscope; also called a microbe.

MRSA (methicillin-resistant *Staphylococcus aureus*): an infection caused by specific bacteria that has become resistant to many antibiotics.

mucous membranes: the membranes that line body cavities that open to the outside of the body, such as the linings of the mouth, nose, eyes, rectum, and genitals.

multidrug-resistant organisms (MDROs): microorganisms, mostly bacteria, that are resistant to one or more antimicrobial agents.

non-communicable disease: a disease not capable of being spread from one person to another.

non-intact skin: skin that is broken by abrasions, cuts, rashes, acne, pimples, lesions, surgical incisions, or boils.

normal flora: the microorganisms that normally live in and on the body and do not cause harm in a healthy person, as long as the flora remain in or at that particular area.

Occupational Safety and Health Administration (OSHA): a federal government agency that makes and enforces rules to protect workers from hazards on the job.

pathogen: microorganisms that are capable of causing infection and disease.

perineal care: care of the genitals and anal area by cleaning.

PPE (personal protective equipment): a barrier between a person and pathogens; includes gloves, gowns, masks, goggles, and face shields.

reinfection: being infected again with the same pathogen.

resistance: the body's ability to prevent infection and disease.

sanitation: ways individuals and communities maintain clean, hygienic conditions that help prevent disease, such as the disposal of sewage and solid waste.

Standard Precautions: a method of infection prevention in which all blood, body fluids, non-intact skin (like abrasions, pimples, or open sores), and mucous membranes (lining of mouth, nose, eyes, rectum, or genitals) are treated as if they were infected with a disease.

sterilization: a measure used to decrease the spread of pathogens and disease by destroying all microorganisms, including those that form spores.

surgical asepsis: method that makes an area or an object completely free of microorganisms; also called sterile technique.

systemic infection: an infection that occurs when pathogens enter the bloodstream and move throughout the body; causes general symptoms, such as chills and fever.

transmission: the way and means by which a disease is spread.

vaccine: a substance prepared from weakened or killed microorganisms that is used to give immunity to disease.

VRE (vancomycin-resistant *enterococcus*): a strain of the bacterium *enterococcus* that is resistant to the powerful antibiotic vancomycin; infections occur when the bacteria enter the bloodstream, urinary tract, or surgical wounds.

2. Define "infection prevention" and discuss types of infections

Individuals and communities strive to maintain clean conditions in order to help prevent the spread of disease. This is known as **sanitation**. In facilities, **infection prevention** is the set of methods used to control and prevent the spread of disease. Infection prevention is the responsibility of all members of the care team. Know your facility's policies and follow them. They help protect you, residents, visitors, and other staff members from disease.

A **microorganism** (**MO**) is a tiny living thing visible only by a microscope. It is also called a **microbe**. Microorganisms are always present in the environment (Fig. 6-1). **Infections** are caused by **pathogens**, which are harmful microorganisms. For infections to develop, pathogens must invade and grow within the human body.

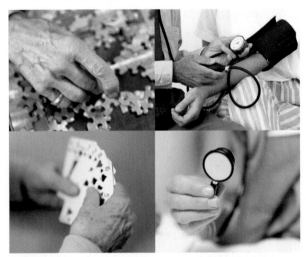

Fig. 6-1. Microorganisms are always present in the environment. They are on almost everything we touch.

There are two main types of infections, localized and systemic. A **localized infection** is limited to a specific part of the body. It has local symptoms, which are near the site of infection. For example, if the eye becomes infected, the area around it might be red, swollen, painful, and warm to the touch. A **systemic infection** occurs when pathogens enter the bloodstream and move throughout the body. It causes general symptoms, such as fever, chills, or mental confusion. AIDS (acquired immune deficiency syndrome) is an example of a systemic infection. You will learn more about AIDS later in this chapter and in Chapter 24.

A special type of infection that can be localized or systemic is a **healthcare-associated infection** (**HAI**), formerly known as "nosocomial infection." A healthcare-associated infection is an infection associated with healthcare delivery in any setting, including long-term care facilities, hospitals, ambulatory settings, and home care. HAIs can be mild or life-threatening.

There are signs and symptoms of infection that you need to know to be able to report them to the nurse. It is important to report these signs promptly. Not reporting immediately can put residents at risk for even greater infections. If you forget to report a resident's symptoms before leaving the facility, by the time you return the next day, the infection might have traveled into the bloodstream and become systemic. Always report the following signs and symptoms right away.

Signs and symptoms of a localized infection include the following:

- Redness

- Swelling

- Pain

- Heat

- **Drainage** (fluid from a wound or cavity)

Signs and symptoms of a systemic infection include the following:

- Fever

- Chills

- Headache

- Change in other vital signs

- Nausea, vomiting, and diarrhea

- Mental confusion

An **infectious disease** is a disease caused by a pathogen. The pathogen will cause an infection if conditions are right. Pathogens grow best in warm, dark, and moist places where food is present, and in hosts who have low resistance. **Resistance** is the body's ability to prevent infection and disease. There are two types of infectious diseases: communicable and non-communicable.

A **communicable disease** is an infectious disease. It is transmitted by direct contact with the infected person or his secretions, or indirectly, by touching objects contaminated by the infected person. An example of a communicable disease is influenza. A **contagious disease** is a type of communicable disease that spreads quickly from person to person. Chickenpox is an example of a contagious disease. A **non-communicable disease** is a disease not capable of being spread from one person to another. For example, a person who has emphysema, a disease of the lungs, is not contagious to others.

By using proper infection prevention methods, you can help prevent residents, visitors, and staff members from acquiring an infection from another person, object, place, or from one part of the body to another. This is called **cross-infection**, or cross-contamination. Infection prevention methods will also help protect a person from being infected again with the same pathogen, called **reinfection**.

3. Discuss terms related to infection prevention

Infection prevention is about breaking the chain of infection, which is discussed in the next learning objective. **Transmission** of disease can be blocked by using proper infection prevention practices, such as handwashing, which are a part of **medical asepsis**. Medical asepsis is used in all healthcare facilities. Before asepsis is explained in more detail, some terms must be understood.

In health care, an object can be called **clean** if it has not been **contaminated** with pathogens. An object that is **dirty** has been contaminated with pathogens.

Measures like disinfection and sterilization decrease the spread of pathogens that could cause disease. **Disinfection** means that only pathogens are destroyed. **Sterilization** means all microorganisms are destroyed, including those that form spores. Spore-forming microorganisms are a special group of organisms that produce a protective covering that is difficult to penetrate. An **autoclave** is a type of special equipment used to sterilize objects and kill pathogens that form spores. This machine creates a hot steam under pressure for a period of time to kill all microorganisms. There are other types of devices used to kill microorganisms. These sterilizing devices use toxic gases, dry heat, strong chemical solutions, or radiation.

The goal of medical asepsis is to prevent the spread of pathogens by keeping a facility as clean as possible. This does not mean that the facility is free from all microorganisms. The only way to make an area or object completely free of microorganisms is to use **surgical asepsis**. Another term for surgical asepsis is sterile technique. Surgical asepsis makes an object or area sterile. This means it is completely free of all microorganisms. There may be times when you will assist a nurse with a procedure that requires sterile technique. You will have special training to help with this type of procedure. Chapter 18 has more information on the sterile field, sterile gloves, and sterile dressings. These are all used in surgical asepsis.

Facilities will have separate areas for clean and dirty items, such as equipment, linen and supplies. They are normally called the "clean" and the "dirty" or "contaminated" utility rooms. Before entering a clean utility room, wash your hands. This helps keep the equipment in this room clean.

The contaminated or dirty utility room is separate from the clean utility room. It is used to store equipment that is not needed by the resident. Supplies in this room, such as trash bags, are not considered clean. A sink is usually in this room. Wash your hands before leaving the dirty utility room so that you do not transfer pathogens to other areas in the facility. After washing your hands, do not touch anything in the dirty utility room, including the door handle. If you do, you must wash your hands again.

Know the location of the clean and dirty utility rooms and what is stored in each. You will learn more about handling linen and equipment in Learning Objective 9 of this chapter.

4. Describe the chain of infection

The chain of infection describes how disease is transmitted from one being to another (Fig. 6-2). There are six links in the chain of infection:

- Link 1: Causative agent

- Link 2: Reservoir

- Link 3: Portal of exit

- Link 4: Mode of transmission

- Link 5: Portal of entry

- Link 6: Susceptible host

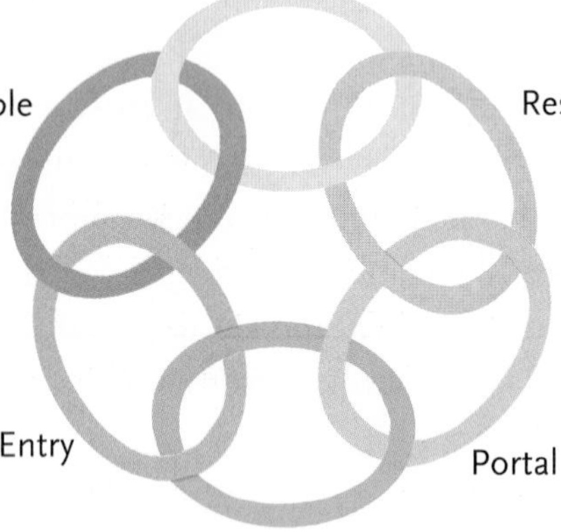

Fig. 6-2. The chain of infection.

If one of the links in the chain of infection is broken, transmission of infection can be prevented.

Chain Link 1: The causative agent is a pathogenic microorganism that causes disease. As you learned, microorganisms are small living bodies that cannot be seen without a microscope. They are everywhere—on skin, in food, in the air, and in water. Causative agents include bacteria, viruses, fungi, and parasites.

Normal flora are the microorganisms that normally live in and on the body without causing harm to a healthy person, as long as the flora remain in or at that particular area. When they enter a different part of the body, they may cause an infection.

There is a waiting period between the time the pathogen enters the body and the time it causes visible signs and symptoms of disease. This period is called an **incubation period**. Some examples of incubation periods include:

- Chickenpox: 10-21 days

- Influenza (flu): 1-3 days

- Measles: 10-21 days

An infection prevention example for Link 1 is vaccines. **Vaccines**, substances prepared from weakened or killed microorganisms, can give **immunity** to a disease without causing physical signs and symptoms of the particular disease. The immunity may not last forever.

Chain Link 2: A reservoir is where the pathogen lives and grows. A reservoir can be a human, an animal, a plant, soil, or a substance. Microorganisms grow best in warm, dark, and moist places where food is present. Some microorganisms need oxygen to survive, while others do not. The blood and the lungs are examples of reservoirs.

There are two main ways of spreading an infection from a reservoir: direct and indirect. **Direct spread** occurs when a person gets a disease directly from another person (reservoir). The human reservoir may be a person with an active disease or a person carrying the disease (a **carrier**). A human carrier "carries" the disease, but usually does not show any signs or symptoms at the time he or she spreads the disease. This carrier may or may not get the disease later.

Indirect spread occurs when a person gets a disease from an object, insect, or animal (reservoir). Objects are also called "fomites." A **fomite** is an object that is contaminated with a pathogen and can now spread the pathogen to another person. Fomites may be things like infected food, water, food utensils, bedpans, or bed linens.

An infection prevention example for Link 2 is to keep surfaces clean and dry.

Chain Link 3: There can be different exit routes, or portals of exit, from a reservoir. The portal of exit is any opening on an infected person allowing pathogens to leave. These include the nose, mouth, eyes, or a cut in the skin (Fig. 6-3). An infection prevention example for Link 3 is covering the nose and mouth when sneezing.

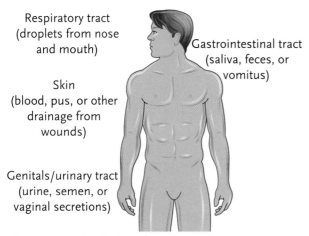

Fig. 6-3. *Portals of exit.*

Chain Link 4: The mode of transmission describes how the pathogen travels. The actual transmission of an infectious disease occurs in different ways. The main routes of transmission are contact, droplet, and airborne transmission. The primary route of disease transmission within the healthcare setting is on the hands of healthcare workers.

Contact transmission occurs through contact with the person's blood or body fluids that are contaminated by the pathogen. **Body fluids** include tears, saliva, sputum (mucus coughed up), urine, feces, semen, vaginal secretions, pus or other wound drainage, and vomit. **Direct contact** happens by touching the infected person or his or her secretions. **Indirect contact** results from touching something contaminated by the infected person, such as a needle, instrument, or dressing.

Droplet transmission occurs when the pathogen travels short distances after being expelled. Droplets normally do not travel more than three feet, but they may travel further. Droplets can be created when the infected person coughs, sneezes, or talks. Laughing, suctioning, singing, and spitting may also transmit droplets. A susceptible host (Link 6) inhales contaminated droplets and may get an infection.

In airborne transmission, the pathogen is transmitted through the air after being expelled. The pathogen is carried a distance, usually more than three feet, on air currents. A pathogen can also be carried by dust. A susceptible host (Link 6) inhales contaminated moisture or dust, which may cause an infection.

An infection prevention example for Link 4 is washing hands.

Chain Link 5: Pathogens enter the human host through different portals of entry. The portal of entry is any body opening on an uninfected person that allows pathogens to enter. This includes the nose, mouth, eyes, and other mucous membranes, cuts in the skin, and cracked skin (Fig. 6-4). **Mucous membranes** are the membranes that line body cavities that open to the outside of the body. These include the linings of the mouth, nose, eyes, rectum, and genitals.

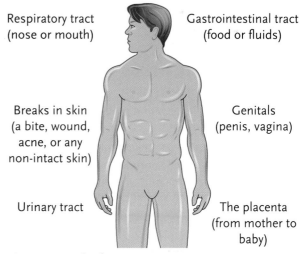

Fig. 6-4. *Portals of entry.*

When a pathogen invades the body, it can cause an infection. Many areas of the body are protected from invading pathogens. A sort of body "armor" works with the immune system to help protect the body from harmful bacteria (Fig. 6-5). The box on the next page describes how the body keeps itself healthy.

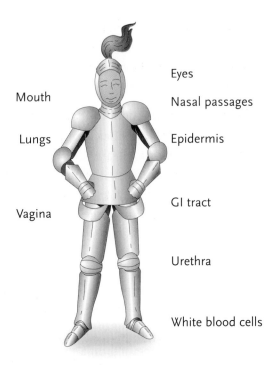

Fig. 6-5. *The human body has a sort of "armor" that helps protect it from harmful bacteria.*

The Human Body's Defensive Armor

Nasal passages: Mucous membranes have cilia, tiny hairs in the nose that trap microorganisms.

Epidermis: As long as skin stays unbroken and undamaged, microorganisms cannot get inside.

Lungs: Cilia move microbes, mucus, and debris up and out of the airways.

Mouth: Saliva has a protein called lactoferrin that blocks the growth of pathogens.

Eyes: The eyes have tears that protect them by cleaning out microorganisms.

GI (gastrointestinal) tract: The GI tract has "good" microorganisms, called "normal flora," that prevent the growth of "bad" microorganisms, or pathogens. In addition, the strong acid environment of the gastrointestinal tract prevents many microorganisms from surviving.

Vagina: The vagina has a low pH of about 3.5 to 4.5, which blocks the growth of pathogens.

Urethra: Urine rinses out pathogens from the urinary tract.

Blood cells: White blood cells defend the body from microorganisms and play a role in the secretion of antibodies.

An infection prevention example for Link 5 is wearing gloves.

Chain Link 6: A susceptible host is an uninfected person who could become ill. A person becomes a susceptible host when his or her resistance to disease decreases. Some reasons for lowered resistance include age, existing illnesses, fatigue, poor nutrition, lack of adequate fluid intake, certain medications, and stress. The elderly have weaker immune systems and lower resistance to pathogens. When a pathogen invades the body, it will start reproducing itself, causing tissue invasion and tissue damage.

An infection prevention example for Link 6 is staying healthy and protecting the elderly and ill from pathogens.

Trivia

The Amazing Discovery of Edward Jenner

In 18th-century England, smallpox was a very common, horribly disfiguring disease. A doctor at that time, Edward Jenner (1749-1823), noticed that people who were exposed to cowpox, such as the milkmaids who milked cows, would develop a small sore and then never get smallpox. He then developed a vaccine from the cowpox sores to give immunity to smallpox. After he injected the matter from the sore into a boy, James Phipps, he tested the vaccine by trying to give James the disease more than once. Each time, Jenner found that little James was immune to the disease.

5. Explain why the elderly are at a higher risk for infection

Residents are at a greater risk of acquiring infections while living in a facility. As people age, multiple changes occur to make the elderly more susceptible to infections (Fig. 6-6). Elderly individuals are hospitalized more often, which increases their chances for acquiring a healthcare-associated infection (HAI). In addition, the elderly may have more serious infections with longer recovery times.

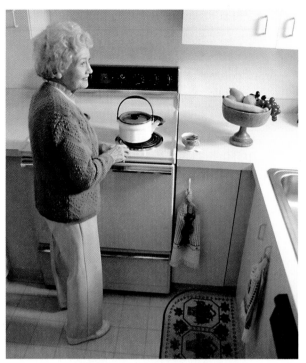

Fig. 6-6. *The elderly are at higher risk for infection due to weaker immune systems, limited mobility, thinner skin, slow wound healing, and many other reasons.*

As people age, their skin becomes less elastic. The skin's oil glands become less productive, leading to dryness and thinning of the skin layers. This can cause skin to tear easily and delays the healing process. Skin changes and limited mobility increase the risk of pressure ulcers and skin infections.

Bones become more brittle and can break more easily. Broken bones increase the risk of infection. Decreased circulation and slow wound healing also contribute to infections in the elderly.

Elderly people may require catheters for urinary elimination. **Catheters** and other types of tubing, such as feeding tubes, can greatly increase the risk of infections.

Older adults are at risk for dehydration and **malnutrition**. A person who is malnourished is not getting the proper nutrition. **Dehydration** occurs when there is an excessive loss of water from the body. Both dehydration and malnutrition are serious problems. They may be caused

by a lack of thirst and appetite, certain illnesses, or medications. When cells do not get proper nutrients and fluids, the chance of infection greatly increases.

One method of reducing infection is to keep residents as healthy as possible by promoting good health habits and using proper infection prevention methods. This is required of all staff members. You will learn more methods on how to keep residents infection-free in Chapter 24.

6. Describe Centers for Disease Control and Prevention (CDC) and explain Standard Precautions

Centers for Disease Control and Prevention (CDC) is a federal government agency that issues guidelines to protect and improve health. It promotes public health and safety through education and tries to control and prevent disease. In 1996, the CDC created new guidelines to protect people in health care from contracting infectious diseases. In 2007, the CDC released some changes to this system.

There are two levels of precautions in the infection prevention system recommended by the CDC. They are Standard Precautions and Transmission-Based, or Isolation, Precautions. To **isolate** means to keep something separate, or by itself.

Standard Precautions must be used with every resident in your care. **Standard Precautions** means treating blood, body fluids, non-intact skin, and mucous membranes as if they were infected. Body fluids include tears, saliva, sputum (mucus coughed up), urine, feces, semen, vaginal secretions, pus or other wound drainage, and vomit. They do not include sweat. Standard Precautions are always followed because you cannot tell by looking at residents or their charts whether or not they have a contagious disease (Fig. 6-7). The guidelines for Standard Precautions are listed below.

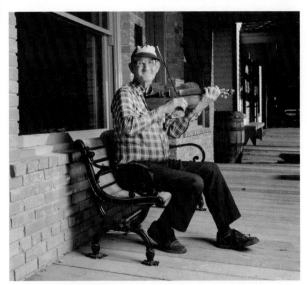

Fig. 6-7. *Standard Precautions must be practiced on every person in your care, no matter how healthy or unhealthy he seems. You cannot tell by looking at a person whether he has an infectious disease or not.*

Guidelines: Standard Precautions

G **Wash your hands** before putting on gloves. Wash them immediately after removing gloves. Do not touch clean objects with contaminated gloves.

G **Wear gloves** if you may come into contact with blood, body fluids, secretions and excretions, broken or open skin, human tissue, or mucous membranes (linings of the eyes, nose, mouth, vagina, penis, or rectum).

G **Immediately wash all skin surfaces that have been contaminated** with blood and body fluids.

G **Wear a disposable gown** if you may come into contact with blood, body fluids, secretions or excretions, or when splashing or spraying blood or body fluids is likely.

G **Wear a mask, protective goggles, and/or face shield** if you may come into contact with blood, body fluids, secretions or excretions, or when splashing or spraying blood or body fluids is likely.

G **Wear gloves and use caution when handling razor blades and other sharps.** Be careful not to cut yourself or nick or cut residents when

using razor blades. Place sharps carefully in a biohazard container for sharps. Biohazard containers used for sharps are hard, leak-proof containers. They are clearly labeled and warn of the danger of the contents inside (Fig. 6-8). There are also biohazard bags that are used for biomedical waste that is not sharp, such as soiled dressings, contaminated tubing, and other items. OSHA recommends disposal of biomedical/biohazard waste at the "point of origin," or where the waste occurs.

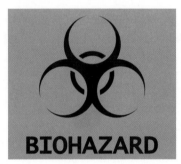

Fig. 6-8. *This label indicates that the material is potentially infectious.*

G **Never attempt to re-cap needles or sharps after use.** You might stick yourself. Dispose of them in an approved container.

G **Bag all disposable contaminated supplies.** Dispose of them according to your facility's policy. Special containers are used for disposal. Place non-disposable contaminated supplies, such as linens and reusable equipment, in the proper container.

G **Clean all surfaces that may be contaminated with infectious waste.** Follow facility policy. Examples of these areas are overbed tables, beds, wheelchairs, and shower chairs.

G **Remember that Standard Precautions must be practiced on every single person in your care.** Standard Precautions help reduce the risk of acquiring disease from those in your care. They also help prevent residents' infections from being passed to other residents.

In addition to Standard Precautions, here are general guidelines for preventing infection in a facility:

Guidelines: Additional Ways to Prevent Infection

G Clean a cut or break in your skin immediately with a facility-approved disinfecting product.

G Cover your mouth and nose with a tissue when coughing or sneezing. If you do not have a tissue, cough or sneeze into your upper sleeve or elbow, not your hands. Immediately wash your hands afterward or clean with an alcohol-based hand rub.

G Keep yourself as healthy as possible.

G Never use one resident's personal items with another resident. Keep all personal items separate and labeled with resident's name and room number.

G Never transfer personal items or any kind of equipment from one room to another. An exception is something like your stethoscope. You must disinfect the part of your stethoscope that touches a resident after each use.

G Hold all equipment, personal care items, and soiled laundry and linens away from your uniform while walking.

G When objects have dropped to the floor, do not use them. Obtain new/clean items.

G Clean all equipment used by residents after use. Follow the facility's guidelines for disinfection.

G Clean all common areas (areas used by more than one resident) after use.

G Remove food or soiled eating utensils in residents' rooms after food trays have been picked up.

G Change and date water cups often. Make sure name and room number are on water cups.

G Clean resident toothbrushes and shaving equipment often, following facility policy. Place in proper container that is clearly labeled following use.

G Never place contaminated items like bedpans or any other dirty items on the overbed table.

You will learn more about resident's unit equipment in Chapter 10.

G When cleaning anything, move from the cleanest to the dirtiest area.

Respiratory Hygiene/Cough Etiquette

Guidelines for all persons entering facilities who show any signs of respiratory illnesses have been developed as a part of Standard Precautions. The guidelines are listed below:

- Covering the nose and mouth with a tissue when coughing or sneezing, or coughing or sneezing into the upper sleeve or elbow, not the hands

- Promptly disposing of the tissues in the nearest no-touch waste container

- Cleaning hands after coughing or sneezing by washing them with soap and water, using an alcohol-based hand rub, or antiseptic handwash

- Wearing special masks and turning the head away from others when coughing

- Encouraging coughing persons to sit at least three feet from others in common waiting areas

7. Define "hand hygiene" and identify when to wash hands

In your work, you will use your hands constantly. Microorganisms are on everything you touch. The single most common transmission of health care-associated infections (HAIs) in a healthcare setting is via the hands of healthcare workers. Washing your hands is the single most important thing you can do to prevent the spread of disease (Fig. 6-9).

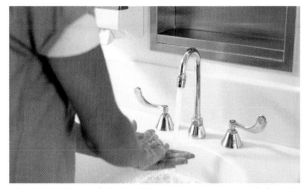

Fig. 6-9. All people in health care must wash their hands often. Washing your hands is the most important thing you can do to prevent the spread of disease.

Hand hygiene is defined by the CDC as washing hands with either plain or antiseptic soap and water or using alcohol-based hand rubs. Alcohol-based hand rubs (often called "**hand rubs**" or "hand sanitizers") include gels, rinses, and foams which do not require the use of water. Alcohol-based hand rubs are not a substitute for frequent and proper handwashing. When hands are visibly soiled, wash them with plain or antimicrobial soap and water. An **antimicrobial** agent destroys, resists, or prevents the development of pathogens.

Keep your nails short and clean. Do not wear artificial nails or extenders because they harbor bacteria, even if you wash your hands often. Rings and other jewelry collect bacteria and can cause infection. Keep them at home.

Use unscented lotions to keep your hands soft and intact. It is dangerous for you to work with cracked, broken skin. Use lotions at home, as well, to minimize or prevent skin dryness and irritation.

You must wash your hands at these times:

- When you first arrive at work
- Whenever they are visibly soiled
- Before, between, and after all contact with residents
- Before putting on gloves and after removing gloves
- Before and after touching meal trays and/or handling food
- Before and after feeding residents
- Before entering a "clean" supply room
- Before getting clean linen
- Before leaving a "dirty" supply room
- Before and after you eat
- After contact with blood or any body fluids, mucous membranes, non-intact skin, or wound dressings
- After handling contaminated items

- After contact with any object, including medical equipment, in the resident's room
- After touching garbage
- After cleaning spills or picking up anything from the floor
- After using the toilet
- After coughing, sneezing, or blowing your nose
- After smoking
- After handling your hair or touching areas on your body, such as your nose, mouth, eyes, and face
- After touching jewelry
- After changing diapers
- After handling animals/pets and after contact with pet care items
- Before leaving work and after you get home from work before touching anything or anyone

Washing hands

Equipment: soap, paper towels

1. Turn on water at the sink. Keep your clothes dry, because moisture breeds bacteria. Do not let your clothing touch the outside portion of the sink or counter.

2. Angle your arms downward, with your fingertips pointing down into the sink. Your hands should be lower than your elbows. Wet your hands and wrists thoroughly (Fig. 6-10).

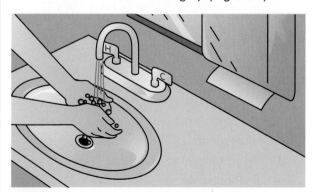

Fig. 6-10.

3.　Apply skin cleanser or soap to your hands.

4.　Rub hands together and fingers between each other to create a lather. Lather all surfaces of your fingers and hands, including your wrists (Fig. 6-11). Use friction for at least 20 seconds.

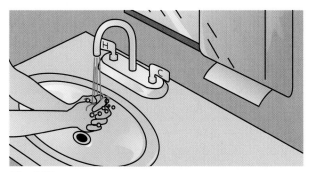

Fig. 6-11.

5.　Clean your nails by rubbing them in the palm of your other hand.

6.　Being careful not to touch the sink, rinse thoroughly under running water. Rinse all surfaces of your hands and wrists. Run water down from wrists to fingertips. Do not run water over unwashed arms down to clean hands.

7.　Use a clean, dry paper towel to dry all surfaces of your hands, wrists, and fingers. Do not wipe towel on unwashed forearms and then wipe clean hands. Dispose of towel without touching wastebasket. If your hands touch the sink or wastebasket, start over.

8.　Use clean, dry paper towel to turn off the faucet. Do not contaminate your hands by touching the surface of the sink or faucet (Fig. 6-12).

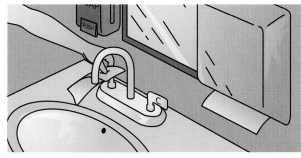

Fig. 6-12.

9.　Dispose of used paper towels in proper waste receptacle after shutting off faucet. Avoid touching doorknobs, if possible, when leaving bathrooms. Use a paper towel to open the door.

8. Discuss the use of personal protective equipment (PPE) in facilities

Personal protective equipment (**PPE**) is a barrier (a block or obstacle) between a person and pathogens. PPE is what you wear to help protect you from contact with potentially infectious material. You will need to know how to put on, or **don**, use, and remove, or **doff**, PPE correctly.

PPE includes gloves, gowns, masks, goggles, and face shields. Gloves protect hands, and gowns protect the skin and clothing. Masks protect the mouth and nose. Goggles protect the eyes, and face shields protect the entire face—the eyes, nose, and mouth.

Your employers will provide you with the proper PPE to wear. The type of PPE you wear depends on what kind of exposure you may encounter. For example, a chance of coming into contact with spraying or splashing blood or body fluids is one type of exposure that requires gown, gloves, and mask and goggles, or face shield. PPE selection also depends on the type of Transmission-Based Precautions that are ordered for a resident. You will learn more about these precautions in Learning Objective 11. PPE use is determined by the type of task you will do. Always perform hand hygiene after removing and disposing of PPE.

Gloves

There are two types of gloves: non-sterile and sterile. Non-sterile gloves are used for basic care in a facility. They come in different sizes and may be made of nitrile, vinyl, or latex. Some people are allergic to latex. If you are, let the nurse know so that alternative gloves can be provided. Gloves should fit your hands comfortably. They should not be too loose or too snug.

When wearing gloves, always work from clean to dirty. This means you should touch clean surfaces or areas before touching contaminated ones.

Always wear gloves when:

- You may come into contact with blood or any body fluids, open wounds, or mucous membranes

- Performing or helping with mouth care or care of any mucous membrane

- Performing or helping with **perineal care** (care of the genitals and anal area)

- Performing care on a resident who has **non-intact skin**—skin that is broken by abrasions, cuts, rashes, acne, pimples, lesions, surgical incisions, or boils

- You have any open sores or cuts on your hands

- Shaving a resident

- Disposing of soiled bed linens, gowns, dressings, and pads

- You will have direct contact with residents who require Contact Precautions (a type of Transmission-Based Precautions; see Learning Objective 11)

- Touching surfaces or equipment or handling equipment that is either visibly contaminated or may be contaminated

If you do have open areas on your hands, cover them first with a bandage, then put on gloves. Disposable gloves cannot be washed or re-used. Wear them only once and then discard them.

Before contact with mucous membranes or broken skin, remove gloves, wash your hands and don new gloves. Change gloves immediately if they become wet, worn, soiled, or torn. Do not contaminate skin or clothing when removing gloves. Wash your hands before putting on new gloves. Do not wear gloves outside the resident's room. Do not touch anything with contaminated gloves that anyone else may touch without wearing gloves.

For example, if you are carrying a used bedpan, do not touch the doorknob or open the door with gloved hands. If you did, the doorknob would be contaminated. Change gloves if your hands will move from a body site that is contaminated to a body site that is not contaminated. Before touching any surface, remove your gloves, wash your hands, and put on new gloves if needed.

Putting on (donning) gloves

1. Wash your hands.

2. If you are right-handed, slide one glove on your left hand (reverse if left-handed).

3. Using your gloved hand, slide the other hand into the second glove.

4. Interlace fingers to smooth out folds and create a comfortable fit.

5. Check for tears, holes, cracks, or discolored spots in the gloves. Replace the glove if needed.

6. Adjust gloves until they are pulled up over the wrist and fit correctly. If wearing a gown, pull the cuff of the gloves over the sleeves of the gown (Fig. 6-13).

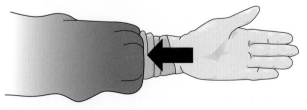

Fig. 6-13.

Infection Prevention

Remove gloves immediately after use and before caring for another resident. Wash your hands. Never touch your face or adjust PPE with clean or dirty gloves.

Removing (doffing) gloves

1. Touch only the outside of one glove. Pull the first glove off by pulling down from the cuff toward the fingers (Fig. 6-14).

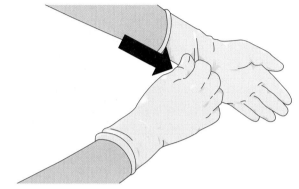

Fig. 6-14.

2. As this glove comes off the hand it should be turned inside out.

3. With the fingertips of your gloved hand, hold the glove you just removed. With your ungloved hand, reach two fingers inside the remaining glove at wrist. Be careful not to touch any part of the outside of the glove (Fig. 6-15).

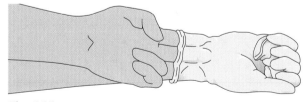

Fig. 6-15.

4. Pull down, turning this glove inside out and over the first glove as you remove it.

5. You should now be holding one glove from its clean inner side. The other glove should be inside it.

6. Drop both gloves into the proper container.

7. Wash your hands.

Gowns

Gowns protect the skin and the clothing from contamination. Wear a gown if you may come into contact with blood, body fluids, secretions or excretions, tissue, or when splashing or spraying blood or body fluids is likely. Wear a gown if your clothing will have direct contact with the resident or any contaminated equipment or surfaces that may have come into contact with the resident. Wear a gown when handling any equipment that is visibly soiled or may have had contact with blood or body fluids.

Gowns should fully cover your torso. They should fit comfortably over your body, and have long sleeves that fit snugly at the wrist. If a gown does not fit you properly, report it to your supervisor. If one gown is too small to safely and completely cover your torso, you may need to wear two gowns. The underlying gown is donned with the opening to the front and the top gown is donned with the opening to the back.

Gowns are usually made of a fluid-resistant material. However, they may still become wet or soiled. If this happens, remove the gown. Check your clothing and put on a new gown. Gowns must be changed immediately if they become wet or soiled. Gowns are used once and disposed of properly. Do not wear gowns outside the resident's room. Remove gown promptly after care. Do not contaminate skin or clothing when removing gowns. After gown removal, avoid touching any surface in the room with your uniform or your skin before exiting the room.

Putting on (donning) gown

1. Wash your hands.

2. Remove watch and place it on a clean paper towel. If wearing long sleeves, push or roll them up.

3. Open the gown. Hold it out in front of you and allow it to open/unfold (Fig. 6-16). Do

not shake gown or touch it to the floor. Slip your arms into the sleeves and pull the gown on.

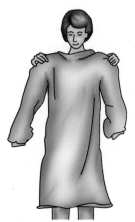

Fig. 6-16.

4. Fasten the neck opening.

5. Reach behind you. Pull the gown until it completely covers your clothing. Secure gown at waist (Fig. 6-17).

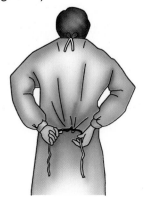

Fig. 6-17.

6. Use gowns only once and then remove and discard. Do not contaminate skin or clothing when removing gowns. Unfasten gown at neck and waist. Hold gown away from body and roll dirty side in. Discard gown in proper container.

7. Put on gloves after putting on a gown.

Masks and Goggles

Masks should be worn when caring for residents who cough or sneeze or have respiratory illnesses. Masks can prevent inhalation of micro-organisms through the nose or mouth. Masks protect the nose and mouth and mucous membranes from contamination during resident care or activities. Wear a mask along with protective goggles if you anticipate that, during resident care or activities, you may come into contact with blood or body fluids.

Goggles are worn with a mask and are used whenever it is likely that blood or body fluids may be splashed or sprayed into your eye area or your eyes. Eyeglasses alone do not provide enough protection. Goggles should fit snugly over and around your eyes or eyeglasses.

Masks should fully cover your nose and mouth and prevent fluid penetration. Masks should fit snugly over the nose and mouth. Masks are worn once and disposed of. Masks that become wet or soiled must be changed immediately. Remove masks after a procedure. Change masks between resident care. Never wear a mask in the hall between resident rooms.

When removing a mask and/or goggles, remove your gloves first and then wash your hands. Be careful to not touch the mask or goggles to your clothing or your skin. The pieces used to secure the mask or goggles to the head are considered clean and can be touched with your ungloved hands. The mask and goggles themselves are considered contaminated. Do not contaminate skin or clothing when removing masks or goggles. Wash hands every time after removing a mask and/or goggles.

Putting on (donning) mask and goggles

1. Wash your hands.

2. Pick up the mask by the top strings or the elastic strap. Do not touch the mask where it touches your face.

3. Adjust the mask over your nose and mouth. Tie top strings, then bottom strings. Never wear a mask hanging from only the bottom strings (Fig. 6-18).

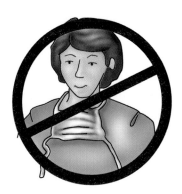

Fig. 6-18.

4. Pinch the metal strip at the top of the mask (if part of the mask) tightly around your nose so that it feels snug. Fit mask snugly around face and below the chin.

5. Put on the goggles. Position them over the eyes. Secure them to the head using the headband or earpieces.

6. Put on your gloves after putting on mask and goggles.

Some respiratory diseases, such as tuberculosis (TB), require special PPE to be worn. More information on TB is in Chapter 20. This equipment helps keep staff safe from this disease. Special masks must be worn because a standard mask does not protect the caregiver from TB. These masks, called respirators, have a filter that protects the face and lungs. An N95 respirator mask is one type of special mask. The caregiver must be fitted for this mask. Each time the person puts the respirator on, a "user-seal check," formerly called a "fit-check," must be done to minimize the leaking of any air from around the respirator. You will be taught how to perform a user-seal check.

Face Shields

Face shields may be worn when contact with blood or body fluids may occur. Face shields are used whenever it is likely that blood or body fluids may be splashed or sprayed into your eye area or your eyes. Face shields can be used instead of goggles and may offer more protection from sprays and splashes than goggles can provide. Face shields may be worn with a mask. Follow facility policy with face shields. The face shield should cover your forehead, go below the chin, and wrap around the side of the head. Secure it on your head using the headband.

Do not wear face shields outside the resident's room. When removing a face shield, remove your gloves first, and wash your hands. Be careful not to touch the shield to your clothing or your skin. The pieces used to secure the shield to the head are considered clean and can be touched with your ungloved hands. The face shield itself is considered contaminated. Do not contaminate skin or clothing when removing face shields. Wash hands every time after removing a face shield.

You are responsible for knowing where the PPE is kept in your facility. If you have questions on what PPE is needed, ask the nurse (Fig. 6-19). When applying PPE, you must follow a specific order. Removing PPE requires a specific order, too. The order depends on what PPE you are wearing and whether special precautions have been ordered.

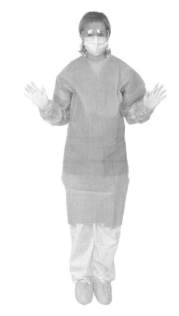

Fig. 6-19. Wear the proper PPE for tasks. Using PPE is an important way to reduce the spread of infection.

Putting on (donning) and removing (doffing) the full set of PPE

Donning:

1. Wash your hands.

2. Put on gown.

3. Put on mask or respirator.

4. Put on goggles or face shield.

5. Put on gloves.

Doffing:

1. Remove and discard gloves.

2. Remove goggles or face shield.

3. Remove and discard gown.

4. Remove and discard mask or respirator.

5. Wash your hands. Performing hand hygiene is always the final step after removing and disposing of PPE.

9. List guidelines for handling linen and equipment

Facilities handle storage and disposal of linen and equipment by following guidelines set by the CDC. As you have learned, facilities have separate areas for clean and dirty items, called the "clean" and the "dirty" or "contaminated" utility rooms. Linen and equipment will be placed in separate containers to be cleaned or discarded.

There will be disposal containers for:

• Linen

• Trash

• Equipment

• Infectious waste

Guidelines: Handling Linen and Equipment

G   Wear gloves when handling, transporting and processing soiled linens.

G   When removing linen, handle it carefully. Check linen to make sure no items are left inside, especially sharps, as you remove it from the bed. Fold or roll linen so that the dirtiest area is inside.

G   Hold and carry dirty linen away from your uniform (Fig. 6-20).

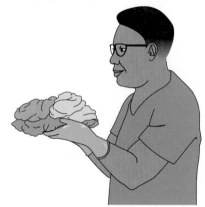

Fig. 6-20. Hold dirty linen away from your uniform.

G   Do not shake dirty linen or clothes.

G   Place or dispose of linen, trash, used equipment, and infectious waste in the proper containers. All sharps must be safely placed in puncture-proof biohazard containers.

G   Do not touch the inside of any disposal container.

G   Do not use "re-usable" equipment again until it has been properly cleaned and reprocessed. Dispose of all single-use, or disposable, equipment properly.

G   Wear gloves when cleaning and disinfecting surfaces. Clean and disinfect beds, bedrails and all bedside equipment. Clean all frequently-touched surfaces, such as doorknobs.

10. Explain how to handle spills

In a healthcare facility, spills are a threat to safety. Spilled blood, body fluids, and other fluids increase the risk of infection, and, in addition, spills put residents and staff at risk for falls. Clean spills using proper equipment and procedures, and follow these guidelines:

G   Don gloves immediately. You may need to use special heavy-duty gloves, depending on the spill.

G   First, absorb the spill with whatever product is used by the facility. It may be an absorbing powder.

G   Scoop up the absorbed spill, and dispose of it in a designated container.

G   Apply the proper disinfectant to the spill area. Allow it to stand wet for the proper length of time, following directions on the label.

G   Be careful if any glass or other sharp objects are in the spill. Get help when picking up and disposing of sharps and other objects. Never pick up broken glass, even with gloved hands. If you do accidentally cut yourself, follow exposure incident guidelines (see Learning Objective 13).

G   For large spills, call for the nurse, and she will follow your facility's policy for large spill clean-up. Dispose of gloves and cleaning supplies according to facility policy.

G   If you spill a substance on your body, immediately wash that area using the proper cleaning agent. Follow exposure incident guidelines.

G   Wash your hands after cleaning spills.

Some facilities have special "spill areas" that have equipment to handle spills. Colored cones are placed to identify the area where the spill occurred. Pads that come in different sizes are placed over the spill. Then the proper department is notified to clean the area.

11. Discuss Transmission-Based Precautions

In 1996, the CDC set forth a second level of precautions beyond Standard Precautions. These guidelines are for persons who are infected or may be infected with certain infectious diseases. They are known as Transmission-Based or Isolation Precautions.

The three categories of Transmission-Based Precautions are Airborne Precautions, Droplet Precautions, and Contact Precautions. The type used depends on what type of disease the person has, or may have, and how it spreads. They may also be used in combination for diseases that have multiple routes of transmission.

Airborne Precautions

Airborne Precautions prevent the spread of pathogens that travel through the air for a distance after being expelled (Fig. 6-21). The pathogens remain floating for some time. They are carried by moisture, by air currents, and by dust. An example of an airborne disease is tuberculosis (TB). TB is a highly contagious lung disease carried on mucous droplets suspended in the air and released by an infected person through talking, coughing, breathing, laughing, or singing. TB can be fatal if not treated. More information on TB is found in Chapter 20. Airborne Precautions include the following:

• Follow all Standard Precautions.

• Residents will be placed in a room called an airborne infection isolation room (AIIR), also called a negative pressure isolation room or acid-fast bacillus (AFB) isolation room. These rooms have a controlled flow of air. All of the air inside the room will be exhausted directly to the outside, or all air will first be recirculated through a special HEPA filter before returning to circulation. Within this ventilation system, air flows into the room from the hallways or other adjacent areas when the door to the room is opened. This helps ensure that contaminated air does not enter other parts of the facility.

Keep windows to these rooms closed. Keep doors to these rooms closed when not going into or out of the room. When entering an airborne infection isolation room, do not open or close the door rapidly. This pulls contaminated room air into the hallway.

- Wear a special mask during resident care. All people entering the room must wear a special mask, such as an N95 respirator mask, prior to entering the AIIR. A standard mask is not safe to use because the TB bacterium is small enough to penetrate a regular mask.

- Follow facility policy on where to remove masks.

- Residents will wear regular surgical masks if they must leave the room and observe Respiratory Hygiene/Cough Etiquette (see earlier box).

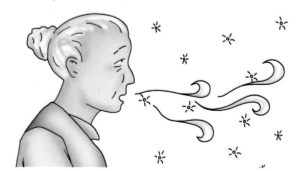

Fig. 6-21. Airborne diseases stay suspended in the air.

Droplet Precautions

Droplet Precautions are used for diseases that are spread by droplets in the air. Droplets normally do not travel further than three feet, but they may travel further. For example, the CDC recommends increasing the droplet distance from three feet to six feet for influenza. Talking, singing, sneezing, laughing, or coughing can spread droplets (Fig. 6-22). An example of a droplet disease is the mumps. Droplet Precautions include the following:

- Follow all Standard Precautions.

- Apply a mask before entering the room. Wear the mask during resident care.

- Facilities should limit transport of residents outside of the room to medical necessities.

Residents must wear masks if they must leave the room and observe Respiratory Hygiene/Cough Etiquette.

- Cover your mouth and nose with a tissue when coughing or sneezing. Ask others to do the same. Dispose of the tissue in a no-touch receptacle. Do not place used tissue in pocket for future use. If you do not have a tissue, cough or sneeze into your upper sleeve or elbow, not your hands. Immediately wash your hands afterward or clean with an alcohol-based hand rub.

- Visits from uninfected people will be restricted.

- Pull the privacy curtain between beds of any residents placed in the same room.

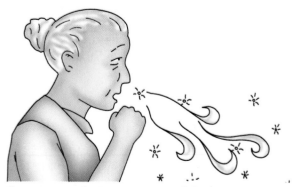

Fig. 6-22. Droplet Precautions are followed when the disease-causing microorganism does not remain in the air.

Contact Precautions

Contact Precautions are used when a resident may spread an infection by direct contact with another person or object. The infection can be spread when a nursing assistant touches a contaminated area on a resident's body or his contaminated blood or body fluids (Fig. 6-23). It may also be spread by touching contaminated personal items, linen, equipment, or supplies. Conjunctivitis (pink eye) and *Clostridium difficile* (*C. diff*) are examples of a contact disease. You will learn more about *C. diff* later in the chapter. Contact Precautions include the following:

- Follow all Standard Precautions.

- Wear proper PPE. Put on gloves before entering a resident's room. Change gloves if they are contaminated with infected material. Remove gloves before leaving the room.

- While still in the room, wash hands with an antimicrobial soap after removing gloves. Do not touch any surface with your hands before exiting.

- Put on a gown before entering a resident's room. Remove and dispose of gown before leaving the room. Do not wear any PPE outside the resident's room. Wash hands after removing gown before leaving. Do not touch any surface in the room with your uniform or your skin before exiting.

- Do not share residents' equipment with other residents. Any equipment that must be used by more than one resident will be disinfected before being used again.

- Do not share residents' towels, bedding, or clothing with other residents.

- Residents will most likely be placed in a private room. If they are not, keep the privacy curtain closed between beds.

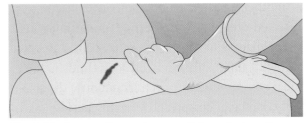

Fig. 6-23. Contact Precautions are followed when the person is at risk of transmitting a microorganism by touching an infected object or person.

When Transmission-Based Precautions are ordered, they are always used in addition to Standard Precautions.

12. Describe care of the resident in an isolation unit

Residents who require Transmission-Based Precautions are referred to as being "in isolation." A sign should be on the door indicating "isolation" or alerting people to see the nurse before entering the room. Tuberculosis and chickenpox are examples of diseases requiring isolation.

Residents in isolation units experience big changes. They cannot move about freely because they are separated from everyone else. Empathize with them. Think about how you would feel if you were in isolation. Spend as much time with the resident as possible. This can help reduce loneliness and gives them a connection to the outside world. Listen to the resident and encourage him or her to talk about feelings and concerns. Reassure the resident that it is the disease, not the person, that is being isolated. Explain why these special steps are being taken. In addition, follow these guidelines:

Guidelines: Residents in Isolation

G   Apply proper PPE before entering the isolation room.

G   Clean and disinfect all equipment properly. Use dedicated (only for use by one resident) equipment when disposable is not an option. Follow facility policy for equipment that belongs to staff and does not stay in the room, such as a stethoscope. Some facilities do not allow staff to take their own items into the room. If so, there will be a stethoscope that stays in the isolation room at all times. Disinfect the stethoscope with alcohol wipes each time before and after using.

G   Dispose of trash in proper containers.

G   Dispose of waste containing blood or body fluids and sharps in biohazard containers.

G   Bag used linen and equipment so that the contaminated items do not touch the outside of the bag. Tie or seal the bag. Should you accidently touch the outside of the bag with the contaminated items, you will need to double-bag the item. This means putting the contaminated bag into another bag.

G   Disinfect all furniture and surfaces (e.g. door-knobs, sinks, other bathroom surfaces) regularly.

G   Assist visitors to put on gowns and masks, as needed.

G   Before you leave the room, make sure the TV, telephone, and radio are all in working order.

G   Encourage reading material that can be disposed of, such as magazines and newspapers. Make sure the resident has access to eyeglasses, if needed.

G   Always place the call light within the resident's reach when leaving the isolation room.

You may assist in setting up an isolation unit. Before doing anything in the isolation area, wash your hands and put on gloves. Follow the nurse's instructions on what to do in the room. Adjust the bed to the proper height. Put away clean towels and other supplies. Leave clean pajamas or gown in an easy-to-reach spot. Check to make sure the following are in working order:

•   The bed controls, including the call light

•   Lights in the room

•   The television and radio controls

•   Telephone

•   Closet and dressers/cabinets

•   Windows and latches

Check bathroom supplies. If the soap or paper towel dispenser needs to be refilled, or trash needs to be emptied, notify the nurse. If anything is damaged or not working properly, tell the nurse immediately.

If asked to set up an isolation cart outside of the resident's room, make sure the cart is stocked with all PPE needed. This includes gloves, gowns, masks, goggles, and face shields. Gather extra plastic bags and laundry bags, too. Some facilities use an anteroom just outside of the isolation room. This anteroom may have a sink. Follow facility policy when using the anteroom. Special steps may need to be taken in that room.

Information on collecting specimens from a resident in isolation will be discussed in Chapter 15.

Residents' Rights

Residents in Isolation

Residents' rights must be protected when they are in isolation. Their dignity, privacy and confidentiality must be maintained at all times. Residents can participate in their care as much as possible. They have the right to choose what care they receive and to file complaints. They have the right to visits from family, friends, or clergy. Visitors must receive training on the safe and proper use of PPE before entering the isolation room.

13. Explain OSHA's Bloodborne Pathogen Standard

Bloodborne pathogens are microorganisms found in human blood that can cause infection and disease. They may also be found in body fluids, draining wounds, and mucous membranes. These pathogens are transmitted by infected blood entering the bloodstream, or if infected semen or vaginal secretions contact mucous membranes. Sharing infected drug needles is another way to spread bloodborne diseases. Infected pregnant women may transmit bloodborne disease to their babies. In health care, contact with infectious blood or body fluids is the most common way to get a bloodborne disease. Infections can be spread by having accidental contact with contaminated blood or body fluids, skin, needles or other sharp objects, or contaminated supplies or equipment.

The **Occupational Safety and Health Administration (OSHA)** is a federal government agency that is responsible for the safety of workers in the U.S. OSHA makes and enforces rules to protect workers from hazards on the job. OSHA conducts workplace inspections to check on worker safety and updates safety standards that are needed at work. OSHA also provides training for employers and employees on workplace safety (Fig. 6-24). The employer is responsible for meeting all safety standards and providing a workplace that is free of hazards. Employees are responsible for doing their job in a way that meets OSHA's safety standards.

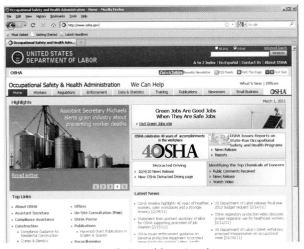

Fig. 6-24. *OSHA's website address is osha.gov.*

OSHA sets standards for equipment use and special techniques to use when working in facilities. One of these standards is the **Bloodborne Pathogen Standard**. This law was passed in 1991. It requires that healthcare facilities protect employees from bloodborne health hazards.

By law, employers must follow these rules to reduce the risk of acquiring infectious diseases. The Standard also guides employers and employees through the steps to follow if exposed to infectious material. Types of waste that are considered infectious are blood, body fluids, and human tissue. Significant exposures include:

- Exposure by injection; a needle stick

- Mucous membrane contact

- Cut from an object containing a potentially infectious body fluid (includes human bites)

- Having non-intact skin (OSHA includes acne in this category)

Guidelines employers must follow include:

- Employers must give in-service training on the risks from bloodborne pathogens and updates on any new safety standards at the time of hire and annually to all employees.

- Employers must have an exposure control plan should an employee accidentally become exposed to any infectious waste. The **exposure control plan** outlines specific work practices to prevent exposure to infectious material and identifies step-by-step procedures to follow when exposures do occur. All employees must be trained on this plan and know its location.

- Employers must give all employees, visitors, and residents proper PPE to wear when needed.

- Employers must place biohazard containers in each resident's room and in other areas in the facility to dispose of equipment and supplies contaminated with infectious waste.

- Biohazard bags are used for biomedical waste. The bag must be sealed tightly before leaving the resident's room. Bags must be safely taken to the proper area for biohazard infectious waste.

- Employers are required to provide a free hepatitis B vaccine to all employees after hire. The hepatitis B vaccine is usually given as a series of three or four shots.

When an employee is exposed to blood or other potentially infectious material, it is called an **exposure incident**. After an exposure incident, specific steps must be taken:

- Immediately follow facility policy regarding a spill, splash, or cut. (More information on skin and eye splashes is in Chapter 7.)

- Report the exposure immediately to your supervisor.

- Fill out an exposure report form. Exposure reports help you get the follow-up care you need after an exposure. They also help employers find ways to prevent future exposures.

- Go to your employer's health service department to get any needed tests.

In 2001, OSHA revised the Bloodborne Pathogens Standard. The revisions address the need for employers to select safer needle devices and to involve employees in choosing these devices. They also require employers to keep a log of injuries from contaminated sharps.

14. Discuss two important bloodborne diseases

Two major groups of bloodborne diseases in the U.S. are HIV (human immunodeficiency virus) and the viral hepatitis family. HIV is the virus that can cause AIDS, or acquired immune deficiency syndrome.

Over time, HIV damages the immune system so that the body cannot fight infections. These types of infections are called "opportunistic infections." In addition to these infections, tumors and central nervous system symptoms may appear. This stage of the disease is known as AIDS, which is the final stage of HIV infection. People with AIDS lose all ability to fight infection. They can die from illnesses that a healthy immune system could fight.

HIV is transmitted by blood, by infected needles, and from mother to fetus. It is also a sexually-transmitted disease. You will learn more about HIV and AIDS in Chapter 24.

Hepatitis is an inflammation of the liver caused by certain viruses and other factors, such as alcohol abuse, some medications, and trauma. Liver function can be permanently damaged by hepatitis. Several different viruses can cause hepatitis, including hepatitis A, B, C, D, and E. The most common are hepatitis A, B, and C. Hepatitis B and C are bloodborne diseases that can cause death. Many more people have hepatitis B (HBV) than HIV. The risk of getting hepatitis is greater than the risk of acquiring HIV.

Hepatitis A is caused by the hepatitis A virus (HAV). It is commonly spread by the fecal-oral route, which means through food or water contaminated by stool from an infected person.

HAV can survive outside the body for months. Symptoms of HAV include fever, loss of appetite, vomiting, jaundice (yellow skin or eyes), dark urine, and joint pain. There is a vaccine available for Hepatitis A.

Hepatitis B (HBV) is a bloodborne form of hepatitis. HBV is spread through sexual contact, by sharing infected needles, from a mother to her baby during delivery, through improperly sterilized needles used for tattoos and piercings, and through grooming supplies, such as razors, nail clippers, and toothbrushes. It is also spread by exposure at work from accidental contact with a used, infected needle or other sharp instrument, or from splashing blood.

The hepatitis B virus can survive outside the body for seven days, and can still cause infection in others during that time. HBV can cause few symptoms or become a severe infection. Some of the symptoms are fatigue, nausea, vomiting, diarrhea, jaundice, lack of appetite, joint pain and abdominal pain. Hepatitis B can lead to serious problems with the liver, such as cirrhosis (liver damage) or liver cancer. In some cases, HBV can be fatal.

HBV poses a serious threat to healthcare workers. It is important to use proper PPE and to handle needles and other sharps carefully to help prevent HBV. Equally important is to get the vaccine for hepatitis B when it is offered. Employers must offer a free vaccine to protect you from hepatitis B. The hepatitis B vaccine is usually given as a series of three or four shots. Talk to your supervisor about getting this vaccine.

Hepatitis C (HCV) is transmitted by blood or body fluids. Many people have no symptoms of Hepatitis C. If symptoms do occur, they include fatigue, nausea, jaundice, dark urine, lack of appetite, and abdominal pain. Hepatitis C can be fatal if it leads to serious illness, such as liver cancer or cirrhosis. A liver transplant may be required. There is no vaccine for hepatitis C.

Hepatitis D (HDV) is transmitted by blood. Hepatitis B (HBV) must be present for the person to get hepatitis D, and HDV worsens HBV. Symptoms of HDV include fatigue, nausea, vomiting, jaundice, dark urine, lack of appetite, joint pain, and abdominal pain.

Hepatitis E (HEV) is spread by a fecal-oral route, mostly through contaminated water. HEV is not common in the United States, but is in other parts of the world. The symptoms are fatigue, nausea, vomiting, jaundice, dark urine, lack of appetite, and abdominal pain. Currently there is no vaccine for hepatitis E.

Residents' Rights

Know the facts.

Do not be afraid of a resident who has HIV or AIDS. Simple touches, handshakes, or hugs cannot spread the HIV virus (Fig. 6-25). It is important to provide emotional support. Do not ignore or avoid residents with HIV or AIDS.

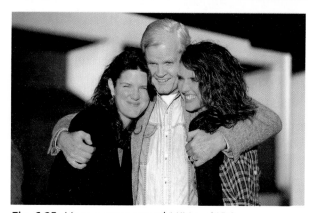

Fig. 6-25. *Hugs cannot spread HIV or AIDS.*

15. Discuss MRSA, VRE, and *C. Difficile*

Multidrug-resistant organisms (**MDROs**) are microorganisms, mostly bacteria, that are resistant to one or more antimicrobial agents. As you learned earlier, an antimicrobial agent destroys, resists, or prevents the development of pathogens. There has been an increase in MDROs in healthcare facilities, and it is a serious problem. Two common types of MDROs are MRSA and VRE.

MRSA stands for methicillin-resistant *Staphylococcus aureus*. *Staphylococcus aureus* is a common type of bacteria that can cause illness. Methicillin is a powerful antibiotic drug. **MRSA** is an antibiotic-resistant infection often acquired in healthcare facilities. This type of MRSA is also known as "HA-MRSA," which stands for "hospital-associated MRSA."

Community-associated methicillin-resistant *Staphylococcus aureus* (CA-MRSA) is a type of MRSA infection that is becoming more common. These infections occur in people who have not recently been admitted to healthcare facilities and who have no past diagnosis of MRSA. Often CA-MRSA manifests as skin infections, such as boils or pimples.

MRSA is mostly spread by direct physical contact with infected people. If a person has MRSA on her skin, especially her hands, and touches someone else, she may spread MRSA. Indirect contact by touching equipment or supplies contaminated by a person with MRSA can also spread MRSA.

Common MRSA infection sites include the respiratory tract, surgical wounds, the perineum, rectum, and the skin. Upon admission, residents may have their nasal passages swabbed to determine if they are colonized with MRSA. Being colonized does not mean the person has active MRSA infection, but the person could spread MRSA to others. Swabbing a wound or testing a body fluid, such as sputum, can indicate if a person has a MRSA infection. Residents with identified MRSA infections may have their infected body site(s) swabbed periodically to determine the progress of the treatment plan.

Symptoms of MRSA infection include drainage, fever, chills, and redness. The single most important way to control MRSA is through proper hand hygiene. Always follow Standard Precautions, along with Transmission-Based Precautions as ordered.

VRE stands for vancomycin-resistant *enterococcus*. *Enterococcus* is a bacterium that lives in the lower intestinal tract. It does not cause problems in healthy people. Vancomycin is a powerful antibiotic used to treat bacterial infections. Vancomycin-resistant *enterococci* are bacteria that have developed resistance to antibiotics as a result of being exposed to vancomycin. VRE is spread through direct and indirect contact.

Symptoms of VRE infection include fever, fatigue, chills, and drainage. VRE infections are often difficult to treat and may require the use of several medications. Preventing VRE is much easier. Proper hand hygiene can help prevent the spread of VRE. Always follow Standard Precautions, along with Transmission-Based Precautions as ordered.

Residents with MRSA may be placed in contact or droplet isolation depending upon the site of the infection. Residents with VRE may be placed in contact isolation.

As with VRE and MRSA, tuberculosis can become resistant to available treatments. This is called multidrug-resistant tuberculosis (MDR-TB). The risk of MDR-TB increases when people do not complete their prescribed course of medications. See Chapter 20 for more information.

Current CDC guidelines state that residents with MRSA or VRE should remain as active as possible. They may be able to eat with others and participate in activities as long as any open sores or wounds are completely covered. All bodily fluids, such as urine, must be properly contained. Residents with MRSA or VRE must follow proper hygienic practices. They should wash their hands often or have staff assist them if they are not able to do this on their own. Some residents with MRSA or VRE will be restricted to their rooms. In addition, all staff members should:

- Wash their hands with soap and water after any physical contact with residents diagnosed with MRSA or VRE.

- After handwashing, discard paper towels immediately in a no-touch waste container.

- Wear disposable gloves when any contact with blood or body fluids may occur.

- Wash linen whenever soiled.

- Clean the resident's room with the proper disinfectant whenever body fluids soil surfaces.

- Alert other caregivers and visitors to take proper precautions prior to any contact with residents with MRSA or VRE.

- Attend all in-service programs on infection prevention methods used with MRSA and VRE residents.

Clostridium difficile is commonly known as "***C. diff***" or "***C. difficile***." It is a spore-forming bacterium which can be part of the normal intestinal flora. When the normal intestinal flora is altered, *C. difficile* can flourish in the intestinal tract. It produces a toxin that causes a watery diarrhea. Enemas, nasogastric tube insertion, and GI tract surgery increase a person's risk of developing the disease. The elderly are at a higher risk of getting *C. difficile*. The overuse of antibiotics may alter the normal intestinal flora and increase the risk of developing *C. difficile* diarrhea. *C. difficile* can also cause colitis, a more serious intestinal condition. It can cause sepsis, a bloodstream infection, which can be fatal. More information about sepsis can be found in Chapter 26.

When released in the environment, *C. difficile* can form a spore that makes it difficult to kill. These spores can be carried on the hands of people who have direct contact with infected residents or with environmental surfaces (floors, bedpans, toilets, etc.) contaminated with *C. difficile*. Touching an object contaminated with *C. difficile* can transmit *C. difficile*. Alcohol-based hand sanitizers are not considered effective on *C. difficile*. Soap and water must be used each time hand hygiene is performed.

Symptoms of *C. difficile* include frequent, foul-smelling, watery stools. Other symptoms include fever, diarrhea that contains blood and mucus, nausea, lack of appetite and abdominal cramps. Proper handwashing with soap and water, especially after using the toilet and before eating or drinking, is vital in preventing the spread of the disease. Contaminated waste should be carefully handled according to facility policy. Additional Transmission-Based Precautions are used with residents who have *C. difficile*. Cleaning surfaces with a facility-approved disinfectant can also help reduce transmission. Limiting the use of antibiotics helps lower the risk of developing *C. difficile* diarrhea.

Residents who have *C. difficile* should have a private room, if possible. They should have dedicated equipment, such as blood pressure monitors. All caregivers and visitors must be advised to take proper precautions before any contact with a resident who has *C. difficile*. They should don gloves and gowns when entering the room of a resident who has *C. difficile*.

There is a quick test that can diagnose *C. difficile*. If you note any of the symptoms, promptly report them to the nurse. The risk of serious illness, along with transmission, increases if the infection is not identified and cared for promptly.

Tip

RSV

If visitors, especially infants or children, are ill, they can cause serious illness and even death in the elderly. The respiratory syncytial virus (RSV) is a potentially dangerous virus that could be transmitted to residents. Staff should discourage visitors with an ill child from visiting until the child recovers completely. RSV is transmitted by droplets and through direct or indirect contact.

Chapter Review

1. What does "infection prevention" mean (LO 2)?

2. How does infection occur (LO 2)?

3. Describe the difference between localized and systemic infections (LO 2).

4. Define communicable disease and non-communicable disease (LO 2).

5. Describe the difference between "clean" and "dirty" in health care (LO 3).

6. What is the difference between sterilization and disinfection (LO 3)?

7. What is surgical asepsis (LO 3)?

8. Describe the six links in the chain of infection and list an infection prevention practice for each link (LO 4).

9. What are mucous membranes (LO 4)?

10. List four reasons the elderly are at a higher risk for infection (LO 5).

11. Under Standard Precautions, what does the term "body fluids" include (LO 6)?

12. On whom should Standard Precautions be practiced (LO 6)?

13. When do Standard Precautions require gloves to be worn (LO 6)?

14. What is hand hygiene (LO 7)?

15. Why should nursing assistants avoid using artificial nails (LO 7)?

16. List ten situations that require handwashing (LO 7).

17. When should gowns be worn (LO 8)?

18. When should a mask and goggles be worn (LO 8)?

19. In what order should PPE be put on and removed (LO 8)?

20. How should soiled linen be carried (LO 9)?

21. When can re-usable equipment be used again (LO 9)?

22. Is it okay to pick up broken glass with gloved hands (LO 10)?

23. List and describe three categories of Transmission-Based Precautions (LO 11).

24. List six guidelines to use for residents in isolation (LO 12).

25. How are bloodborne diseases transmitted (LO 13)?

26. List five guidelines employers must follow to meet the Bloodborne Pathogen Standard (LO 13).

27. What is hepatitis (LO 14)?

28. What does HIV do to the immune system (LO 14)?

29. How is Hepatitis B (HBV) spread (LO 14)?

30. What is one of the best ways to prevent the spread of MRSA and VRE (LO 15)?

31. What are two ways to help prevent the spread of *C. difficile* (LO 15)?

7
Safety and Body Mechanics

The Great Chicago Fire and Daisy the Cow

Legend has it that a cow named Daisy kicked over a lantern and started the Great Chicago Fire of October 8, 1871. That fire killed more than 300 people and left 100,000 more homeless, including patients at Deaconess Hospital of Chicago (later Passavant Memorial Hospital), who were forced to flee for their lives as the fires burned out of control.

Two weeks after the fire, Reverend Passavant arrived in Chicago to survey the damage and assist the homeless and destitute. He observed that "ruin reigns supreme." In fact, the remains of the hospital were sold for the pathetic sum of $8.50.

If the story of Daisy the Cow is true, then the fire that devastated the nation's fourth-largest city in 1871 didn't have to happen. It could have been prevented with a little care and caution.

**Adapted from *To Be a Nurse*
by Susan M. Sacharski**

"The biggest problem in the world could have been solved when it was small."

**Witter Bynner, 1881-1968,
*The Way of Life According to Laotzu***

"When you see a rattlesnake poised to strike, you do not wait until he has struck before you crush him."

Franklin Delano Roosevelt, 1882-1945

1. Define important words in this chapter

aspiration: the inhalation of food, fluid, or foreign material into the lungs.

atrophy: weakening or wasting of muscles.

body mechanics: the way the parts of the body work together when a person moves.

chemical restraint: medications used to control a person's behavior.

combustion: the process of burning.

cyanosis: blue or pale skin and/or mucous membranes due to decreased oxygen in the blood.

dysphagia: difficulty in swallowing.

flammable: easily ignited and capable of burning quickly.

hoarding: collecting and putting things away in a guarded manner.

Material Safety Data Sheet (MSDS): sheet that provides information on the safe use of and hazards of chemicals, as well as emergency steps to take in the event chemicals are splashed, sprayed or ingested.

PASS: acronym for use of a fire extinguisher; stands for Pull-Aim-Squeeze-Sweep.

RACE: acronym for steps taken during a fire; stands for Remove-Activate-Contain-Extinguish.

restraint: a physical or chemical way to restrict voluntary movement or behavior.

restraint alternatives: measures used instead of physical or chemical restraints.

restraint-free care: an environment in which restraints are not kept or used for any reason.

scalds: burns caused by very hot liquids.

slip knot: a quick-release knot used to tie restraints.

suffocation: the stoppage of breathing from a lack of oxygen or excess of carbon dioxide in the body that may result in unconsciousness or death; also known as asphyxia.

2. List common accidents in facilities and ways to prevent them

There are many accidents that can occur in a long-term care facility. Always be on your guard to try to keep residents, other staff, visitors, and yourself safe. Being proactive is the goal. Being proactive means trying to *prevent* an accident from occurring. It is much better than being reactive. Reacting or responding to an accident means that it has already taken place. You can change policy, but you cannot change that an accident happened after it has occurred. Prevention is the key to safety.

Maintaining safety is also a way to protect your residents' rights. Residents have the legal right to be safe and secure.

Some common resident accidents include:

- Falls

- Failing to identify residents before performing procedures or serving food

- Burns and scalds

- Poisoning

- Choking

- Cuts

Fall Prevention

Most of the accidents in a facility are related to falls. Many things increase the risk of falls. Unsafe environments, a person's loss of abilities, diseases, and medications raise the risk for falls. Conditions that put a person at risk for falls include problems with walking, muscle weakness, poor vision, and disorientation, which is confusion about person, place, or time. Follow these guidelines to help prevent falls:

Guidelines: Preventing Falls

G   Identify residents who may be at risk and guard against falls. Report residents who seem unsteady to the nurse.

G   Some medications cause unsteadiness or problems with movement. Nurses should let you know to be especially watchful of residents taking those medications.

G   Respond to call lights promptly. Never wait to respond.

G   Wipe up spills immediately.

G   Remove clutter from walkways. Pick up anything that has fallen on the floor right away. If you see loose electrical cords or wires, notify the nurse. Make sure purse or bag straps are not dangling or on the floor.

G   Get help when moving a resident. Never assume you can handle it alone. When in doubt, ask for help.

G   Lock bed wheels before giving care (Fig. 7-1). Lock bed wheels before moving a resident into or out of bed.

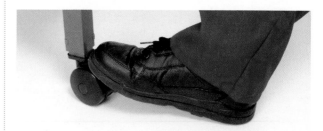

Fig. 7-1. *Always lock the bed wheels before helping a resident into or out of bed and before giving care.*

G   Lock wheelchair wheels before helping residents into or out of them (Fig. 7-2).

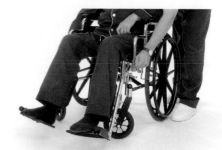

Fig. 7-2. *Always lock wheelchairs before a resident transfers into or out of them.*

G   If side rails are ordered, check to make sure they are raised before leaving the room. Return beds to their lowest position when you are finished with care.

G Residents should wear clothing that fits properly. For example, it should not be too long. Residents must be wearing non-skid shoes at all times when out of bed. Make sure shoelaces are tied. Report if you think a resident needs safer shoes.

G Use non-skid mats or rugs to prevent slipping. Always report any rugs that move. Use non-skid mats in the bath or shower each time residents bathe. If allowed, stay with residents while they are showering or in the tub.

G Report loose hand rails in halls or rooms immediately. Report cracks or holes in floors, tile, walls, furniture, bathrooms, ceilings, or stairwells.

G Report damage to outdoor furniture or benches, walkways, or ramps in outdoor common areas.

G Use brightly colored tape to mark uneven areas on stairs or the floor.

G Keep frequently-used items close to the bedside or chair and in easy reach in the room, especially call lights.

G Keep walkers and canes close by residents. Allow residents to sit for short periods before getting up to prevent lightheadedness.

G Do not move furniture without an order from the nurse. Tell the resident before moving furniture.

G Offer trips to the bathroom often. Respond to residents' requests promptly.

G Keep night light on in room if approved by facility and resident. Keep halls and other areas well-lit. Report any problems with lighting.

G Make sure resident has eyeglasses within reach and that they are not damaged.

G If a resident begins to fall, do not try to stop it or to catch him. Use your body to slide him

to the floor safely (Fig. 7-3). You or the resident may be injured if you try to stop the fall.

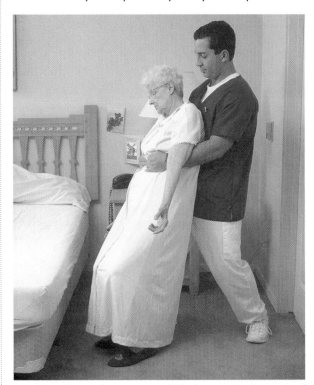

Fig. 7-3. *If a resident starts to fall, do not try to stop the fall. Bring the resident's body close to you to break the fall. Bend your knees and support the resident as you gently lower her to the floor.*

Tip

Safety with Wheelchairs
Lock wheelchairs before moving residents into or out of them. Push wheelchairs slowly and carefully. This helps to ensure safety, as well as making residents feel more secure.

Resident Identification

Residents must always be identified before providing care or serving food. Not doing so can result in serious problems, illnesses, and even death. There is never an excuse for not checking identification. Do it each time you see a resident before providing care or serving food.

Most people are used to seeing armbands as a form of ID on patients in hospitals (Fig. 7-4). However, residents in a facility may not wear name bracelets or armbands. Sometimes photos are placed above the bed or outside the door to identify residents.

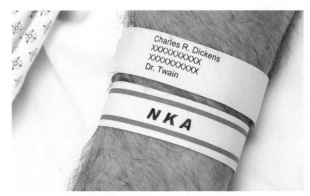

Fig. 7-4. *Identify all residents before giving care. This is an armband, which may or may not be used at your facility to identify residents. The abbreviation "NKA" means "no known allergies."*

For disoriented or confused residents, some facilities use special bands that have alarms on them. The alarm will sound when a resident tries to leave the facility. If a resident wears an alarm band, check alarm often to make sure it is turned on.

Regardless of which method the facility uses, identify each resident before giving care and serving food. Check the resident's identification and call the resident by name. Check diet cards against the resident's identification. Do this every time you see a resident.

Burn/Scald Prevention

Burns and scalds are a common concern in facilities. **Scalds** are burns caused by very hot liquids, such as coffee or tea. It does not take long for a serious burn to occur. When the temperature of a liquid reaches 140°F, it can take five seconds or less to cause a burn.

Burns are extremely painful. They can require surgery. They can cause a resident's condition to deteriorate quickly, depending on his or her physical state prior to the burn. Elderly people and people who have a loss of sensation due to paralysis are at the greatest risk for burns. Follow these guidelines to help prevent burns:

Guidelines: Preventing Burns and Scalds

G   Check water temperature before giving a resident a bath or shower. Temperature should not be over 105°F. Do not allow a resident to get into a bath or shower without checking the water temperature first.

G   Check for proper temperature of warm water applications, such as warm packs. A resident's skin is fragile. Warm or cold water applications may only be applied for 20 minutes at a time. (See Chapter 18 for more information.)

G   Use low settings on hair dryers.

G   Spills can cause burns. Residents may spill drinks on themselves if they are unsteady. Drinking hot liquids can also cause burns. Make sure the drink has cooled before encouraging the resident to drink.

G   Serve residents drinks only when they are seated.

G   Tell residents when you are about to pour or set down hot liquids.

G   Use lids on hot liquids, if possible. Keep hot drinks away from edges of tables.

G   Pour hot liquids away from residents.

G   If plate warmers are used to keep food warm, check the plates carefully. They may be hot. Warn residents if they are hot.

G   Make sure anything that was left in the sun, such as a wheelchair, has cooled off completely before letting a resident sit in it. Residents themselves should not be left out in the sun too long. Use sunscreen and hats when residents are going outside.

G   Tell residents about smoking precautions. Smoking may be allowed in specific areas. Serious burns, and even fires, can occur if a resident falls asleep with a cigarette, pipe, or cigar burning.

Poisoning Prevention

There are many poisonous items in a facility that should not be eaten. Cleaning products, glue, soaps, perfumes, and paints are some examples. These items might be of interest to or be consumed by a confused person. Medication can also be poisonous if taken in the wrong amount and/or by the wrong person. Follow these guidelines to help prevent poisoning:

Guidelines: Preventing Poisoning

G   Keep fresh flowers or plants away from disoriented residents. Store or lock away items like nail polish remover, soaps, perfumes, or hair products. Lock up cleaning products and paints. Do not leave cleaning products in residents' rooms. All of these items may be eaten by a disoriented person. The number of the poison control center should be posted by all telephones.

G   Check dates of foods to ensure that they are fresh.

G   Check bedside table drawers for food that was hoarded and has spoiled. Residents who are confused or have dementia may hoard items; **hoarding** is collecting and putting things away in a guarded manner.

G   Residents can be overcome by fumes when using chemical products. Make sure there is proper ventilation. Always report to the nurse any situation that you believe to be risky.

Choking Prevention

Residents must be watched closely during meals for signs of choking. Residents who are weak or who have dysphagia are at a high risk for choking. **Dysphagia** means difficulty in swallowing. Residents who have swallowing problems may have special diets consisting of thickened liquids. Thickened liquids are easier to swallow.

Swallowing problems cause a high risk for choking on food or drink. Inhaling food, fluid, or foreign material into the lungs is called **aspira-**

tion, which can cause pneumonia or death. You will learn more about dysphagia, thickened liquids, and aspiration in Chapter 14. Follow these guidelines to help prevent choking:

Guidelines: Preventing Choking

G   Residents should be sitting up straight while eating (Fig. 7-5). This is true whether the resident is in bed or in a chair.

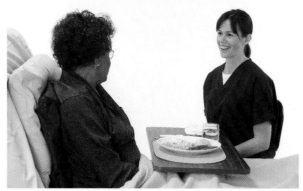

Fig. 7-5. *Residents must be sitting up straight when eating, whether in a bed or a chair.*

G   Assist with feeding slowly. Never rush a resident during a meal.

G   Cut food into small pieces.

G   If you believe a resident would be helped by softer foods or thickened liquids, report this to the nurse.

G   Make sure dentures are in place and fit properly.

G   Know any swallowing precautions residents have.

Cuts and Other Injuries

Cuts, tears, and scrapes can happen quickly. Follow these guidelines to help prevent injuries:

Guidelines: Preventing Cuts, Scrapes, and Other Injuries

G   Do not leave any sharp objects out. Put away residents' supplies, such as razors, after use.

G When approaching doors, move slowly. If there is a window in the door, look on the other side before opening.

G When moving residents in wheelchairs or stretchers, protect their arms and legs. Hands and feet can be hit or bumped into walls or doors. Fingers may be caught in a wheelchair. Make sure arms and legs are inside of the chair or stretcher (gurney).

G Push wheelchairs forward; do not pull them behind you. When entering elevators, turn the chair around so that residents are facing forward. Watch for doors closing before arms and legs are inside.

In addition to the all of the guidelines listed above, here are some general safety guidelines:

- Do not run in a facility. Pay attention to your environment. Look for wet areas or things that you might trip over. Wipe up spilled liquids right away. Remove clutter from walkways.
- Do not stick your hand into a bed or anywhere else without looking first. Be on the lookout for sharp objects or needles.
- Ask for help any time you feel you need it when lifting or assisting residents. Follow facility guidelines on lifting. Use proper equipment provided for lifting.
- Know which residents are combative and watch them closely. Learn the triggers of this behavior. If a resident tries to hit you, protect yourself with your arm or step out of the way. Do not hit back.
- Follow facility policy if a skin splash occurs. Immediately rinse your skin with large amounts of water.
- Follow facility policy if an eye splash occurs. If no eye wash station is available, immediately rinse with large amounts of water at a sink. If an eye wash station is available, follow directions listed there. If you need to use an emergency eye wash, flip the cup lid open. Open your eyelid with your thumb and index finger. Press cup against eye and squeeze bottle repeatedly. Notify the nurse as soon as possible and get checked by a doctor.
- Report all injuries immediately.

3. Explain the Material Safety Data Sheet (MSDS)

The Occupational Safety and Health Administration (OSHA) is responsible for the safety of employees at work. OSHA requires that all dangerous chemicals have a **Material Safety Data Sheet (MSDS)** (Fig. 7-6). These sheets are placed where all staff can access them.

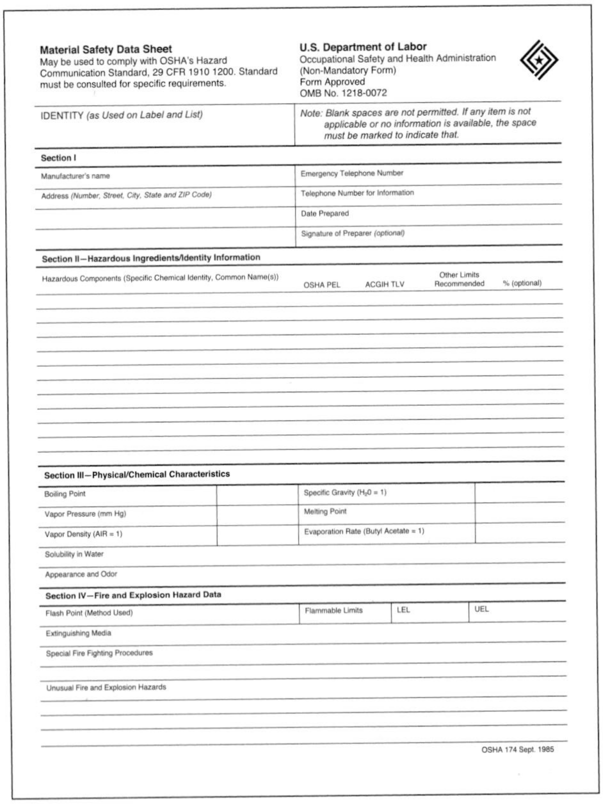
Material Safety Data Sheet
May be used to comply with OSHA's Hazard Communication Standard, 29 CFR 1910 1200. Standard must be consulted for specific requirements.

U.S. Department of Labor
Occupational Safety and Health Administration
(Non-Mandatory Form)
Form Approved
OMB No. 1218-0072

IDENTITY *(as Used on Label and List)*	*Note: Blank spaces are not permitted. If any item is not applicable or no information is available, the space must be marked to indicate that.*

Section I

Manufacturer's name	Emergency Telephone Number
Address *(Number, Street, City, State and ZIP Code)*	Telephone Number for Information
	Date Prepared
	Signature of Preparer *(optional)*

Section II—Hazardous Ingredients/Identity Information

Hazardous Components (Specific Chemical Identity, Common Name(s))	OSHA PEL	ACGIH TLV	Other Limits Recommended	% (optional)

Section III—Physical/Chemical Characteristics

Boiling Point		Specific Gravity (H_20 = 1)	
Vapor Pressure (mm Hg)		Melting Point	
Vapor Density (AIR = 1)		Evaporation Rate (Butyl Acetate = 1)	
Solubility in Water			
Appearance and Odor			

Section IV—Fire and Explosion Hazard Data

Flash Point (Method Used)	Flammable Limits	LEL	UEL
Extinguishing Media			
Special Fire Fighting Procedures			
Unusual Fire and Explosion Hazards			

OSHA 174 Sept. 1985

Fig. 7-6. *A Material Safety Data Sheet.*

The following important information may be found on the MSDS:

- The chemical ingredients of the product
- The dangers of the product
- The protective items to wear when using the chemical

- The correct method of using and cleaning up a chemical

- The emergency response actions to be taken when a chemical is splashed, sprayed, or ingested by a person

- The safe handling procedures for the product

Some facilities use a toll-free number to access MSDS information. Your employer will have an MSDS for every chemical used, and they must be easily accessible. You must know where they are located and how to read them. If you do not know how to read them, ask for help. Some facilities will have an annual MSDS class. Attend this class when it is offered.

4. Describe safety guidelines for sharps and biohazard containers

As you learned in Chapter 6, sharps and biohazard containers are the containers that hold sharp objects and infectious waste. Follow these safety guidelines when using these containers:

Guidelines: Safe Use of Sharps and Biohazard Containers

G　Always wear gloves before touching a sharps container.

G　When dropping an object into the sharps or biohazard container, keep your hands above the opening at the top (Fig. 7-7).

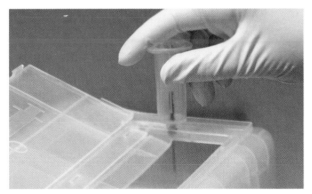

Fig. 7-7. Wear gloves and keep your fingers above the opening of a sharps container.

G　When touching a sharps container, touch the bottom of the container only. If you need to carry the container, carry it by the bottom. Be sure it is closed.

G　Replace the sharps container when it is ¾ full (or follow your facility policy). Ask the nurse about your facility's guidelines for replacing these containers.

G　Remove gloves and wash your hands after putting anything into the sharps container.

G　Use a biohazard container or bag for anything contaminated with infectious waste (blood, body fluids, or human tissue), except for anything sharp.

G　Always wear gloves when disposing of infectious waste.

G　Remove gloves and wash your hands after putting anything into the biohazard container or bag.

5. Explain the principles of body mechanics and apply them to daily activities

Back and body injuries are serious problems that nursing assistants face. They are common risks of working in a facility. Preventing injury by using proper techniques is very important. Every time you move, lift, or transfer a resident, you will need to use good body mechanics.

Body mechanics is the way the parts of the body work together when a person moves. Good body mechanics help save energy and prevent injury and muscle strain. When muscles are used correctly to push and lift objects or people, it reduces the risk of injury. Basic principles of body mechanics will help keep you and your residents safe.

Alignment: Alignment is based on the word "line." When you stand up straight, a vertical line could be drawn right through the center of your body and your center of gravity (Fig. 7-8).

When the line is straight, the body is in alignment. Whether standing, sitting, or lying down, try to have your body in alignment. This means that the two sides of the body are mirror images of each other, with body parts lined up naturally and properly supported. Maintain correct body alignment when lifting or carrying an object by keeping it close to your body. Point your feet and body in the direction you are moving. Do not twist at the waist.

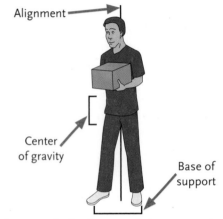

Fig. 7-8. *Proper body alignment is important when standing or when sitting.*

Base of Support: The base of support is the foundation that supports an object. Something that has a wide base of support is more stable than something with a narrow base of support. The feet are the body's base of support. Standing with your legs shoulder-width apart gives a greater base of support. You will be more stable than someone standing with his feet together.

Center of Gravity: The center of gravity in your body is the point where the most weight is concentrated (Fig. 7-9). The location of this point will depend on the position of the body. When you stand, your weight is centered in your pelvis. A low center of gravity gives a more stable base of support. Bending your knees when lifting an object lowers your pelvis. It lowers your center of gravity. This gives you more stability and makes you less likely to fall. It also makes you less likely to strain your muscles. If you are moving or transferring a resident, the center of gravity

includes the resident. When you are transferring a resident, the resident needs to be as close to your body as possible.

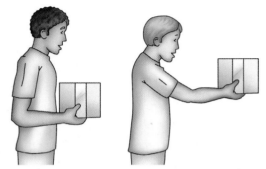

Fig. 7-9. *Holding things close to you moves weight toward your center of gravity. In this illustration, who is more likely to strain his back muscles?*

Consider some activities that require moving or lifting something:

- Lifting a resident

- Picking up a resident's bag of laundry

- Carrying a new resident's luggage

- Taking heavy trash bags to the appropriate site

- Cleaning a floor

- Moving a resident's bed into another room

Each task could cause serious injury if done without using proper body mechanics. Even a simple task, such as picking up something light from the floor, could cause injury to your back. By applying the principles of body mechanics to daily activities, you can avoid injury and use less energy. Here are ways to use proper body mechanics:

Guidelines: Using Proper Body Mechanics

G   Raise beds to a safe working level before making them. This is usually waist high.

G   Stand close to the object.

G   Stand with a wide base of support.

G   Push or slide objects rather than lifting them.

G   Use the largest muscles of your upper arms and upper thighs to lift.

G   Bend at your knees (squat) instead of at your waist (Fig. 7-10).

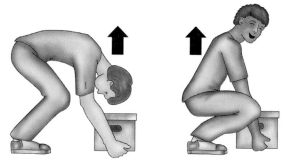

Fig. 7-10. *In this illustration, which person is lifting correctly?*

G   Avoid twisting or choppy movements; keep movements smooth. Face the object or person you are moving. Pivot your feet instead of twisting at the waist.

G   Do not try to lift with just one hand. Use both arms and hands to lift, push, or carry objects.

G   Hold objects close to your body when you are lifting or carrying them (Fig. 7-11).

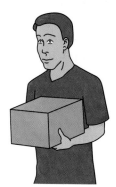

Fig. 7-11. *Keeping objects close while carrying them decreases stress on the back.*

G   Avoid bending and reaching.

G   Get help from co-workers when lifting or helping residents.

G   Talk to residents before moving them. Let them know what will be happening so that they can help if possible. Agree on a signal, such as counting to three. Lift or move on three so that everyone moves together.

Tip

Bend your knees for ease.

When preparing to move or position a resident in bed, always bend your knees. You should be able to feel the bed with your knees before you begin the procedure. If you do not bend your knees properly, you can seriously injure your back.

6. Define two types of restraints and discuss problems associated with restraints

A **restraint** is a physical or chemical way to restrict voluntary movement or behavior. Common physical restraints are the vest restraint, belt restraint, wrist/ankle restraint, and mitt restraint. Side rails and special chairs, such as geriatric chairs, are also considered physical restraints (Fig. 7-12 and 7-13).

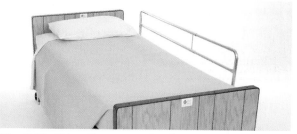

Fig. 7-12. *Side rails are considered restraints because they restrict movement.*

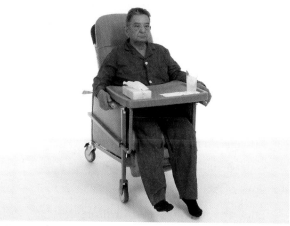

Fig. 7-13. *When the tray table is attached, a geriatric chair, or geri-chair, is considered a restraint.*

Chemical restraints are medications used to control a person's behavior. Overuse of chemical restraints was once a common problem. In the past, residents were routinely restrained for different reasons. They were restrained to prevent falls and to keep confused persons from wandering. Residents were also commonly restrained to keep them from hurting themselves or others and to keep them from pulling out tubing. Restraints were often overused by caregivers. This abuse led to new laws restricting their use. Today, the use of both physical and chemical restraints in facilities has greatly decreased.

Restraints can never be used without a doctor's order. It is against the law to apply restraints for staff convenience or to discipline residents. Residents who are restrained must be continually monitored. This is important. Residents have been severely injured and have died due to improper restraint use and lack of monitoring. You will learn more about what to do if a resident is restrained in Learning Objective 8.

There are many complications of restraint use. These are some negative effects of restraint use:

- Bruises and cuts
- Pressure ulcers
- Pneumonia
- Reduced blood circulation
- Risk of suffocation (**suffocation** is the stoppage of breathing from a lack of oxygen or excess of carbon dioxide in the body that may result in unconsciousness or death)
- Stress on the heart
- Incontinence
- Constipation
- Muscle **atrophy** (weakening or wasting of muscles)
- Loss of bone mass
- Poor appetite and malnutrition
- Depression
- Sleep disorders
- Loss of dignity
- Loss of independence
- Stress and anxiety
- Increased agitation
- Loss of self-esteem
- Severe injury
- Death

7. Define the terms "restraint free" and "restraint alternatives" and list examples of restraint alternatives

The use of restraints is being dramatically reduced in facilities. State and federal agencies encourage facilities to take steps to create restraint-free environments. **Restraint-free care** means that restraints are not kept or used for any reason. Creative ideas that help avoid the need for restraints are being used instead. These creative ideas are called **restraint alternatives**.

Studies have shown that restraints are not truly needed. People tend to respond better to the use of creative ways to reduce tension, pulling at tubes, wandering, and boredom. If you have ideas about ways to avoid using restraints, tell the nurse. You may be able to think of successful restraint alternatives. Examples of restraint alternatives are outlined below:

- Answer call lights immediately. Make sure call lights are within reach.
- Improve lighting to prevent falls and other accidents.
- Use postural devices to support and protect residents.
- Take the resident on a walk. Add more exercise into the care plan.
- Let confused residents wander in designated safe areas.
- Give frequent help with toileting. Make sure residents are clean, dry, and comfortable.
- Encourage independence with all tasks. Provide meaningful activities.

- Encourage participation in social activities. Escort the resident to social activities when needed.

- Get the resident involved in hobbies.

- Create activities for those who wander at night.

- Offer reading materials, such as a newspaper. Read to the resident if needed.

- Offer backrubs.

- Increase visits and social interaction.

- Increase the number of familiar caregivers. Use more volunteers when possible.

- Get the family involved. Family members may decrease tension just by being with residents.

- Offer snacks or drinks.

- Redirect the resident's interest.

- Decrease the noise level.

- Use soothing music. Music has been shown to have a calming effect on some people.

- Report complaints of pain to the nurse immediately.

Bed or body alarms are other examples of restraint alternatives. They can be used in place of side rails. They can also be used with wheelchairs or chairs. They help prevent falls by alerting staff when residents attempt to leave the bed or chair. Alarms can also be used for confused residents who wander. If a resident is ordered to have a body alarm (bed or chair), make sure it is placed properly on the resident and turned on.

In addition to alarms, there are several types of pads, wheelchair inserts, and special chairs that may be used instead of restraints (Fig. 7-14):

- Saddle cushion

- Wedge cushion

- Self-releasing belt

- Lap-top pillow or cushion

- Lap tray

- Foam body support

- Safety sensors

- Wheelchair positioner cushion

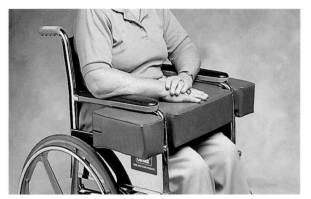

Fig. 7-14. *A lap-top cushion is one type of restraint alternative that helps with positioning.* (PHOTOS COURTESY OF NORTH COAST MEDICAL, INC., WWW.NCMEDICAL.COM, 800-821-9319)

Hot Topic

Music soothes.

"Music that gentlier on the spirit lies,
Than tir'd eyelids upon tir'd eyes;
Music that brings sweet sleep down
from the blissful skies."

Alfred Lord Tennyson (1809-1892), *The Lotus Eaters*

Some people use music to relax. Residents may also respond to music in a positive way. Their tastes will vary. Some may prefer classical or reggae, while others may like country, rhythm and blues, jazz, rock, or rap music. When new residents are admitted, ask them the type of music they prefer. It may help guide the staff in choosing soothing music.

8. Identify what must be done if a restraint is ordered

OBRA sets specific rules for restraint use. Restraints are used only after everything else has been ruled out and only with a doctor's order. Restraints cannot be used for staff convenience or discipline. Do not use a restraint unless the nurse has told you to do so and you have been trained to use it. When restraints have been ordered, follow these guidelines:

Guidelines: Restraints

G   Know your state's laws and facility rules regarding applying restraints. Make sure there is a written doctor's order for a restraint before applying one.

G   Follow manufacturer's instructions when applying restraints.

G   Use the correct size and style of restraint. Ask the nurse for help if needed.

G   Always use a slip knot. A **slip knot** is a quick-release knot used to tie restraints so that they can be removed quickly when needed.

G   Never tie the restraint to side rails. Only tie the restraint to the movable part of a bed frame.

G   Check to make sure the restraint is not too tight. You should be able to place your hand in a flat position between the resident and the restraint. This helps to ensure that the device fits properly and is comfortable.

G   Apply vest or belt style restraint over clothing. Be careful not to catch the resident's breasts or skin in the restraint. The criss-cross in a vest restraint must be placed on the front of the body.

G   Place the call light within the resident's reach. Residents with mitt restraints will not be able to press regular call lights. They will need a special "easy touch" call light. An "easy touch" call light is a soft, vinyl, air-filled bulb that when slightly depressed will activate the call light system.

G   Document the following when restraints are used:

   •   Type of restraint and time applied

   •   Each time of removal

   •   Care given when released

   •   Any circulation, skin, or other problems

When a resident is physically restrained, he must be monitored regularly. Complications that can occur with the use of physical restraints must be prevented.

The physician's order for physical restraints may need to be renewed frequently throughout a 24-hour period or just once a day. There are two kinds of standards for care with physical restraints. There are standards that apply to persons who are not in a behavioral health situation, who are not considered violent or self-destructive. There are also standards that apply to persons receiving behavioral health care, who are considered violent and self-destructive. These sets of standards may be classified under different names, depending upon the state and type of facility.

Residents in physical restraints require care at least every two hours. The restraint must be released for at least 15 minutes, and they must be given appropriate care. Provide help with elimination and related hygiene needs, food and/or fluids, skin care, and range of motion exercises. Take vital signs. Offer comfort measures, as needed. Persons who are in behavioral health situations and who are considered violent and self-destructive must be checked and assessed at least every 15 minutes.

Check for blue-tinged, gray, or pale skin (**cyanosis**), which could mean lack of oxygen in the blood. With dark-skinned residents, the skin color may darken or appear purple. In addition, notify the nurse if redness or swelling is noted in any area of the body.

Applying a physical tie restraint safely

Equipment: correct size and type of restraint

1.   Identify yourself by name. Identify the resident. Greet the resident by name.

2.   Wash your hands.

3.   Explain procedure to the resident. Speak clearly, slowly, and directly. Maintain face-to-face contact whenever possible.

4. Provide for the resident's privacy with a curtain, screen, or door.

5. Apply the restraint carefully. Follow manufacturer's directions and facility policy. For each type of restraint, make sure that it is not too tight.

   CHEST or BELT-STYLE RESTRAINTS: Make sure you do not catch breasts or skin in the restraints. Double-check before actually tying together or attaching buckle.

   VEST: The criss-cross in the vest restraint must be placed on the front of the body.

   MITT: Place a rolled-up washcloth or commercial hand roll in the mitt restraint. This helps the hand stay in proper alignment and helps prevent contractures (permanent and painful shortening of a muscle).

   WRIST/ANKLE: Make sure the restraint will not slide off the wrist or ankle.

6. Use a slip knot to tie the restraint. Make sure it is not too tight. If restraint is used on a resident who is in bed, tie it to the movable part of the bed frame. Do not tie it to the side rail.

7. Make resident comfortable.

8. Leave call light within resident's reach.

9. Wash your hands.

10. Be courteous and respectful at all times.

11. Report any changes in the resident to the nurse. Document procedure using facility guidelines.

9. List safety guidelines for oxygen use

Oxygen is used by residents who have breathing problems. Oxygen use is prescribed by a doctor. Nursing assistants do not turn off or adjust oxygen levels. This is the nurse's responsibility. You will learn more about oxygen in Chapter 20.

Working with oxygen requires special safety precautions because oxygen is a dangerous fire hazard. Oxygen makes other things burn; however, oxygen itself does not burn. It merely supports combustion. **Combustion** means the process of burning. There are strict safety rules that must be followed when working around oxygen.

Guidelines: Safety with Oxygen

G Post "No Smoking" and "Oxygen in Use" signs. These should be posted on each door and over the resident's bed. **Do not** allow smoking anywhere around oxygen equipment. If you find smoking materials in a room where oxygen is in use or on a resident who is using oxygen, report to the nurse immediately.

G Remove fire hazards from the room. This includes electrical equipment, such as electric razors and hair dryers. Tell the nurse if residents do not want fire hazards removed.

G Remove flammable liquids from the area. **Flammable** means easily ignited and capable of burning quickly. Examples of flammable liquids are alcohol and nail polish remover. Read the label on liquids if you are unsure. If it says "flammable," remove them from the area.

G Do not allow candles, lighters, or matches around oxygen.

G Check the nasal area and behind the ears often and report signs of irritation from the tubing from the nasal cannula or face mask (Fig. 7-15).

G Make sure that the resident is not lying on the oxygen tubing and that there are no kinks in it. Make sure nothing is pressing on the tubing.

G Learn how to turn oxygen off in case of a fire. Never adjust oxygen levels.

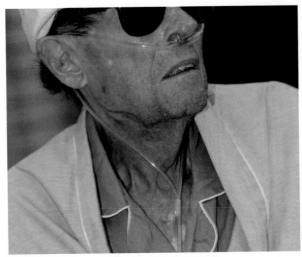

Fig. 7-15. *A resident with a nasal cannula.*

Tip

Watch for flammables!

Do you know anyone who smokes while polishing her nails or using nail polish remover? If so, advise her to stop this practice. Nail polish and nail polish remover are flammable and are dangerous when around sparks or flames. Lighting a cigarette or smoking a cigarette near flammable liquids can cause the product to explode. This can cause injury or even a fire.

10. Identify safety guidelines for intravenous (IV) lines

"IV" is an abbreviation for "intravenous," which means into a vein. A resident with an IV is receiving medication, nutrition, or fluids through a vein (Fig. 7-16). When caring for residents who have IVs, follow these guidelines:

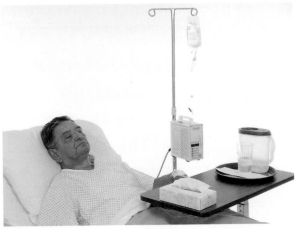

Fig. 7-16. *A resident with an IV.*

Guidelines: IVs

G Always wear gloves if you have to touch the IV area.

G Do not do any of the following when caring for a resident with an IV:

- Take blood pressure on an arm with an IV.
- Get the IV site wet.
- Pull on or catch the tubing on anything, such as clothing, during positioning.
- Leave the tubing kinked.
- Lower the IV bag below the IV site.
- Touch the clamp.
- Disconnect IV from pump or turn off alarm.

G Report to the nurse if any of the following occurs:

- The needle or catheter has fallen out or moves out of the vein. If an IV catheter comes out of the vein, it can cause an infiltration. An infiltration is the administration of fluids into surrounding tissue. Symptoms of infiltration include tissue swelling, cool or cold skin, red or warm skin, pain, tenderness, bleeding, and leaking of fluid from IV site.
- The armboard or handboard (device taped to the arm or hand, used to help keep the IV catheter properly positioned inside the vein) becomes loose.
- The tubing is disconnected.
- Blood appears in the tubing.
- The IV fluid in the bag or container is gone or almost gone.
- The IV fluid is not dripping, is leaking, or the bag breaks.
- The IV pump is beeping.
- The resident complains of pain, has difficulty breathing, or has a fever. Pain and fever may indicate phlebitis, which is inflammation of a vein.

- The resident pulls out or attempts to pull out the IV.

Oxygen and IVs

Residents who use oxygen or have IVs have the continued right to freedom of movement. They must be kept safe from the hazards of oxygen use and from the risks of having an IV.

11. Discuss fire safety and explain the "RACE" and "PASS" acronyms

There are many causes of fire. For a fire to occur, it must have these three things:

1. Heat: makes the flame
2. Fuel: the object that burns
3. Oxygen: gas that will keep the fire burning

There are many potential causes of a fire in facilities, including:

- Smoking
- Frayed or damaged electrical cords
- Electrical equipment in need of repair
- Overloaded electrical plugs
- Oxygen use
- Careless cooking
- Flammable liquids or rags with oils on them
- Stacks of newspapers or other clutter

Ways to prevent fires from occurring include:

- Stay with a resident who is smoking at all times.
- Check ashtrays for lit cigarettes or matches. Put out burning cigarettes.
- Make sure cigarettes or other smoking materials have not fallen on an area where a fire may start.
- If emptying an ashtray, make sure there are no hot ashes, matches, or cigarette butts in the ashtray.

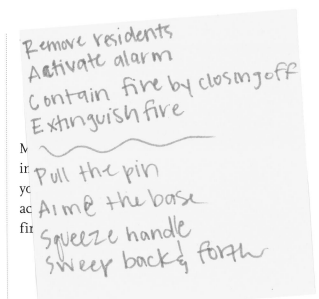

M[...]
in[...]
yo[...]
ac[...]
fir[...]

handwritten note:
Remove residents
Activate alarm
Contain fire by closing off
Extinguish fire

Pull the pin
Aime the base
Squeeze handle
Sweep back & forth

Contain the fire by closing all doors and windows, if possible.

Extinguish the fire, or fire department will extinguish. Evacuate if instructed to do so.

There will be many fire extinguishers at every facility (Fig. 7-17). Learn where they are located. In order to understand how to use an extinguisher, follow the **PASS** acronym:

Pull the pin.

Aim at the base of the fire when spraying.

Squeeze the handle.

Sweep back and forth at the base of the fire.

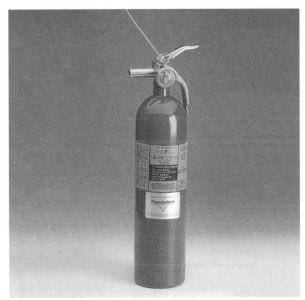

Fig. 7-17. *Know the location of your facility's fire extinguishers and how to use them.*

All facilities have fire safety plans. Learn your facility's plan. It will help you know what to do in the event of a fire. Here are general guidelines to follow in case of a fire:

Guidelines: What to Do in Case of Fire

G   Call for immediate help.

G   Know the location of the fire evacuation plan.

G   Remain calm. Do not panic.

G   Remove all persons in the immediate area of the fire (see RACE acronym).

G   If a door is closed, always check it for heat before opening it.

G   Stay low in a room when trying to escape a fire.

G   Use wet towels to block doorways to prevent smoke from entering a room.

G   Use a covering over the face to reduce smoke inhalation.

G   If clothing is on fire, remember to stop, drop, and roll to put out fire.

G   Never get into an elevator during a fire unless directed to do so by the fire department.

In case of fire, nursing assistants may be asked to turn off all oxygen and electrical equipment in the area, if possible. Follow your facility's policies.

12. List general safety steps to protect yourself and residents in a facility

Living or working in a facility may sometimes put a person at risk of crime. Many people go in and out of a facility during the day. Delivery people, visitors, clergy, temporary workers, and others may enter facilities regularly. Unfortunately, not everyone is honest and trustworthy. It is best to watch for any suspicious behavior. If you notice any suspicious behavior, report it immediately. In addition, follow these safety guidelines:

Guidelines: Safety in a Facility

G   Keep valuable personal items at home.

G   Ask the nurse to lock up residents' valuable items.

G   If any visitor or staff member makes you uneasy, do not leave a resident alone with the person.

G   Follow guidelines for the number of visitors allowed at one time in a resident's room.

G   Do not share your personal information with anyone. Do not share residents' or other staff members' information with anyone.

G   Report any situation or person who makes you feel unsafe or concerned to your supervisor.

Chapter Review

1. List each of the six common resident accidents in facilities and list two ways to prevent each one (LO 2).

2. In what position should a resident be placed for eating (LO 2)?

3. What is the important information the MSDS provides about chemicals (LO 3)?

4. What should be disposed of in a biohazard container or bag (LO 4)?

5. Define "body mechanics" (LO 5).

6. Should objects be held close to the body or far away from the body when lifting or carrying them (LO 5)?

7. How should legs be positioned when standing to give a better base of support (LO 5)?

8. When lifting, is it better to bend at the waist or at the knees (LO 5)?

9. Define "restraint" (LO 6).

10. Why was restraint use restricted (LO 6)?

11. List 12 complications of restraint use (LO 6).

12. List ten examples of restraint alternatives (LO 7).

13. What does a "restraint-free" environment mean (LO 7)?

14. When can a restraint be applied (LO 8)?

15. How can a nursing assistant check to make sure that a restraint is not too tight (LO 8)?

16. Should restraints be tied to side rails (LO 8)?

17. When a resident is restrained, how often does he or she require care (LO 8)?

18. List four guidelines for working safely around oxygen (LO 9).

19. List six signs to report to a nurse about an IV (LO 10).

20. What three things need to be present for a fire to occur (LO 11)?

21. Identify what the acronyms "RACE" and "PASS" stand for (LO 11).

22. If a fire has started, what should the nursing assistant do before opening a closed door (LO 11)?

23. List two general safety steps to protect residents in a facility (LO 12).

8
Emergency Care, First Aid, and Disasters

Emergency Transfer of Victims During the 1500s

Compare the rescue of a traveler in ancient times to the care our emergency squads give today. "The misfortune befell me in the manner which follows: wishing to pass across the water and trying to make my hackney enter a boat, I struck [the horse] . . . with a riding crop [and] the animal gave me such a kick that she broke entirely the two bones of my left leg . . . . I was quickly carried into the boat to cross to the other side in order to have me treated. But its shaking almost made me die, because the ends of the broken bones rubbed against the flesh, and those who were carrying me could not give it fit posture. From the boat, I was carried into a house of the village with greater pain than I had endured in the boat . . . . Finally, however, they placed me on a bed to regain my breath a little . . . while my dressing was being made . . ."

Ambroise Paré, 1510-1590,
from *Ten Books of Surgery*, published by the
University of Georgia Press.

"It is by presence of mind in untried emergencies that the native metal of a man is tested."

James Russell Lowell, 1819-1891

" . . . the truly noble and resolved spirit raises itself, and becomes more conspicuous in times of disaster and ill fortune."

Plutarch, A.D. 46-120

1. Define important words in this chapter

abdominal thrusts: a method of attempting to remove an object from the airway of someone who is choking.

cardiac arrest: the medical term for the stopping of the heartbeat.

code team: group of people chosen for a particular shift to respond to resident emergencies.

conscious: the state of being mentally alert and having awareness of surroundings, sensations, and thoughts.

CPR (cardiopulmonary resuscitation): refers to medical procedures used when a person's heart and lungs have stopped working.

diabetic ketoacidosis: a life-threatening complication of diabetes that can result from undiagnosed diabetes, not enough insulin, eating too much, not getting enough exercise, and stress; also known as ketoacidosis or hyperglycemia.

dyspnea: difficulty breathing.

emesis: the act of vomiting, or ejecting stomach contents through the mouth and/or nose.

epistaxis: a nosebleed.

expressive aphasia: inability to express oneself to others through speech or written words.

fainting: loss of consciousness; also called syncope.

first aid: care given by the first people to respond to an emergency.

hemiparesis: weakness on one side of the body.

hemiplegia: paralysis of one side of the body.

hyperglycemia: a life-threatening complication of diabetes that can result from undiagnosed diabetes, not enough insulin, eating too much, not getting enough exercise, and stress; also known as diabetic ketoacidosis (DKA) or ketoacidosis.

hypoglycemia: a life-threatening complication of diabetes that can result from either too much insulin or too little food; also known as insulin reaction and insulin shock.

insulin reaction: a life-threatening complication of diabetes that can result from either too much insulin or too little food; also known as hypoglycemia or insulin shock.

myocardial infarction: a condition in which blood flow to the heart is blocked and muscle cells die; also called a heart attack.

obstructed airway: a condition in which the tube through which air enters the lungs is blocked.

receptive aphasia: inability to understand what others are communicating through speech or written words.

respiratory arrest: the medical term for the stopping of breathing.

shock: a condition in which there is decreased blood flow to organs and tissues.

syncope: loss of consciousness; also called fainting.

2. Demonstrate how to respond to medical emergencies

Medical emergencies can happen when you least expect them (Fig. 8-1). Choking, diabetic emergencies, falls, poisoning, heart attacks, strokes, stab wounds, and gunshot wounds are all medical emergencies. The most serious medical emergencies involve these situations:

- The person is unconscious
- The person is not breathing
- The person has no pulse
- The person is bleeding severely

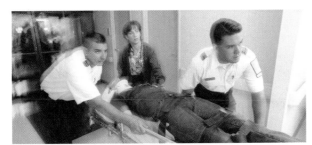

Fig. 8-1. *Medical emergencies can happen at any time. Being calm and prepared is the best way to respond to emergencies.*

When an emergency happens, try to remain calm. Act quickly and communicate clearly. Take two pairs of gloves and a barrier face mask with you. Look around to make sure the area is safe. Make sure you are safe before providing care. Once you have your gloves on, follow these steps:

- **Assess the situation.** Notice the time. Try to find out what has happened.

- **Assess the victim.** Ask the injured or ill person what has happened. If the person cannot respond, he may be unconscious. Being **conscious** means being mentally alert and having awareness of surroundings, sensations, and thoughts. Determine whether the person is conscious. Tap the person and ask if he is all right. Speak loudly. Use the person's name if you know it. If there is no response, assume that the person is unconscious. This is an emergency. Call for help right away, or send someone else to call.

If a person is conscious and able to speak, then he is breathing and has a pulse. Talk with the person about what happened and check him for injury. Look for these things:

- Severe bleeding
- Changes in consciousness
- Irregular breathing
- Unusual color or feel to the skin
- Swollen places on the body
- Medical alert tags
- Anything the person says is painful

If any of these exist, you may need professional medical help. Always get help. Call the nurse before doing anything else. If the injured or ill person is conscious, he may be frightened. Listen to the person. Tell him what is being done to help him. Be calm and confident. Reassure him that he is being taken care of.

After the emergency, while still on duty, document the emergency in your notes. You may need to complete an incident report. Try to remember as many details as you can. Remember, only report the facts, not opinions. If you think a resident suffered a heart attack, write only the signs and symptoms you observed. Record the actions you took. Knowing what information you will have to document will help you remember the important facts. For example, it is especially important to remember the time a person became unconscious.

Tip

PPE SCC

Performing first aid is something for which many people are not prepared. If you have to perform first aid, remember this acronym: PPE SCC.

- **PPE**: Grab and apply personal protective equipment.
- **S**afety first! Are you safe?
- **C**all for help or point to person and say: "You, get help now!"
- **C**are for victims.

Trivia

"Flying Ambulances"

Napoleon invaded Italy in 1796. During that invasion, Dominique Jean Larrey (1766-1842) developed "flying ambulances." These were horse-drawn vehicles that were able to quickly remove the wounded from the front lines for treatment. During the American Civil War, around 1863, "ambulance trains" similar to the legendary wagon trains of western lore appeared.

3. Demonstrate knowledge of first aid procedures

Emergency situations can happen to anyone at any time. When a person is involved in a serious accident, such as drowning or choking, respiratory arrest can occur. **Respiratory arrest** means that breathing stops. If the person is not helped quickly, cardiac arrest may soon follow. **Cardiac arrest** is when the heart stops. When respiratory arrest occurs, rescue breathing must be initiated. When respiratory arrest and cardiac arrest occur, **cardiopulmonary resuscitation (CPR)** is necessary. CPR refers to medical procedures used when the heart and lungs have stopped working and is used until medical help arrives.

Quick action is necessary. The first few minutes of any emergency can determine the victim's ability to survive the incident. CPR must be started immediately to help prevent or minimize brain damage. Brain damage can occur within four to six minutes after breathing stops and the heart stops beating.

Only properly trained people should perform CPR. In an emergency situation, never do anything that is beyond your ability or training. Give basic first aid until the emergency medical team arrives. **First aid** is the care given by the first people to respond to an emergency.

If your employer does not arrange for you to be trained in CPR, the American Heart Association and the American Red Cross, among others, offer courses in CPR. Keep your CPR certification current. A separate first aid course, to stay up-to-date on life-saving methods, is also available.

Some facilities do not allow nursing assistants to begin CPR without the direction of a nurse, even if they have been trained. This is due, in part, to residents' advance directives. Some residents have made the decision that they do not want CPR. Know your facility's policies on whether you can initiate CPR if you have been trained.

The AED

An automated external defibrillator, or AED, may be used for a cardiac arrest. The AED is a computerized device that can restart the heart by giving it an electrical shock. When using this device, a clear, computerized voice takes the user through each step that must be performed. Lights and text messages may also relay instructions.

AEDs are available at healthcare facilities and are also located in airplanes, offices, malls, and many other places. AED training will be given during CPR classes. Care must be taken when using this device near oxygen. Fires can occur due to sparks.

AEDs must be properly maintained for best performance. Regular checks should be scheduled at your facility to ensure the AED is in proper working order.

Choking

Residents who have difficulty chewing or swallowing, are confused, or have poor vision may be at risk of choking. When something is blocking the tube through which air enters the lungs, the person has an **obstructed airway**. When people are choking, they usually put their hands to their throats and cough (Fig. 8-2). As long as the person can speak, cough, or breathe, do nothing. Encourage her to cough as forcefully as possible to get the object out. Ask someone to get a nurse. Stay with the person until she stops choking or can no longer speak, cough, or breathe.

If a person can no longer speak, cough, or breathe, or turns blue, call for help immediately. Time is of extreme importance. Use the call light or emergency cord to notify someone that you need help. Do not leave a choking victim to call for help. **Abdominal thrusts** are a method of attempting to remove an object from the airway of someone who is choking. These thrusts work to remove the blockage upward, out of the throat.

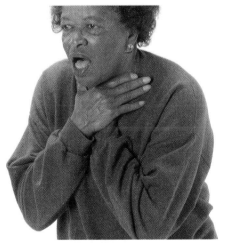

Fig. 8-2. *A common sign of choking is when a person puts her hands to her throat and coughs.*

The procedure for giving abdominal thrusts is described below. Follow your facility's procedure

for clearing an obstructed airway. For obese people or women in the later stages of pregnancy, training on chest thrusts will be provided. Keep any first aid certifications current.

Make sure the person needs help before giving abdominal thrusts. The person must show signs of a severely obstructed airway. These include poor air exchange, an increase in trouble breathing, silent coughing, blue-tinged skin (cyanosis), or inability to speak, cough or breathe. You must ask the person, "Are you choking?"

If the person nods her head "Yes," she has a severe airway obstruction and needs immediate help. Give abdominal thrusts. Do this only if your facility allows you to perform this procedure. Do not perform this procedure on a person who is not choking. This risks serious injury.

Performing abdominal thrusts for the conscious person

1. Stand behind the person. Bring your arms under her arms. Wrap your arms around the person's waist.

2. Make a fist with one hand. Place the flat, thumb side of the fist against the person's abdomen, above the navel but below the breastbone.

3. Grasp the fist with your other hand. Pull both hands toward you and up (inward and upward), quickly and forcefully (Fig. 8-3).

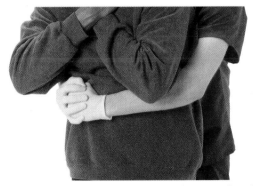

Fig. 8-3. *Pull both hands toward you and up (inward and upward), quickly and forcefully.*

4. Repeat until the object is pushed out.

If the person becomes unconscious while choking, stop what you are doing. Help her to the floor gently. Lie her on her back on a hard surface. Activate emergency medical services (EMS) and begin proper CPR for an unconscious person. Make sure help is on its way. The person may have a completely blocked airway and needs professional medical help immediately. Stay with the victim until help arrives.

Shock

Shock occurs when organs and tissues in the body do not receive an adequate blood supply. Bleeding, heart attack, severe infection, and falling blood pressure can lead to shock. Shock can become worse when the person is frightened or in severe pain.

Shock is a dangerous, life-threatening situation. Signs of shock include pale or cyanotic (bluish) skin, staring, increased pulse and respiration rates, decreased blood pressure, and extreme thirst. Always call for help if you suspect a person is in shock. To treat shock, do the following:

Responding to shock

1. Notify the nurse immediately. Victims of shock should always receive medical care as soon as possible.

2. If controlling bleeding, put on gloves first. The next procedure will explain how to do this.

3. Have the person lie down on her back. If the person is bleeding from the mouth or vomiting, place her on her side (unless you suspect that the neck, back, or spinal cord is injured).

4. Check pulse and respirations if possible (Chapter 13). Begin CPR if breathing and pulse are absent.

5. Keep the person as calm and comfortable as possible. Loosen clothing or ties around the neck and any belts or waist strings.

6. Maintain normal body temperature. If the weather is cold, place a blanket around the person. If the weather is hot, provide shade.

7. Elevate the feet unless the person has a head, neck, back, spinal or abdominal injury, breathing difficulties, or fractures (Fig. 8-4). Never elevate a body part if a broken bone exists or if it causes pain.

8. Do not give the person anything to eat or drink.

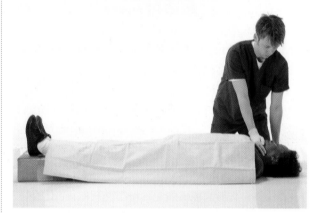

Fig. 8-4. *Elevate the feet, unless the person has head, neck, back, spinal, or abdominal injuries, breathing problems, or fractures.*

Bleeding

Severe bleeding can cause death quickly and must be controlled. Follow these steps to control bleeding:

Controlling bleeding

1. Notify the nurse immediately.

2. Put on gloves. Always take time to do this. If the person is able, he can hold his bare hand over the wound until you can put on gloves.

3. Hold a thick sterile pad, clean cloth, handkerchief, or towel against the wound.

4. Press down hard directly on the bleeding wound until help arrives (Fig. 8-5). Do not decrease pressure. Put additional pads over the first pad if blood seeps through. Do not remove the first pad.

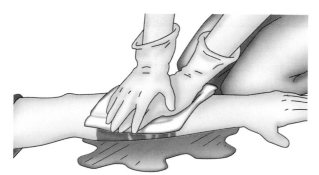

Fig. 8-5. *Press down hard directly on the bleeding wound; do not decrease pressure.*

5. If you can, raise the wound above the level of the heart to slow down the bleeding. If the wound is on an arm, leg, hand, or foot, and there are no head, neck, back, spinal, or abdominal injuries or fractures, prop up the limb. Use towels or other absorbent material.

6. When bleeding is under control, secure the dressing to keep it in place. Check the person for symptoms of shock (pale skin, staring, increased pulse and respiration rates, decreased blood pressure, and extreme thirst). Stay with the person until help arrives.

7. Remove gloves and wash hands thoroughly when finished.

Burns

You learned about preventing burns and scalds in Chapter 7. Care of a burn depends on its depth, size, and location. There are three types of burns: first-degree (superficial), second-degree (partial-thickness), and third-degree (full thickness) burns. You will learn more about burns in Chapter 18. If a resident is burned, call or have someone call for the nurse immediately.

Treating burns

To treat a minor burn:

1. Notify the nurse immediately. Put on gloves.

2. Use cool, clean water to decrease the skin temperature and prevent further injury (Fig.

8-6). Do not use ice or ice water, as ice may cause further skin damage. Dampen a clean towel with cool water, and place it over the burn.

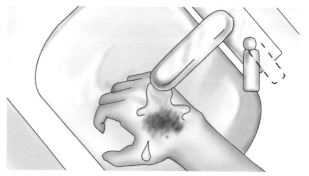

Fig. 8-6. *Use cool, clean water, not ice, on burned skin.*

3. Once the pain has eased, you may cover the area with a dry, clean dressing or non-adhesive sterile bandage.

4. Never use any kind of ointment, water, salve, or grease on a burn.

For more serious burns:

1. If clothing has caught fire, have the person stop, drop, and roll, or smother the fire with a blanket or towel. Use water to help put out the fire, if possible. Protect yourself from the source of the burn.

2. Notify the nurse immediately. Put on gloves.

3. Check for breathing, pulse, and severe bleeding. If the person is not breathing, begin rescue breathing. If the person is not breathing and has no pulse, begin CPR. Do not put pillows under the head, as this may obstruct the airway.

4. Do not use any type of ointment, water, salve, or grease on the burn.

5. Do not try to pull away any clothing from burned areas. Cover the burn with a clean cloth, a dry, non-adhesive sterile bandage, or a clean sheet. Apply the cloth, bandage, or sheet lightly. Take care not to rub the burned area.

6. Take steps to prevent shock.

7. Do not give the person food or fluids.

8. Monitor vital signs and wait for emergency medical help.

9. Remove gloves and wash hands.

Fainting (Syncope)

Fainting, or **syncope**, occurs as a result of decreased blood flow to the brain, causing a loss of consciousness. Fainting may be the result of hunger, fear, pain, fatigue, standing for a long time, poor ventilation, pregnancy, or overheating. Signs and symptoms of fainting include dizziness, nausea, perspiration, pale skin, weak pulse, shallow respirations, and blackness in the visual field. If someone appears likely to faint, follow these steps:

Responding to fainting

1. Notify the nurse immediately.

2. Have the person lie down or sit down before fainting occurs.

3. If the person is in a sitting position, have her bend forward and place her head between her knees (Fig. 8-7). If the person is lying flat on her back, elevate the legs.

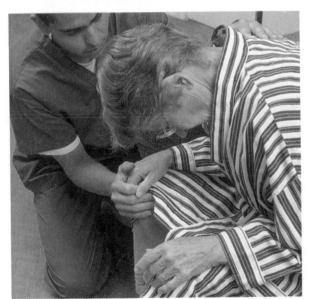

Fig. 8-7. *Have the person bend forward and place her head between her knees if she is sitting.*

4. Loosen any tight clothing.

5. Have the person stay in this position for at least five minutes after symptoms disappear.

6. Help the person get up slowly. Continue to observe her for symptoms of fainting. Assist her to sit down if needed. Stay with her until she feels better. If you need help but cannot leave the person, use the call light.

If a person does faint, lower her to the floor or other flat surface. Position her on her back. If she has no head, neck, back or spinal injuries, elevate her legs 8 to 12 inches. If unsure about injuries, leave her flat on her back. Check to make sure the person is breathing. She should recover quickly, but keep her lying down for several minutes. Report the incident to the nurse immediately. Fainting may be a sign of a more serious medical condition.

Poisoning

As you learned in Chapter 7, facilities contain many harmful substances that should not be swallowed. Always have the poison control center phone number available. Suspect poisoning when a resident suddenly collapses, vomits, and has heavy, difficult breathing. If you suspect poisoning, take the following steps:

Responding to poisoning

1. Notify the nurse immediately.

2. Put on gloves. Look for a container that will help you determine what the person has taken or eaten. With your gloves on, carefully open mouth and look inside to check the mouth for chemical burns. Do not place your fingers inside the mouth. Note breath odor.

3. The nurse may have you call a poison control center. Follow these instructions.

4. Remove gloves and wash your hands.

Emergency Care, First Aid, and Disasters

Nosebleed

A nosebleed can occur suddenly when the air is dry, when injury has occurred, or when a person has taken certain medications. The medical term for a nosebleed is **epistaxis**. If a resident has a nosebleed, take the following steps:

Responding to a nosebleed

1. Notify the nurse immediately.

2. Elevate the head of the bed, or tell the person to remain in a sitting position, leaning forward slightly. Offer tissues or a clean cloth to catch the blood. Do not touch blood or bloody clothes, tissues, or cloths without gloves.

3. Put on gloves. Apply firm pressure over the bridge of the nose. Squeeze the bridge of the nose with your thumb and forefinger (Fig. 8-8). You can have the person do this until you are able to put on gloves.

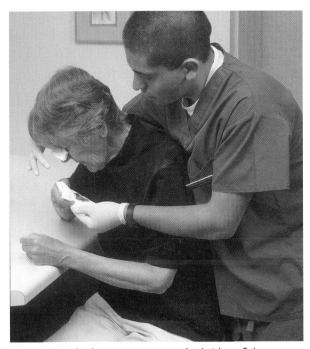

Fig. 8-8. With gloves on, squeeze the bridge of the nose with your thumb and forefinger.

4. Apply pressure until the bleeding stops.

5. Use a cool cloth or ice wrapped in a cloth on the back of the neck, the forehead, or the upper lip to slow the flow of blood. Never apply ice directly to skin.

6. Keep person still and calm until help arrives.

7. Remove gloves and wash hands.

Vomiting

Vomiting, or **emesis**, is the act of ejecting stomach contents through the mouth and/or nose. It can be a sign of a serious illness or injury. Because you may not know when a resident is going to vomit, you may not have time to explain what you will do ahead of time. Talk to the resident soothingly as you help him clean up. Tell him what you are doing to help him. If a resident has vomited, take the following steps:

Responding to vomiting

1. Notify the nurse immediately.

2. Put on gloves.

3. Place an emesis basin under the chin. If an emesis basin is not nearby, use the wash basin. Remove it when vomiting has stopped.

4. Remove soiled linens or clothes and set aside. Replace with fresh linens or clothes.

5. Note amount, color, and consistency of vomitus. Look for blood in vomitus, blood-tinged vomitus, or medication (pills) in vomitus. Find out if a specimen should be sent to the laboratory. Show the nurse the vomitus before discarding or if blood or pills are noted.

6. Flush vomitus down the toilet and wash and store the basin.

7. Remove and discard gloves.

8. Wash your hands.

9. Put on fresh gloves.

10. Provide comfort to the person. Wipe his face and mouth (Fig. 8-9). Position him comfortably, and offer a drink of water or a sip to swish in the mouth and spit. Provide oral

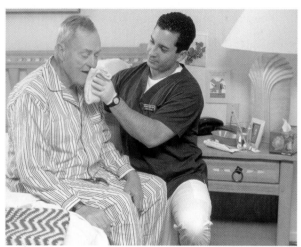

care (see Chapter 12). It helps get rid of the vomit taste in the mouth.

Fig. 8-9. Be calm and comforting when helping a resident who has vomited.

11. Put the soiled linen in proper containers.

12. Remove and discard gloves.

13. Wash your hands again.

14. Document time, amount, color, odor and consistency of vomitus.

Myocardial Infarction or Heart Attack

When blood flow to an area of the heart is blocked, oxygen and nutrients fail to reach its cells. Waste products are not removed and the muscle cells die. This is called a **myocardial infarction** (MI), or heart attack. The area of dead tissue may be large or small. This depends on the artery or arteries involved. A myocardial infarction is an emergency that can result in serious heart damage or death. The following are signs and symptoms of MI:

• Sudden, severe pain in the chest, usually on the left side or in the center, behind the breastbone

• Pain or discomfort in other areas of the body, such as one or both arms, the back, neck, jaw, or stomach

• Indigestion or heartburn

• Nausea and vomiting

• **Dyspnea**, or difficulty breathing

• Dizziness

• Pale, gray, or cyanotic skin color or mucous membranes, indicating lack of oxygen

• Perspiration

• Cold and clammy skin

• Weak and irregular pulse rate

• Low blood pressure

• Anxiety and a sense of doom

• Denial of a heart problem

The pain of a heart attack is commonly described as a crushing, pressing, squeezing, stabbing, piercing pain, or, "like someone is sitting on my chest." The pain may go down the inside of the left arm. A person may also feel it in the neck and/or in the jaw. The pain usually does not go away.

As with men, chest pain or discomfort is the most common symptom in women. But women are somewhat more likely than men to have shortness of breath, nausea/vomiting, and back, shoulder, or jaw pain. Some women's symptoms seem more flu-like, and women are more likely to deny that they are having a heart attack.

You must take immediate action if a resident experiences any of these symptoms. Follow these steps:

Responding to a myocardial infarction

1. Call or have someone call the nurse.

2. Place the person in a comfortable position. Encourage him to rest. Reassure him that you will not leave him alone.

3. Loosen clothing around the person's neck (Fig. 8-10).

4. Do not give the person food or fluids.

5. Monitor the person's breathing and pulse. If the person stops breathing, perform rescue breathing. If the person has no pulse, begin CPR if trained and allowed to do so.

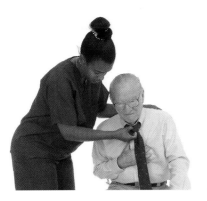

Fig. 8-10. *Loosen the clothing around the person's neck if you suspect he is having an MI.*

6. Stay with the person until help has arrived.

See Chapter 19 for more information on myocardial infarctions.

Insulin Reaction and Diabetic Ketoacidosis

Insulin reaction and diabetic ketoacidosis are complications of diabetes that can be life-threatening. **Insulin reaction**, or **hypoglycemia**, can result from either too much insulin or too little food. It occurs when insulin is given and the person skips a meal or does not eat all the food required. Even when a regular amount of food is eaten, additional physical activity may cause the body to rapidly absorb the food. This causes too much insulin in the body. Vomiting and diarrhea may also lead to insulin reaction in people with diabetes.

The first signs of insulin reaction include feeling weak or different, nervousness, dizziness, and perspiration. These signal that the resident needs food. The food should be in a form that can be rapidly absorbed. A lump of sugar, a hard candy, or a glass of orange or grape juice should be consumed right away. A diabetic may have other quick sources of sugar handy, such as glucose tablets. Call the nurse if the resident has shown signs of insulin reaction. Other signs and symptoms of insulin reaction include:

*   Hunger
*   Weakness
*   Rapid pulse
*   Headache
*   Low blood pressure
*   Cold, clammy skin
*   Confusion
*   Trembling
*   Blurred vision
*   Numbness of the lips and tongue
*   Unconsciousness

Having too little insulin in the body causes **diabetic ketoacidosis** (DKA), also known as ketoacidosis or **hyperglycemia**. It can result from infection (especially a urinary tract infection), undiagnosed diabetes, not enough insulin, eating too much, not getting enough exercise, or physical and emotional stress.

The signs of onset of diabetic ketoacidosis include increased thirst or urination, abdominal pain, deep or difficult breathing, and breath that smells sweet or fruity. Call the nurse immediately if you observe signs of DKA. Other signs and symptoms include:

*   Nausea and vomiting
*   Loss of appetite
*   Headache
*   Blurred vision
*   Rapid, weak pulse
*   Low blood pressure
*   Shortness of breath or air hunger (person gasping for air and being unable to catch his breath)
*   Dry skin, dry mouth
*   Flushed cheeks
*   Drowsiness
*   Confusion
*   Weakness
*   Unconsciousness

If left untreated, DKA can lead to diabetic coma and death. See Chapter 23 for more information.

Seizures

Seizures are involuntary, often violent, contractions of muscles. They can involve a small area or the entire body. Seizures are caused by an abnormality in the brain. They can occur in young children who have a high fever. Older children and adults who have a serious illness, fever, or head injury may also have seizures.

The main goal of a caregiver during a seizure is to make sure the resident is safe. During a seizure, a person may shake severely and thrust arms and legs uncontrollably. He may clench his jaw, drool, and be unable to swallow. Most seizures last a short amount of time. Take the following measures if a resident has a seizure:

Responding to seizures

1. Note the time. Put on gloves.

2. Lower the person to the floor. Cradle and protect his head. Loosen clothing to help with breathing. Attempt to turn his head to one side to lower the risk of choking. This may not be possible during a violent seizure.

3. Have someone call the nurse immediately or use the call light. Do not leave the person unless you must do so to get medical help.

4. Move furniture away to prevent injury. If a pillow is nearby, place it under his head.

5. Do not try to stop the seizure or restrain the person.

6. Do not force anything between the person's teeth. Do not place your hands in his mouth for any reason. You could be bitten.

7. Do not give the person food or fluids.

8. When the seizure is over, note the time. Gently turn the person to his left side if you do not suspect a head, neck, or spinal injury. This reduces the risk of choking on vomit or saliva. If the person begins to choke, get help immediately. Check for adequate breathing and pulse. If the person stops breathing, perform rescue breathing. If the person has no pulse, begin CPR if trained and allowed to do so. Do not begin CPR during a seizure.

9. Report the length of the seizure and your observations to the nurse.

10. Remove gloves and wash hands.

Types of General Seizures

Absence or Petit Mal: Absence, or petit mal, seizures are brief episodes of staring in which the levels of awareness and responsiveness are limited. Usually people do not realize when they have had this type of seizure. There is no warning beforehand, and being alert afterward is common.

Myoclonic: Myoclonic seizures are brief jerks of a muscle or a group of muscles. They usually do not last more than a few seconds.

Atonic: With atonic seizures (also called "drop attacks" or "drop seizures"), the muscles suddenly lose strength, which can cause drooping of the eyelids and nodding of the head. The person may drop things and fall to the ground. The person usually remains conscious while having this seizure. The seizure usually lasts less than 15 seconds.

Tonic: In tonic seizures, muscle tone is greatly increased temporarily, and the body, arms, or legs can suddenly stiffen. The person usually remains conscious. Tonic seizures most often occur during sleep. They usually last less than 20 seconds.

Clonic: Clonic seizures consist of rhythmic jerking of the arms and legs. This can occur on one or both sides of the body. The length of time this seizure lasts varies.

Tonic-Clonic: During a tonic-clonic seizure (formerly known as a "grand mal" seizure), all the muscles stiffen. The person may groan and lose consciousness, falling to the floor. He may bite his tongue or cheek and may turn blue. The arms and legs may make rhythmic jerking and bending movements. The person may lose control of his bladder and/or bowels. These seizures usually last one to three minutes. After the jerking stops, consciousness returns slowly. The person may be confused, tired, or agitated.

CVA or Stroke

The medical term for a stroke is cerebrovascular accident (CVA). A CVA, or stroke, occurs when the blood supply to a portion of the brain is cut off (Fig. 8-11). A clot, a ruptured blood vessel, or pressure from a tumor compressing a vessel may cause a stroke.

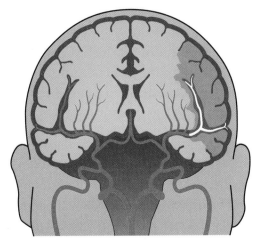

Fig. 8-11. *A CVA, or stroke, occurs when the blood supply to the brain is suddenly cut off.*

Symptoms that a stroke is beginning include dizziness, ringing in the ears, blurred vision, headache, nausea, vomiting, slurring of words, and loss of memory. These signs and symptoms should be reported immediately. A quick response to a suspected stroke is critical. Tests and treatment need to be given within a short time of the stroke's onset (ideally within an hour). Early treatment may be able to reduce the severity of the stroke.

A transient ischemic attack, or TIA, is a warning sign of a CVA. It is the result of a temporary lack of oxygen in the brain. Symptoms may last up to 24 hours. They include tingling, weakness, or some loss of movement in an arm or leg. These symptoms should not be ignored. Report them to the nurse immediately. These are also signs that a TIA or stroke is occurring:

* Dizziness
* Confusion
* Loss of consciousness
* Seizures

* Shaking or trembling
* Redness in the face
* Facial droop, inability to smile
* Drooping of one eyelid or eye
* Sudden loss of sight in one eye
* Pupil of one eye is larger
* Blurred vision
* Trouble with hearing or ringing in the ears
* Intense headache that will not go away
* Nausea and vomiting
* Loss of bowel or bladder control
* Numbness or tingling on one side of the body
* Paralysis on one side of the body, called **hemiplegia**
* Weakness on one side of the body, called **hemiparesis**
* Inability to express oneself to others through speech or written words, called **expressive aphasia**
* Inability to understand what others are communicating through speech or written words, called **receptive aphasia**
* Use of strange words
* Noisy breathing
* Elevated blood pressure
* Slow pulse rate

More information on CVAs can be found in Chapter 22.

4. Explain the nursing assistant's role on a code team

Facilities often use codes to inform staff of emergencies without alarming residents and visitors. For example, "Code Red" usually means fire, and "Code Blue" usually means cardiac arrest. Know the codes for your facility.

When staff are given their assignments at the beginning of shifts, some facilities also assign positions on the "code team." The **code team** is the team chosen for that shift to respond in case of a resident emergency. Staff on the code team may be asked to get a special cart or other emergency equipment, such as a suction machine, CPR equipment, oxygen, or other items. Although nursing assistants will not do many of the code team procedures, they may be asked to do chest compressions during CPR. If your facility uses code teams, note whether or not you are on this team at the start of your shift.

Should a code be called during your shift, respond from wherever you are in the facility. Respond calmly. Do not panic when you hear a code announced. If you are caring for a resident, get another staff member to take over. After the resident is secured, respond to the code.

Annual classes to update proper responses to codes may be held in your facility.

Responding to Codes

When a resident goes into respiratory or cardiac arrest, it can be difficult for staff, other residents, and visitors. When a code occurs, the staff's main concern is the victim's survival. Sometimes staff do not consider the impact of a code on other people in a facility.

Be aware of the people who are near the emergency. Staff not involved in responding to the code can move these people away from the area until the problem has been resolved. In some facilities a "Code Watcher" team is established to respond to a code and deal only with the emotional concerns of residents, staff, and visitors. This team is made up of nursing staff, social workers, trained volunteers, unit clerks, and administrative staff.

When a code occurs, do not leave a roommate in his room or close to where the code is occurring. Unconscious residents may also be aware of everything that is happening. Reassure unconscious residents, too, during emergency situations.

5. Describe guidelines for responding to disasters

A disaster can occur during your shift at a facility. Disasters can include fire, flood, earthquake,

hurricane, tornado, or severe weather. Acts of terrorism are also considered disasters.

Nursing assistants are expected to respond calmly and skillfully to disasters. You need to be responsible and efficient. Facilities will have an area-specific disaster plan available for employees to learn. Know where the plan is located and what to do in the event of disasters. There will be general guidelines, as well as specific guidelines for the area in which you work. For example, NAs working where hurricanes occur, such as Florida, need to know guidelines for hurricanes, as well as other disasters.

During an emergency, a nurse or the administrator will give directions. Listen carefully to all directions. Know what your responsibilities are, and follow instructions. Know the locations of all exits and stairways. Know where the fire alarms and extinguishers are located. Emphasize that everyone should remain calm in an emergency.

Being educated and prepared for emergencies helps decrease panic and ensure the appropriate response in a timely fashion. This helps to protect you and your residents.

Classes on disasters and disaster drills are held at facilities so that staff can prepare for disasters ahead of time. Take advantage of these sessions. Pay close attention to the instructions.

For more information on disaster preparedness, see the Federal Emergency Management Agency's (FEMA) website at fema.gov.

Blackouts

If a blackout occurs, emergency generators should automatically begin working. If a generator fails, emergency battery packs may be needed for some electrical equipment, such as ventilators and IV pumps. Supplies like flashlights, portable radios and portable clocks with extra batteries should be readily available.

Tip

Evacuation Carries

If an evacuation is required, be familiar with different types of evacuation carries. An evacuation carry is a method of removing an immobile resident safely from a dangerous situation. Make sure you attend emergency care and disaster plan in-services at your facility. Practice evacuation carries during disaster drills. Contact your local fire department for information and/or training.

Chapter Review

1. When an emergency occurs, what should a nursing assistant take with him or her (LO 2)?

2. List the two steps to follow in an emergency after making sure the area is safe and putting on gloves (LO 2).

3. When checking a person for injury, what should a nursing assistant look for (LO 2)?

4. What is the difference between respiratory and cardiac arrest (LO 3)?

5. How soon can brain damage occur after the heart stops beating and breathing stops (LO 3)?

6. When a person is choking, but can speak, cough, or breathe, what should the nursing assistant do (LO 3)?

7. In what position should a person be placed if he is in shock (LO 3)?

8. List a reason why gloves should always be put on before helping a person who is bleeding (LO 3).

9. If blood seeps through the first pad over a wound, should the first pad be removed before applying a second pad (LO 3)?

10. What should never be applied to a burn (LO 3)?

11. Why should ice not be applied to burns (LO 3)?

12. If a person feels faint and is sitting down, what should the nursing assistant do (LO 3)?

13. When should a nursing assistant suspect a person has been poisoned (LO 3)?

14. After putting on gloves, what should a nursing assistant do for a person who has a nosebleed (LO 3)?

15. What is a medical term for vomiting (LO 3)?

16. Explain why a nursing assistant should give oral care to a resident who has vomited (LO 3).

17. List ten general signs or symptoms of a myocardial infarction (MI) (LO 3).

18. What symptoms are women more likely to experience than men if they are having an MI (LO 3)?

19. What causes insulin reaction (LO 3)?

20. What causes diabetic ketoacidosis (LO 3)?

21. What are three things a nursing assistant should never do when a person is having a seizure (LO 3)?

22. What is a transient ischemic attack (TIA) (LO 3)?

23. List eight signs that a stroke is occurring (LO 3).

24. What does the term "Code Blue" usually stand for during an emergency (LO 4)?

25. List five types of disasters. Give one example of a disaster that occurred in your area within the last two years (LO 5).

9 Admission, Transfer, Discharge, and Physical Exams

"A Walk Through a Ward of the Eighteenth Century" by Grace Goldin

The old ward of St. John's Hospital, Bruges, housed patients continuously from the 12th century, when its first section was built, until the 20th . . . . A division was customary in medieval times. . . forming two wards side by side with separate entrances; or two wards built one above the other to separate the sexes . . . . The . . . hospital of the 18th century was a dangerous place, mortality there was higher than among patients nursed at home, and therefore it catered only to wretches with no alternative; but among these, many got better. The bonneted beldame at the rear of the center aisle, being shown out the door with a pat on the shoulder, is very likely being discharged "cured."

Excerpt from "A Walk Through a Ward of the Eighteenth Century" by Grace Goldin. From *Journal of the History of Medicine and Allied Sciences*, Volume XXII, Number 2, 1967. Reprinted with permission of Oxford University Press.

"Where we love is home,
Home that our feet may leave,
but not our hearts."
Oliver Wendell Holmes, 1809-1894

"The best thing we can do is to
make wherever we're in look as
much like home as we can."
Christopher Fry, 1907-2005

1. Define important words in this chapter

abdominal girth: a measurement of the circumference around the abdomen at the umbilicus (navel).

admission pack: personal care items supplied upon a resident's admission.

baseline: initial value that can be compared to future measurements.

bedridden: confined to bed.

contracture: the permanent and often painful shortening of a muscle, usually due to a lack of activity.

dorsal recumbent: position in which a person is flat on her back with knees flexed and slightly separated and her feet flat on the bed.

kilogram: a unit of mass equal to 1000 grams; one kilogram equals 2.2 pounds.

knee-chest: position in which a person is lying on his abdomen with knees pulled up towards the abdomen and with legs separated; arms are pulled up and flexed and the head is turned to one side.

lithotomy: position in which a person is on her back with her hips at the edge of the exam table; legs are flexed and feet are in padded stirrups.

metric: system of weights and measures based upon the meter.

pound: a unit of weight equal to 16 ounces.

2. List factors for families in choosing a facility

Choosing the right facility for a loved one can be a challenging, emotional, and difficult process. To help guide their choice, family and friends may look at information from federal agencies, such as the Centers for Medicare & Medicaid Services (CMS). They may ask for recommendations from friends. Families may review facilities' results from past state surveys or inspections. They may check to see if the facility has been accredited by the Joint Commission.

Early in the process, families usually visit each facility they are considering (Fig. 9-1). In some cases, a single visit is enough to decide if a facility is right or not. For example, if a strong smell of urine is present, they may not return again to see if it was an isolated incident. These are some questions considered before placing a loved one in a facility:

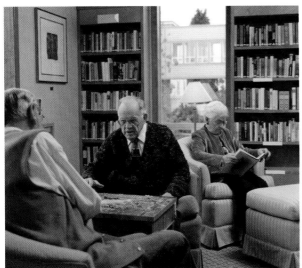

Fig. 9-1. Before choosing a facility for a loved one, families may tour the facility. They may observe the environment, how the residents look, and what types of activities are offered.

- Do the staff seem courteous and friendly?
- Do most of the staff speak the resident's native language? Is an interpreter available?
- Are there enough staff members on duty at the facility? What is the ratio of nurses and nursing assistants to residents? How is the facility staffed on evenings and weekends?
- Are foul odors present?
- What is the food like at the facility? Is attention paid to individual food preferences? Is a dietician available for meetings?
- Are residents up and dressed in the morning?
- Do staff interact positively with the residents?

- Do staff speak courteously to other staff members?
- Do residents look groomed, taken care of, and happy?
- How are residents' complaints resolved?
- Is the facility licensed?
- Have the state survey and other inspection results been satisfactory?
- Does the facility explain Residents' Rights?
- Does the facility provide assistance with activities of daily living (ADLs)? If so, how is it provided, and what are the associated fees?
- Are physical, occupational, and speech therapists available?
- How often do falls, infections, and pressure ulcers occur?
- Do volunteers work with residents? If so, are their interactions positive?
- How involved can the family be in creating the resident's care plan?
- Does the facility provide the level of care the resident needs? What about future needs?
- Is the environment safe, functional, and homelike?
- Is there an activities department? What kinds of activities are offered?
- What are the steps to take if a resident wants to move out of the facility?
- What policies does the facility have on advance directives and end-of-life decisions?

These are only some factors families consider when choosing a facility for a loved one.

3. Explain the nursing assistant's role in the emotional adjustment of a new resident

Moving into a facility requires a big adjustment. New residents may have been independent for a long time. They may be moving from a family member's home. Either way, there is a huge emotional adjustment to be made.

Think about some of the life-altering changes residents have had to make. They had to leave their homes and get rid of some of their personal belongings (Fig. 9-2). The move may have been sudden due to health reasons. They may have had to give away beloved pets. Loved ones may have died. Due to all of these things, new residents are experiencing many losses and emotions, such as fear, anger, and uncertainty, along with a decline in health and independence.

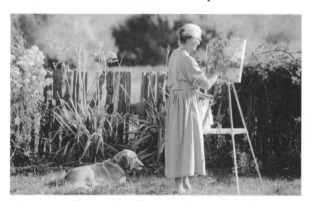

Fig. 9-2. *Understand and be empathetic to the fact that many residents had to leave familiar places. They may have had to give away personal items and beloved pets.*

Nursing assistants should empathize with new residents. Think about how you would feel if you had to give up many of your things to move into an unfamiliar place full of strangers. Understanding some of what residents are going through will help you provide compassionate care. Your residents will need it during those early days and weeks in their new home.

Nursing assistants are the team members most involved with residents on a daily basis. You will have an important role in helping new residents feel comfortable in the facility. Other guidelines to help new residents adjust follow:

Guidelines: Helping New Residents Adjust

G   Have a positive attitude. New residents, like most people, want to be near others who are nice and pleasant. Residents want to feel

comfortable around staff who provide their care. Residents should not feel as though they are a burden to staff.

G   Be tactful. Think before you speak.

G   Communicate clearly. Giving a simple reminder about meal times helps the resident feel more connected.

G   Show respect for residents' belongings. New residents may be frightened of their new surroundings. They may feel very protective of their personal items. Treat items carefully. Show that you are trustworthy.

G   Be responsible. If you make a mistake with resident care, report it to the nurse immediately. People respect and trust you more when you admit mistakes.

G   Be honest. Do not make promises you cannot keep. If you tell residents you are coming by to visit, they will look for you. If you forget, apologize, and reschedule the visit as soon as possible.

G   Listen to residents if they want to talk. New residents may want to express their feelings about what they are going through (Fig. 9-3). They may want to share some of their stories and backgrounds. Make time to listen.

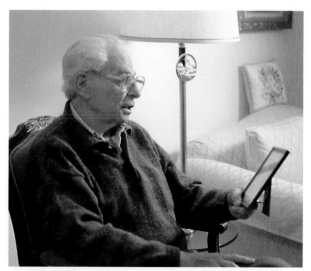

Fig. 9-3. *New residents must leave familiar places and personal items. They are experiencing many losses, such as the death of someone close to them. Be supportive; listen if they want to share their feelings.*

G   Pay attention to residents' wishes. For example, if a resident wants to be alone instead of joining others for an activity, let him do that. You can say, "Maybe next time," and leave him alone. Residents have the right to make choices about what to do and how to spend their time. If they choose to be alone, honor this decision.

G   Respect residents' privacy. The right to privacy is a legal right, and it is always important. It can be especially important when residents are first admitted. Take care to make sure residents have as much privacy as possible.

G   Be patient and kind. A new resident might have a good day followed by a not-so-good day. Allow residents to adapt at their own pace. Everyone is different. The process of adjusting may take some time. Dealing with multiple losses initiates the grieving process.

Tip

The Welcome Committee

To assist new residents with the transition into a facility, a "Welcome Committee" can be helpful. Team members from each department can be chosen to greet the new resident. Each department can make or buy a card for the resident. The special cards can be brought to the resident's new room one by one or as a group. This idea can be expanded to include other niceties, such as having flowers waiting for a resident in her new room. Small ways of showing care and warmth can help new residents feel better about the transition to a facility.

4. Describe the nursing assistant's role in the admission process

Admission is often the first time you meet new residents. Staff will be told the approximate time that the new resident will arrive. When the resident arrives, give him a good first impression of the staff and the facility. Welcome him in a friendly manner. Introduce yourself to the resident and all family members. Answer any questions residents and their family members

have. Ask questions to get information on the resident's personal preferences, history, rituals, and routines. Family members are great sources of information about the resident; take time to ask them questions.

The facility will have specific procedures for admitting new residents. Follow these general guidelines to help make the experience pleasant and successful:

Guidelines: Admission

G   Wash your hands. Then gather any necessary equipment to bring to the resident's room. This equipment may include:

- An **admission pack** or kit contains personal care items for the resident (Fig. 9-4). The pack usually has a wash basin, bedpan, urinal (for male residents), toothpaste, soap, and a water pitcher and cup. Other items may be in the pack, such as a toothbrush, comb, special lotions or soaps.

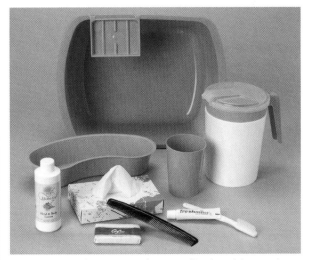

Fig. 9-4. An admission pack is usually placed in a resident's room before he or she is admitted. It may contain personal care items that the resident will need. (REPRINTED WITH PERMISSION OF BRIGGS CORPORATION, 800-247-2343, WWW.BRIGGSCORP.COM)

- A stethoscope and a sphygmomanometer (used to measure blood pressure; you will learn about this in Chapter 13) (Fig. 9-5).

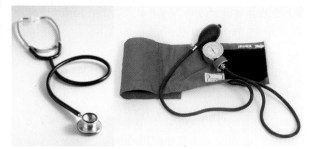

Fig. 9-5. a) A stethoscope and b) one type of sphygmomanometer.

- A thermometer
- A facility gown or pajamas, depending upon the resident

G Prepare the resident's room before the resident arrives to help make him feel welcome. Know the resident's condition. Know if he or she is bed-bound or is able to walk.

G Prepare the bed according to the nurse's instructions. Open the curtains or blinds.

G If a roommate is in the room, notify him or her of the new resident's arrival.

G When the resident arrives, introduce yourself. State your position. Call the person by his formal name until he tells you what he wants to be called.

G Do not rush the process or the resident. He should not feel as if he is an inconvenience. Make sure that he feels welcome and wanted.

G Introduce the new resident to his roommate and other residents in the rooms on either side and across the hall. This helps the resident feel more comfortable. It may also help the family feel better.

G Explain day-to-day life in the facility. Offer to take him and his family on a facility tour. Show them the dining room, chapel, and all other important areas, such as the activity room. If available, show them activity schedules. Point out information about menus. During the tour, introduce residents to all staff and residents you see (Fig. 9-6).

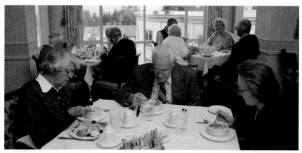

Fig. 9-6. Take new residents on a tour of the facility and introduce them to all residents and staff you see.

G Show the resident how to work the bed controls.

G Make sure the call light is close to the bed. Show the resident how to work the call light and explain its use.

G Explain how to work the television and the telephone.

G Handle all of the resident's personal items with care and respect. These are the items he has chosen to bring with him to the facility. Treat them carefully. Help the resident unpack everything. Ask him where he wants the items placed and how he would like the room set up (Fig. 9-7).

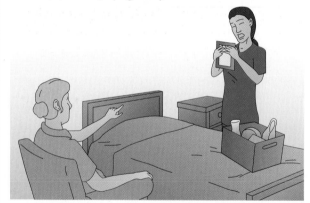

Fig. 9-7. Handle a resident's personal items carefully. Set up the room according to her preference.

Admitting a resident

Equipment: may include admission paperwork (checklist and inventory form), gloves, and vital signs equipment

1. Identify yourself by name. Identify the resident. Greet the resident by name.

2. Wash your hands.

3. Explain procedure to the resident. Speak clearly, slowly, and directly. Maintain face-to-face contact whenever possible.

4. Provide for the resident's privacy with a curtain, screen, or door. Ask the family to step outside until the initial admission process is complete. Show them where they may wait and let them know approximately how long they will have to wait. Tell them where they can get refreshments.

5. If instructed, do these things:

   Take the resident's height, weight, and vital signs. (Height and weight procedures follow; vitals signs are in Chapter 13.) Most facilities require baseline height, weight, and vital sign measurements. **Baseline** signs are initial values that can be compared to future measurements. Document on admission form and elsewhere per facility policy.

   Obtain a urine specimen if required (see Chapter 16).

   Complete the paperwork. Take an inventory of all of the personal items. Help the resident put personal items away. Label each item if it is facility policy. If the resident has valuables, ask the nurse for instructions.

   Fill the water pitcher with fresh water. Add ice if requested.

6. When the initial portion of the admission is complete, locate the family and let them know they may return to the resident's room.

7. Show the resident the room and bathroom. Explain how to work the bed controls and the call light. Point out the lights, telephone, and television and how to work them. Give the resident information on menus, dining times, and activity schedules.

8. Introduce the resident to his roommate, if there is one. Introduce other residents and staff.

9. Make resident comfortable. Remove privacy measures.

10. Leave call light within resident's reach.

11. Wash your hands.

12. Be courteous and respectful at all times. Let the resident know when you are leaving. Ask if he needs anything else.

13. Document procedure using facility guidelines.

Residents' weight and height will be checked when they are admitted. Nursing assistants also check weight as part of regular care. Height is usually not checked as often as weight. Report weight loss or gain, no matter how small, promptly to the nurse. Changes in a resident's weight can be a sign of illness.

Weight will be measured using **pounds** or kilograms. **Kilograms** are units of **metric** measurement. Bedridden residents will need to be weighed, too. Being **bedridden** means that residents are unable to get out of bed.

Measuring and recording weight of an ambulatory resident

Equipment: standing/upright scale, pen and paper to record your findings

1. Identify yourself by name. Identify the resident. Greet the resident by name.

2. Wash your hands.

3. Explain procedure to the resident. Speak clearly, slowly, and directly. Maintain face-to-face contact whenever possible.

4. Provide for the resident's privacy with a curtain, screen, or door.

5. Make sure resident is wearing non-skid shoes before walking to scale.

6. Start with the scale balanced at zero. If you do not know how to balance the scale, ask the nurse.

7. Help the resident step onto the center of the scale, facing the scale. Once on the scale, his arms must hang free.

8. Determine resident's weight. This is done by balancing the scale by making the balance bar level. Move the small and large weight indicators until the bar balances. Read the two numbers shown (on the small and large weight indicators) when the bar is balanced. Add these two numbers together. This is the resident's weight (Fig. 9-8).

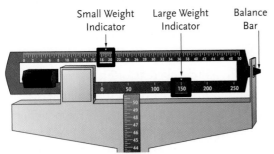

Small Weight Indicator   Large Weight Indicator   Balance Bar

Fig. 9-8. *Move the small and large weight indicators until the bar balances. The weight shown in the illustration is 169 pounds.*

9. Help the resident off the scale before recording weight.

10. Record the resident's weight.

11. Remove privacy measures.

12. Leave call light within resident's reach.

13. Wash your hands.

14. Be courteous and respectful at all times.

15. Report any changes in the resident to the nurse. Document procedure using facility guidelines.

When residents are not able to get out of wheelchairs easily, they are weighed using a special wheelchair scale. With this scale, wheelchairs are rolled directly onto the scale (Fig. 9-9). With some wheelchair scales, you will need to subtract the weight of the wheelchair from the resident's weight. If the weight of the wheelchair is not listed on the chair, weigh the empty wheelchair first. Then subtract the wheelchair's

weight from the total. Some scales automatically adjust for the wheelchair's weight.

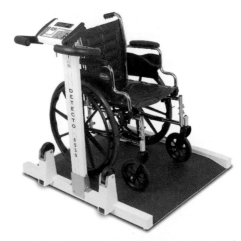

Fig. 9-9. *Wheelchairs can be rolled directly onto wheelchair scales to determine weight.* (PHOTO COURTESY OF DETECTO, WWW.DETECTO.COM, 800-641-2008)

When residents cannot get out of bed, they are weighed on special bed scales (Fig. 9-10). Before using a bed scale, know how it works and how to use it properly and safely. Follow your facility's procedure and any manufacturer's instructions. This is a general procedure for weighing someone on a bed scale.

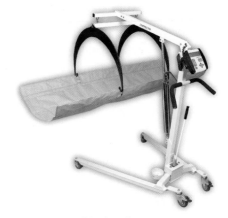

Fig. 9-10. *A type of bed scale.* (PHOTO COURTESY OF DETECTO, WWW.DETECTO.COM, 800-641-2008)

Measuring and recording weight of a bedridden resident

Equipment: scale, pen and paper to record findings

Have another co-worker assist you.

1. Identify yourself by name. Identify the resident. Greet the resident by name.

2. Wash your hands.

3. Explain procedure to the resident. Speak clearly, slowly, and directly. Maintain face-to-face contact whenever possible.

4. Provide for the resident's privacy with a curtain, screen, or door.

5. Adjust the bed to a safe level, usually waist high. Lock the bed wheels.

6. Start with the scale balanced at zero. If you do not know how to balance the scale, ask the nurse.

7. Examine the sling, straps, chains, and/or pad for any damage. Do not use the scale if you find damage.

8. Turn linen down so that it is off the resident.

9. Turn resident to one side away from you (Chapter 11) or if flat pad scale is used, slide resident onto pad using a helper. If a sling is used, remove from the scale and place underneath the resident without wrinkling it.

10. When using a sling, turn the resident back on his back and straighten sling.

11. Attach the sling to the scale or, if using a flat pad scale, position resident securely on the pad.

12. Check the straps or other connectors, and raise the sling or the pad until the resident is clear of the bed. With some scales, you can keep the resident directly over the bed while weighing him. With others, you have to move the scale away from the bed. Secure the resident before moving the scale.

13. For digital scales, turn them on and note reading. With other scales, move the weights until you get a reading. Note the weight.

14. Lower the resident back down on the bed. If using a sling, turn resident to both sides to remove the sling. If using a pad scale, carefully slide the resident back onto the bed.

15. Record the resident's weight.

16. Make resident comfortable. Replace bed linens.

17. Return bed to lowest position. Remove privacy measures.

18. Leave call light within resident's reach.

19. Wash your hands.

20. Be courteous and respectful at all times.

21. Report any changes in the resident to the nurse. Document procedure using facility guidelines.

For measuring height, the rod measures in inches and fractions of inches. Record the total number of inches. If you have to change inches into feet, remember that there are 12 inches in a foot, and 60 inches equal five feet.

Measuring and recording height of an ambulatory resident

Equipment: standing/upright scale, pen and paper to record your findings

1. Identify yourself by name. Identify the resident. Greet the resident by name.

2. Wash your hands.

3. Explain procedure to the resident. Speak clearly, slowly, and directly. Maintain face-to-face contact whenever possible.

4. Provide for the resident's privacy with a curtain, screen, or door.

5. Help the resident to step onto scale, facing away from the scale.

6. Ask the resident to stand straight, if possible. Help as needed.

7. Pull up measuring rod from back of scale. Gently lower measuring rod until it rests flat on the resident's head (Fig. 9-11).

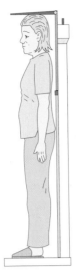

Fig. 9-11. *To determine height on a standing scale, gently lower measuring rod until it rests flat on resident's head.*

8.   Determine resident's height.

9.   Help the resident off scale before recording height. Make sure measuring rod does not hit resident in the head while helping resident off the scale.

10. Record height.

11. Remove privacy measures.

12. Leave call light within resident's reach.

13. Wash your hands.

14. Be courteous and respectful at all times.

15. Report any changes in the resident to the nurse. Document procedure using facility guidelines.

Measuring and recording height of a bedridden resident

Equipment: measuring tape (Fig. 9-12), pencil, pen and paper to record your findings

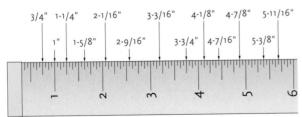

Fig. 9-12. *A tape measure.*

1.   Identify yourself by name. Identify the resident. Greet the resident by name.

2.   Wash your hands.

3.   Explain procedure to the resident. Speak clearly, slowly, and directly. Maintain face-to-face contact whenever possible.

4.   Provide for the resident's privacy with a curtain, screen, or door.

5.   Adjust the bed to a safe level, usually waist high. Lock the bed wheels.

6.   Turn linen down so it is off the resident.

7.   Position resident lying straight in the supine (back) position. Be sure the bed sheet is smooth underneath the resident.

8.   Using a pencil, make a small mark on the bottom sheet at the top of the resident's head.

9.   Make another pencil mark at the resident's heel (Fig. 9-13).

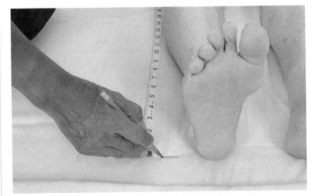

Fig. 9-13. *Make marks on the sheet at the resident's head and heel.*

10. Using the tape measure, measure the area between the pencil marks. This is the resident's height.

11. Record the resident's height.

12. Make resident comfortable. Replace bed linen.

13. Return bed to lowest position. Remove privacy measures.

14. Leave call light within resident's reach.

15. Wash your hands.

16. Be courteous and respectful at all times.

17. Report any changes in the resident to the nurse. Document procedure using facility guidelines.

Some residents cannot lie straight due to contractures. A **contracture** is the permanent and often painful shortening of a muscle. Some facilities require that a tape measure be used to follow the curves of the spine and legs. The number of inches is totaled and recorded. This is the least accurate way of measuring height.

Another method used on residents with contractures is called the demi-span. Using this method, you measure the distance from the middle of the top of the chest, called the sternal notch, to the tip of the middle finger. Ideally, the left arm is used. The arm is held up straight out from the shoulder. Once this measurement is obtained, a calculation is done for females and males. The final height is recorded in centimeters. You will receive special training if you are required to use this procedure.

Abdominal girth is a measurement of the circumference around the abdomen at the umbilicus (navel). This measurement is required for some residents and may need to be included on an admission checklist form.

Measuring abdominal girth

Equipment: measuring tape, pen and paper to record your findings

1. Identify yourself by name. Identify the resident. Greet the resident by name.

2. Wash your hands.

3. Explain procedure to the resident. Speak clearly, slowly, and directly. Maintain face-to-face contact whenever possible.

4. Provide for the resident's privacy with a curtain, screen, or door.

5. Adjust the bed to a safe level, usually waist high. Lock the bed wheels.

6. Position resident lying straight in the supine (back) position.

7. Turn linen down and raise gown or top enough to expose only the abdomen. Keep all areas covered that do not need to be exposed. Promote resident's right to dignity and privacy.

8. Gently wrap measuring tape around the resident's abdomen at the level of the navel.

9. Read the number where the ends of the tape meet (Fig. 9-14).

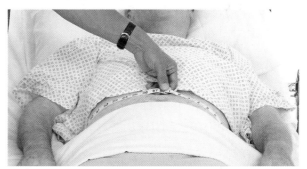

Fig. 9-14. *After wrapping the measuring tape around the resident's abdomen, read the number where the ends of the tape meet.*

10. Carefully remove the tape measure. Record abdominal girth measurement.

11. Make resident comfortable. Replace clothing and bed linen.

12. Return bed to lowest position. Remove privacy measures.

13. Leave call light within resident's reach.

14. Wash your hands.

15. Be courteous and respectful at all times.

16. Report any changes in the resident to the nurse. Document procedure using facility guidelines.

5. Explain the nursing assistant's role during an in-house transfer of a resident

Residents may be transferred to another room within a facility. Residents may need to be transferred to a different unit that offers more skilled care. Whatever the reason for the transfer, it may be a difficult time for the resident. Change is always hard, but this is especially true if the resident has an illness or his condition has worsened. Nursing assistants should try to make the transfer as smooth as possible for residents.

Notifying residents as soon as possible of the transfer can help lessen the stress. Explain all the details you know, including where, when, and why the transfer is happening. Refer any questions to the nurse. Residents have the right to be notified of any room or roommate change.

Nursing assistants are usually responsible for packing all of the resident's belongings. Packing all of the items may take some time. Pack personal items carefully so that nothing breaks, is damaged, or is lost.

The resident may be transferred in a bed, in a stretcher, or in a wheelchair. Find out the method of transfer from the nurse so that you can plan the move.

When you arrive at the new unit, introduce the resident to everyone. If you unpack the resident's belongings, do it carefully. Try to re-create the way the belongings were set up in the former room. It is a good idea to check on the resident later in the day to make sure he is settled. After that, it is nice to stop in sometimes to say hello. This helps the resident feel that staff members care about him.

When you leave the resident's room, report to the nurse in charge of that resident. At that point, you will have formally transferred responsibility to the new unit.

Transferring a resident

Equipment: may include wheelchair or stretcher, cart for belongings, all of the resident's personal care items

1. Identify yourself by name. Identify the resident. Greet the resident by name.

2. Wash your hands.

3. Explain procedure to the resident. Speak clearly, slowly, and directly. Maintain face-to-face contact whenever possible.

4. Provide for the resident's privacy with a curtain, screen, or door.

5. Collect the items to be moved onto the cart, and ask another staff member to help take them to the new location.

6. Lock wheelchair or stretcher wheels. Help the resident into the wheelchair or onto the stretcher. Take him or her to the new area.

7. Introduce the resident to the new residents and staff.

8. Lock wheelchair or stretcher wheels. Transfer the resident to the new bed, if needed.

9. Unpack all belongings. Help the resident to put personal items away.

10. Make resident comfortable. Remove privacy measures.

11. Leave call light within resident's reach.

12. Wash your hands.

13. Be courteous and respectful at all times.

14. Report any changes in the resident to the nurse. Document procedure using facility guidelines.

6. Explain the nursing assistant's role in the discharge of a resident

A discharge is official after the doctor writes the discharge order that releases the resident to leave the facility to go home or to another facility. The nurse will then complete instructions for the resident to follow after discharge. These instructions may include future doctor appointments, medications, ambulation instructions, and special dietary requirements (Fig. 9-15). They may also contain special exercises for the resident to do and community resources for the resident.

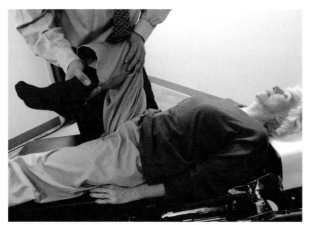

Fig. 9-15. *After a resident is discharged, she may continue to receive physical therapy and have other medical appointments.*

Your responsibility is to collect the resident's belongings and to pack them carefully. You may need to ask a nurse to obtain valuables from a secure area. Check each item against the inventory list done at admission. This helps make sure everything is included.

A resident who is going home may be happy, although he may be unsure if he is ready for this important change. Be positive and reassuring. If he has additional questions, inform the nurse.

Know the resident's condition and whether or not he will need a wheelchair or stretcher for discharge. You are responsible for him until he is safely in the vehicle. Stay with the resident until he and his belongings are in the vehicle. Residents have the right to a safe and secure discharge. Your responsibility does not end until the doors of the vehicle are closed.

Discharging a resident

Equipment: may include a wheelchair or stretcher, cart for belongings, the discharge paperwork, including the inventory list done on admission, all of the resident's personal care items

1. Identify yourself by name. Identify the resident. Greet the resident by name.

2. Wash your hands.

3. Explain procedure to the resident. Speak clearly, slowly, and directly. Maintain face-to-face contact whenever possible.

4. Provide for the resident's privacy with a curtain, screen, or door.

5. Compare the inventory list to the items being packed. Ask the resident to sign if all items are there.

6. Carefully put the items to be taken onto the cart, and ask another staff member to help transport items to the pick-up area.

7. Help the resident dress in clothing of his choice. Make sure the nurse has removed all dressings, IVs and tubes that need to be removed prior to discharge.

8. Lock wheelchair or stretcher wheels. Help him safely into the wheelchair or onto the stretcher (Chapter 11).

9. Help the resident say his goodbyes to other residents and the staff.

10. Take him to the pick-up area. Lock wheelchair or stretcher wheels. Help the resident into the vehicle. Transfer personal items into the vehicle.

11. Say goodbye to the resident. You are responsible for the resident until he or she is safely in the vehicle and the door is closed.

12. Wash your hands.

13. Document procedure using facility guidelines.

7. Describe the nursing assistant's role during physical exams

Some residents need a physical exam when arriving at a facility. Others need a physical exam after they have been there for a while. Know your role during a physical exam so the process runs smoothly. Doctors or nurses will do part or all of the exam. Nursing assistants may be asked to help.

You can help residents with their emotional needs by being there for them. Exams can make people anxious. They may fear what the examiner will do or what he or she will find. Exams can cause discomfort and embarrassment. Help residents by listening to them, talking to them, or even holding their hands.

Nursing assistants are often responsible for gathering equipment for the nurse or doctor. The equipment you might collect includes:

- Sphygmomanometer (for blood pressure)
- Stethoscope
- Alcohol wipes
- Flashlight
- Thermometer
- Tongue depressor
- Eye chart for vision screening
- Tuning fork (tests hearing with vibrations)
- Reflex hammer (taps body parts to test reflexes)
- Otoscope (lighted instrument that examines the outer ear and eardrum)
- Ophthalmoscope (lighted instrument that examines the eye)
- Specimen containers
- Lubricant
- Hemoccult® card (tests for blood in stool)
- Vaginal speculum for females (opens the vagina so that it and the cervix can be examined)
- Gloves
- Drape

During the exam, the nursing assistant will place the resident in the correct position and stay with the resident as needed. The NA may help drape the resident for privacy and comfort. Expose only the body part being examined.

Some positions are embarrassing and uncomfortable. You can help by explaining why the position is needed. Explain how long the resident can expect to stay in the position.

Common positions used during physical exams include the following:

- The **dorsal recumbent** position is used to examine the breasts, chest, abdomen, and perineal area. A person in this position is flat on her back. The knees are flexed and feet are flat on the bed. The drape is put over the resident, covering her body. Her head remains uncovered (Fig. 9-16).

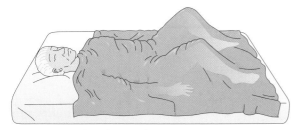

Fig. 9-16. *The dorsal recumbent position.*

- The **lithotomy** position is used to examine the vagina. The resident lies on her back and her hips are brought to the edge of the exam table. Her legs are flexed and her feet are in padded stirrups. The drape is put over the resident, covering her body. Her head remains uncovered. The drape is also brought down to cover the perineal area (Fig. 9-17).

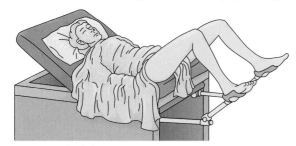

Fig. 9-17. *The lithotomy position.*

- The **knee-chest** position may be used to examine the rectum or the vagina. A resident in the knee-chest position is lying on his or her abdomen. The knees are pulled towards the abdomen and legs are separated. Arms are pulled up and flexed. The head is turned to one side. In the knee-chest position, the resident will be wearing a gown and possibly socks. The drape should be applied in a diamond shape to cover the back, buttocks and thighs (Fig. 9-18).

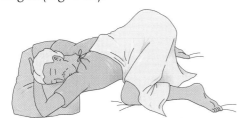

Fig. 9-18. *The knee-chest position.*

More information on different body positions is in Chapter 11.

In addition to helping with equipment, positioning and draping, the nursing assistant should:

- Wash her hands before and after the exam.
- Provide other privacy measures throughout the exam, such as closing the privacy screen or curtain and closing the door. Let the resident know that he or she will not be exposed more than necessary during the exam.
- Provide enough light for the doctor or nurse.
- Ask the resident to urinate before the exam. Collect any urine needed for a specimen at this time. Gather and label specimens as needed.
- Listen to the resident throughout the exam. Try to help him or her remain calm.
- Follow any of the doctor's or nurse's instructions.
- Make sure the resident does not fall.
- Put instruments in the proper place for the doctor or nurse. Hand instruments to the doctor or nurse as needed.
- Follow Standard Precautions.

After the exam, help the resident clean up and get dressed. Help the resident safely back to his or her room. Dispose of any trash and disposable equipment in the exam area. Bring all reusable equipment to the proper cleaning room. Clean and store reusable equipment according to facility policy. Label and bring any specimens to the proper place so that they can go to the lab.

Residents' Rights

Knock first, and then wait for permission to enter.

At some point in your life, you may have had a healthcare provider knock on the door to an examination room and not wait to hear you say "come in." That might have made you uncomfortable. When a resident is in an examination room, not waiting for permission to enter may expose him not only to you, but also to people walking through the hallway. Respect your residents' rights to privacy and dignity. Knock and wait to hear "come in" before you enter an examination room.

Chapter Review

1. Name ten factors families may consider when choosing a facility (LO 2).

2. Why is moving into a facility a big emotional adjustment for new residents (LO 3)?

3. Name seven ways nursing assistants can help new residents adjust to a facility (LO 3).

4. Why is it a good idea for nursing assistants to ask family members questions about residents upon admission (LO 4)?

5. Why do you think it is important to introduce new residents to all other staff and residents in the area during admission (LO 4)?

6. What should the scale be balanced at before measuring a resident's weight (LO 4)?

7. Why might a transfer be difficult for a resident (LO 5)?

8. During discharge of a resident, when does a nursing assistant's responsibility for the resident end (LO 6)?

9. List and describe three common positions used during physical exams (LO 7).

10. How can a nursing assistant provide privacy for a resident during an exam (LO 7)?

11. List ten examples of equipment nursing assistants may collect for physical exams (LO 7).

10 Bedmaking and Unit Care

Alcmaeon: One Theory About the Nature of Sleep

In the 6th century, medicine was taught in places where teachers, students, and philosophers gathered together. Crotona was one of these places, or "medical schools." Crotona was in Sicily, south of Italy. Alcmaeon was one of the teachers at the Crotona school. He believed that harmony in the body maintained health, and that disease was caused by a change in the body's harmony. He also had interesting ideas about sleep. He thought that sleep was something that occurred when the blood vessels in the brain were filled. When the blood drained out of the brain, the person would awaken.

"Oh it's nice to get up in the mornin'/But it's nicer to lie in bed."

Sir Harry Lauder, 1870-1950

"Egyptian Proverb:
The worst things:
To be in bed and sleep not
To want for one who comes not
To try to please and please not."

F. Scott Fitzgerald, 1896-1940

1. Define important words in this chapter

biorhythms: natural rhythms or cycles related to bodily functions.

circadian rhythm: the 24-hour day-night cycle.

closed bed: bed completely made with the bedspread and blankets in place.

depressant: a substance that causes calmness and drowsiness.

disposable: only to be used once and then discarded.

draw sheet: an extra sheet placed on top of the bottom sheet; used for moving residents.

incontinence: the inability to control the bladder or bowels, which leads to an involuntary loss of urine or feces.

insomnia: the inability to fall asleep or remain asleep.

occupied bed: a bed made while the person is in the bed.

open bed: bed made with linen folded down to the foot of the bed.

parasomnias: sleep disorders.

sleep: natural period of rest for the mind and body during which energy is restored.

stimulant: a drug that increases or quickens actions of the body.

surgical bed: bed made so that a person can easily move onto it from a stretcher.

unoccupied bed: a bed made while no person is in the bed.

2. Discuss the importance of sleep

Sleep is a natural period of rest for the mind and body during which energy is restored. Sleep and rest are two basic needs, as described in Chapter 5. The human body cannot survive long without sleep. Sleep is needed to replace old cells with new ones and provide new energy to organs. Sleep is vital to proper physical and mental development. Deep sleep helps the body to renew.

The study of the rhythms of the body is called biorhythmology. **Biorhythms** are the natural rhythms or cycles related to body functions that occur due to daily, monthly or yearly changes. Light and darkness, gravity, and temperature changes are examples of changes that can affect living organisms.

The most famous biorhythm is the circadian rhythm. The **circadian rhythm** is the 24-hour day-night cycle. It usually appears in infants when they are about three weeks old. The circadian rhythm can affect the body in many ways. In addition to sleep patterns, other changes in the body can occur during the 24-hour cycle. These include variations in blood pressure and body temperature.

Tip

Sleep cycles in your genes?

Have you ever wondered why two children in the same family have different sleep cycles? During non-school times, one child wakes up early in the morning and falls asleep at 10:00 p.m., while the other wakes up after noon and stays up well past midnight. The early riser is often called a "lark," and the person who stays up late is called an "owl." These are common terms given to people who have different body clocks, or circadian rhythms. Some believe that this is due to genetics—that sleep cycles are in our genes.

3. Describe types of sleep disorders

The inability to fall asleep or to remain asleep is called **insomnia**. A person may have difficulty falling asleep, may not stay asleep through the night, or may wake up too early in the morning. There are many different causes of insomnia. Some of the reasons that people develop sleep disorders, or **parasomnias**, are illness, anxiety, fear, stress, medications, trouble breathing, noise, hunger or thirst. Some common sleep disorders are described in the following box:

Parasomnias

Somnambulism is sleepwalking. With this sleep disorder, the person performs activities that people normally perform while awake. In most cases, the episodes do not result in injury.

Sleeptalking is talking during sleep. This usually occurs without the person being aware of what he is saying, or even that he was talking. Episodes are usually brief and do not occur often.

Bruxism is grinding and clenching the teeth. It can cause headaches, jaw problems and pain, neck aches, and can loosen teeth.

REM sleep behavior disorder is talking, often along with violent movements, during REM (dreaming) sleep. The person may be acting out his dreams. This disorder is more common among elderly people who have illnesses affecting the nervous system, such as Parkinson's or Alzheimer's disease. (See Chapter 22.)

4. Identify factors affecting sleep

Many elderly people, especially those living away from their homes, have sleep problems (Fig. 10-1). Many factors can affect residents' sleep. The more you pay attention to these factors and try to improve conditions, the better residents will sleep.

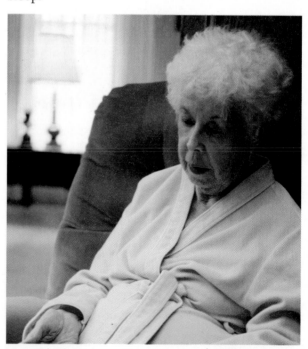

Fig. 10-1. *Living away from home can interfere with quality sleep.*

Factors affecting residents' sleep include:

Environment: Residents may have been used to sleeping with a mate or alone when they lived at home. Adjusting to a new place and a roommate is very difficult. Even if married residents are in the same room at a facility, sleep can be difficult because they are no longer in their home. Ways to help with environmental issues include:

- Listen to residents if they wish to talk. Be compassionate and reassuring.

- Have enough pillows and blankets.

- Make sure mattresses fit properly and are not damaged or lumpy. If a mattress does not fit properly, report it to the nurse or proper department.

Noise level and/or lighting can affect a resident's ability to sleep. Keeping the room dark is very important to some residents. Other residents prefer to sleep with a light or a night-light on. Ways to help address noise level and/or lighting include:

- Keep the noise level low, especially during shift changes, which are often noisy times. Closing doors at night may help.

- Keep your voice low.

- Do not bang equipment or meal trays.

- Use blinds or shades to help darken a room for sleep. Keep light controls within residents' reach.

Problems with odors and inadequate ventilation can cause a person to have difficulty sleeping. Residents may be **incontinent** (unable to control the bladder or bowels, which leads to an involuntary loss of urine or feces) which can cause odors. Vomit and wound drainage can cause odors. Certain diseases cause odors as well. Body odors can be offensive, too. Ways to help with odors and ventilation include:

- Change incontinent briefs often.

- Keep equipment and supplies clean.

- Give personal care often to help avoid breath and body odors.

- Change soiled bed linens and clothing as soon as possible.

- Open a window to help eliminate odors.

- Housekeeping may have a spray deodorizer available for persistent odors.

Temperature problems can affect sleep. Some people will want the room to be cooler; others like a warmer temperature for sleep. This may be due to normal changes of aging or just personal preference. Ways to help with temperature include:

- Help find a comfortable temperature for residents.

- Report to the nurse if the temperature is a problem.

- Layer clothing and bed covers for warmth.

Anxiety: The resident may be anxious about sleeping alone in a private room. He may have anxiety about sleeping in a new environment with a roommate. He may be worried about illness and a decline in independence. If the resident has lost a mate and/or friends and family, he may be sad. Ways to help with anxiety include:

- Sit with residents and listen if they want to talk. Visits from family, friends, or clergy may also help.

- Use touch and soothing words.

- Offer to give a back rub.

- Report to the nurse if a resident is anxious. If anxiety is prolonged, the resident may benefit from talking with a mental health professional.

Illness: Some illnesses or diseases cause chronic or occasional pain and discomfort. For example, arthritis can cause chronic pain in different areas of the body. Arthritis is a disease that refers to inflammation, or swelling, of the joints. It causes stiffness, pain, and decreased mobility.

Ways to help with illness, pain, and discomfort include:

- Make sure residents are clean and comfortable before bed.

- Observe and report signs of pain promptly to the nurse. The nurse may give the resident medication or you may be asked to help by giving a back rub or a bath. Signs of pain and measures to reduce pain are found in Chapter 13.

Aging changes: Sleep patterns are different for elderly people than for younger people. They may sleep a similar number of hours, but those hours may be spread out over the 24-hour day. The elderly may take frequent naps during the day, which affects sleep at night. They take longer to fall asleep. Elderly people may get up more often during the night to go the bathroom and have a hard time falling asleep again. Hormonal changes can cause difficulty sleeping. A lack of regular, moderate exercise affects sleep as well. Ways to help with aging changes include:

- Assist residents to the bathroom just before bedtime.

- Honor fluid restrictions in the evening, if they are ordered.

- Use music or reading to help the resident fall asleep.

- Provide naps as needed throughout the day.

- Encourage residents to exercise, if it is in their care plan. Exercise often helps people sleep longer and more soundly.

- Encourage residents to wear day wear instead of night clothes during the day.

Dietary habits: Drinking or eating products with caffeine, such as soda or chocolate, can prevent sleep (Fig. 10-2). Eating heavy meals before bedtime can cause restlessness or discomfort. Sugar can cause a person to be excited and anxious. This can make it harder to fall asleep or can cause wakefulness during the night. Ways to help with dietary habits include:

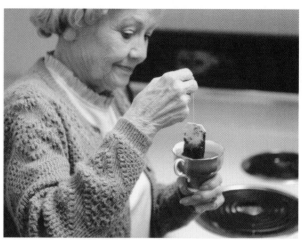

Fig. 10-2. *Caffeinated drinks, such as coffee or some teas, can prevent sleep.*

- Limit caffeine intake. Offer herbal teas or warm milk instead.

- Avoid serving heavy meals before bedtime. Serve meals earlier in the evening, not late at night.

Medications, alcohol, and cigarettes: Some medications cause wakefulness and interfere with sleep. For example, antihistamines can either cause a person to become very sleepy or to be unable to fall asleep. Antihistamines are medications used to treat allergic reactions or allergies. Alcoholic drinks, including beer and wine, are depressants and can cause problems with sleep (Fig. 10-3). A **depressant** is a substance that causes calmness and drowsiness. Smoking can also cause problems with sleeping. Nicotine, which is found in cigarettes, is a stimulant. A **stimulant** is a drug that increases or quickens actions of the body. Ways to help with medications, alcohol, and cigarettes include:

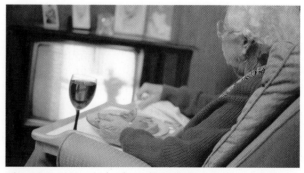

Fig. 10-3. *Wine and other alcoholic beverages can prevent a person from sleeping well.*

- Report if residents are not taking medications ordered for sleep.

- Report any evidence of unusual sleepiness or sudden inability to fall asleep.

- Discourage smoking and drinking alcohol before bedtime.

Not sleeping well can cause many problems, such as decreased mental function, reduced reaction time, decreased immune system function, and irritability. It is important to observe and report residents' complaints of lack of sleep.

A care conference may be planned to correct a resident's sleeping problems. Family members may participate. The nurse or doctor will assess the resident's medications to see if they are affecting sleep. Offer any suggestions you have to help improve a resident's ability to sleep.

5. Describe a standard resident unit and equipment

Residents' units are their living spaces. They contain their beds, other furniture and personal items. These units must be kept clean and neat, while also honoring residents' personal choices. As you learned earlier, this room is the resident's home. You must always knock and wait for permission before entering.

Residents' belongings are very important to them. Treat their personal items with respect. Once personal items are in place within a room or unit, do not move them without the resident's permission. If a safety hazard exists, inform the nurse, and let him or her handle the situation.

Each unit may have slightly different equipment, because residents may bring furniture or other belongings from home. Personal items that bring the resident happiness should be encouraged. Resident rooms should be personal and home-like.

Standard unit equipment includes the following:

- Bed
- Bedside stand and possibly a dresser
- Overbed table
- Chair
- Bath basin
- Emesis basin
- Bedpan
- Urinal for males
- Water pitcher and cup
- Privacy screen or curtain
- Call light

The bedside stand is used for storing equipment like emesis basins, bath basins, urinals, and bedpans. Facility policy may require these items to be placed in plastic bags to promote infection prevention. Soap, toothbrushes, toothpaste, combs and brushes, and other items may also be placed in the bedside stand but have to be kept separate from basins, urinals, and bedpans. Personal articles are usually kept in the top drawer. Basins are generally placed on the top shelf, and bedpans and urinals are on the lower shelf in the section underneath. A telephone and/or a radio, along with other personal items, may be placed on the top of the stand.

The overbed table may be used for residents' meals or personal care. It is a clean area and must be kept clean and free of clutter. Bedpans, urinals and soiled linen should not be placed on overbed tables because these tables are used for food (Fig. 10-4). Right before mealtime, clear these tables so that the meal tray may slide smoothly onto it. A water pitcher and cup are routinely kept on the overbed table.

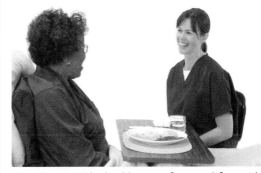

Fig. 10-4. *Overbed tables are often used for residents' meals; they must be kept clean. Do not place bedpans, urinals, or soiled linens on overbed tables.*

Residents' Rights

Making fun is *not* funny!

Making fun of any resident's personal items is inappropriate and cruel. Treat residents' belongings with respect.

6. Explain how to clean a resident unit and equipment

General care of the unit must be done whenever needed throughout the day. You should clean up spills promptly. Bedpans and urinals must be emptied and cleaned immediately after use. Bed linens should be straightened before leaving the resident's room.

You will be taught how to use many different types of equipment. Make sure that you use and care for equipment properly. This prevents infection and injury.

There are many types of equipment that will be used one time and then discarded. This is called **disposable** equipment. Some types of disposable equipment are cups, tissues, gloves, paper gowns, masks, disposable razors, and pads. Disposable equipment prevents the spread of microorganisms. Dispose of this equipment in the proper container. Wear gloves when using or disposing of some types of equipment, such as razors and pads.

Some equipment, such as urinals and bedpans, is cleaned after each use. You must wear gloves when handling this equipment. You may need to clean and disinfect this equipment, or place it in the proper area for cleaning. Follow facility policy.

If equipment is to be re-used, it may need to be sterilized in the autoclave. Follow facility policy for this type of equipment. Do not use a piece of reusable equipment on another resident if it has not been properly sterilized.

Guidelines: Resident's Unit

G   Keep residents' units neat and clean. Clean the overbed table after use. Use a paper towel or cloth and facility-approved cleaning fluid. When cleaning, move the damp paper towel or cloth away from you to avoid wiping dirt or dust onto your uniform. Place the table within the resident's reach before leaving.

G   Keep the call light within the resident's reach (Fig. 10-5). Make sure it is within reach before you leave the room. Report to the nurse immediately if the call light is not working.

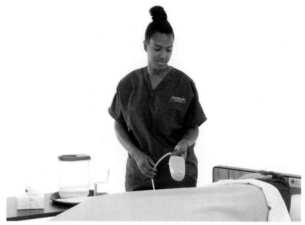

Fig. 10-5. *Always leave the call light within the resident's reach before you leave the room.*

G   Straighten bed linens and remove crumbs from the bed after meals and before leaving.

G   Restock all resident supplies daily, including facial tissues, bathroom tissue, paper towels, soap, or any other needed item. If this is not your responsibility, write out a supply order for the appropriate department.

G   If the bathroom needs to be cleaned, notify the housekeeping department. If the toilet, sink, or tub/shower are not working, report this promptly to the proper department.

G   Check equipment daily to make sure it is working properly and not damaged in any way. Cords may be frayed or cracked; TVs or radios may not work. Report these situations immediately to the proper department.

G   Refill water pitchers regularly unless resident has a fluid restriction. Promptly report to a nurse if a resident is not drinking fluids.

Bedmaking and Unit Care

G Remove anything that might cause odors or safety hazards, like trash, clutter, or spills. Dispose of any disposable supplies. Clean up spills promptly. If trash needs to be emptied, notify the housekeeping department. Discard any old or spoiled food you see.

G Report signs of insects or pests immediately.

G Leave residents' belongings where you find them. Do not throw away residents' personal items.

After providing care, leave the unit neat and tidy. Put away equipment after it has been properly cleaned and disinfected. Make sure the call light is within the resident's reach.

If you notice other equipment that is damaged, such as wheelchairs, IV poles, canes, crutches, or walkers, promptly report it. If you wait, a resident may become injured when using broken equipment.

Depending on the facility, nursing assistants may be responsible for more thorough unit cleaning. When a resident is transferred, discharged, or dies, the unit will have to be completely cleaned and disinfected. If this is your responsibility, you will need to use special heavy-duty gloves. Follow facility policy. General guidelines for doing this type of thorough unit cleaning are listed below:

Guidelines: Unit Cleaning After Transfer, Discharge, or Death

G Wash your hands before doing unit cleaning.

G Wear gloves and the proper PPE as required by your facility.

G Remove and dispose of equipment and supplies carefully. These may include oxygen tubing, suction canisters, tissue boxes, water pitchers, and cups. Also remove towels, washcloths, and equipment that will be sent for cleaning. If you find any of the resident's personal items, take them to the new unit, or inform the nurse so that they can be sent to the resident or the family.

G Raise the bed to a safe working level, and remove soiled linen. Roll dirty linens away from you, watching for personal items. Wash all surfaces of the bed, including both sides of the mattress, with the facility-approved disinfectant. Allow to dry completely. Remove gloves, wash your hands, and then make a neat, wrinkle-free bed. See Learning Objective 7 for more information on bedmaking guidelines and the procedures for making a bed.

G Make sure the area is well-ventilated when using strong cleaning solutions. Clean all other unit items and equipment following facility policy. These may include items such as the telephone, TV and bed controls, bedside stand, overbed table, chairs, bathrooms, windows and window sills, and door handles.

G Write repair orders for any damaged or broken furniture.

G Remove all PPE and wash your hands.

G Place new equipment and supplies in the room for a new resident.

Tip

Central Supply (CS) or Supply, Processing and Distribution (SPD)

The CS or SPD department is responsible for ordering, processing, and delivering equipment to units and other departments in a facility. Residents usually bring items from home; however, they may need additional items that CS can obtain. If you are responsible for ordering new supplies, you will be trained in the proper procedure.

7. Discuss types of beds and demonstrate proper bedmaking

The resident's bed is a place in which he or she will spend a great deal of time. Neat, well-made beds help residents sleep better each night. In addition, careful bedmaking prevents infection. A clean, neat, dry bed helps prevent skin breakdown and odors and promotes good health and overall comfort. Skin breakdown and pressure ulcers are serious problems for the elderly and are covered in detail in Chapter 18.

Many facilities have electric beds for residents. Electric beds can be raised at the head and knee area (Fig. 10-6). Some electric beds have a safety lock that helps prevent the resident or visitor from accidentally moving the bed up or down.

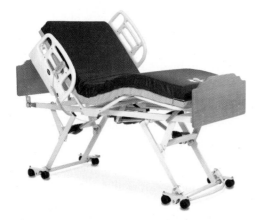

Fig. 10-6. *One type of electric bed.* (PHOTO COURTESY OF INVACARE CONTINUING CARE, 1-800-668-2337, WWW.INVACARE-CC.COM)

The controls on electric beds vary. Generally, a person controls the electric bed by pressing buttons on a control panel. There will be a button to move the entire bed, one for the head of the bed, and another for the bottom of the bed (Fig. 10-7). There may also be controls for the bed to move into special doctor-ordered positions. These controls should only be used by the nurses. Residents and families will be taught how to use the bed control on admission.

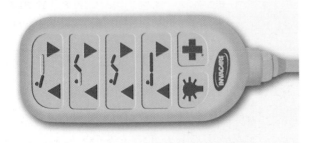

Fig. 10-7. *Controls for an electric bed.* (PHOTO COURTESY OF INVACARE CONTINUING CARE, 1-800-668-2337, WWW.INVACARE-CC.COM)

Beds can be equipped with a variety of functions. Some beds have built-in weight scales for weighing bedridden residents so that they do not have to be transferred to a scale.

Alternating pressure mattresses are used for residents who are at risk for pressure ulcers or who have pressure ulcers. They are able to alternate the pressure inside the mattress so that one area of the body does not rest on a spot for too long. This type of mattress helps prevent pressure ulcers.

There are special beds for residents who weigh more than the average person. These beds are called bariatric beds. They are for residents who weigh from 350 to 600 pounds. Special step stools help larger residents move from the bed to the floor. These stools are wider, longer and closer to the floor than standard step stools.

Beds should remain locked in their lowest positions whenever residents are in the beds. Special floor cushions or pads may be placed on the floor by the bed to protect residents if they should fall. If ordered by the doctor, special pads can also be placed along the length of the bed on both sides to prevent falls. These pads may be used with side rails.

Guidelines: Bedmaking

G   Bed linens must be changed when they are wet, soiled, or when they are too wrinkled for comfort. Residents can develop pressure ulcers when left in wet, wrinkled, or soiled linens. Make sure to remove and change disposable pads whenever they become soiled or wet (Fig. 10-8).

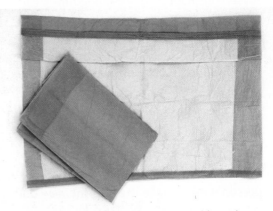

Fig. 10-8. *One type of absorbent disposable pad.*

G Before getting clean linen, wash your hands. Always use proper infection prevention procedures. Wear gloves when removing soiled linens.

G Gather linen in order of placement on the bed. This means first pick up mattress pad, then all sheets, blankets, bedspreads, and pillowcases.

G Carry clean linen away from your uniform. If it touches your uniform, the linen becomes contaminated (Fig. 10-9).

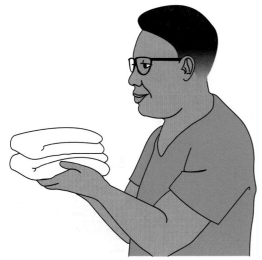

Fig. 10-9. *Carry clean linen away from your uniform.*

G Bring linen into one resident's room at a time. Put it down after flipping the stack of linen so that the first item to be placed on the bed (mattress pad) is now on the top of the stack.

G Never pick up linen from one room and transfer it to another room.

G Place clean linen on a facility-approved spot, such as a chair, overbed table, or bedside stand. Do not place clean linen on the floor or on a contaminated area.

G Use proper body mechanics when making beds. Bend your knees, use a good stance, and raise the bed height to a safe working level.

G Look at linens closely for any personal items, such as dentures, hearing aids and batteries,

glasses, rings, watches, and money, before removing them.

G Roll dirty linen away from you as you remove it from the bed. Rolling puts the dirtiest surface of the linen inward, which lessens contamination.

G Do not shake linen because it may spread airborne contaminants.

G Place used linen in proper container. Do not place used linen on the floor or on any piece of furniture in the room.

G To save energy, make one side of the bed first. Then go to the other side of the bed to complete bedmaking.

G Keep beds wrinkle-free and free of all crumbs. Remove lumps of any kind in the bed, such as from pads, etc. If a lumpy mattress cannot be smoothed out, inform the nurse. Lumps, crumbs, and wrinkles increase the risk of pressure ulcers.

G Wash your hands after handling linen.

Residents' Rights

Give prompt and compassionate care.

Some residents have episodes of incontinence while in bed. When a bed is wet or soiled, change the sheets, pads, and all clothing immediately. Be compassionate and respectful while doing this. Act professionally; this may help lessen embarrassment or discomfort. Do not draw attention to the resident or tell other residents what happened. Clean the resident and make him or her comfortable again. Leaving residents in soiled beds can cause skin breakdown and infection. It is also considered neglectful or abusive behavior.

There are four basic types of beds: closed, open, occupied, and surgical (also called postoperative, post-op, recovery, gurney, or stretcher bed). A **closed bed** is usually made for a resident who will be out of bed all day. It is a bed completely made with the bedspread, blankets, and pillows in place. A closed bed is turned into an **open bed** by folding the linen down to the foot of the bed. This makes it easier for a resident to get into the bed in the afternoon for a nap or at bedtime. You will also open a bed when a new resident has been assigned to that room.

Making a closed bed

Equipment: clean linen—mattress pad, fitted or flat bottom sheet, waterproof bed protector if needed, cotton **draw sheet**, *flat top sheet, blanket(s), bedspread (if used), pillowcase(s), gloves*

1. Wash your hands.

2. If resident is in the room, identify yourself by name. Identify the resident. Greet the resident by name.

3. Explain procedure to the resident. Speak clearly, slowly, and directly. Maintain face-to-face contact whenever possible.

4. Place clean linen on clean surface within reach (e.g., bedside stand, overbed table, or chair).

5. Adjust bed to safe working level, usually waist high. Put bed in flattest position. Lock bed wheels.

6. Put on gloves.

7. Loosen soiled linen and roll soiled linen (soiled side inside) from head to foot of bed. Avoid contact with your skin or clothes. Place it in a hamper or linen bag. Do not place on overbed table, chair, or floor.

8. Remove and discard gloves. Wash your hands.

9. Remake the bed. Place the mattress pad (if used) on the bed, attaching elastic at corners as necessary.

10. Place bottom sheet on bed without shaking linen. If using a flat sheet with seams, this sheet must be placed with the crease in the center of the mattress. The seams on both ends must be placed down. If using a fitted bottom sheet, place right-side up and tightly pull over all four corners of the bed.

11. Make hospital, or mitered, corners to keep bottom sheet wrinkle-free (Fig. 10-10).

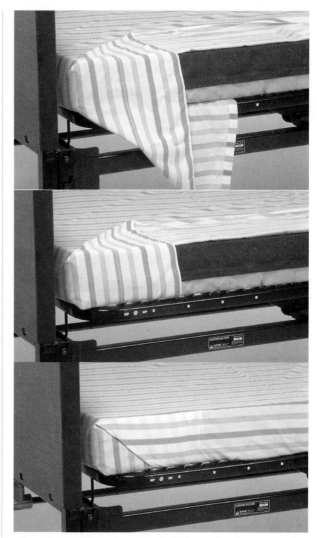

Fig. 10-10. *Hospital corners help keep the sheet smooth under the resident.*

12. Put on waterproof bed protector and then the draw sheet, if used. Place them in the center of the bed on the bottom sheet. Smooth, and tightly tuck the bottom sheet and draw sheet together under the sides of bed. Move from the head of the bed to the foot of the bed.

13. Place the top sheet over the bed and center it. The seam must be up.

14. Place blanket over the bed and center it.

15. Place the bedspread over the bed and center it.

16. Tuck top sheet and blanket under the foot of the bed and make hospital corners.

17. Fold down the top sheet to make a cuff of about six inches over the blanket.

18. Take a pillow, and with one hand, grasp the clean pillowcase at the closed end. Turn it inside out over your arm. Next, using the hand that has the pillowcase over it, grasp the one narrow edge of the pillow. Pull the pillowcase over it with your free hand (Fig. 10-11). Do the same for any other pillows. Place them at the head of the bed with open end away from the door. Make sure zippers or tags are on the inside.

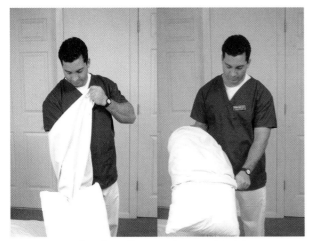

Fig. 10-11. *After the pillowcase is turned inside out over your arm, grasp one end of the pillow. Pull the pillowcase over the pillow.*

19. Return bed to lowest position.

20. Leave call light within resident's reach.

21. Wash your hands.

22. Take laundry bag or hamper to proper area.

23. Document procedure using facility guidelines.

Tip

Seams and the Skin

Residents' skin may be very fragile. Seams rubbing against an elderly person's skin can cause the skin to tear or crack. Remember to follow these rules for placing linens properly on beds:

Bottom Sheet: Seam Down = Bottom Down

Top Sheet: Seam Up = Top Up

Making an open bed

Equipment: clean linen—mattress pad, fitted or flat bottom sheet, waterproof bed protector if needed, cotton draw sheet, flat top sheet, blanket(s), bedspread (if used), pillowcase(s), gloves

1. Wash your hands.

2. Make a closed bed, as described in previous procedure.

3. Stand at the head of the bed. Grasp the top sheet and blanket, and bedspread, and fold them down to the foot of the bed. Then bring them back up the bed to form a large cuff.

4. Bring the cuff on the top linens to a point where it is one hand-width above the linen underneath. This way, when the resident gets into bed, he will not pull all the linen out at the foot of the bed.

5. Make sure all linen is wrinkle-free.

6. Wash your hands.

7. Document procedure using facility guidelines.

An **occupied bed** is a bed made while the resident is in the bed. A resident may have a doctor's order to stay in bed at all times. These orders are called "absolute bedrest (ABR)," "strict bedrest," or "complete bedrest (CBR)." This type of bed may be completed more safely if you are able to work with a co-worker. Remember to lock the bed wheels, and bend your knees while making the bed. Raise the height of the bed to a safe working level.

Making an occupied bed gives you an opportunity to observe a resident's skin for signs of breakdown. Bedbound residents are at great risk for pressure ulcers.

An **unoccupied bed** is a bed made while no resident is in the bed. If the resident can be safely moved out of bed, making the bed will be easier.

Bedmaking and Unit Care

Side Rails

The use of side rails has become uncommon because they are considered restraints and can put residents at risk for injury. If side rail use is ordered by a doctor, they must be raised and lowered for resident care. Only one side rail should be lowered on the working side of the bed when one person is giving care. If care is being given by two caregivers, both side rails may be lowered, as long as both caregivers stay at the bedside. Side rails must be raised, and the bed lowered, when care is completed before caregivers leave the resident's bedside.

Making an occupied bed

Equipment: clean linen—mattress pad, fitted or flat bottom sheet, waterproof bed protector if needed, cotton draw sheet, flat top sheet, blanket(s), bedspread (if used), bath blanket, pillowcase(s), gloves

1. Wash your hands.

2. Identify yourself by name. Identify the resident. Greet the resident by name.

3. Explain procedure to the resident. Speak clearly, slowly, and directly. Maintain face-to-face contact whenever possible.

4. Provide for the resident's privacy with a curtain, screen, or door.

5. Place clean linen on clean surface within reach (e.g., bedside stand, overbed table, or chair).

6. Adjust bed to safe working level, usually waist high. Lower head of bed. Lock bed wheels.

7. Put on gloves.

8. Loosen top linen from the end of the bed on the working side.

9. Unfold the bath blanket over the top sheet and remove the top sheet. Keep resident covered at all times with the bath blanket.

10. You will make the bed one side at a time. Raise side rail (if bed has them) on far side of bed. After raising side rail, go to the other side of the bed. Gently help resident to turn onto her side slowly, moving away from you,

toward raised side rail (see Procedure: Turning a Resident in Chapter 11) (Fig. 10-12).

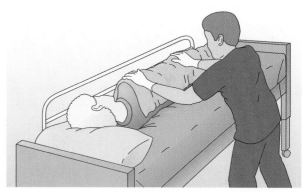

Fig. 10-12. *Turn resident onto her side, toward raised side rail.*

11. Loosen bottom soiled linen, mattress pad, and protector, if present, on the working side.

12. Roll bottom soiled linen toward resident and center of bed, soiled side inside. Tuck it snugly against resident's back.

13. Place the mattress pad (if used) on the bed, attaching elastic at corners on working side.

14. Place clean bottom linen or fitted bottom sheet with the center crease in the center. If flat sheet is used, tuck in at top and on working side. Make hospital corners to keep bottom sheet wrinkle-free. If fitted sheet is used, tightly pull two fitted corners on working side.

15. Smooth the bottom sheet out toward the resident. Be sure there are no wrinkles in the mattress pad. Roll the extra material toward the resident. Tuck it under the resident's body (Fig. 10-13).

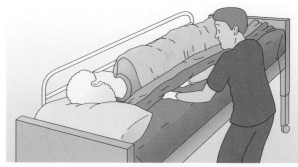

Fig. 10-13. *Tuck extra material under the resident's body.*

16. If using a waterproof bed protector, unfold it and center it on the bed. Smooth it out toward the resident.

17. If using a draw sheet, place it on the bed. Tuck in on your side, smooth, and tuck as you did with the other bedding.

18. Raise side rail nearest you. Go to the other side of the bed. Lower side rail on the working side. Help resident roll or turn onto clean bottom sheet (Fig. 10-14). Explain that he will be moving over a roll of linen. Protect the resident from any soiled matter on the old linens.

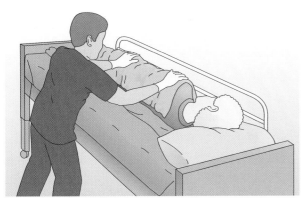

Fig. 10-14. *While helping the resident turn onto the clean linen, try to avoid contact with soiled matter on dirty linen.*

19. Loosen soiled linen. Look for personal items. Roll linen from head to foot of bed, avoiding contact with your skin or clothes. Do not shake soiled linen. Place it in a hamper or linen bag. Do not place on overbed table, chair, or floor.

20. Pull the clean linen through as quickly as possible. Start with the mattress pad and wrap around corners. Pull and tuck in clean bottom linen, just like the other side. Pull and tuck in waterproof bed protector and draw sheet, if used. Make hospital corners with bottom sheet. Finish with bottom sheet free of wrinkles.

21. Place resident on his back. Keep resident covered and comfortable, with a pillow under his head.

22. Unfold the top sheet. Place it over the resident and center it. Ask the resident to hold the top sheet and pull the bath blanket out from underneath (Fig. 10-15). Put it in the hamper/bag.

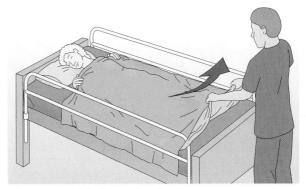

Fig. 10-15. *With the resident holding on to the top sheet, pull the bath blanket out.*

23. Place the blanket over the top sheet and center it. Place the bedspread over the blanket and center it. Tuck the top sheet, blanket and bedspread under the foot of the bed and make hospital corners on each side. Loosen the top linens over the resident's feet.

24. At the top of the bed, fold down the top sheet to make a cuff of about six inches over the blanket.

25. Gently hold and lift resident's head and remove pillow. Do not hold it near your face. Remove the soiled pillowcase by turning it inside out. Place it in the hamper/bag.

26. Remove and discard gloves. Wash your hands.

27. With one hand, grasp the clean pillowcase at the closed end. Turn it inside out over your arm. Next, using the hand that has the pillowcase over it, grasp the center of the end of the pillow. Pull the pillowcase over it with your free hand. Do the same for any other pillows. Place them gently under resident's head with open end away from the door. Make sure zippers or tags are on the inside.

28. Make sure bed is wrinkle-free. Make resident comfortable.

29. Return bed to lowest position. Return side rails to ordered position. Remove privacy measures.

30. Leave call light within resident's reach.

31. Be courteous and respectful at all times.

32. Wash your hands.

33. Take laundry bag or hamper to proper area.

34. Report any changes in the resident to the nurse. Document procedure using facility guidelines.

A **surgical bed** is made so that it can easily accept residents who must return to bed on stretchers or gurneys. Residents on stretchers are usually returning from treatment or hospital visits. Use caution when transferring residents from stretchers to beds. The bed and stretcher wheels must be locked, and the bed and stretcher must be close together during the transfer.

Discuss the preparation for the arrival of a resident on a stretcher with the nurse. When preparing the room, you may need to set up equipment in the room. Check with the nurse for instructions on gathering any extra equipment/supplies.

Making a surgical bed

Equipment: clean linen (see Procedure: Making a closed bed), gloves

1. Wash your hands.

2. Place clean linen on clean surface within reach (e.g., bedside stand, overbed table, or chair).

3. Adjust bed to safe working level, usually waist high. Lock bed wheels.

4. Put on gloves.

5. Remove all soiled linen, rolling it (soiled side inside) from head to foot of bed. Avoid con-

tact with your skin or clothes. Place it in a hamper or linen bag.

6. Remove and discard gloves.

7. Wash your hands.

8. Make a closed bed. Do not tuck top linens under the mattress.

9. Fold top linens down from the head of the bed and up from the foot of the bed (Fig. 10-16).

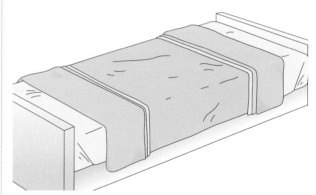

Fig. 10-16. *Fold linens down from the head of the bed and up from the foot of the bed.*

10. Form a triangle with the linen. Fanfold the linen triangle into pleated layers and position opposite the stretcher side of the bed (Fig. 10-17). Fanfolding means folding several times into pleats. After fanfolding, form a tiny tip with the end of the linen triangle. The tip can be grasped quickly and pulled over the returning resident. This step quickly provides much-needed warmth to the resident.

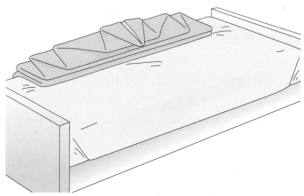

Fig. 10-17. *Fanfold the linen so that it is in pleated layers and position linen opposite the stretcher side of bed.*

11. Put on clean pillowcases. Place the clean pillows on a clean surface off the bed, such as on the bedside stand or chair.

12. Leave bed in its locked position. Leave both side rails down.

13. Move all furniture to make room for the stretcher.

14. Do not place call light on bed. That is placed after the resident returns to bed.

15. Wash your hands.

16. Take laundry bag or hamper to proper area.

17. Document procedure using facility guidelines.

Chapter Review

1. List three functions that sleep performs (LO 2).

2. List six reasons that residents can develop parasomnias (LO 3).

3. List five factors that can affect a resident's ability to sleep. For each item listed, describe one thing that can be done to help promote better sleep (LO 4).

4. What is usually stored in the bedside stand (LO 5)?

5. What is the overbed table used for? Can a bedpan be placed on it (LO 5)?

6. Where should the call light always be placed (LO 6)?

7. Define disposable equipment (LO 6).

8. List three ways that careful bedmaking and clean, neat, and dry beds help residents (LO 7).

9. Why is it important that linen always be changed when it is wet, damp, wrinkled, or soiled (LO 7)?

10. Why should nursing assistants carry clean linen away from their uniforms (LO 7)?

11. Why should linen never be shaken (LO 7)?

12. Describe the difference between a closed bed and an open bed (LO 7).

13. While making an occupied bed, what should be observed by a nursing assistant (LO 7)?

14. When is a surgical bed made (LO 7)?

11 Positioning, Moving, and Lifting

A View from the Past: "Falling into Life"

"Having lost the use of my legs during the polio epidemic that swept across the eastern United States during the summer of 1944, I was soon immersed in a process of rehabilitation that was . . . as much spiritual as physical. That was a full decade before the discovery of the Salk vaccine ended polio's reign as the disease most dreaded by America's parents and their children. Treatment of the disease had been standardized by 1944: following the initial onslaught of the virus, patients were kept in isolation for a period of ten days to two weeks. Following that, orthodox medical opinion was content to subject patients to as much heat as they could stand. Stiff paralyzed limbs were swathed in heated, coarse woolen towels known as 'hot packs.' As soon as the hot packs had baked enough pain and stiffness out of a patient's body so that he could be moved on and off a stretcher, the treatment was ended, and the patient faced a series of daily immersions in a heated pool. I would ultimately spend two full years at the appropriately named New York State Reconstruction Home. . . . We would learn during our days in the New York State Reconstruction Home to confront the world that was . . . My future had arrived."

Leonard Kriegel

"Take her up tenderly/Lift her with care..."

Thomas Hood, 1798-1845

1. Define important words in this chapter

ambulation: walking.

dangle: to sit up with the legs over the side of the bed in order to regain balance.

ergonomics: the science of designing equipment, areas and tasks to make them safer and to suit the worker's abilities.

Fowler's: position in which a person is in a semi-sitting position (45 to 60 degrees).

gait belt: a belt made of canvas or other heavy material used to help people who are weak, unsteady, or uncoordinated to stand, sit, or walk; also called a transfer belt.

lateral: position in which a person is lying on either side.

logrolling: moving a person as a unit, without disturbing the alignment of the body.

mechanical lift: special equipment used to lift and move or lift and weigh a person; also called hydraulic lift.

MSDs: acronym that stands for work-related musculoskeletal disorders.

positioning: the act of helping people into positions that will be comfortable and healthy for them.

posture: the way a person holds and positions his body.

prone: position in which a person is lying on his or her stomach.

shearing: rubbing or friction resulting from the skin moving one way and the bone underneath it remaining fixed or moving in the opposite direction.

Sims': position in which a person is in a left side-lying position with the upper knee flexed and raised toward the chest.

supine: position in which a person is lying flat on his or her back.

transfer belt: a belt made of canvas or other heavy material used to help people who are weak, unsteady, or uncoordinated to stand, sit, or walk; also called a gait belt.

2. Explain body alignment and review the principles of body mechanics

The positioning of the body plays an important part in the proper functioning of the body. Whether standing, sitting, or lying down, the body should be in correct alignment and exhibiting good posture. **Posture** is the way a person holds and positions his body.

Correct body alignment helps the body achieve balance without causing muscle or joint strain. In addition, good body alignment allows the body to function at its highest level. The lungs are able to expand and contract, blood circulation is more efficient, digestion is easier, and the kidneys are able to better clean the body of wastes. Also, good body alignment helps prevent complications of immobility, such as contractures and atrophy. Contractures are the permanent and often painful stiffening of a joint and muscle. Atrophy is the weakening or wasting of muscles.

You first learned about body mechanics in Chapter 7. When you do not move and position residents using good body mechanics, you and residents can be injured. These guidelines will help you remember to use proper body mechanics:

Guidelines: Using Proper Body Mechanics

G **Assess the load.** Before lifting, assess the weight of the load to determine if you can safely move the object without help. Know the lift policies at your facility. Never attempt to lift someone you are not sure you can lift.

G **Think ahead, plan, and communicate the move.** Check for any objects in your path or any potential risks, such as a wet floor. Make sure the path is clear. Watch for hazards, like high-traffic areas, combative residents, or a loose toilet seat. Decide exactly what you are going to do together and agree on the instructions you will use before attempting to transfer, or move the resident from one place to another.

G **Check your base of support and be sure you have firm footing.** Use a wide but balanced stance to increase support, and keep this stance when walking. Have enough room to maintain a wide base of support. Make sure you and the resident are wearing non-skid shoes with the laces tied.

G **Face what you are lifting.** Your feet should always face the direction you are moving. This enables you to move your body as one unit and keeps your back straight. Twisting at the waist increases the likelihood of injury.

G **Keep your back straight.** Keeping your head up and shoulders back will keep the back in the proper position. Taking a deep breath will help you regain correct posture.

G **Begin in a squatting position, and lift with your legs.** Bend at the hips and knees, and use the strength of your leg muscles to stand and lift the object (Fig. 11-1). You will need to push your buttocks out to accomplish this. Before you stand with the object you are lifting, remember that your legs, not your back, will enable you to lift. You should be able to feel your leg muscles as they work. Lift with the large leg muscles to decrease stress on the back.

G **Tighten your stomach muscles when beginning the lift.** This will help to take weight off the spine and maintain alignment.

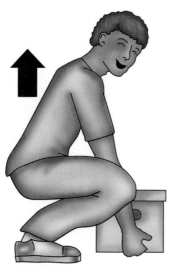

Fig. 11-1. *To lift an object, you will bend your knees slightly and lift with your legs.*

G **Keep the object close to your body.** This decreases stress on your back. Lift objects only to your waist. Carrying them any higher can affect your balance (Fig. 11-2).

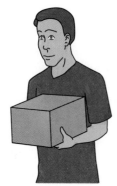

Fig. 11-2. *Keeping objects close while carrying them decreases stress on your back.*

G **Do not twist.** Turn and face the area you are moving the object to and then set the object down. Twisting increases the stress on your back and should always be avoided.

G **Push when possible rather than lifting.** When you lift an object, you must overcome gravity to balance the load. When you push an object, you only need to overcome the friction between the surface and the object. Use your body weight to move the object, rather than your lifting muscles. Stay close to the object. Use both arms and tighten your stomach muscles.

3. Explain why position changes are important for bedbound residents and describe basic body positions

Residents who are bedbound or who spend a lot of time in bed often need help getting into comfortable positions. They also need to change positions periodically. Residents need to be turned often so that pressure on skin surfaces alternates from one side to the other. Too much pressure on one area for too long can cause a decrease in circulation. This increases the risk of pressure ulcers and other problems like muscle contractures. Constant pressure causes the greatest risk of pressure ulcers, a major problem in long-term care. To try to prevent these sores from occurring, many facilities have established turning schedules. You will learn more about pressure ulcers and prevention in Chapters 12 and 18.

Positioning means the act of helping residents into positions that promote comfort and good health. You will reposition bedbound residents at least every two hours. Follow posted turn schedules and care plans carefully. You may have several residents who require frequent turning. Every time you position a resident, you must document the position and time. When positioning residents, use proper body mechanics to help prevent injury. Check the resident's skin for whiteness, redness, or warm spots, especially around bony areas, each time you reposition a resident.

You first learned about body positions in Chapter 9. Here are five basic body positions you may use for residents:

Supine: In this position, the resident lies flat on his back. To maintain correct body position, support the head and shoulders with a pillow (Fig. 11-3). You may also use pillows, rolled towels, or washcloths to support his arms (especially a weak or immobilized arm) or hands. The heels need to be raised so they do not touch the bed. Place a pillow under the calves. Use footboards, padded boards placed against the resident's feet, to keep them positioned properly, as needed.

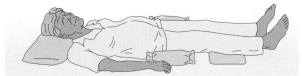

Fig. 11-3. *A person in the supine position is lying flat on his or her back.*

Lateral/side: A resident in the lateral position is lying on either side (Fig. 11-4). There are many ways to do this. Pillows can support the arm and leg on the upper side, the back, and the head. Ideally, the knee on the upper side of the body should be flexed. The leg is brought in front of the body and supported on a pillow. There should be a pillow under the bottom foot, and the toes should not touch the bed. If the top leg cannot be brought forward, it should be placed slightly behind the bottom leg, never resting directly on it. Pillows should be used between the two legs to help relieve pressure and avoid skin breakdown.

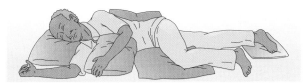

Fig. 11-4. *A person in the lateral position is lying on his side.*

Prone: A resident in the prone position is lying on the abdomen, or front side of the body (Fig. 11-5). This is not comfortable for many people, especially elderly people. Never leave a resident in a prone position for very long. In this position, the arms are either placed at the sides, raised above the head, or one raised and one by the side. The head is turned to one side. A small pil-

low may be used under the head and under the legs. This keeps the feet from touching the bed.

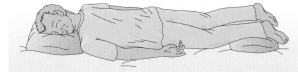

Fig. 11-5. *A person lying in the prone position is lying on his abdomen.*

Fowler's: A resident in the Fowler's position is in a partially-reclined sitting position (45 to 60 degrees) (Fig. 11-6). The head and shoulders are elevated and the resident's knees may be flexed and elevated. Use a pillow or rolled blanket as a support. The feet may be supported using a footboard or other support. The spine should be straight. In a high-Fowler's position, the upper body is sitting nearly straight up (60 to 90 degrees). In a semi-Fowler's position, the upper body is not raised as high (30 to 45 degrees).

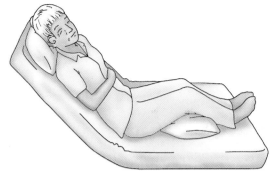

Fig. 11-6. *A person lying in the Fowler's position is partially reclined.*

Sims': The Sims' position is a left side-lying position (Fig. 11-7). The lower arm is behind the back. The upper knee is flexed and raised toward the chest, using a pillow as support. There should be a pillow under the bottom foot so that the toes do not touch the bed.

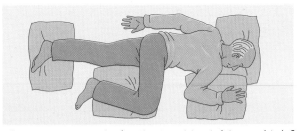

Fig. 11-7. *A person in the Sims' position is lying on his left side with one leg drawn up.*

The Trendelenburg and Reverse Trendelenburg positions are used with residents who have special needs. For example, Trendelenburg may be used for a resident who has gone into shock and has poor blood flow (Fig. 11-8). Reverse Trendelenburg may be used for a resident who needs a faster emptying of the stomach due to a digestive problem (Fig. 11-9). These positions always require a doctor's order. Some electric beds have buttons or levers that place the bed in these two positions.

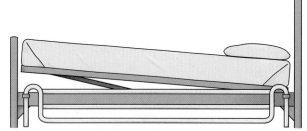

Fig. 11-8. *The Trendelenburg position is only used with a doctor's order.*

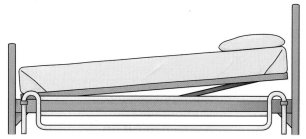

Fig. 11-9. *The Reverse Trendelenburg position is only used with a doctor's order.*

Many positioning devices are available to help make residents more comfortable and safe in different body positions. See Chapter 25 for a list of these devices.

Residents' Rights

Communicate.

Any time you assist residents, discuss with them what you would like to do. Promote their independence by allowing them to do what they can. You must work together, especially during transfers.

Helping a resident sit up using the arm lock

1. Identify yourself by name. Identify the resident. Greet the resident by name.

2. Wash your hands.

3. Explain procedure to resident. Speak clearly, slowly, and directly. Maintain face-to-face contact whenever possible.

4. Provide for the resident's privacy with a curtain, screen, or door.

5. Adjust the bed to a safe level, usually waist high. Lock the bed wheels.

6. Move the pillow to the head of the bed.

7. Stand at the side of the bed and face the head of bed.

8. Spread feet shoulder-width apart and slightly bend the knees to protect your back.

9. Place your arm under the resident's arm and grasp the resident's shoulder. Have the resident grasp your shoulder in the same manner. This hold is called the arm lock or lock arm (Fig. 11-10).

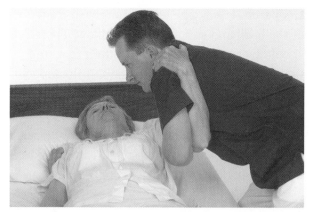

Fig. 11-10. *Gently grasp the resident's shoulder, while she grasps your shoulder.*

10. Reach under the resident's head and place your other hand on the resident's far shoulder.

11. At the count of three, rock yourself backward and pull the resident to a sitting position. Use pillows or a bed rest to support the resident in the sitting position.

12. Check the resident for dizziness or weakness.

13. Replace pillow. Make resident comfortable.

14. Return bed to lowest position. Remove privacy measures.

15. Leave call light within resident's reach.

16. Wash your hands.

17. Be courteous and respectful at all times.

18. Report any changes in the resident to the nurse. Document procedure using facility guidelines.

Use draw sheets under residents who cannot help with turning, lifting, or moving up in bed. A draw sheet, or turning sheet, is an extra sheet placed on top of the bottom sheet (Fig. 11-11). Draw sheets help prevent skin damage caused by shearing. **Shearing** is rubbing or friction resulting from the skin moving one way and the bone underneath it remaining fixed or moving in the opposite direction.

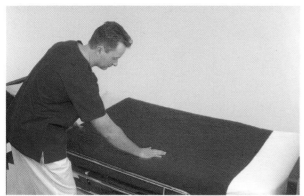

Fig. 11-11. A draw sheet is a special sheet (or a regular bed sheet folded in half) used to move residents in bed without causing shearing.

Assisting a resident to move up in bed

1. Identify yourself by name. Identify the resident. Greet the resident by name.

2. Wash your hands.

3. Explain procedure to resident. Speak clearly, slowly, and directly. Maintain face-to-face contact whenever possible.

4. Provide for the resident's privacy with a curtain, screen, or door.

5. Adjust the bed to a safe level, usually waist high. Lock the bed wheels.

6. Lower the head of bed to make it flat. Move the pillow to the head of bed.

7. If the bed has side rails, raise the rail on the far side of the bed.

8. Stand by bed with feet shoulder-width apart. Face the resident.

9. Place one arm under the resident's shoulder blades. Place the other arm under the resident's thighs.

10. Ask resident to bend knees, brace feet on the mattress, and push feet and hands on the count of three.

11. Keep your back straight. At the count of three, shift body weight to move resident while resident pushes with her feet (Fig. 11-12).

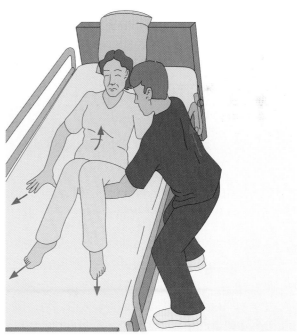

Fig. 11-12. Keep your back straight and your knees bent.

12. Replace pillow under the resident's head.

13. Make resident comfortable.

14. Return bed to lowest position. Return side rails to ordered position. Remove privacy measures.

15. Leave call light within resident's reach.

16. Wash your hands.

17. Be courteous and respectful at all times.

18. Report any changes in the resident to the nurse. Document procedure using facility guidelines.

If a co-worker is available, ask her to help you move residents. Always get help if you feel it is not safe to move the resident by yourself.

Assisting a resident to move up in bed with assistance (using draw sheet)

Equipment: draw sheet

1. Identify yourself by name. Identify the resident. Greet the resident by name.

2. Wash your hands.

3. Explain procedure to resident. Speak clearly, slowly, and directly. Maintain face-to-face contact whenever possible. Encourage resident to assist if possible.

4. Provide for the resident's privacy with a curtain, screen, or door.

5. Adjust the bed to a safe level, usually waist high. Lock the bed wheels.

6. Lower the head of bed to make it flat. Move the pillow to the head of bed.

7. Stand on the opposite side of the bed from your helper. Each of you should be turned slightly toward the head of the bed. For each of you, the foot that is closest to the head of the bed should be pointed in that direction. Stand with feet about shoulder-width apart. Bend your knees. Keep your back straight.

8. Roll the draw sheet up to the resident's side. Have your helper do the same on his side of the bed. Grasp the sheet with your palms up at the resident's shoulders and hips. Have your helper do the same.

9. Shift your weight to your back foot (the foot closer to the foot of the bed). Have your helper do the same (Fig. 11-13). On the count of three, you and your helper both shift your weight to your forward feet. Slide the resident toward the head of the bed (Fig. 11-14).

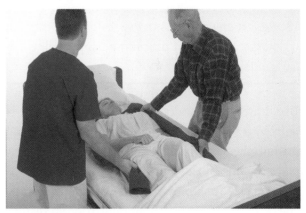

Fig. 11-13. Both workers shift their weight to their back feet and prepare to move.

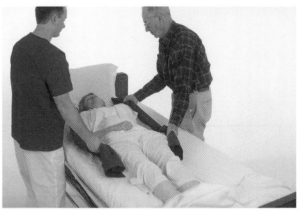

Fig. 11-14. On the count of three, both workers shift their weight to their forward feet and slide the resident toward the head of the bed.

10. Replace pillow under the resident's head.

11. Make resident comfortable. Unroll the draw sheet. Leave it in place for the next repositioning.

12. Return bed to lowest position if raised. Remove privacy measures.

13. Leave call light within resident's reach.

14. Wash your hands.

15. Be courteous and respectful at all times.

16. Report any changes in the resident to the nurse. Document procedure using facility guidelines.

Moving a resident to the side of the bed

1. Identify yourself by name. Identify the resident. Greet the resident by name.

2. Wash your hands.

3. Explain procedure to resident. Speak clearly, slowly, and directly. Maintain face-to-face contact whenever possible. Encourage resident to assist if possible.

4. Provide for the resident's privacy with a curtain, screen, or door.

5. Adjust the bed to a safe level, usually waist high. Lock the bed wheels.

6. Lower the head of bed.

7. Stand on the same side of the bed to which you are moving the resident.

8. Stand with feet about shoulder-width apart. Bend your knees. Keep your back straight.

9. Gently slide your hands under the resident's head and shoulders and move them toward you (Fig. 11-15).

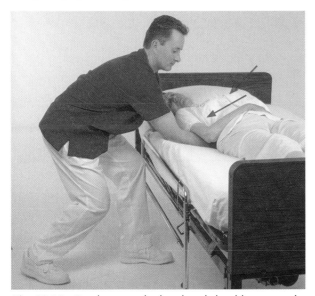

Fig. 11-15. *Gently move the head and shoulders toward you.*

10. Gently slide your hands under the resident's midsection and move it toward you.

11. Gently slide your hands under the resident's hips and legs and move them toward you (Fig. 11-16).

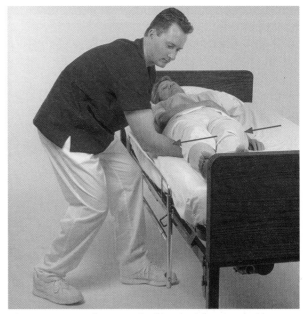

Fig. 11-16. *Gently move the hips and legs toward you.*

12. Make resident comfortable.

13. Return bed to lowest position. Remove privacy measures.

14. Leave call light within resident's reach.

15. Wash your hands.

16. Be courteous and respectful at all times.

17. Report any changes in the resident to the nurse. Document procedure using facility guidelines.

Moving a resident to the side of the bed with assistance (using draw sheet)

Equipment: draw sheet

1. Identify yourself by name. Identify the resident. Greet the resident by name.

2. Wash your hands.

3. Explain procedure to resident. Speak clearly, slowly, and directly. Maintain face-to-face con-

tact whenever possible. Encourage resident to assist if possible.

4. Provide for the resident's privacy with a curtain, screen, or door.

5. Adjust the bed to a safe level, usually waist high. Lock the bed wheels.

6. Lower the head of bed. Move the pillow to the head of bed.

7. Stand on the opposite side of the bed from your helper. Each of you should be facing each other. Stand up straight, facing the side of the bed, with feet shoulder-width apart. Point feet toward the side of the bed. Bend your knees.

8. Roll the draw sheet up to the resident's side. Have your helper do the same on his side of the bed. Grasp the sheet with your palms up at the resident's shoulders and hips. Have your helper do the same (Fig. 11-17).

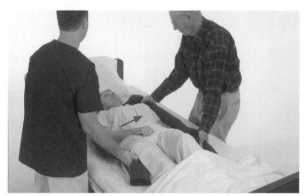

Fig. 11-17. *Both workers grasp the draw sheet at the resident's shoulders and hips and prepare to move.*

9. On the count of three, slide the resident toward the side of the bed. Your weight should be equal on each foot because you are moving the person to the side of the bed, not to the head of the bed.

10. Replace pillow under the resident's head.

11. Make resident comfortable. Unroll the draw sheet. Leave it in place for the next repositioning.

12. Return bed to lowest position. Remove privacy measures.

13. Leave call light within resident's reach.

14. Wash your hands.

15. Be courteous and respectful at all times.

16. Report any changes in the resident to the nurse. Document procedure using facility guidelines.

Turning a resident away from you

1. Identify yourself by name. Identify the resident. Greet the resident by name.

2. Wash your hands.

3. Explain procedure to resident. Speak clearly, slowly, and directly. Maintain face-to-face contact whenever possible.

4. Provide for the resident's privacy with a curtain, screen, or door.

5. Adjust the bed to a safe level, usually waist high. Lock the bed wheels.

6. Lower the head of bed.

7. Stand on side of bed opposite to where resident will be turned. The far side rail should be raised (if bed has one). Lower side rail nearest you if it is up.

8. Move resident to side of bed nearest you, using previous procedure.

9. Cross resident's arm over his or her chest. Move arm on side resident is being turned to out of the way. Cross leg nearest you over the far leg (Fig. 11-18).

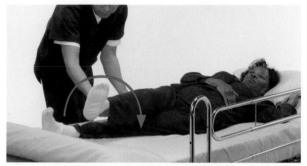

Fig. 11-18. *Cross leg nearest you over the far leg.*

10. Stand with feet shoulder-width apart. Bend your knees.

11. Place one hand on the resident's shoulder. Place the other hand on the resident's nearest hip.

12. While supporting the body, gently push onto side as one unit, toward the other side of bed (toward raised side rail). Shift your weight from your back leg to your front leg (Fig. 11-19). Make sure resident's face is not covered by the pillow.

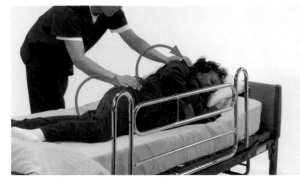

Fig. 11-19. Gently push resident toward other side of bed while shifting your weight from your back leg to your front leg.

13. Position resident properly in good alignment:

   • Head supported by pillow

   • Shoulder adjusted so resident is not lying on arm

   • Top arm supported by pillow

   • Back supported by supportive device

   • Hips properly aligned

   • Top knee flexed

   • Supportive device between legs with top knee flexed; knee and ankle supported

14. Cover resident with top linens. Make resident comfortable.

15. Return bed to lowest position. Return side rails to ordered position. Remove privacy measures.

16. Leave call light within resident's reach.

17. Wash your hands.

18. Be courteous and respectful at all times.

19. Report any changes in the resident to the nurse. Document procedure using facility guidelines.

Turning a resident toward you

1. Identify yourself by name. Identify the resident. Greet the resident by name.

2. Wash your hands.

3. Explain procedure to resident. Speak clearly, slowly, and directly. Maintain face-to-face contact whenever possible.

4. Provide for the resident's privacy with a curtain, screen, or door.

5. Adjust the bed to a safe level, usually waist high. Lock the bed wheels.

6. Lower the head of bed.

7. Stand on side of bed opposite to where resident will be turned. The far side rail should be raised (if bed has one). Lower side rail nearest you if it is up.

8. Move resident to side of bed nearest you using previous procedure.

9. Cross resident's arm over his or her chest. Move arm on side resident is being turned to out of the way. Cross leg furthest from you over the near leg.

10. Stand with feet shoulder-width apart. Bend your knees.

11. Place one hand on the resident's far shoulder. Place the other hand on the resident's far hip.

12. While supporting the body, gently roll the resident toward you (Fig. 11-20). The goal is

to block the resident to prevent her from rolling out of bed. Make sure resident's face is not covered by the pillow.

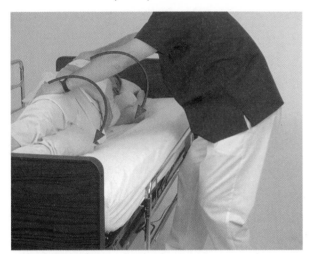

Fig. 11-20. *Gently roll the resident toward you.*

13. Position resident properly in good alignment:

- Head supported by pillow
- Shoulder adjusted so resident is not lying on arm
- Top arm supported by pillow
- Back supported by supportive device
- Hips properly aligned
- Top knee flexed
- Supportive device between legs with top knee flexed; knee and ankle supported

14. Cover resident with top linens and straighten. Make resident comfortable.

15. Return bed to lowest position. Return side rails to ordered position. Remove privacy measures.

16. Leave call light within resident's reach.

17. Wash your hands.

18. Be courteous and respectful at all times.

19. Report any changes in the resident to the nurse. Document procedure using facility guidelines.

Logrolling allows you to turn a resident as a unit, while keeping the spine straight. The alignment of the body is not disturbed; the head, back and legs are kept in a straight line. Logrolling may be necessary if the resident has neck or back problems, head or spinal cord injuries, or has had neck, back, or hip surgeries. Use a draw sheet to perform this procedure. Be very careful when logrolling a resident. You will need at least one co-worker to assist.

Logrolling a resident with assistance

Equipment: draw sheet

1. Identify yourself by name. Identify the resident. Greet the resident by name.

2. Wash your hands.

3. Explain procedure to resident. Speak clearly, slowly, and directly. Maintain face-to-face contact whenever possible.

4. Provide for the resident's privacy with a curtain, screen, or door.

5. Adjust the bed to a safe level, usually waist high. Lock the bed wheels.

6. Lower the head of bed.

7. Both co-workers stand on the same side of the bed. One person stands at the resident's head and shoulders. The other stands near the resident's midsection.

8. Place a pillow under the resident's head to support the neck during the move.

9. Place the resident's arms across his or her chest. Place a pillow between the knees.

10. Stand with feet shoulder-width apart. Bend your knees.

11. Grasp the draw sheet on the far side (Fig. 11-21).

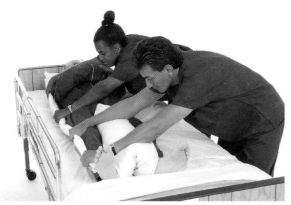

Fig. 11-21. Both workers should grasp the draw sheet on the far side.

12. On the count of three, gently roll the resident toward you. Turn the resident as a unit (Fig. 11-22). The goal is to block the resident to prevent him from rolling out of bed.

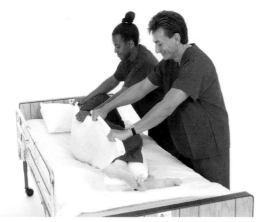

Fig. 11-22. On the count of three, both workers should roll the resident towards them, turning the person as a unit.

13. Reposition resident comfortably in good alignment. Place pillow under head. Cover resident with top linens and straighten.

14. Return bed to lowest position. Remove privacy measures.

15. Leave call light within resident's reach.

16. Wash your hands.

17. Be courteous and respectful at all times.

18. Report any changes in the resident to the nurse. Document procedure using facility guidelines.

To **dangle** means to sit up on the side of the bed with the legs hanging over the side. This helps residents regain balance before standing up, equalizes blood flow in the body, and returns blood flow to the head. It helps prevent dizziness and lightheadedness that can cause fainting. Residents who cannot walk may have an order to dangle their legs for a few minutes regularly.

Assisting a resident to sit up on side of bed: dangling

1. Identify yourself by name. Identify the resident. Greet the resident by name.

2. Wash your hands.

3. Explain procedure to resident. Speak clearly, slowly, and directly. Maintain face-to-face contact whenever possible.

4. Provide for the resident's privacy with a curtain, screen, or door.

5. Adjust the bed to the lowest position. Lock the bed wheels.

6. Raise the head of bed to sitting position. Fold linen to the foot of the bed.

7. Stand at the side of the bed with feet shoulder-width apart. Bend your knees. Keep your back straight. Help resident slowly move toward the side of the bed on which you are standing.

8. Place one arm under resident's shoulder blades. Place the other arm under resident's thighs (Fig. 11-23).

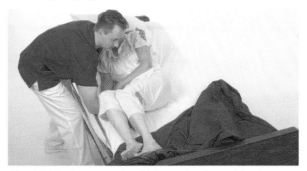

Fig. 11-23. One arm should be under the resident's shoulder blades, and the other arm should be under the thighs.

9. On the count of three, gently and slowly turn resident into sitting position with legs dangling over the side of bed (Fig. 11-24).

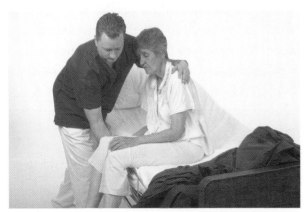

Fig. 11-24. *The weight of the resident's legs hanging down from the bed helps the resident sit up.*

10. Ask resident to sit up straight and push both fists into the edge of mattress. Assist resident to put on non-skid shoes, if she is going to get out of bed.

11. Have resident dangle as long as ordered. The care plan may direct you to allow the resident to dangle for several minutes and then return her to lying down, or it may direct you to allow the resident to dangle in preparation for walking or a transfer. Follow the care plan. Place a pillow or other supporting device behind resident's back during dangle. Stay with the resident at all times. Check for dizziness. If resident feels dizzy or faint, help her lie down again and make sure she is secure. Tell the nurse immediately.

12. Take vital signs as ordered (Chapter 13).

13. Remove shoes.

14. Gently assist resident back into bed. Place one arm around resident's shoulders. Place the other arm under resident's knees. Slowly move resident's legs onto bed.

15. Make resident comfortable. Cover resident with top linens and straighten. Replace pillow under the resident's head.

16. Return bed to lowest position. Remove privacy measures.

17. Leave call light within resident's reach.

18. Wash your hands.

19. Be courteous and respectful at all times.

20. Report any changes in the resident to the nurse. Document procedure using facility guidelines.

4. Describe how to safely transfer residents

Transfers allow residents to move from one place to another. Examples include transfers from bed to chair or wheelchair to toilet or vehicle.

With transferring, it is important to know that some residents have a strong side and a weak side. The weak side is called the "involved" or "affected" side. You must plan the move so that the strong side moves first and the weak side follows. It is difficult for a resident to move a weak arm and leg first and be able to bear enough weight to allow for the move.

Safety is one of the most important concerns during resident transfers. OSHA has set specific ergonomic guidelines to help avoid injuries during transfers. **Ergonomics** is the science of designing equipment, areas, and tasks to make them safer and to suit the worker's abilities. One goal of ergonomics is to reduce stress on the body to avoid potential injury.

Certain parts of the body, such as the back, are more prone to injury. OSHA's ergonomic guidelines address ways to help avoid these work-related musculoskeletal disorders, or **MSDs**. OSHA states that manual lifting and transferring of residents should be reduced and eliminated when possible.

This means that proper equipment should be available in facilities. Staff should be trained how to use this equipment and should use it whenever possible to avoid injury. Follow your facility's policies, and always get enough help when moving and lifting residents.

To reduce risks of pain and injury, some facilities have adopted "zero lift," "lift-free," or "safe lifting" programs, which means that there are strict guidelines in place for lifting and transferring residents. Manual lifting may be prohibited entirely, and equipment might always be required to lift and move residents.

Bariatric Residents

Due to a dramatic increase in the number of obese and morbidly obese people, healthcare facilities need to be able to accommodate bariatric residents. A person who is overweight has a BMI (body mass index) of 25 to 29. A person who is considered obese has a BMI of 30 to 39. A person who is considered morbidly obese has a BMI of 40 or higher.

Obese people have a higher risk of having certain diseases, such as diabetes, hypertension, and heart disease.

There are many practical issues that need to be considered in order to care for bariatric residents, including the following:

- Special bariatric beds, wheelchairs, and stretchers that can hold heavier people will need to be provided. Doorways may need to be widened.

- Oversized chairs with a higher weight capacity may be needed in resident rooms, dining areas and other areas, such as lobbies.

- Mechanical lifts made for bariatric residents will be used, and two to three caregivers will be needed to safely transfer a bariatric resident using a lift.

- If regular weight scales—whether standing or bed scales—cannot accommodate obese residents, special scales will be used.

- Sturdier toilets, larger showers and shower areas, heavy-duty hand bars, and wider spaces between the toilet and the wall may be necessary.

When evaluating residents for transfers, staff may determine that residents require a transfer belt or gait belt for safety. A **transfer belt** is a safety device used to transfer residents who are weak, unsteady, or uncoordinated. It is called a **gait belt** when it is used to help residents walk. The belt is made of canvas or other heavy material, and it has a strong buckle and cloth handles. It fits around the resident's waist, over his clothes, and then it is secured. The transfer belt gives you something firm to hold onto when assisting with transfers. These belts are generally not used if a resident has fragile bones or recent fractures. A transfer belt may also not be used when a resident has difficulty breathing, has had abdominal surgery, or any type of surgical removal of a part of the intestines. Follow the care plan and the nurse's instructions.

Applying a transfer belt

Equipment: transfer belt

1. Identify yourself by name. Identify the resident. Greet the resident by name.

2. Wash your hands.

3. Explain procedure to resident. Speak clearly, slowly, and directly. Maintain face-to-face contact whenever possible.

4. Provide for the resident's privacy with a curtain, screen, or door.

5. Adjust bed to lowest position. Lock bed wheels.

6. Supporting the back and hips, assist resident to a sitting position with feet flat on the floor.

7. Put on and properly fasten non-skid footwear on resident.

8. Place the belt over the resident's clothing below the rib cage and above the waist. Do not put it over bare skin.

9. Tighten the buckle until it is snug. Leave enough room to insert three fingers into the belt. The fingers should fit comfortably under the belt. The belt must not interfere with circulation or breathing.

10. Check to make sure that breasts are not caught under the belt.

11. Position the buckle slightly off-center in the front or back for comfort.

Sliding or transfer boards help residents transfer from one sitting position to another (Fig. 11-25). These boards can be used for transferring from wheelchairs or chairs to beds, vehicles, shower chairs, and other areas. Sliding boards are used for people who have weak legs or cannot bear any weight on their legs. Sliding or transfer boards are made out of sturdy material, such as wood, so they can hold the resident's weight.

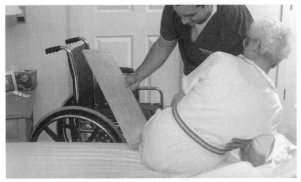

Fig. 11-25. *A sliding or transfer board can help with bed-to-chair transfers.*

Wheelchairs and Geriatric Chairs

Wheelchairs must always be locked before transferring residents to or from the wheelchair (Fig. 11-26). Here are some general guidelines for wheelchair use:

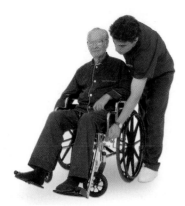

Fig. 11-26. *You must always lock the wheelchair before a resident gets into or out of it.*

Guidelines: Wheelchairs and Geriatric Chairs

G   To open a standard wheelchair, pull on both sides to make the armrests separate and the seat flatten. To close the wheelchair, lift the center of the seat and pull upward until the sides of the chair fold inward.

G   To remove an armrest on a standard wheelchair, press a button by the armrest, and lift it off. To attach an armrest, line up the button, and slip into place until the button clicks.

G   To remove the footrest, locate the lever, pull back, and pull the footrest off the knobs (Fig. 11-27). To re-attach the footrest, line up the knobs, and slide footrest into place until it clicks.

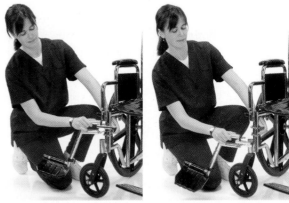

Fig. 11-27. *To remove footrests, pull back the lever, and pull the footrest off the knobs.*

G   To lift or lower footrest, support the leg or foot, squeeze lever, and pull up or push down.

G   If there is a pocket in the back of the wheelchair, it can be used to temporarily store a resident's chart during the transport.

G   When moving down a ramp, go down backwards, with the resident facing the top of the ramp, also going down backwards. The wheelchair could get away from you if the wheelchair heads down first.

G   When using an elevator, turn the chair around before entering it, so the resident faces forward in the elevator.

G   When positioning a resident in a wheelchair, make sure his hips are at the very back of the chair. To do this, lock the wheelchair wheels. Stand in front of the wheelchair and ask the resident to grasp the armrests while his feet are flat on the floor. Brace your knees against the resident's knees. On the count of three, ask the resident to push with his feet into the floor and move himself toward the back of the chair. Gently assist as needed. Help him get into a comfortable position.

G   An alternate method of positioning a resident properly is to get behind him while he pushes. First go to the back of the chair and reach forward and down under the resident's arms (but not in the armpits). The resident can put his feet flat on the floor and push up with his feet. Gently pull the resident up in the chair while the resident pushes. You may need a co-worker to help you do this safely.

G   A geriatric chair, or geri-chair, is a special chair that reclines. A tray table can be attached to it. This chair helps residents who are mostly bedbound avoid staying in bed all day. The chair helps keep residents in proper alignment, which reduces pressure on the skin.

G   Lock the wheels on both sides before moving a resident into or out of a geri-chair. The tray tables on geri-chairs can be heavy. Use caution when handling the tray table. Do not catch your fingers or the resident's fingers in the tray when attaching or releasing it. When the tray table is attached, geri-chairs are considered restraints. See Chapter 7 for more information.

Tip

The strong arm transfers.
When transferring a resident with one weak side, remember that the strong arm transfers.

Transferring a resident from bed to a chair or wheelchair

Equipment: wheelchair, transfer belt, non-skid footwear

1.   Identify yourself by name. Identify the resident. Greet the resident by name.

2.   Wash your hands.

3.   Explain procedure to resident. Speak clearly, slowly, and directly. Maintain face-to-face contact whenever possible.

4.   Provide for the resident's privacy with a curtain, screen, or door.

5.   Remove wheelchair footrests close to the bed.

6.   Place wheelchair near the head of the bed with arm of the wheelchair almost touching the bed. Wheelchair should be facing the foot of the bed. It should be placed on resident's stronger, or unaffected, side.

7.   Lock wheelchair wheels.

8.   Raise the head of the bed. Adjust bed level. The height of the bed should be equal to or slightly higher than the chair. Lock bed wheels.

9.   Assist resident to a sitting position with feet flat on the floor. Let resident sit for a few minutes.

10. Put non-skid footwear on resident and fasten securely.

11. ***With transfer belt***:

a.   Stand in front of resident.

b.   Stand with feet about shoulder-width apart. Bend your knees. Keep your back straight.

c.   Place belt below the rib cage and above the waist. Do not put it over bare skin. Check to make sure that breasts are not caught under the belt. Grasp belt securely on both sides.

Without transfer belt:

a.   Stand in front of resident.

b.   Stand with feet about shoulder-width apart. Bend your knees. Keep your back straight.

c.   Place your arms around the resident's torso under the arms, but not in the armpits. Repeated pressure in the axilla may cause nerve damage. Do not allow resident to grasp your shoulders or your neck. This may cause you to lose your balance.

12. Provide instructions to allow resident to help with transfer. Instructions may include: "When you start to stand, push with your hands against the bed." "Once standing, if you're able, you can take small steps in the direction of the chair." "Once standing, reach for the chair with your stronger hand."

13. With your legs, brace resident's lower legs to prevent slipping. This can be done by placing both of your knees in front of the resident's knees.

14. On the count of three, slowly help resident to stand.

15. Tell the resident to take small steps in the direction of the chair while turning her back toward the chair. If more help is needed, help resident pivot toward front of wheelchair, placing back of resident's legs against wheelchair (Fig. 11-28).

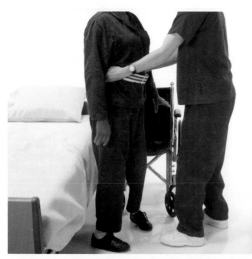

Fig. 11-28. *Help her pivot to the front of the wheelchair. Pivoting is safer than twisting.*

16. Ask resident to put hands on wheelchair armrests, if able. When the resident's legs touch the back of the chair, help her lower herself into the chair.

17. Reposition resident with hips touching back of wheelchair. See previous guidelines on how to do this. Remove transfer belt, if used.

18. Attach footrests. Place resident's feet on footrests. Check that resident is in good alignment.

19. Make resident comfortable.

20. Remove privacy measures.

21. Leave call light within resident's reach.

22. Wash your hands.

23. Be courteous and respectful at all times.

24. Report any changes in the resident to the nurse. Document procedure using facility guidelines.

To transfer back to bed from a wheelchair, follow these steps:

1. Perform steps 1 through 7 above.

2. Adjust bed level to a low position. The height of the bed should be equal to or slightly lower than the chair. Lock bed wheels.

3. Perform steps 11 through 14 above.

   The resident should be allowed to stand until he feels stable enough to move toward the bed. If the transfer belt is used, do not let go of it during this time.

4. Help resident pivot to bed with back of resident's legs against bed. When he feels the bed, he should slowly sit down on the side of the bed.

5. Make resident comfortable. Remove transfer belt, if used.

6. Return bed to lowest position. Remove privacy measures.

7. Leave call light within resident's reach.

8. Wash your hands.

9. Be courteous and respectful at all times.

10. Report any changes in the resident to the nurse. Document procedure using facility guidelines.

Stretchers

Stretchers, also called gurneys, are a way to transport residents from place to place within a facility. They are also used to transfer a resident to a vehicle. Residents who are unable to walk or sit in a wheelchair may need to be moved on a stretcher. People who are severely ill and must be transported by ambulance will need to be moved on a stretcher.

Stretchers have safety straps that are used when the resident is on the stretcher. Nursing assistants must secure the safety belts on the stretcher before moving residents. Lock the brakes on the stretcher when it is not in motion.

Keep residents properly covered at all times for warmth and privacy while on a stretcher. Residents should never be left alone on a stretcher. If riding with a resident who is being transported, make sure to formally transfer the care to the nurse at the new facility. The chart and any equipment or belongings must also be transferred to the nurse.

A draw sheet is used to transfer a resident to a stretcher. The procedure below shows a transfer to a stretcher from a bed using four workers. At least three workers are necessary to safely transfer a resident to a stretcher.

Transferring a resident from bed to stretcher with assistance

Equipment: stretcher, bath blanket

1. Identify yourself by name. Identify the resident. Greet the resident by name.

2. Wash your hands.

3. Explain procedure to resident. Speak clearly, slowly, and directly. Maintain face-to-face contact whenever possible.

4. Provide for the resident's privacy with a curtain, screen, or door.

5. Lower the head of bed so that it is flat. Lock bed wheels.

6. Fold linens to foot of the bed. Cover resident with bath blanket. Do not expose resident during the procedure.

7. Move the resident to the side of the bed. Have your co-workers help you do this. Refer back to the procedure "Moving a resident to the side of the bed" earlier in this chapter.

8. Place stretcher solidly against the bed. Lock stretcher wheels. Bed height should be equal to or slightly above the height of the stretcher. Move stretcher safety belts out of the way.

9. Two workers should be on the side of the bed opposite the stretcher. Two more workers should be on the other side of the stretcher.

10. Each worker should roll up the sides of the draw sheet and prepare to move the resident (Fig. 11-29). Protect the resident's arms and legs during the transfer. If facility policy permits, two workers may actually get up on the bed on their knees to protect their backs.

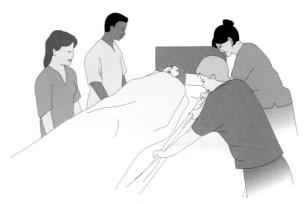

Fig. 11-29. With two workers on each side, roll up the sides of the draw sheet and prepare to move the resident.

11. On the count of three, the workers should lift and move the resident to the stretcher. All should move at once (Fig. 11-30). Make sure the resident is centered on the stretcher.

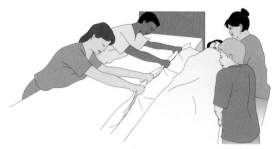

Fig. 11-30. *On the count of three, all workers should lift and move at once.*

12. Raise the head of the stretcher or place a pillow under the resident's head. Make sure bath blanket still covers the resident.

13. Place safety straps across the resident. Raise side rails on stretcher.

14. Unlock stretcher's wheels. Take resident to proper site. Stay with the resident until another team member takes over responsibility of the resident.

15. Wash your hands.

16. Be courteous and respectful at all times.

17. Report any changes in the resident to the nurse. Document procedure using facility guidelines.

To transfer back to bed from stretcher:

The bed height should be equal to or slightly below the stretcher when transferring the resident back to bed.

Mechanical Lifts

Mechanical lifts are types of equipment that are used to lift and move residents. They help prevent injury and help protect staff and residents. Learn to use the lifts available at your facility. Know how to explain their use to residents to ease their fears of them.

There are many different types of mechanical lifts (Fig. 11-31). Some common names of these lifts include "hydraulic," "power," "standing," "heavy duty," and "pool and bath." You must be trained on the specific lift you will be using.

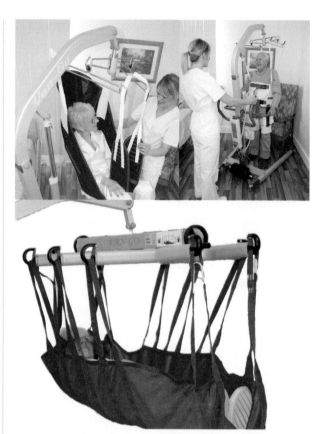

Fig. 11-31. *There are many different types of lifts for transferring both completely dependent residents and residents who can bear some weight.* (PHOTOS COURTESY OF VANCARE INC., VANCARE.COM, 800-694-4525)

This is a basic procedure for transferring a resident using a mechanical lift. Other lifts may have different procedures. If you are unsure how to perform this procedure, ask for more training. Do not operate lifts if you have not been trained in their use. Do not use the lift if it is broken or does not appear to be functioning properly. Many facilities require two or more people to perform the following procedure. Follow your facility's policy.

Transferring a resident using a mechanical lift with assistance

Equipment: wheelchair or chair, mechanical or hydraulic lift, washcloth

Before performing this procedure, check the weight limit of the lift to make sure the resident is within the weight limit. Make sure you know how to use the lift.

1. Identify yourself by name. Identify the resident. Greet the resident by name.

2. Wash your hands.

3. Explain procedure to resident. Speak clearly, slowly, and directly. Maintain face-to-face contact whenever possible.

4. Provide for the resident's privacy with a curtain, screen, or door.

5. Lock bed wheels.

6. Remove wheelchair footrests close to the bed. Position wheelchair next to bed. Lock wheelchair brakes.

7. The farthest side rail should be raised (if bed has one). Lower side rail nearest you if it is up. Help the resident turn to one side of the bed, away from you. Pad the sling where the neck will rest with a washcloth for resident's comfort. A sheet may be used over the sling to protect it from soiling. Position the sling under the resident, with the edge next to the resident's back. Fanfold if possible. Make the bottom of the sling even with the resident's knees (some slings only come to the top of the buttocks). Help the resident roll to his opposite side. Spread out the fanfolded edge of the sling, then roll him back to the middle of the bed.

8. Roll the mechanical lift to bedside. Make sure the base is opened to its widest point. Push the base of the lift under the bed. Lock lift wheels.

9. Place the overhead bar directly over the resident. Be careful so the bar does not hit anyone.

10. With the resident lying on his back, attach one set of straps to each side of the sling. Attach one set of straps to the overhead bar (Fig. 11-32). Have a co-worker support the resident at the head, shoulders, and knees while being lifted. The resident's arms should be folded across his chest. If the device has

"S" hooks, they should face away from resident. Make sure all straps are connected properly.

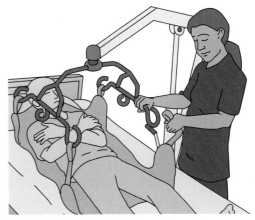
Fig. 11-32. Attach straps to overhead bar.

11. Following manufacturer's instructions, raise the resident two inches above the bed. Pause a moment for the resident to regain stability or balance. Unlock lift wheels.

12. Have co-worker support and guide the resident's body (Fig. 11-33). You can then move the lift so that the resident is positioned over the chair or wheelchair.

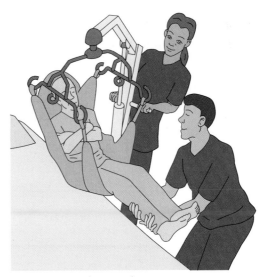
Fig. 11-33. Make sure that one person supports and guides the resident's body to help prevent injury.

13. Slowly lower the resident into the chair or wheelchair. Push down gently on the resident's knees to help the resident into a sitting position.

14. Undo the straps from the overhead bar. Leave the sling in place for transfer back to bed (some slings can be easily removed when resident is seated).

15. Be sure the resident is seated comfortably and correctly in the chair or wheelchair. Put non-skid footwear on resident and fasten. Replace footrests. Cover the resident with a lap cover or robe if he requests it.

16. Remove privacy measures.

17. Leave call light within resident's reach.

18. Wash your hands.

19. Be courteous and respectful at all times.

20. Report any changes in the resident to the nurse. Document procedure using facility guidelines.

Toilet Transfers

The toilet is better than a bedpan or a urinal for eliminating urine. The bladder tends to empty more completely when using the toilet or portable commode because of the position of the person over the toilet. Chapter 15 has more information on bedpan and urinal use.

Ask residents often if they need to use the bathroom. Take them to the bathroom as soon as they request a trip. When a call light is pressed, respond immediately.

For a resident to be able to use a toilet, he must be able to bear some weight on his legs. Falls can occur on the way to the bathroom, during toileting, or on the way back to bed or chair. Do not leave residents alone if you feel it is unsafe or if residents require assistance.

Transferring a resident onto and off a toilet

Equipment: gloves, toilet tissue, wheelchair, non-skid shoes

1. Identify yourself by name. Identify the resident. Greet the resident by name.

2. Wash your hands.

3. Explain procedure to resident. Speak clearly, slowly, and directly. Maintain face-to-face contact whenever possible.

4. Provide for the resident's privacy with a curtain, screen, or door.

5. Position wheelchair at a right angle to the toilet to face the hand bar/wall rail. Place wheelchair on the resident's stronger side.

6. Remove wheelchair footrests. Lock wheels. Put non-skid footwear on resident. Fasten securely.

7. Put on gloves. Ask resident to push against the armrests of the wheelchair and stand, reaching for and grasping the hand bar with her stronger arm (Fig. 11-34). Move wheelchair out of the way.

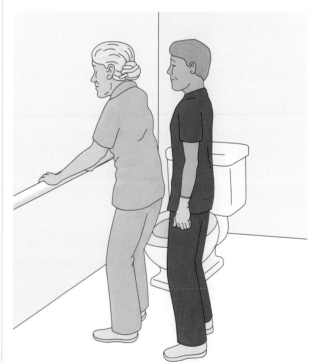

Fig. 11-34. *Ask the resident to push up using the armrests of the wheelchair, stand and grasp the hand bar. Stand behind her in case she needs help.*

8. Ask resident to pivot her feet and back up so that she can feel the front of the toilet with the back of her legs (Fig. 11-35).

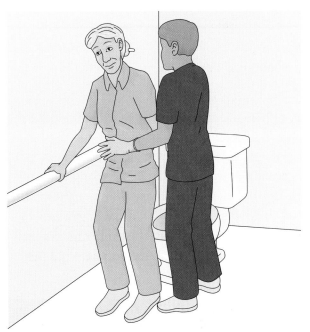

Fig. 11-35. Have the resident pivot and feel the toilet with the back of her legs. Assist as needed.

9. Help resident to pull down underwear and pants.

10. Help resident to slowly sit down onto the toilet. Allow privacy unless resident cannot be left alone. Ask resident to pull on the emergency cord if she needs help. Close bathroom door. Stay near the door until resident is finished.

11. When the resident is finished, assist with perineal care as necessary (see Chapters 12 and 16). Ask her to stand and reach for the hand bar.

12. Use toilet tissue or damp cloth to clean the resident. Make sure she is clean and dry before pulling up clothing. Remove and discard gloves.

13. Help resident to the sink to wash hands.

14. Wash your hands.

15. Help resident back into wheelchair. Be sure the resident is seated comfortably and correctly in the wheelchair. Replace footrests.

16. Help resident to leave the bathroom.

17. Leave call light within resident's reach.

18. Wash your hands.

19. Be courteous and respectful at all times.

20. Report any changes in the resident to the nurse. Document procedure using facility guidelines.

Vehicle Transfers

When a resident is discharged from a facility, you may need to help him or her into a vehicle. The front seat of the vehicle is wider and is usually easier to get into. Remember that your responsibility does not end until the resident is safely inside the vehicle and the door is closed.

Transferring a resident into a vehicle

Equipment: wheelchair, cart with personal belongings, co-worker

1. Identify yourself by name. Identify the resident. Greet the resident by name.

2. Wash your hands.

3. Explain procedure to resident. Speak clearly, slowly, and directly. Maintain face-to-face contact whenever possible.

4. Place wheelchair close to the vehicle at a 45-degree angle. Open the door on the resident's stronger side, if possible.

5. Lock wheelchair.

6. Ask the resident to push against the arm rests of the wheelchair and stand.

7. Ask the resident to stand, grasp the vehicle or dashboard, and pivot his foot so the side of the seat touches the back of the legs.

8. The resident should then sit in the seat and lift one leg, and then the other, into the vehicle (Fig. 11-36).

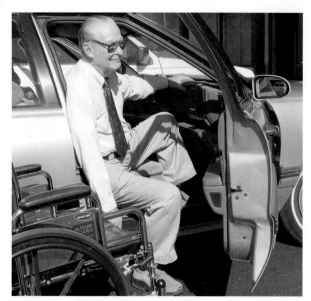

Fig. 11-36. *After resident sits in the vehicle seat, he should put his legs in one at a time.*

9. Position the resident comfortably in the vehicle. Help fasten seat belt.

10. Have co-worker place belongings in vehicle. Safely shut the door(s).

11. Return the wheelchair to the appropriate place for cleaning.

12. Wash your hands.

13. Document procedure using facility guidelines.

For more information on transferring residents recovering from a hip replacement or stroke, see Chapters 21 and 22.

5. Discuss ambulation

Ambulation means walking. A resident who is ambulatory can get out of bed and walk. Residents should ambulate to maintain independence and prevent problems. Regular ambulation and exercise are very important and help to improve these things:

- Quality and health of the skin
- Circulation
- Strength
- Sleep and relaxation
- Appetite
- Elimination
- Oxygen level

Residents should only walk for short distances, especially if the person is just starting to ambulate. Over time, the distance may be increased. Residents may require a transfer or gait belt and/or more than one staff member to ambulate safely. Follow the nurse's instructions and the care plan.

Assisting a resident to ambulate

Equipment: gait belt, non-skid footwear

1. Identify yourself by name. Identify the resident. Greet the resident by name.

2. Wash your hands.

3. Explain procedure to resident. Speak clearly, slowly, and directly. Maintain face-to-face contact whenever possible.

4. Provide for the resident's privacy with a curtain, screen, or door.

5. Adjust the bed to the lowest position so that the resident's feet are flat on the floor. Lock the bed wheels.

6. Put non-skid footwear on resident. Fasten securely.

7. Help resident move to a dangling position, as described in earlier procedure.

8. Stand in front of and face the resident. Stand with feet about shoulder-width apart. Bend your knees. Keep your back straight.

9. *With gait belt*: Place belt below the rib cage and above the waist. Do not put it over bare skin. Check to make sure that breasts are not caught under the belt. Grasp the belt on both sides.

Without gait belt: Place arms around the resident's torso under the arms, but not in the armpits.

10. With your legs, brace resident's lower legs to prevent slipping. This can be done by placing both of your knees in front of the resident's knees.

11. On the count of three, slowly help resident to stand.

12. **With gait belt**: Walk slightly behind and to one side of resident for the full distance, while holding onto the gait belt (Fig. 11-37). If the resident has a weaker side, stand on the weaker side. Ask resident to look forward, not down at floor, during ambulation. If resident becomes dizzy or faint, help him to a nearby seat and call nurse for help.

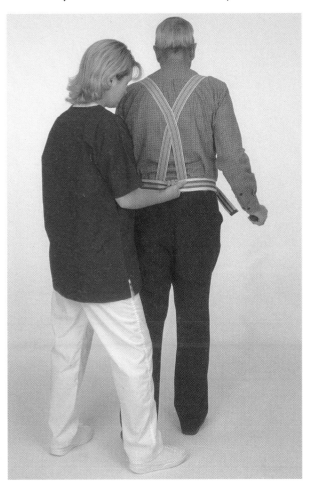

Fig. 11-37. Walk slightly behind, standing on the weaker side, when assisting a resident to ambulate. Hold onto the gait belt, if used, for the full distance.

Without gait belt: Walk slightly behind and to one side of resident for the full distance. Support resident's back with your arm. Ask resident to look forward, not down at floor, during ambulation. If resident becomes dizzy or faint, help him to a nearby seat and call nurse for help.

13. After ambulation, make resident comfortable. Remove gait belt, if used.

14. Return bed to lowest position. Remove privacy measures.

15. Leave call light within resident's reach.

16. Wash your hands.

17. Be courteous and respectful at all times.

18. Report any changes in the resident to the nurse. Document procedure using facility guidelines.

When helping a visually-impaired resident walk, let the person walk beside and slightly behind you, as he rests a hand on your elbow. Walk at a normal pace. Let the person know when you are about to turn a corner, or when a step is approaching. Tell him whether you will be stepping up or down.

For more information on assisting with ambulation for a resident using a walker, cane, or crutches, see Chapter 25.

Chapter Review

1. How does proper body alignment benefit the human body (LO 2)?

2. Why should a nursing assistant face what she is lifting (LO 2)?

3. In what position should a nursing assistant be before lifting an object (LO 2)?

4. Should objects be lifted by using muscles in the legs or the back (LO 2)?

5. Explain why objects should be kept close to the body when carrying them (LO 2).

6. Why should regular turning schedules always be maintained (LO 3)?

7. Briefly describe what each of the following positions are: supine, lateral, prone, Fowler's, and Sims' (LO 3).

8. What is the benefit of using a draw sheet when repositioning (LO 3)?

9. Define "logrolling" (LO 3).

10. During dangling, what should the nursing assistant do if the resident feels faint (LO 3)?

11. For a resident with one weak side and one strong side, which side should move first and why (LO 4)?

12. What is a transfer, or gait, belt (LO 4)?

13. When moving a resident down a ramp in a wheelchair, in which direction should the resident be facing (LO 4)?

14. Why is it important to use mechanical lifts if they are available (LO 4)?

15. What must a resident be able to do in order to use the toilet (LO 4)?

16. List six benefits of regular ambulation (LO 5).

12
Personal Care

1. Define important words in this chapter

additive: a substance added to another substance, changing its effect.

axilla: underarm or armpit area.

bridge: a type of dental appliance that replaces missing or pulled teeth.

dandruff: excessive shedding of dead skin cells from the scalp.

dentures: artificial teeth.

edema: swelling in body tissues caused by excess fluid.

edentulous: lacking teeth; toothless.

gingivitis: an inflammation of the gums.

grooming: practices to care for oneself, such as caring for fingernails and hair.

halitosis: bad-smelling breath.

hygiene: methods of keeping the body clean.

partial bath: bath that includes washing the face, underarms, hands, and perineal area.

pediculosis: an infestation of lice.

plaque: a substance that accumulates on the teeth from food and bacteria.

tartar: hard deposits on the teeth that are filled with bacteria; may cause gum disease and loose teeth if they are not removed.

2. Explain personal care of residents

Good hygiene is important to good health. **Hygiene** is the term used to describe methods of keeping the body clean. Good grooming helps keep a person clean and healthy as well. **Grooming** includes practices like fingernail, foot, and hair care. Hygiene and grooming, along with other personal care tasks, are called activities of daily living (ADLs). ADLs include grooming, dressing, bathing, eating and drinking, transferring, and elimination. Nursing assistants help residents every day with their ADLs.

The type of daily care you provide for residents depends on what shifts you work at the facility. Care will vary according to what time of day it is. Bathing usually happens in the morning; however, it can be done in the evening, depending on residents' preferences and facility policy. Care done in the mornings is called "a.m. care" and care done in the evenings is "p.m. care."

Assisting with a.m. care includes the following:

- Taking resident to the bathroom, offering a bedpan, urinal, or an incontinent brief change, helping with perineal care, if needed, and washing resident's hands

- Helping with mouth care or denture care before and/or after breakfast, as the resident prefers

- Assisting with washing face and hands in bed, shower room, or in bathroom

- Changing resident's gown, pajamas, or clothing

- Providing breakfast and fluids

- Assisting with bathing, as the resident prefers

- Helping resident with shaving, hair care, hand and fingernail care, foot care, and cosmetics (Fig. 12-1)

- Making the bed and tidying resident's room

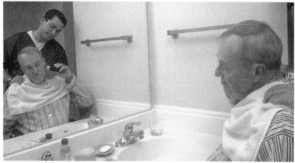

Fig. 12-1. Assisting residents with grooming, such as shaving, is part of a.m. care.

Assisting with p.m. care includes the following::

- Taking resident to the bathroom, offering bedpan or urinal, or an incontinent brief change and assisting with handwashing

- Helping with mouth care or denture care after lunch and dinner, as the resident prefers

- Providing lunch, dinner, snacks, and fluids; giving fresh drinking water

- Assisting the resident with bathing, if evening is preferable

- Giving a back massage

- Changing into resident's gown or pajamas

- Helping resident with hair care

- Assisting with washing face and removing makeup as needed

- Changing linens as needed and preparing the bed for the resident's return

- Tidying resident's room

The personal care you provide will depend upon the resident's needs and ability to care for himself. The way that you go about providing this care is important to residents' self-esteem and dignity. Promote self-care as much as possible. Encourage residents to perform tasks independently whenever they can. This may make some tasks, such as getting dressed, take longer. Be patient; residents should do as much as they are able to do, no matter how long it takes. In addition to promoting dignity and independence, doing self-care also helps keep the body functioning well.

It is very difficult to give up all or part of one's independence. Residents may never have needed help with bathing, dressing, or eating during their adult lives. Being required to accept help with these activities can cause anger, frustration, and sadness. Residents may be embarrassed by having someone, especially a member of the opposite sex, provide personal care. Be empathetic to the emotions residents are experiencing. Explain the care you are going to provide, and answer any questions the resident has. Let the resident make as many choices as possible about the care you will be performing (Fig. 12-2). Always provide privacy when giving personal care.

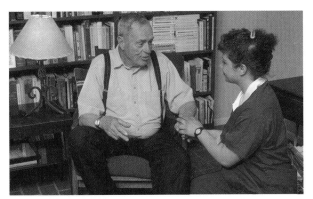

Fig. 12-2. Talk with residents about the care you are going to perform. Let them make as many decisions as possible about personal care.

Here are additional ways to provide respect and dignity when performing personal care tasks:

- Allow residents enough time to use the bathroom. Do not rush or interrupt them. It is a good idea to ask if a resident wants to use the bathroom or bedpan before beginning personal care.

- Assist with dressing as needed, but allow as much independence as possible. Provide for personal choice throughout care. Residents have the right to choose what they will wear, including jewelry. They can choose to wear cosmetics. Be patient while they make these decisions.

- Be patient while they perform care tasks. Encourage residents to do whatever they can for themselves.

- Be respectful if residents are using the phone or talking with visitors. Leave the room if they want privacy.

- Keep residents covered whenever possible when dressing and bathing.

- Promote residents' safety. Do not leave them alone during bathing. Do not rush them during care, as it may cause falls or other injuries. Always ask for help to perform personal care when you need it.

- Take the time to talk with residents during personal care. Report any changes, concerns, or problems you notice to the nurse.

3. Describe different types of baths and list observations to make about the skin during bathing

There are four basic types of baths: a partial bath, a shower, a tub bath, and a complete bed bath. The type of bath given is determined first by the resident's needs and abilities and then by the resident's preference.

A **partial bath**, also called a set-up bath, includes washing the face, underarms, hands, and the perineal (genital and anal) area. It is best suited to a resident who:

- Has drier, fragile, and more sensitive skin

- Should not have daily full baths

- Is unable to get up to take a shower or tub bath

- Wants a quick bath before a meal and plans on taking a shower or bath later in the day

A shower is best suited to a resident who:

- Is able to stand during a shower

- Is able to safely sit in a shower chair

A tub bath can take place in a regular bathtub or in a special tub, such as a whirlpool. It is best suited to a resident who:

- Is able to transfer into and out of a tub

- Has a doctor's order for a special bath using an **additive**—a substance added to another substance, changing its effect—to the tub water; examples of bath additives are bran, oatmeal, sodium bicarbonate, and epsom salts

A complete bed bath is best suited to a resident who:

- Is unable to get out of bed to shower or bathe and requires a full bath

The decision about which bath to give a resident rests first with the doctor or nurse, then with the resident. For example, a doctor may write an order for "no shower" until a wound has healed. Some residents are confined to bed, which prevents them from getting up for a tub bath or a shower. Some residents do not shower for personal reasons; they may simply prefer a tub bath because they have always taken baths at home. Discuss residents' preferences and decisions regarding bathing with the nurse prior to giving care.

Personal care and bathing give you the opportunity to carefully observe for changes in residents or their skin (Fig. 12-3). This is especially important in the prevention of pressure ulcers, a serious skin wound caused by skin breakdown. You will learn more about pressure ulcers and prevention in Chapter 18.

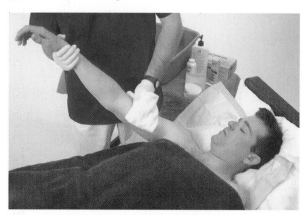

Fig. 12-3. *Every time you bathe residents, closely observe their skin for any changes. Report changes promptly to the nurse.*

Residents may discuss health problems and issues during personal care. They may also bring up personal concerns regarding staff, family, or friends. Listen to residents closely and report concerns or observations to the nurse.

Some of the things to observe for and report during personal care and bathing include:

Observing and Reporting: Personal Care and Bathing

- O/R Change in size of one or both pupils
- O/R Difference in appearance from one eye to another
- O/R Yellow or red color in whites of the eyes

- O/R Changes in vision, ability to hear, and sense of smell
- O/R Drooping on one side of the face
- O/R Weight loss
- O/R Drainage coming from any area, including eyes, ears, nipples, or genitals
- O/R Foul odors from any body area
- O/R Pale, blue-tinged (cyanotic), white, reddened, or purple areas on the skin
- O/R Dry, flaky, broken, or cracked skin
- O/R Lumps or bumps on the skin
- O/R Moles or spots on the skin, especially those that are red, white, yellow, dark brown, gray, or black
- O/R Rashes or any skin discoloration
- O/R Bruises
- O/R Blisters
- O/R Cuts, scrapes, or scratches
- O/R Open sores or ulcers on any area of the body
- O/R Changes in open sore, wound, or ulcer (color, size, drainage, odor, overall depth of sore)
- O/R Swelling/edema of any area, especially the knuckles, fingers, groin, abdomen, legs, ankles, or feet (**edema** is swelling in body tissues caused by excess fluid)
- O/R Poor condition of fingernails or toenails
- O/R Nails in need of trimming
- O/R Dry, cracked, or broken skin in between toes or toenails
- O/R Itching or scratching
- O/R Change in emotional state
- O/R Change in level of mobility
- O/R Complaints of pain or discomfort
- O/R Stiff neck
- O/R Numbness, burning, warmth, or tingling in the extremities or other areas of the body

4. Explain safety guidelines for bathing

Safety must be the highest priority when bathing residents. Many accidents happen in the bathroom or shower room. Assess the area for any risks before bathing a resident. Follow these guidelines for safety:

Guidelines: Safety for Bathing

G   Make sure you can perform this procedure alone. If you need help, ask for it. Do not try to bathe a resident alone if you do not believe you can handle the task safely.

G   Know any special orders for bathing. Follow the care plan.

G   Clean showers, tubs, and all equipment before and after use, per facility policy.

G   Make sure the floor in the shower or tub room is dry. Wipe up any spills or wet areas.

G   Place nonslip mats in regular tubs. A slippery tub may cause falls.

G   Check to see that hand rails and grab bars are secure and in proper working order. Encourage weak and unsteady residents to use safety bars to get into and out of tubs or showers.

G   Gather all needed equipment before entering the shower area. Be organized. Place needed items within easy reach.

G   Bath oils, gels, and talcum powder can create slippery surfaces and can put residents at risk of falling. Avoid using these items.

G   Make sure that water temperature is not too hot for residents. Comfortable temperature varies for each person. Water temperature should not be over 105°F. Check water temperature with a bath thermometer or on your wrist. Then have the resident test water himself.

G   Put away electrical appliances when they are not in use. Do not use electrical appliances near a water source.

G   Do not leave residents alone while bathing or showering.

5. List the order in which body parts are washed during bathing

When bathing a person, it is important to follow a specific order. This reduces the risk of transferring microorganisms from a dirty area to a clean area of the body. The general rule is to wash from cleanest to dirtiest. For example, you will wash the face before washing the buttocks. The correct order of washing parts of the body is listed below and shown in the illustration (Fig. 12-4):

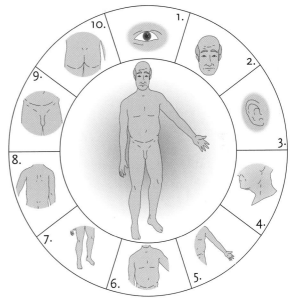

Fig. 12-4. *The parts of the body have corresponding numbers that show the exact order to complete a bed bath. Following this order helps prevent the transfer of microorganisms from a dirty area to a clean area of the body.*

1.   Eyes

2.   Face

3.   Ears

4.   Neck

5.   Arms, **axilla** (axillae), and hands

6. Chest and abdomen

7. Legs and feet

8. Back

9. Perineal area

10. Buttocks

6. Explain how to assist with bathing

Regular bathing provides many benefits. It promotes good health and hygiene. Bathing increases circulation, especially for bed-bound residents. Bathing also provides an opportunity to observe the skin.

The face, underarms, hands, and perineal area should be bathed every day. Perineal care is care of the genital and anal area. People with fragile, dry skin may not be bathed every day. Bathing only a couple of times per week will help prevent further dryness. In some facilities, complete baths are done on certain days of the week. Follow bathing schedules and care plans carefully. In addition, follow these guidelines:

Guidelines: Bathing

G   If using a tub or shower room for bathing, clean and prepare the room, and gather all equipment before moving the resident there.

G   Make sure the room is warm enough before starting a bath or shower.

G   Make sure the water temperature is comfortable. The resident should help choose a proper and comfortable water temperature. Comfortable temperature is different for each person.

G   Wear gloves while bathing a resident and change gloves before performing perineal care.

G   Make sure all soap residue is removed. This prevents further drying and irritation of the skin.

G   When preparing to do perineal care, make sure residents understand the care you are going to provide. Get a translator if necessary. More information on perineal care is in Chapter 16.

G   During the bath, you will have the chance to observe residents closely. You should check the skin carefully every time you bathe residents. Review the list of items to observe and report in Learning Objective 3.

Giving a complete bed bath

Equipment: bath blanket, bath basin, soap, bath thermometer, 2-4 washcloths, 2-4 bath towels, clean gown or clothes, 2 pairs of gloves, lotion, deodorant, orangewood stick or emery board

1. Identify yourself by name. Identify the resident. Greet the resident by name.

2. Wash your hands.

3. Explain procedure to resident. Speak clearly, slowly, and directly. Maintain face-to-face contact whenever possible.

4. Provide for the resident's privacy with a curtain, screen, or door. Be sure the room is at a comfortable temperature and there are no drafts.

5. Adjust bed to safe working level, usually waist high. Lock bed wheels.

6. Place a bath blanket or towel over resident. Ask him to hold onto it as you remove or fold back top bedding (Fig. 12-5). Remove gown, while keeping resident covered with bath blanket (or top sheet).

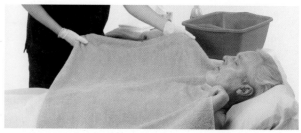

Fig. 12-5. Cover the resident with a bath blanket before removing top bedding.

7. Fill the basin with warm water. Test water temperature with thermometer or your wrist and ensure it is safe. Water temperature should not be over 105°F. It cools quickly. Have resident check water temperature. Adjust if necessary. Change the water when it becomes too cool, soapy, or dirty.

8. Put on gloves.

9. Ask the resident to participate in washing. Help him do this whenever needed.

10. Uncover only one part of the body at a time. Place a towel under the body part being washed.

11. Wash, rinse, and dry one part of the body at a time. Start at the head. Work down, and complete the front first. When washing, use a clean area of the washcloth for each stroke.

   Eyes, Face, Ears, Neck: Wash face with wet washcloth (no soap). Begin with the eye farther away from you. Wash inner area to outer area (Fig. 12-6). Use a different area of the washcloth for each eye. Wash the face from the middle outward. Use firm but gentle strokes. Wash the ears and behind the ears and the neck. Rinse and pat dry with blotting motion.

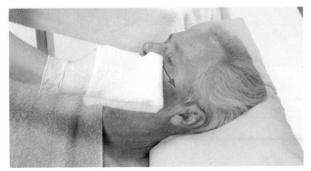

Fig. 12-6. Wash the eye from the inner part to the outer part.

   Arms and Axillae: Remove one arm from under the towel. With a soapy washcloth, wash the upper arm and underarm. Use long strokes from the shoulder to the wrist (Fig. 12-7). Rinse and pat dry. Repeat for the other arm.

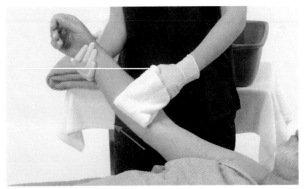

Fig. 12-7. Support the wrist while washing the shoulder, arm, underarm, and elbow.

   Hands: Wash the hand in a basin. Clean under the nails with an orangewood stick or nail brush (Fig. 12-8). Rinse and pat dry. Make sure to dry between the fingers. Give nail care (see procedure later in this chapter) if it has been assigned. Repeat for the other hand. Put lotion on the resident's elbows and hands if ordered.

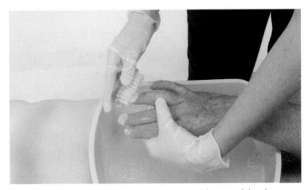

Fig. 12-8. Wash the hand in a basin. Thoroughly clean under the nails with a nail brush.

   Chest: Place the towel across the resident's chest. Pull the bath blanket down to the waist. Lift the towel only enough to wash the chest. Rinse it and pat dry. For a female resident, wash, rinse, and dry breasts and under breasts. Check the skin in this area for signs of irritation.

   Abdomen: Keep towel across chest. Fold the bath blanket down so that it still covers the genital area. Wash the abdomen, rinse, and pat dry. Cover with the towel. Pull the bath blanket up to the resident's chin. Remove the towel.

Legs and Feet: Expose one leg. Place a towel under it. Wash the thigh. Use long, downward strokes. Rinse and pat dry. Do the same from the knee to the ankle (Fig. 12-9).

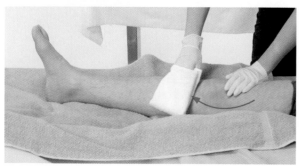

Fig. 12-9. *Use long, downward strokes when washing the legs.*

Place another towel under the foot. Move the basin to the towel. Place the foot into the basin. Wash the foot and between the toes (Fig. 12-10). Rinse foot and pat dry. Dry between toes. Give nail care if it has been assigned. Do not give nail care for a diabetic resident. Never clip a resident's toenails. Apply lotion to the foot if ordered, especially at the heels. Do not apply lotion between the toes. Repeat steps for the other leg and foot.

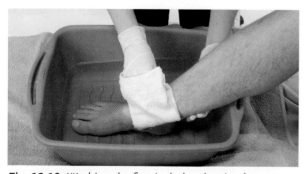

Fig. 12-10. *Washing the feet includes cleaning between the toes.*

Back: Help resident move to the center of the bed. Ask resident to turn onto his side so his back is facing you. If the bed has rails, raise the rail on the far side for safety. Fold the blanket away from the back. Place a towel lengthwise next to the back. Wash the back, neck, and buttocks with long, downward strokes (Fig. 12-11). Rinse and pat dry. Apply lotion if ordered.

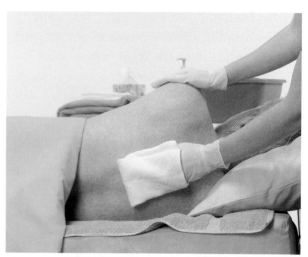

Fig. 12-11. *Wash the back with long, downward strokes.*

12. Place the towel under the buttocks and upper thighs. Help the resident turn onto his back. If the resident is able to wash his or her perineal area, place a basin of clean, warm water and a washcloth and towel within reach. Hand items to the resident as needed. If the resident wants you to leave the room, remove and discard gloves. Wash your hands. Leave supplies and the call light within reach. If the resident has a urinary catheter in place, remind him not to pull on it.

13. If the resident cannot provide perineal care, you will do so. Remove and discard your gloves. Wash your hands. Put on clean gloves. Make sure to provide privacy at all times.

14. **Perineal area and buttocks**: Change bath water. Wash, rinse, and dry perineal area. Work from front to back (clean to dirty).

For a female resident: Use water and a small amount of soap, and clean from front to back (Fig. 12-12). Use single strokes. Do not wash from the back to the front, as this may cause infection. Use a clean area of washcloth or clean washcloth for each stroke.

First separate the labia majora, the outside folds of perineal skin that protect the urinary meatus and the vaginal opening. The meatus is the opening of the female urethra that is above the vaginal opening. Clean from front to back on one side with a clean washcloth, using a single stroke. Using a clean area of washcloth, clean the other side. Clean the perineum (area between genitals and anus) last with a front to back motion. Rinse the area thoroughly in the same way. Make sure all soap is removed.

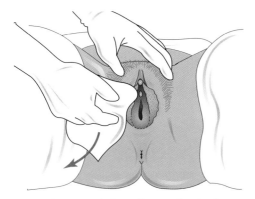

Fig. 12-12. Always work from front to back when performing perineal care. This helps prevent infection.

Dry entire perineal area. Move from front to back. Use a blotting motion with towel. Ask resident to turn on her side. Wash, rinse, and dry buttocks and anal area. Clean the anal area without contaminating the perineal area.

For a male resident: If the resident is uncircumcised, pull back the foreskin first. Gently push skin towards the base of penis. Hold the penis by the shaft. Wash in a circular motion from the tip down to the base (Fig. 12-13). Use a clean area of washcloth or clean washcloth for each stroke.

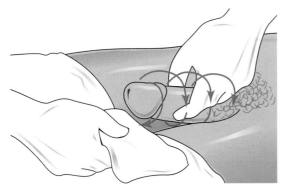

Fig. 12-13. Wash the penis in a circular motion from the tip down to the base.

Thoroughly rinse the penis. If resident is uncircumcised, gently return foreskin to normal position. Then wash the scrotum and groin. The groin is the area from the pubis (area around the penis and scrotum) to the upper thighs. Rinse thoroughly and pat dry. Ask the resident to turn on his side. Wash, rinse, and dry buttocks and anal area. Clean the anal area without contaminating the perineal area.

15. Empty, rinse, and dry bath basin. Place basin in designated dirty supply area or return to storage, depending on facility policy.

16. Place soiled clothing and linens in proper containers.

17. Remove and discard gloves.

18. Wash your hands.

19. Provide deodorant.

20. Put clean gown or clothes on resident. Assist with brushing or combing resident's hair (see procedure later in the chapter).

21. Remove bath blanket. Replace bedding. Make resident comfortable.

22. Return bed to lowest position. Remove privacy measures.

23. Leave call light within resident's reach.

24. Wash your hands.

25. Be courteous and respectful at all times.

26. Report any changes in the resident to the nurse. Document procedure using facility guidelines.

Partial Bath

A partial bath is performed on days when a complete bed bath, tub bath, or shower is not done. It usually includes washing the face, underarms, hands, and the perineal area. However, for testing purposes, nursing assistants are often asked to give a partial bath that may include other body parts than those listed here. Follow your facility's guidelines.

Shampooing a resident's hair in bed

Equipment: shampoo, hair conditioner (if requested), 2 bath towels, washcloth, bath thermometer, pitcher or handheld shower or sink attachment, waterproof pad, bath blanket, gloves, trough and catch basin, comb and brush, hair dryer

1. Identify yourself by name. Identify the resident. Greet the resident by name.

2. Wash your hands.

3. Explain procedure to resident. Speak clearly, slowly, and directly. Maintain face-to-face contact whenever possible.

4. Provide for the resident's privacy with a curtain, screen, or door. Be sure the room is at a comfortable temperature and there are no drafts.

5. Adjust bed to safe working level, usually waist high. Lock bed wheels.

6. Lower the head of bed. Remove pillow.

7. Test water temperature with thermometer or your wrist. Ensure it is safe. Water temperature should not be over 105°F. Have resident check water temperature. Adjust if necessary.

8. Put on gloves.

9. Place the waterproof pad under the resident's head and shoulders. Cover the resident with the bath blanket. Fold back the top sheet and regular blankets.

10. Place the trough under resident's head. Connect trough to catch basin. Place one towel across the resident's shoulders.

11. Protect resident's eyes with dry washcloth.

12. Use pitcher or attachment to wet hair thoroughly. Apply a small amount of shampoo, usually the size of a quarter.

13. Lather and massage scalp with fingertips. Use a circular motion from front to back (Fig. 12-14). Do not scratch the scalp.

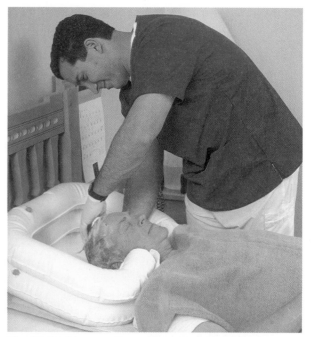

Fig. 12-14. *Use your fingertips to work shampoo into a lather. Be gentle so that you do not scratch the scalp.*

14. Rinse hair until water runs clear. Apply conditioner. Rinse as directed on container. Be sure to rinse the hair thoroughly to prevent the scalp from getting dry and itchy.

15. Wrap resident's hair in a clean towel. Dry his face with washcloth used to protect eyes. Gently rub the scalp and hair with the towel.

16. Remove trough and waterproof covering.

17. Empty, rinse, and wipe bath basin/pitcher. Return to proper storage.

18. Place soiled linen in proper container.

19. Remove and discard gloves. Wash your hands.

20. Raise head of bed.

21. Dry and comb resident's hair as he or she prefers. See procedure later in the chapter. Return hair dryer and comb/brush to proper storage.

22. Make resident comfortable.

23. Return bed to lowest position. Remove privacy measures.

24. Leave call light within resident's reach.

25. Wash your hands.

26. Be courteous and respectful at all times.

27. Report any changes in the resident to the nurse. Document procedure using facility guidelines.

Shampooing at the Sink

Some residents will have their hair shampooed at a sink. Seat the resident in a chair that is the correct height for the sink. Pad the edge of the sink so that the neck is comfortable. The resident's head should be tilted back slightly; the head should not be sharply extended beyond its normal range. Carefully spray water over the hair, taking care that the water and shampoo/conditioner do not get into the eyes. Rinse the hair thoroughly.

When assisting a resident on a stretcher with shampooing hair, bring the stretcher to the sink and adjust the height of the stretcher to be even with the sink. Lock the stretcher wheels and fasten safety straps. Raise one side rail on the side farthest from you. Follow the same guidelines as listed above.

Before giving a tub bath or shower, check the room for cleanliness and clean if needed. Pre-fill the tub with warm water and place all needed clean supplies and equipment in the room. Be sure to keep the door closed and the resident covered whenever possible (Fig. 12-15).

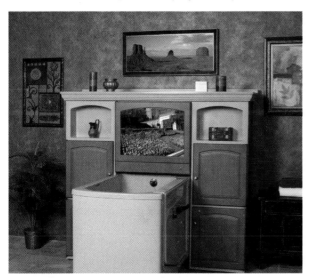

Fig. 12-15. *A common style of tub used in long-term care facilities.* (PHOTO COURTESY OF LEE PENNER OF PENNER TUBS)

Giving a shower or tub bath

Equipment: bath blanket, soap, shampoo, bath thermometer, 2-4 washcloths, 2-4 bath towels, clean gown and robe or clothes, non-skid footwear, 2 pairs of gloves, lotion, deodorant

1. Wash your hands.

2. Place equipment in shower or tub room. Put on gloves. Clean shower or tub area and shower chair.

3. Remove and discard gloves.

4. Wash your hands.

5. Go to resident's room. Identify yourself by name. Identify the resident. Greet the resident by name.

6. Explain procedure to resident. Speak clearly, slowly, and directly. Maintain face-to-face contact whenever possible.

7. Provide for the resident's privacy with a curtain, screen, or door.

8. Help resident to put on non-skid footwear. Transport resident to shower or tub room.

For a shower:

9. If using a shower chair, place it into position and lock its wheels. Safely transfer resident into shower chair (Fig. 12-16).

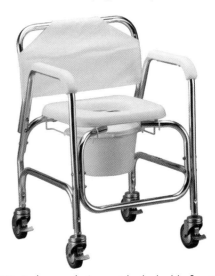

Fig. 12-16. *A shower chair must be locked before transferring a resident into it.* (PHOTO COURTESY OF NOVA MEDICAL PRODUCTS, WWW.NOVAMEDICALPRODUCTS.COM)

10. Turn on water. Test water temperature with thermometer. Water temperature should be no more than 105°F. Have resident check water temperature. Adjust if necessary. Check water temperature frequently throughout the shower.

For a tub bath:

9. Safely transfer resident onto chair or tub lift.

10. Fill the tub halfway with warm water. Test water temperature with thermometer. Water temperature should be no more than 105° F. Have resident check water temperature.

Remaining steps for either procedure:

11. Put on clean gloves.

12. Help resident remove clothing and shoes.

13. Help the resident into shower or tub. Put shower chair into shower and lock wheels.

14. Stay with resident during the entire procedure.

15. Let resident wash as much as possible on his or her own. Help to wash his or her face.

16. Help resident shampoo hair. The resident's head should be tilted back slightly for the shampoo. The head should not be extended beyond its normal range. Carefully spray water over the hair, taking care that the water and shampoo/conditioner do not get into the eyes. Rinse the hair thoroughly.

17. Help to wash and rinse the entire body. Move from head to toe (clean to dirty).

18. Turn off water or drain the tub. Cover resident with bath blanket until the tub drains.

19. Unlock shower chair wheels if used. Roll resident out of shower, or help resident out of tub and onto a chair.

20. Give resident towel(s) and help to pat dry. Remember to pat dry under the breasts, between skin folds, in the perineal area, and between toes.

21. Place soiled clothing and linens in proper containers.

22. Remove and discard gloves.

23. Wash your hands.

24. Apply lotion and deodorant as needed. Help resident dress and comb hair before leaving shower or tub room (see procedures later in this chapter). Put on non-skid footwear. Return resident to room.

25. Make resident comfortable.

26. Leave call light within resident's reach.

27. Wash your hands.

28. Be courteous and respectful at all times.

29. Report any changes in the resident to the nurse. Document procedure using facility guidelines.

After returning resident to his room, return to shower room, and clean and disinfect the shower or tub area, as well as the shower chair. Wear heavy-duty gloves and follow facility policy. After this is complete, remove and discard gloves and wash your hands.

Some residents will have whirlpool baths. These baths are special baths in which the water moves around the tub. The water movement helps clean the body, improve circulation, and promote wound healing. To take a whirlpool bath, the resident must first be covered and kept warm. He will need to be safely transported to the whirlpool bath site. The resident will be placed in a chair lift and lowered into the whirlpool bath.

If you assist with this bath, do not leave a resident alone, even for a few seconds. Whirlpool baths can cause a person to become dizzy or feel faint. If this happens, you may need to remove the resident from the bath.

Help as needed during the bath, and do not rush the resident. Afterwards, safely transport the resident back to his room, assist with dressing, and make sure he is comfortable. Then return to the bath site and clean and disinfect the chair and the whirlpool bath using heavy-duty gloves. Remove gloves. Wash your hands.

7. Describe how to perform a back rub

Back rubs help relax tired, tense muscles and improve circulation. Back rubs are often given after bathing or prior to going to bed at night. They may also be given regularly to relieve pain or discomfort. Sometimes back rubs should not be given due to conditions or illnesses. Follow the care plan. If the resident has broken or open skin on his back, apply gloves before giving a back rub.

Giving a back rub

Equipment: bath blanket or towel, lotion

1. Identify yourself by name. Identify the resident. Greet the resident by name.

2. Wash your hands.

3. Explain procedure to resident. Speak clearly, slowly, and directly. Maintain face-to-face contact whenever possible.

4. Provide for the resident's privacy with a curtain, screen, or door.

5. Adjust bed to safe working level, usually waist high. Lower the head of the bed. Lock bed wheels.

6. Position resident lying on his side (lateral position) or his stomach (prone position). Many elderly residents find lying on their stomachs uncomfortable. If so, have him lie on his side. Cover with a bath blanket. Expose back to the top of the buttocks. Back rubs can also be given with the resident sitting up.

7. Warm lotion by putting bottle in warm water for five minutes. Run your hands under warm water. Pour lotion on your hands. Rub them together. Always put lotion on your hands rather than directly on resident's skin.

8. Place hands on each side of upper part of the buttocks. Use the full palm of hand. Make long, smooth upward strokes with both hands. Move along each side of the spine, up to the shoulders (Figs. 12-17 and 12-18). Circle hands outward. Move back along outer edges of the back. At buttocks, make another circle. Move hands back up to the shoulders. Without taking hands from resident's skin, repeat this motion for three to five minutes.

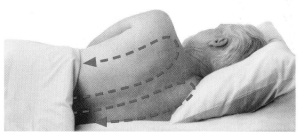

Fig. 12-17. *A resident can be placed on his side or on his stomach for a back rub.*

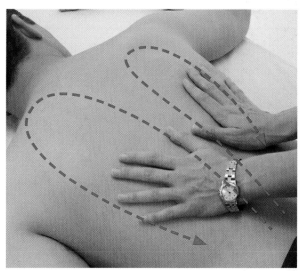

Fig. 12-18. *Long upward strokes help release muscle tension.*

9. Knead with the first two fingers and thumb of each hand. Place them at base of the spine. Move upward together along each side of the spine. Apply gentle downward pressure with fingers and thumbs. Follow same direction as with the long smooth strokes, circling at shoulders and buttocks.

10. Gently massage bony areas (spine, shoulder blades, hip bones). Use circular motions of fingertips. Do not massage any pale, white, or red areas.

11. Finish with long, smooth strokes.

12. Dry the back if it has extra lotion remaining.

13. Remove bath blanket. Help the resident to get dressed. Make resident comfortable.

14. Return bed to lowest position. Remove privacy measures.

15. Store supplies. Place soiled clothing and linens in proper containers.

16. Leave call light within resident's reach.

17. Wash your hands.

18. Be courteous and respectful at all times.

19. Report any changes in the resident to the nurse, including pale, white or red areas. Document procedure using facility guidelines.

8. Explain guidelines for performing good oral care

The methods used to care for the mouth, teeth, and gums are called oral care. Oral care must be provided at least twice a day, but some residents will need or want this care more often. Oral care consists of brushing the teeth, tongue, and gums, flossing, caring for lips, and caring for dentures (Fig. 12-19). Care for the lips includes applying lip moisturizer and observing and reporting any problems with the lips. You will learn more about dentures in the next learning objective.

Regular oral care helps prevent gum disease and bad-smelling breath, or **halitosis**. A healthy mouth also promotes a healthy appetite, which can prevent unintended weight loss, a serious problem with the elderly. Oral care may also reduce the risk of certain respiratory infections.

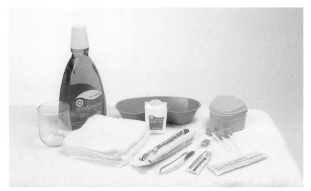

Fig. 12-19. *Some supplies needed for oral care.*

Plaque is a substance that accumulates on the teeth from food and bacteria. Plaque can turn into hard deposits, called tartar, if left on the teeth too long. **Tartar** is filled with bacteria and may cause gum disease and loose teeth if they are not removed by a dentist. **Gingivitis** is an inflammation of the gums. This can lead to periodontal disease when the areas supporting the teeth, such as the gums, become diseased. When you give oral care, observe the resident's mouth and teeth to help prevent these and other problems.

Sometimes a problem that is discovered in the mouth is a sign that a bigger problem exists elsewhere in the body. For example, a person who has fruity breath may have diabetes (see Chapter 23). Observing and reporting signs and symptoms is very important in treating illnesses and preventing them from getting worse.

During oral care, observe the mouth carefully.

Observing and Reporting: Oral Care

Report any of the following to the nurse:

O/R Dry, cracked, bleeding, or chapped lips

O/R Cold sores on the lips

O/R Raised areas

O/R Swollen, irritated, red, bleeding, or whitish gums

O/R Loose, cracked, chipped, broken, or decayed teeth

○/ᴿ Yellow-filled or red sores, such as canker sores inside the mouth

○/ᴿ White spots inside the mouth

○/ᴿ Pus or drainage

○/ᴿ Coated or swollen tongue

○/ᴿ Bad breath or fruity-smelling breath

○/ᴿ Change in the resident's ability to drink, suck on a straw, or swallow

○/ᴿ Gagging or choking

○/ᴿ Resident reports mouth pain

Always wear gloves when giving oral care. Keep toothbrushes and toothpaste separate and labeled. Do not share these items between residents. Follow Standard Precautions.

Tip

Gum Health

Take care of your residents' gums (and your own) by giving proper, regular oral care. Studies have shown a possible link between gum disease and the risk of having heart disease, a stroke, and diabetes. In addition, cranberries have been shown to reduce bacterial growth on gum tissue and to limit gum disease. Cranberry extract is being added to some toothpastes.

Providing oral care

Equipment: toothbrush, toothpaste, emesis basin, gloves, towel, glass of water

Maintain clean technique with placement of toothbrush throughout procedure.

1. Identify yourself by name. Identify the resident. Greet the resident by name.

2. Wash your hands.

3. Explain procedure to resident. Speak clearly, slowly, and directly. Maintain face-to-face contact whenever possible.

4. Provide for the resident's privacy with a curtain, screen, or door.

5. Adjust bed to safe working level, usually waist high. Lock bed wheels. Make sure resident is sitting upright.

6. Put on gloves.

7. Place towel across resident's chest.

8. Wet brush. Apply toothpaste.

9. Clean entire mouth (including tongue and all surfaces of teeth and the gumline) using gentle strokes. First brush inner, outer and chewing surfaces of the upper teeth, then do the same with the lower teeth. Use short strokes. Brush back and forth.

10. Hold emesis basin to the resident's chin.

11. Have resident rinse mouth with water and spit into emesis basin (Fig. 12-20).

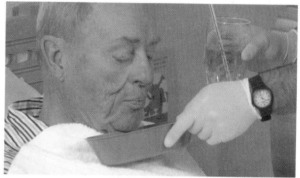

Fig. 12-20. *Rinsing and spitting removes food particles and toothpaste.*

12. Wipe resident's mouth and remove towel.

13. Empty, rinse and wipe emesis basin. Rinse toothbrush. Return supplies to proper storage.

14. Dispose of soiled linen in the proper container.

15. Remove and discard gloves. Wash your hands.

16. Make resident comfortable.

17. Return bed to lowest position. Remove privacy measures.

18. Leave call light within resident's reach.

19. Wash your hands.

20. Be courteous and respectful at all times.

21. Report any changes in the resident to the nurse. Report any problems with teeth, mouth, tongue, or lips to nurse. This includes odor, cracking, sores, bleeding, and any discoloration. Document procedure using facility guidelines.

Tip

Edentulous Residents

The term for lacking teeth or being toothless is **edentulous**. Giving oral care to an edentulous resident is similar to caring for a resident who has teeth. You will clean the outside and inside of the mouth, including the lips, top and bottom gums and gumlines, and the inside of the mouth with a moistened swab. Make sure to clean the tongue, too. Change swabs as needed.

A resident who can brush his own teeth will only need a little assistance. The nursing assistant may need to do the following:

- Collect and set up supplies
- Cover the overbed table
- Raise the head of bed
- Provide a bath towel for the chest
- Pour fresh water and mouthwash
- Help with cleaning the face and neck
- Remove the towel, overbed table cover, and all supplies
- Empty, clean, and store supplies

Encourage the resident to do as much self-care as possible. Only help the resident with what he cannot do on his own. Remove your gloves and wash your hands when you are finished.

Flossing teeth

Equipment: floss, cup with water, emesis basin, gloves, towel

1. Identify yourself by name. Identify the resident. Greet the resident by name.

2. Wash your hands.

3. Explain procedure to resident. Speak clearly, slowly, and directly. Maintain face-to-face contact whenever possible.

4. Provide for the resident's privacy with a curtain, screen, or door.

5. Adjust bed to safe working level, usually waist high. Lock bed wheels. Make sure resident is in an upright sitting position.

6. Put on gloves.

7. Wrap the ends of floss securely around each index finger (Fig. 12-21).

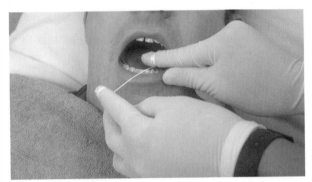

Fig. 12-21. *Before beginning, wrap floss securely around each index finger.*

8. Starting with the back teeth, place floss between teeth. Move it down the surface of the tooth. Use a gentle sawing motion (Fig. 12-22).

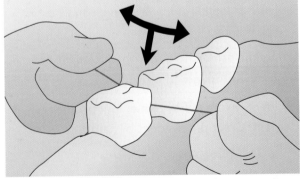

Fig. 12-22. *Floss teeth gently. Being gentle protects the gums.*

Continue to the gum line. At the gum line, curve the floss. Slip it gently into the space between the gum and tooth. Then go back up, scraping that side of the tooth (Fig. 12-23). Repeat on the side of the other tooth.

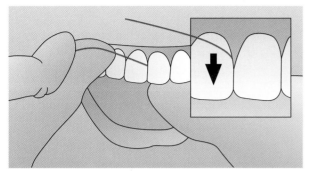

Fig. 12-23. *Floss gently in the space between the gum and tooth. This removes food and prevents tooth decay.*

9. After every two teeth, unwind floss from your fingers. Move it so you are using a clean area. Floss all teeth.

10. Offer water to rinse the mouth. Ask the resident to spit it into the basin.

11. Offer resident a face towel when done.

12. Discard floss. Empty basin into the toilet. Clean and store basin and supplies.

13. Dispose of soiled linen in the proper container.

14. Remove and discard gloves. Wash your hands.

15. Make resident comfortable.

16. Return bed to lowest position. Remove privacy measures.

17. Leave call light within resident's reach.

18. Wash your hands.

19. Be courteous and respectful at all times.

20. Report any changes in the resident to the nurse. Report any problems with teeth, mouth, tongue, or lips to nurse. This includes odor, cracking, sores, bleeding, and any discoloration. Document procedure using facility guidelines.

9. Define "dentures" and explain care guidelines

Dentures are artificial teeth. There are different types of dentures. A person may have a full set of dentures, a top or bottom set of dentures, a partial plate, or a bridge. A **bridge** is a type of dental appliance that replaces missing teeth. A bridge may be permanently placed in the mouth or it may be removable for cleaning.

Dentures are very expensive and time-consuming for a specialist to make. Handle dentures carefully. They are important to residents. If residents' dentures break, they cannot eat.

Always wear gloves when cleaning dentures. The type of cleaning product used will depend on the resident's preference or facility policy. After cleaning dentures, store them in a covered denture cup with the resident's name on it. Make sure you match the dentures to the correct resident. Dentures must always be stored in lukewarm water so that they do not dry out and warp. Dentures may crack if left uncovered.

Cleaning and storing dentures

Equipment: denture brush or toothbrush, denture cleanser or tablet, labeled denture cup with cover, 2 towels, gauze squares, gloves, cup with water, emesis basin, denture cream or adhesive (if replacing dentures in mouth)

Maintain clean technique with placement of dentures and toothbrush throughout procedure.

1. Identify yourself by name. Identify the resident. Greet the resident by name.

2. Wash your hands.

3. Explain procedure to resident. Speak clearly, slowly, and directly. Maintain face-to-face contact whenever possible. Encourage resident to assist if possible.

4. Provide for the resident's privacy with a curtain, screen, or door.

5. Adjust bed to safe working level, usually waist high. Lock bed wheels. Make sure resident is in an upright sitting position.

6. Put on gloves.

7. Line sink/basin with a towel(s) and partially fill sink with water. This prevents dentures from breaking if dropped. Handle dentures carefully.

8. If you are allowed to do so, and if a resident cannot remove dentures, you will do it.

9. Remove the lower denture first. The lower denture is easier to remove because it floats on the gum line of the lower jaw. Grasp the lower denture with a gauze square (for a good grip) and remove it. The upper denture is sealed by suction. Firmly grasp the upper denture with a gauze square. Give a slight downward pull to break the suction. Turn it at an angle to take it out of the mouth.

10. Rinse dentures in tepid/lukewarm running water before brushing them. Do not use hot water. Hot water may warp or damage dentures.

11. Apply toothpaste or cleanser to toothbrush.

12. Brush the dentures on all surfaces (Fig. 12-24). This includes the inner, outer, and chewing surfaces of the upper and lower dentures.

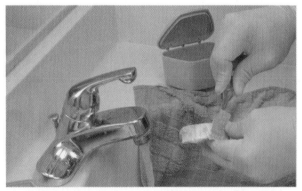

Fig. 12-24. Brush dentures on all surfaces to properly clean them.

13. Rinse all surfaces of dentures under tepid/lukewarm running water. Do not use hot water.

14. Offer water to rinse the resident's mouth. Ask the resident to spit it into the emesis basin.

15. Rinse denture cup if placing clean dentures inside it.

16. Place dentures in clean denture cup with special solution or lukewarm water and cover. Make sure cup is labeled with resident's name. Return denture cup to storage.

17. Some residents will want to wear their dentures all of the time. They will only want them removed for cleaning. If replacing dentures in resident's mouth, make sure resident is still sitting upright. Apply denture cream or adhesive to the dentures, if needed. When the resident's mouth is open, place upper denture into the mouth by turning it at an angle. Straighten it. Press it onto the upper gum line firmly and evenly (Fig. 12-25). Insert the lower denture onto the gum line of the lower jaw. Press firmly.

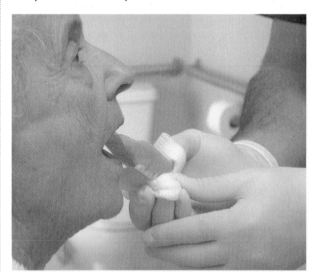

Fig. 12-25. Press upper denture onto the upper gum line firmly and evenly.

18. Clean, dry, and return the equipment to proper storage.

19. Dispose of soiled linen in the proper container and drain sink.

20. Remove and discard gloves. Wash your hands.

21. Make resident comfortable.

22. Return bed to lowest position. Remove privacy measures.

23. Leave call light within resident's reach.

24. Wash your hands.

25. Be courteous and respectful at all times.

26. Report any changes in the resident or the appearance of dentures to the nurse. Document procedure using facility guidelines.

10. Discuss guidelines for performing oral care for an unconscious resident

Oral care must be done frequently when a person is unconscious. The mouth becomes dry due to lack of oral fluids, breathing through the mouth, and oxygen therapy. Crusts called sordes can develop on the lips, gums, and teeth. These contain microorganisms, certain types of cells, mucus, and food. Good oral care keeps the mouth clean and moist and removes sordes.

Aspiration is the primary risk for unconscious residents. Aspiration is the inhalation of food, fluid, or foreign material into the lungs; it can cause pneumonia or death. Using as little liquid as possible during oral care is the best way to prevent aspiration. Turning unconscious residents on their side before beginning oral care can also help prevent aspiration. In addition, only swabs soaked in tiny amounts of fluid should be used to clean the mouth. Follow the care plan. Chapter 14 has more information on aspiration.

Providing oral care for the unconscious resident

Equipment: sponge swabs, tongue depressor, towel, emesis basin, gloves, lip lubricant, cleaning solution (check the care plan)

1. Identify yourself by name. Identify the resident. Greet the resident by name. Even residents who are unconscious may be able to hear you. Always speak to them as you would to any resident.

2. Wash your hands.

3. Explain procedure to resident. Speak clearly, slowly, and directly. Maintain face-to-face contact whenever possible.

4. Provide for the resident's privacy with a curtain, screen, or door.

5. Adjust bed to a safe level, usually waist high. Lock bed wheels.

6. Put on gloves.

7. Turn resident on his side or turn head to the side. Place a towel under his cheek and chin. Place an emesis basin next to the cheek and chin for excess fluid.

8. Hold mouth open with tongue depressor. Do not use your fingers to open the mouth or keep it open.

9. Dip swab in cleaning solution. Squeeze excess solution to prevent aspiration. Wipe inner, outer, and chewing surfaces of the upper and lower teeth, gums, tongue, and inside surfaces of mouth (Fig. 12-26). Change swab often. Repeat until the mouth is clean.

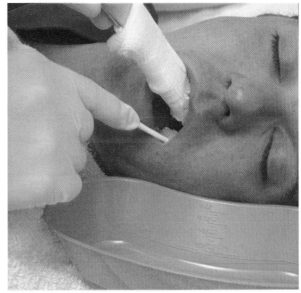

Fig. 12-26. *Wipe all inside surfaces of the mouth to clean the mouth, stimulate the gums, and remove mucus.*

10. Rinse with clean swab dipped in water. Squeeze swab first to remove excess water.

11. Remove the towel and basin. Pat lips or face dry. Apply lip lubricant.

12. Clean and return supplies to proper storage.

13. Dispose of soiled linen in the proper container.

14. Remove and discard gloves. Wash your hands.

15. Make resident comfortable.

16. Return bed to lowest position. Remove privacy measures.

17. Leave call light within resident's reach.

18. Wash your hands.

19. Be courteous and respectful at all times.

20. Report any changes in the resident to the nurse. Report any problems with teeth, mouth, tongue, or lips to nurse. This includes odor, cracking, sores, bleeding, and any discoloration. Document procedure using facility guidelines.

Unconscious Residents

Even when people are unconscious they still may be able to hear what is going on around them. Unconscious people have been known to regain consciousness and relate many of the things they heard while they were unconscious. Limit your discussions to the care you are providing. Speak respectfully and explain what you are doing. Do not talk to others while giving care. Speak to unconscious residents as you would to any resident.

An unconscious resident's eyes require special care because they can become dry. The blink reflex is usually absent, leading to drier eyes. The air around the person also contributes to dryness. If you assist in eye care for an unconscious resident, follow these guidelines:

Guidelines: Eye Care for Unconscious Residents

G Use gloves when bathing the eyes.

G If using a washcloth, rinse it thoroughly before cleaning the opposite eye. If using cotton balls, use a clean cotton ball for one eye and then dispose of it. Do not use the same cotton ball to clean both eyes.

G Wipe from the inner area of the eye to the outer area of the eye when cleaning (Fig. 12-27). This helps prevent harmful deposits from being pushed into the tear duct at the inner corner of the eye.

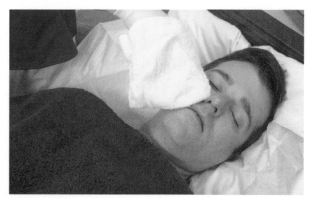

Fig. 12-27. When cleaning the eyes, move from the inner area to the outer area.

G Use moist compresses on the eyes, as directed.

G Special lubricant may need to be applied to the eyes. Follow the care plan.

11. Explain how to assist with grooming

Grooming is a very important part of the activities of daily living (ADLs). Each day, some residents will require help with brushing and styling their hair, shaving, dressing, caring for fingernails, and applying makeup and jewelry.

Appearance has a great deal to do with the way people feel about themselves. Good grooming can have a positive effect on self-esteem, attitude, and independence (Fig. 12-28). A well-groomed person is also likely to feel better physically because she is clean and neatly dressed.

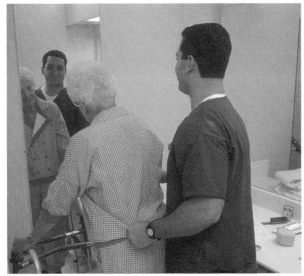

Fig. 12-28. A well-groomed appearance helps people feel good about themselves.

When assisting residents with grooming, make sure they do whatever they can for themselves. Promote self-care and independence whenever possible. Follow their preferences and routines, as well as the care plan. Residents may be depressed, angry, or embarrassed about the help they need to perform these tasks. Be sensitive and empathetic.

Shaving

Shaving is a very important part of the daily grooming routine. Wear gloves when shaving residents due to the risk of bleeding. Glove use promotes infection prevention. Follow Standard Precautions and avoid nicks and cuts.

Guidelines: Shaving

G   Some residents will not want to be shaved. Respect personal preferences for shaving.

G   Wash and comb beards and mustaches every day after asking the resident how he would like it done. Never trim or shave a beard or mustache without the resident's permission.

G   Always wear gloves when shaving.

G   When using safety or disposable razors, soften hair on face first with a warm, wet cloth.

G   Always shave in the direction of the hair growth.

G   Use shaving products, such as after-shave, only with resident's permission.

G   Carefully discard any disposable shaving products in the biohazard container.

G   Razors must never be used on more than one resident. Do not share razors.

Types of razors are electric razors, disposable razors, and safety razors. An electric razor is the safest and easiest type of razor to use. It does not require soap or shaving cream and may help prevent nicks and cuts. Do not use an electric razor near water or any water source, where oxygen is in use, or on a resident who has a pacemaker.

A safety razor requires that shaving cream, lotion or soap be used. These razors are usually very sharp. Safety razors have a special safety casing to help prevent cuts. The blades need to be changed periodically. When changing blades, handle them carefully. Dispose of the old blade in a sharps container.

Disposable razors are used with shaving cream, lotion, or soap. They can be extremely sharp and must be used carefully. Discard disposable razors in a sharps container after use. Do not try to reapply the caps on these razors, as it can cause cuts.

Shaving a resident

Equipment: razor, basin filled halfway with warm water (if using a safety or disposable razor), washcloth, 2 towels, mirror, shaving cream or soap, gloves, after-shave lotion

1.   Identify yourself by name. Identify the resident. Greet the resident by name.

2.   Wash your hands.

3. Explain procedure to resident. Speak clearly, slowly, and directly. Maintain face-to-face contact whenever possible.

4. Provide for the resident's privacy with a curtain, screen, or door.

5. Adjust bed to safe working level, usually waist high. Lock bed wheels.

6. Raise head of bed so resident is sitting up. Place towel across the resident's chest, under his chin.

7. Put on gloves.

Shaving using a safety or disposable razor:

8. Soften the beard with a warm, wet washcloth on the face for a few minutes before shaving. Lather the face with shaving cream or soap and warm water.

9. Hold skin taut. Shave in direction of the hair growth. Shave beard in short, downward, and even strokes on face and upward strokes on neck (Fig. 12-29). Rinse the blade often in warm water to keep it clean and wet.

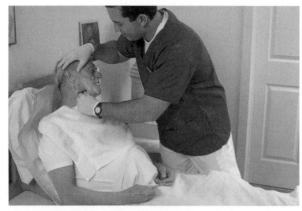

Fig. 12-29. *Holding the skin taut, shave in downward strokes on face and upward strokes on neck.*

10. When you have finished, wash, rinse, and dry the resident's face with a warm, wet washcloth. If he is able, let him use the washcloth himself. Offer mirror to resident.

Shaving using an electric razor:

8. Use a small brush to clean razor, if necessary. Do not use an electric razor near any water

source, when oxygen is in use, or if resident has a pacemaker.

9. Turn on the razor and hold skin taut. Shave with smooth, even movements. Shave beard with back and forth motion in direction of beard growth with foil shaver. Shave beard in circular motion with three-head shaver. Shave the chin and under the chin.

10. Offer mirror to resident.

Final steps:

11. Apply after-shave lotion as resident wishes.

12. Remove the towel and place towel and washcloth in proper container.

13. Clean equipment and store it. **For safety razor**: rinse the razor and store it. **For disposable razor**: dispose of it in a sharps container. Do not recap razor. **For electric razor**: clean head of razor. Remove whiskers from razor. Recap shaving head. Return razor to case.

14. Remove and discard gloves. Wash your hands.

15. Make sure that there are no loose hairs. Make resident comfortable.

16. Return bed to lowest position. Remove privacy measures.

17. Leave call light within resident's reach.

18. Wash your hands.

19. Be courteous and respectful at all times.

20. Report any changes in the resident to the nurse. Document procedure using facility guidelines.

If assisting a woman with shaving, do not shave any facial or body hair she wants to keep. For example, some women do not shave their underarms or legs. Do not judge a resident's personal preferences for shaving. When shaving underarms, be gentle. Be careful to avoid nicks and cuts. Shave in the direction of hair growth.

Nail Care

Proper grooming includes regular nail care. Fingernails can collect and harbor microorganisms. In addition, long and ragged nails can easily scratch residents, visitors, and staff. Washing and cleaning the nails is a part of the bathing process.

Fingernail care usually requires the use of an orangewood stick. These small sticks are made of wood and help clean under the nails. If you use an orangewood stick, be gentle to avoid injuring the resident. Emery boards are used for filing the nails. Nail files can tear fragile skin around the nail and must be used carefully.

Do not cut a resident's toenails. Problems with circulation can lead to a serious infection if skin is accidentally cut while caring for the nails. For a resident who has diabetes (Chapter 23), an infection can lead to a severe wound or even amputation. Follow the care plan. Never use the same nail equipment on more than one resident.

Providing fingernail care

Equipment: orangewood stick, emery board, basin, soap, gloves, washcloth, 2 towels, bath thermometer

1. Identify yourself by name. Identify the resident. Greet the resident by name.

2. Wash your hands.

3. Explain procedure to resident. Speak clearly, slowly, and directly. Maintain face-to-face contact whenever possible.

4. Provide for the resident's privacy with a curtain, screen, or door.

5. If the resident is in bed, adjust bed to safe working level, usually waist high. Lock bed wheels.

6. Fill the basin halfway with warm water. Test water temperature with thermometer or your wrist. Ensure it is safe. Water temperature should not be over 105°F. Have resident check water temperature. Adjust if neces-

sary. Place basin at a comfortable level for resident.

7. Put on gloves.

8. Soak the resident's nails in the basin of water. Soak all 10 fingertips for at least five minutes.

9. Remove hands. Wash hands with soapy washcloth. Rinse. Pat hands dry with towel, including between fingers. Remove the hand basin.

10. Place resident's hands on the towel. Gently clean under each fingernail with orangewood stick (Fig. 12-30).

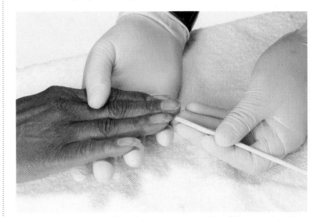

Fig. 12-30. *Be gentle when removing dirt from under the nails with an orangewood stick.*

11. Wipe orangewood stick on towel after each nail. Wash resident's hands again. Dry them thoroughly, especially between fingers.

12. Shape nails with file or emery board. File in a curve. Finish with nails smooth and free of rough edges.

13. Empty, rinse, and wipe basin. Place basin in proper area for cleaning or clean and store it according to policy.

14. Dispose of soiled linen in the proper container.

15. Remove and discard gloves. Wash your hands.

16. Make resident comfortable.

17. Return bed to lowest position. Remove privacy measures.

18. Leave call light within resident's reach.

19. Wash your hands.

20. Be courteous and respectful at all times.

21. Report any changes in the resident to the nurse. Document procedure using facility guidelines.

Tip

Cosmetics

Cosmetics or makeup are items used to enhance beauty or clean and improve the face, skin, hair, and nails. Women usually use them more, although some men use them. Help to apply cosmetics as residents request. The application of makeup, including type and amount, should be based on residents' wishes. However, if staff note too much makeup on a resident, gentle suggestions may be offered.

Information on foot care is in the section on diabetes in Chapter 23.

Hair Care

Daily hair care affects the way residents look and feel about themselves. NAs help keep residents' hair clean and styled. It is important to allow residents to choose their own hairstyles. Use hair ornaments only as requested. Do not comb or brush residents' hair into childish styles.

Be very gentle when handling residents' hair. Hair usually thins as people age. Pieces of hair can be pulled out of the head while combing or brushing the hair. Also, the skin on an elderly person's head is fragile. Be careful when working with hair.

Do not cut residents' hair. Many facilities have a barber, beautician, and/or professional hairstylist available to residents. If residents make a hair appointment, help them get ready to go.

Dandruff is a skin condition in which dry, white flakes appear on the scalp and hair due to shedding of dead skin from the scalp. Itching can accompany the white flakes. Causes of dandruff include the following:

- Climate, especially dry, cold areas

- Stress

- Excessive sweating

- A type of fungus

- Hormonal changes

- Some types of dermatitis (inflammation of the skin)

Dandruff can be controlled by using a medicated dandruff shampoo regularly.

Combing or brushing hair

Equipment: comb, brush, towel, mirror, hair care items requested by resident

Use hair care products that the resident prefers for his or her type of hair.

1. Identify yourself by name. Identify the resident. Greet the resident by name.

2. Wash your hands.

3. Explain procedure to resident. Speak clearly, slowly, and directly. Maintain face-to-face contact whenever possible.

4. Provide for the resident's privacy with a curtain, screen, or door.

5. If the resident is in bed, adjust bed to safe working level, usually waist high. Lock bed wheels.

6. Raise head of bed so resident is sitting up. Place a towel under the head or around the shoulders.

7. Remove any hair pins, hair ties and clips.

8. Remove tangles first by dividing hair into small sections. Gently comb out from ends

of hair to roots. Be careful not to break hair or cause any discomfort.

9. After tangles are removed, brush two-inch sections of hair at a time. Brush from ends to roots (Fig. 12-31).

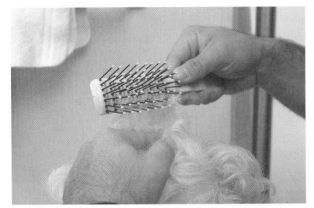

Fig. 12-31. Gently brush hair after tangles are removed.

10. Neatly style hair as resident prefers. Avoid childish hairstyles. Each resident may prefer different styles and different hair products. Offer mirror to resident.

11. Make resident comfortable.

12. Return bed to lowest position. Remove privacy measures.

13. Return supplies to proper storage. Clean hair from brush/comb. Clean comb and brush.

14. Dispose of soiled linen in the proper container.

15. Leave call light within resident's reach.

16. Wash your hands.

17. Be courteous and respectful at all times.

18. Report any changes in the resident to the nurse. Document procedure using facility guidelines.

Pediculosis is the medical term for an infestation of lice. Lice are tiny parasites that attach their eggs to the skin or the hair. Lice are very hard to see with the eye alone. Parts of the body that may have lice infestation include the head, the pubic area (area on and around the genitals), and other areas of the body, such as the underarms.

Symptoms of lice include intense itching, scratching, and scratch marks or rashes on the scalp, neck, or body. Lice eggs can be seen on the hair, behind the ears, and on the neck. The eggs are small and round. They are brown before they hatch and white to light brown after hatching. Lice droppings may be visible on sheets or pillows. They look like a fine black powder.

If you note any of these symptoms, report them to the nurse immediately. Lice can spread very quickly. The resident's roommates, spouse, partner, and family and friends may also need to be checked for lice.

Lice can be transmitted through sharing personal items, such as combs, brushes and clothing. They can also be transmitted by sexual contact or sleeping in the same bed with someone who has lice. Do not share residents' combs, brushes, clothing, hats, scarves, caps, wigs, and hairpieces. Lice can be eliminated by using special shampoo, creams, lotions and sprays. Hot water must be used on bed linens and clothing to remove lice. Many items that cannot be washed can be put into a large plastic bag that is tightly sealed. After two weeks, the items can be removed, cleaned, and reused.

Another common skin infestation is scabies. See Chapter 18 for more information on scabies.

Dressing and Undressing

Dressing and undressing residents is an important part of daily care. Residents may have one side of the body that is weaker than the other side due to stroke or injury. This side is called the "weaker," "affected," or "involved" side. Do not refer to it as the "bad side" or use the terms "bad leg" or "bad arm." When dressing residents, always begin with the weaker side of the body to reduce the risk of injury.

The acronym POW can be used to help you remember to put clothing on the weak side first.

Put

On

Weak

Do the opposite when removing clothing. Begin with the stronger, or unaffected, side first when undressing.

Treat residents' clothing carefully when dressing and/or undressing residents. They may have clothing that is very meaningful to them.

Guidelines: Dressing

G   Encourage residents to be as independent as possible when dressing and undressing. Dressing and undressing can increase muscle strength, stimulate circulation, and may help promote self-esteem.

G   Additional time is needed when residents dress themselves. Do not rush them through this process.

G   Make sure all clothing is marked with the resident's name, if policy at your facility.

G   Be careful when handling residents' clothing. Request that clothing be mended when rips or tears are noted.

G   Allow residents to choose their own clothing. Encourage use of regular clothing during the day, not nightwear or pajamas.

G   Clothing should fit the resident well. Report if clothing is too tight, too loose, or too long. Clothing that is too long can get caught under a resident's feet and increases the risk of falls.

G   Always provide privacy when dressing or undressing residents. Cover residents at all times. Do not expose any more than what is necessary.

G   Apply clothing to the weaker, or affected side first (Fig. 12-32).

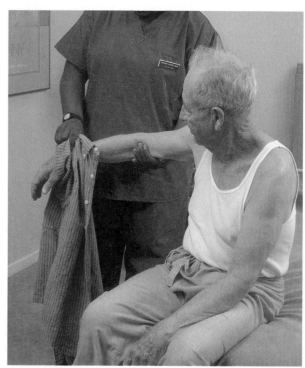

Fig. 12-32. When dressing residents, start with the affected (weaker) side first.

G   Be gentle with the feet and legs when applying socks or stockings. Report to the nurse if socks are too tight. Smooth both socks to remove wrinkles and twists.

G   Bras should fit female residents properly. Breasts should fit inside the bra cups. Assist females with putting on bras if needed. A bra that fastens in the front can be easier for residents to put on by themselves. Bras that fasten in the back can be applied more easily if wrapped around the waist, fastened and then rotated around to the proper position. Put arms through straps last.

G   Slacks, pants, and skirts that have elastic waists are easier to get on and off. Waistbands should fit comfortably and not be twisted. Belts, if used, should not be too tight.

G   Use special dressing aids, called assistive or adaptive devices, whenever needed. These help residents dress themselves (Fig. 12-33). See Chapter 25 for more information on assistive devices.

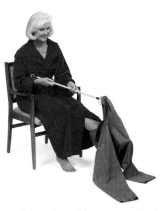

Fig. 12-33. *Special dressing aids promote independence by helping residents dress themselves.* (PHOTO COURTESY OF NORTH COAST MEDICAL, INC., WWW.NCMEDICAL.COM, 800-821-9319)

Dressing a resident

Equipment: clean clothes of resident's choice, non-skid footwear

When putting on all items, move resident's body gently and naturally. Avoid force and over-extension of limbs and joints.

1. Identify yourself by name. Identify the resident. Greet the resident by name.

2. Wash your hands.

3. Explain procedure to resident. Speak clearly, slowly, and directly. Maintain face-to-face contact whenever possible.

4. Provide for the resident's privacy with a curtain, screen, or door.

5. Ask resident what she would like to wear (Fig. 12-34). Dress her in outfit of choice.

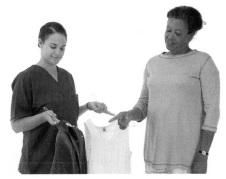

Fig. 12-34. *Encourage residents to choose what they want to wear. This promotes their independence, as well as their legal right to choose.*

6. Remove resident's gown. Do not completely expose resident. Take clothes off stronger, or unaffected, side first when undressing. Then remove from weaker side.

7. Gather up sleeve to ease pulling over affected arm. Insert your hand through sleeve and grasp resident's hand to support arm while dressing. Assist resident to put the affected/ weaker arm through the sleeve of the shirt, sweater, or slip before placing garment on the unaffected/stronger arm.

8. Help resident to put on skirt, pants, or dress. Put the affected/weak leg through skirt or pants first. Raise the buttocks or turn resident from side to side to draw pants over the buttocks up to waist.

9. Place bed at the lowest position. Lock bed wheels.

10. Have resident sit down. Pull up socks until they are both smooth and without wrinkles. Put on non-skid footwear. Fasten securely.

11. Finish with resident dressed appropriately. Make sure clothing is right-side out and zippers/buttons are fastened. Make sure skirt, pants, or dress is not caught under resident's shoes.

12. Make resident comfortable. Remove privacy measures.

13. Place gown in soiled linen container.

14. Leave call light within resident's reach.

15. Wash your hands.

16. Be courteous and respectful at all times.

17. Report any changes in the resident to the nurse. Document procedure using facility guidelines.

Remember when undressing residents to remove clothing from the stronger, or unaffected, side first.

Tip

Dressing Residents with IVs

When a resident has an IV, you may need to help him or her dress and undress. Remove the clothing starting with the stronger, or unaffected, side. In this case, the unaffected side is the side without the IV. Slowly pull off clothing, sliding it over the tubing. Lift the IV bag off the hook and pull the garment over the bag (Fig. 12-35). Do not pull on or catch the tubing in the clothing. Keep the IV bag above the IV site at all times. Hang the bag back on the hook.

Put on clothing by starting with the weaker, or affected side. In this case the affected side is the side with the IV. Lift the bag off of the hook, and slide the clean clothing over the bag. Hang the bag back on the hook. Gently pull the clothing over the tubing and the arm. Pull the clothing over the other arm and secure clothing. Check to make sure that the tubing is not kinked after you are finished. If you note the IV is not dripping, report to the nurse immediately. Ask the nurse to check the IV if you have concerns.

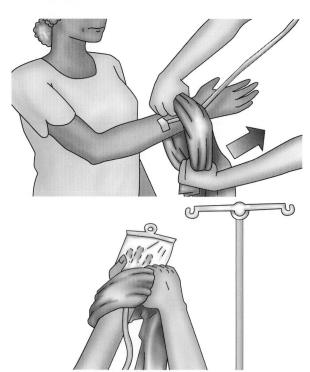

Fig. 12-35. *Pull clothing off slowly, and slide it over the tubing and then the bag.*

Chapter Review

1. Define the terms "hygiene" and "grooming" (LO 2).

2. List three ways nursing assistants can help promote residents' dignity when performing personal care (LO 2).

3. Explain what a partial bath is and list two reasons why it may be suitable for certain residents (LO 3).

4. Which serious skin wound can nursing assistants help prevent by observing residents' skin closely (LO 3)?

5. List 20 things that are important to observe for and report during personal care and bathing (LO 3).

6. In general, what should the water temperature be for bathing residents (LO 4)?

7. Why should the use of bath oils and gels be avoided when bathing residents (LO 4)?

8. List the correct order of washing parts of the body (LO 5).

9. How often should the perineal area be bathed (LO 6)?

10. Why should residents be involved in choosing a comfortable water temperature (LO 6)?

11. In the procedure "Giving a complete bed bath," step 9 states that nursing assistants should ask the resident to participate in washing. Why (LO 6)?

12. List three benefits of a whirlpool bath (LO 6).

13. What are two benefits of back rubs (LO 7)?

14. How often should oral care be performed (LO 8)?

15. List ten items to observe and report about oral care (LO 8).

16. Why is it important to handle dentures carefully (LO 9)?

17. Explain why hot water should not be used when cleaning dentures (LO 9).

18. What is the best way to prevent aspiration when performing oral care on unconscious residents (LO 10)?

19. Why should nursing assistants explain what they are doing when working with unconscious residents (LO 10)?

20. Should nursing assistants wear gloves when shaving residents? Why or why not (LO 11)?

21. In what circumstances should an electric razor not be used (LO 11)?

22. Why should nursing assistants not cut residents' toenails (LO 11)?

23. Why should nursing assistants be gentle when handling residents' hair (LO 11)?

24. In the section on hair care, it reads, "Do not comb or brush residents' hair into childish styles." Why should nursing assistants not do that (LO 11)?

25. Why is it important not to share personal items with residents who have lice (LO 11)?

26. When dressing and undressing residents, how should nursing assistants refer to the weaker side (LO 11)?

27. When dressing a resident, on which side should a nursing assistant start? When undressing a resident, on which side should a nursing assistant start (LO 11)?

13
Vital Signs

The Invention of the Stethoscope

In 1816, René Théophile Hyacinthe Laën-nec had difficulty hearing the heartbeat of a large-sized woman. He solved the problem creatively. Using a rolled-up piece of paper, he placed his ear to one end of the paper and placed the other end over the heart. He realized he could actually hear her heartbeat. This ability to hear the heartbeat so clearly was the beginning of what we now call the stethoscope.

"The same heart beats in every human breast."

Matthew Arnold, 1822-1888

"Once Antigones was told his son was ill, and went to see him. At the door he met some young beauty. Going in, he sat down by the bed and took his pulse. 'The fever,' said Demetrius, 'has just left me.' 'Oh, Yes,' replied the father, 'I met it going out at the door.'"

Plutarch, A.D. 46-120

1. Define important words in this chapter

apical pulse: the pulse on the left side of the chest, just below the nipple.

apnea: the absence of breathing.

BPM: the medical abbreviation for "beats per minute."

brachial pulse: the pulse inside the elbow; about 1 to 1½ inches above the elbow.

bradycardia: a slow heart rate—under 60 beats per minute.

Celsius: the centigrade temperature scale in which the boiling point of water is 100 degrees and the freezing point of water is 0 degrees.

Cheyne-Stokes respiration: type of respiration with periods of apnea lasting at least 10 seconds, along with alternating periods of slow, irregular respirations and rapid, shallow respirations.

diastolic: second measurement of blood pressure; phase when the heart relaxes.

dilate: to widen.

dyspnea: difficulty breathing.

eupnea: normal respirations.

expiration: the process of exhaling air out of the lungs.

Fahrenheit: a temperature scale in which the boiling point of water is 212 degrees and the freezing point of water is 32 degrees.

hypertension: high blood pressure, measuring 140/90 or higher.

hypotension: low blood pressure, measuring 100/60 or lower.

hypothermia: a condition in which body temperature drops below the level required for normal functioning; severe sub-normal body temperature.

inspiration: the process of inhaling air into the lungs.

orthopnea: shortness of breath when lying down that is relieved by sitting up.

orthostatic hypotension: a sudden drop in blood pressure that occurs when a person stands or sits up; also called postural hypotension.

prehypertension: a condition in which a person has a systolic measurement of 120–139 mm Hg and a diastolic measurement of 80–89 mm Hg; indicator that the person is likely to have high blood pressure in the future, even though he or she does not have it now.

radial pulse: the pulse on the inside of the wrist, where the radial artery runs just beneath the skin.

respiration: the process of inhaling air into the lungs (inspiration) and exhaling air out of the lungs (expiration).

sphygmomanometer: a device that measures blood pressure.

stethoscope: an instrument used to hear sounds in the human body, such as the heartbeat or pulse, breathing sounds, or bowel sounds.

systolic: first measurement of blood pressure; phase when the heart is at work, contracting and pushing blood out of the left ventricle.

tachycardia: a fast heartbeat—over 100 beats per minute.

tachypnea: rapid respirations—over 20 breaths per minute.

thermometer: a device used for measuring the degree of heat or cold.

vital signs: measurements (body temperature, pulse, respirations, blood pressure, and pain level) that monitor the function of the vital organs of the body.

2. Discuss the relationship of vital signs to health and well-being

The **vital signs** consist of body temperature, pulse, respirations, blood pressure, and pain level. Vital signs are important readings that monitor the function of the vital organs of the body. They can indicate whether the person is healthy or ill.

Checking residents' vital signs periodically during the day is an important nursing assistant task. Medical providers are always watching for signs of illness. The first sign that a person is ill may be a change in his or her vital signs. When one or more of the vital signs is too high or too low, it signals a potential health problem. This is why it is so important to accurately report changes in vital signs to the nurse.

You will learn more about how to take vital signs and factors that affect vital sign readings later in this chapter. See the box below for a list of ranges for vital signs.

Ranges for Adult Vital Signs

Temp. Site	Fahrenheit	Celsius
Oral	97.6° - 99.6°	36.5° - 37.5°
Rectal	98.6° - 100.6°	37.0° - 38.1°
Axillary	96.6°- 98.6°	36.0° - 37.0°

Normal Pulse Rate: 60-100 beats per minute
Normal Respiratory Rate: 12-20 respirations per minute

Blood Pressure
Normal
       Systolic: 100-119
       Diastolic: 60-79

Low
       Below 100/60

Prehypertensive
       Systolic: 120-139
       Diastolic: 80-89

High
       140/90 or above

Residents' Rights

Never guess on vital signs.

Vital sign measurements may be difficult to obtain. If you cannot get a measurement, do not guess. If you record a guess, it is not only illegal, but it may put a resident's life in danger. Nurses and doctors make decisions about care based on your reports. If you cannot obtain a proper reading, tell the nurse. Always be truthful and accurate in your reporting.

3. Identify factors that affect body temperature

Body temperature is controlled by the hypothalamus in the brain. The hypothalamus regulates body temperature by balancing the amount of heat the body makes with the amount of heat the body loses.

Body temperature averages 98.6°F (Fahrenheit) or 37°C (Celsius). A normal temperature is a sign of well-being. A high or low temperature may indicate a problem or an illness.

There are many factors that affect body temperature, including the following:

- **The person's age**: As a person ages, protective fatty tissue is lost. Elderly people are less able to prevent heat loss and may feel colder. Reduced blood circulation may also cause changes in body temperature (Fig. 13-1).

- **Amount of exercise**: Exercise helps increase body temperature due to the contraction of muscles that produce heat.

- **The circadian rhythm**: You first learned about the circadian rhythm, which is the 24-hour day-night cycle, in Chapter 10. Average temperature readings change during a 24-hour day. People may have lower average temperatures in the morning and higher temperatures in the late afternoon and evening.

- **Stress**: When a person is experiencing stress, certain hormones are released into the body. This hormonal shift may increase body temperature.

- **Illnesses**: Illnesses, such as infections, can increase body temperature. Some infections also cause dehydration, which is a serious condition in which a person does not have enough fluid in the body. When fluid levels are too low, body temperature may increase in response. Other illnesses, like diabetes, cause poor circulation and also affect body temperature.

- **Environment**: The temperature inside and outside influences body temperature. The elderly may become chilled or overheated easily. Adjusting the room temperature, layering clothing, and using blankets can help.

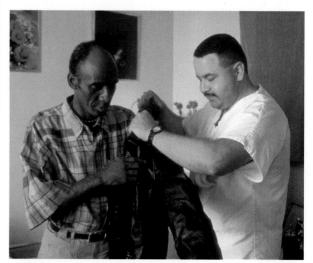

Fig. 13-1. *Elderly people usually have less fat and decreased circulation, which may make them feel colder.*

People may have body temperatures that are below normal. Sub-normal body temperatures are temperatures below 97°F. Some causes of sub-normal body temperature are infection, alcohol usage, diabetes, problems with the thyroid gland, or exposure to extreme cold. Severe sub-normal body temperature is called hypothermia. **Hypothermia** is a condition in which body temperature drops below the level required for normal functioning. It is a dangerous condition and can lead to death if not treated. Signs and symptoms of hypothermia must be reported to the nurse immediately:

- Shivering
- Numbness
- Quick and shallow breathing
- Slow movements
- Mild confusion
- Changes in mental status
- Pale and/or bluish (cyanotic) skin

Hypothermia is treated with specific warming techniques. Report sub-normal body temperatures to the nurse promptly.

An increase in body temperature may indicate an infection or disease. Signs and symptoms of a fever, in addition to the temperature reading, include headache, fatigue, muscle aches, and chills. Skin may feel warm and look flushed. Residents with darker skin tones who have a fever may show more subtle skin color changes.

If you suspect a fever, always take a temperature (see next Learning Objective). Fevers can develop quickly. It is possible to detect an infection early and prevent complications from occurring. Report fevers to the nurse immediately.

4. List guidelines for taking body temperature

Thermometers measure heat or cold in either degrees **Fahrenheit** (F) or **Celsius** (C). Fahrenheit and Celsius are two different scales that are used to measure temperature. The Fahrenheit scale is more common in the United States. In degrees Fahrenheit (F), each long line represents one degree and each short line represents two-tenths of a degree. In degrees Celsius (C), the long lines represent one degree and the short lines represent one-tenth of a degree (Fig. 13-2). In most other countries, the Celsius scale is used, along with the metric system of measurement.

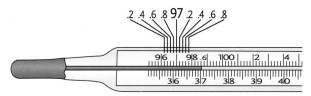

Fig. 13-2. This shows a normal temperature reading: 98.6°F and 37°C.

There are four main sites on the body for measuring a temperature: the mouth (oral), the rectum (rectal), the armpit (axillary), and the ear (tympanic). Taking a temperature orally is most common. A rectal temperature is considered to be the most accurate, while an axillary temperature is considered to be the least accurate.

Common types of thermometers are:

- Mercury-free
- Digital
- Electronic
- Disposable
- Tympanic
- Temporal artery

The mercury-free thermometer can be used to take an oral, rectal, or axillary temperature. Thermometers are usually color-coded to tell you which is an oral and which is a rectal thermometer. Oral thermometers are usually green or blue. Rectal thermometers are usually red (Fig. 13-3).

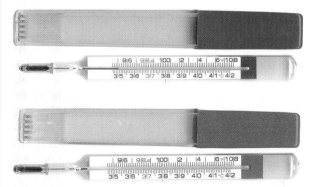

Fig. 13-3. A mercury-free oral thermometer and a mercury-free rectal thermometer. Oral thermometers are usually green or blue; rectal thermometers are usually red.
(PHOTOS COURTESY OF RG MEDICAL DIAGNOSTICS OF WIXOM, MI, RGMD.COM)

Digital thermometers can be used to take an oral, rectal, or axillary temperature. This thermometer displays results digitally. A digital thermometer usually takes two to 60 seconds to show the temperature. The thermometer will usually flash or beep when the temperature has registered. These models are battery-operated and require that the battery be replaced periodically. A digital thermometer requires the use of a disposable plastic sheath used to cover the probe (Fig. 13-4). This helps prevent infection. The sheath is used once and then disposed of in a facility-approved container.

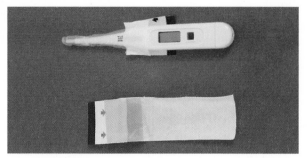

Fig. 13-4. *A digital thermometer with a disposable sheath cover underneath it.*

The electronic thermometer is battery-operated and is stored in a wall unit for recharging when not in use (Fig. 13-5). It can be used to take an oral, rectal, or axillary temperature. An electronic thermometer registers the temperature digitally in two to 60 seconds. The thermometer flashes or makes a sound when the temperature is displayed. The probe on an electric thermometer must have a probe cover applied before use. The probe cover is used on only one person and is then disposed of properly. The probe cover cannot be used on more than one resident.

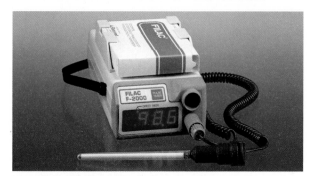

Fig. 13-5. *An electronic thermometer.*

A disposable thermometer can be used to take oral or axillary temperatures. This type of thermometer is for single use, meaning it is used once and then disposed of in the proper container. It does not require the use of a disposable sheath. A disposable thermometer helps reduce the risk of infection, since it is only used on one resident. These types of thermometers are often used on residents who are in isolation. The temperature reading registers in approximately 60 seconds. A disposable thermometer is made of rigid plastic and must be removed slowly to avoid causing tears in the mouth.

A tympanic thermometer is used to measure the temperature reading in the ear (Fig. 13-6). It registers the temperature in seconds. When using this thermometer, it is important to follow instructions to get as accurate a reading as possible. Ear wax may cause an inaccurate reading. Ear injury is possible with this thermometer. Hearing aids may need to be removed before taking a temperature this way.

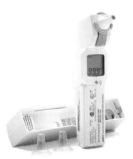

Fig. 13-6. *A tympanic thermometer.*

Another type of thermometer is the temporal artery thermometer (Fig. 13-7). This is an infrared thermometer that measures the temperature of the temporal artery, the artery under the skin of the forehead, in about three seconds. The probe on the thermometer is moved straight across the forehead to obtain a reading. It is non-invasive, meaning it does not require a probe to be inserted into the ear, the mouth, under the arm, or in the rectum. Clothing does not need to be removed in order to take a temperature. If temporal artery thermometers are used at your facility, you will be trained how to use them.

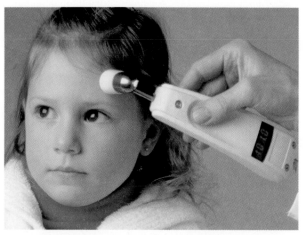

Fig. 13-7. *A temporal artery thermometer.* (PHOTO COURTESY OF EXERGEN CORPORATION, 800-422-3006, WWW.EXERGEN.COM)

Temperatures are often taken orally. Do not take an oral temperature on a person who:

- Is unconscious

- Is using oxygen

- Is confused or disoriented

- Is paralyzed from stroke

- Has facial trauma

- Is likely to have a seizure

- Has a nasogastric or orogastric tube (Chapter 26)

- Is younger than six years old

- Has sores, redness, swelling, or pain in the mouth

- Has an injury to the face or neck

Measuring and recording oral temperature

Equipment: clean mercury-free, digital, or electronic thermometer, gloves, disposable sheath/cover for thermometer, tissues, pen and paper

Do not take an oral temperature on a resident who has smoked, eaten or drunk fluids, chewed gum, or exercised within the last 10–20 minutes.

1. Identify yourself by name. Identify the resident. Greet the resident by name.

2. Wash your hands.

3. Explain procedure to resident. Speak clearly, slowly, and directly. Maintain face-to-face contact whenever possible.

4. Provide for the resident's privacy with a curtain, screen, or door.

5. Put on gloves.

6. *Mercury-free thermometer*: Hold thermometer by stem. Before inserting thermometer in resident's mouth, shake thermometer down to below the lowest number (at least below 96°F or 35°C). To shake thermometer down, hold it at the end opposite the bulb with the thumb and two fingers. With a snapping mo-

tion of the wrist, shake the thermometer (Fig. 13-8). Stand away from furniture and walls while doing so.

Digital thermometer: Put on disposable sheath. Turn on thermometer. Wait until "ready" sign appears.

Electronic thermometer: Remove probe from base unit. Put on probe cover.

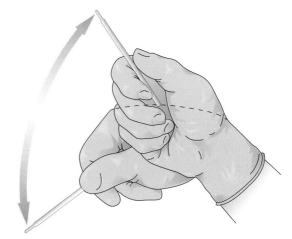

Fig. 13-8. Shake thermometer down to below the lowest number before inserting in a resident's mouth.

7. *Mercury-free thermometer*: Put on disposable sheath, if applicable. Gently insert bulb end of thermometer into resident's mouth. Place it under tongue and to one side (Fig. 13-9). Resident should breathe through his or her nose.

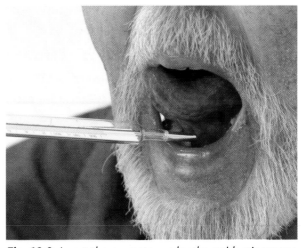

Fig. 13-9. Insert thermometer under the resident's tongue and to one side.

Digital thermometer: Insert end of digital thermometer into resident's mouth. Place under tongue and to one side.

Electronic thermometer: Insert the covered probe into resident's mouth. Place under tongue and to one side.

8. *Mercury-free thermometer*: Tell resident to hold thermometer in mouth with lips closed. Assist as necessary. Ask the resident not to bite down or to talk. Leave thermometer in place for at least three minutes.

   Digital thermometer: Leave in place until thermometer blinks or beeps.

   Electronic thermometer: Leave in place until you hear a tone or see a flashing or steady light.

9. *Mercury-free thermometer*: Remove the thermometer. Wipe with tissue from stem to bulb or remove sheath. Dispose of tissue or sheath. Hold thermometer at eye level. Rotate until line appears, rolling the thermometer between your thumb and forefinger. Read temperature. Remember the temperature reading.

   Digital thermometer: Remove the thermometer. Read temperature on display screen. Remember the temperature reading.

   Electronic thermometer: Read the temperature on the display screen. Remember the temperature reading. Remove the probe.

10. *Mercury-free thermometer*: Clean thermometer according to facility policy. Return it to plastic case or container.

    Digital thermometer: Using a tissue, remove and discard sheath. Clean thermometer according to facility policy. Replace thermometer in case.

    Electronic thermometer: Press the eject button to discard the cover (Fig. 13-10). Return the probe to the holder.

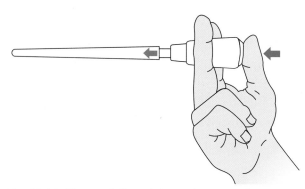

Fig. 13-10. Eject and discard the probe cover after use.

11. Remove and discard gloves. Wash your hands.

12. Make resident comfortable. Remove privacy measures.

13. Leave call light within resident's reach.

14. Wash your hands.

15. Be courteous and respectful at all times.

16. Report any changes in the resident to the nurse. Document procedure using facility guidelines. Record the resident's name, temperature, date, time and method used (oral).

Tip

Mercury Glass Thermometers

Using glass bulb or mercury thermometers to take oral, rectal, or axillary temperatures is no longer common because mercury is a dangerous, toxic substance. Many healthcare facilities now discourage the use of mercury, and some states have passed laws to ban the sale of mercury thermometers.

If your facility uses mercury glass thermometers, use cool water when rinsing them. Do not use hot water because it can heat the mercury and break the thermometer. If a mercury thermometer breaks, tell the nurse immediately. Do not touch the mercury or the broken glass. Procedures have to be followed to clean and dispose of mercury safely and properly.

Taking rectal temperatures may be necessary for unconscious residents, residents with poorly-fitting dentures or missing teeth, or residents who have difficulty breathing through the nose, have a seizure disorder or have been vomiting. Rectal thermometers should be lubricated and inserted carefully one-half inch to one inch for adults. Explain clearly what you will be doing before starting this procedure. When taking a rectal temperature, you must stay with the resident for the entire time the thermometer is in place. You must also hold the thermometer in place the entire time it is in the rectum. Ask the resident to be very still during this procedure, and explain that it will only take a few minutes.

Measuring and recording rectal temperature

Equipment: clean rectal mercury-free, digital or electronic thermometer, lubricant, gloves, tissue, disposable sheath/cover, pen and paper

1. Identify yourself by name. Identify the resident. Greet the resident by name.

2. Wash your hands.

3. Explain procedure to resident. Speak clearly, slowly, and directly. Maintain face-to-face contact whenever possible. Remind resident that the procedure will take only a few minutes.

4. Provide for the resident's privacy with a curtain, screen, or door.

5. Adjust bed to safe working level, usually waist high. Lock bed wheels.

6. Help the resident to left-lying (Sims') position (Fig. 13-11).

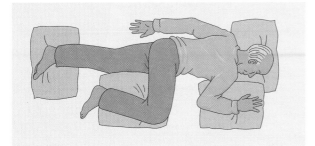

Fig. 13-11. *The resident must be in the left-lying (Sims') position.*

7. Fold back linens to expose only rectal area.

8. Put on gloves.

9. **Mercury-free thermometer**: Hold thermometer by stem. Shake thermometer down to below the lowest number. Put on disposable sheath.

   Digital thermometer: Put on disposable sheath. Turn on thermometer. Wait until "ready" sign appears.

   Electronic thermometer: Remove probe from base unit. Put on probe cover.

10. Apply a small amount of lubricant to tip of bulb or probe cover (or apply pre-lubricated cover).

11. Separate the buttocks. Gently insert thermometer one-half to one inch into rectum (Fig. 13-12). Stop if you meet resistance. Do not force the thermometer into the rectum.

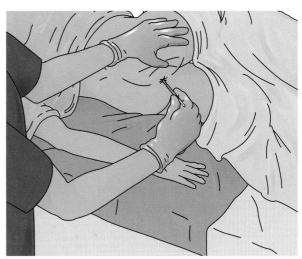

Fig. 13-12. *Gently insert a rectal thermometer one-half to one inch into the rectum. Do not force it into the rectum.*

12. Replace sheet over buttocks while holding on to the thermometer. Hold onto the thermometer at all times.

13. **Mercury-free thermometer**: Hold thermometer in place for at least three minutes.

    Digital thermometer: Hold thermometer in place until thermometer blinks or beeps.

    Electronic thermometer: Leave in place until you hear a tone or see a flashing or steady light.

14. Gently remove the thermometer. Wipe with tissue from stem to bulb or remove sheath or cover. Dispose of tissue or sheath.

15. Read thermometer at eye level as you would for an oral temperature. Remember the temperature reading.

16. **Mercury-free thermometer**: Clean thermometer according to facility policy. Return it to plastic case or container.

    Digital thermometer: Clean thermometer according to facility policy. Replace thermometer in case.

    Electronic thermometer: Press the eject button to discard the cover. Return the probe to the holder.

17. Remove and discard gloves.

18. Wash your hands.

19. Make resident comfortable.

20. Return bed to lowest position. Remove privacy measures.

21. Leave call light within resident's reach.

22. Wash your hands.

23. Be courteous and respectful at all times.

24. Report any changes in the resident to the nurse. Document procedure using facility guidelines. Immediately record the resident's name, temperature, date, time and method used (rectal).

Tympanic thermometers take fast temperature readings. When taking a tympanic temperature, let the resident know that you will be placing the tip of the thermometer in his ear and that it should be painless. The tip of the thermometer will only go into the ear one-quarter to one-half inch. Follow the manufacturer's instructions, as models vary.

Measuring and recording tympanic temperature

Equipment: tympanic thermometer, gloves, disposable sheath/cover, pen and paper

1. Identify yourself by name. Identify the resident. Greet the resident by name.

2. Wash your hands.

3. Explain procedure to resident. Speak clearly, slowly, and directly. Maintain face-to-face contact whenever possible.

4. Provide for the resident's privacy with a curtain, screen, or door.

5. Put on gloves.

6. Put a disposable sheath over earpiece of the thermometer.

7. Position the resident's head so that the ear is in front of you. Straighten the ear canal by gently pulling up and back on the outside edge of the ear (Fig. 13-13). Insert the covered probe into the ear canal. Press the button.

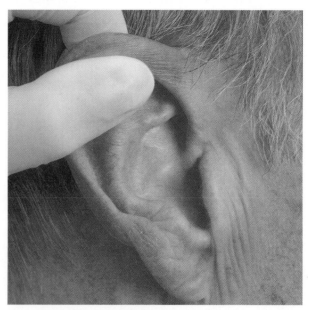

Fig. 13-13. *Gently pull up and back on the outside edge of the ear to straighten the ear canal.*

8. Hold thermometer in place until thermometer blinks or beeps.

9. Read temperature. Remember the temperature reading.

10. Dispose of sheath. Return thermometer to storage or to the battery charger if thermometer is rechargeable.

11. Remove and discard gloves. Wash your hands.

12. Make resident comfortable. Remove privacy measures.

13. Leave call light within resident's reach.

14. Wash your hands.

15. Be courteous and respectful at all times.

16. Report any changes in the resident to the nurse. Document procedure using facility guidelines. Immediately record resident's name, temperature, date, time, and method used (tympanic).

Axillary temperatures are not as accurate as temperatures taken at other sites. Make sure the axillary area is clean and dry before taking a temperature reading. The arm should be placed over the chest to hold the thermometer in place.

Measuring and recording axillary temperature

Equipment: clean mercury-free, digital or electronic thermometer, gloves, tissues, disposable sheath/cover, pen and paper

1. Identify yourself by name. Identify the resident. Greet the resident by name.

2. Wash your hands.

3. Explain procedure to resident. Speak clearly, slowly, and directly. Maintain face-to-face contact whenever possible.

4. Provide for the resident's privacy with a curtain, screen, or door.

5. Adjust bed to safe working level, usually waist high. Lock bed wheels.

6. Put on gloves.

7. Remove resident's arm from sleeve of gown. Wipe axillary area with tissues.

8. **Mercury-free thermometer**: Hold thermometer by stem. Shake thermometer down to below the lowest number. Put on disposable sheath, if applicable.

   Digital thermometer: Put on disposable sheath. Turn on thermometer. Wait until "ready" sign appears.

   Electronic thermometer: Remove probe from base unit. Put on probe cover.

9. Position thermometer (bulb end for mercury-free) in center of the armpit. Fold resident's arm over chest.

10. **Mercury-free thermometer**: Hold thermometer in place, with the arm close against the side, for eight to ten minutes (Fig. 13-14).

    Digital thermometer: Hold thermometer in place until thermometer blinks or beeps.

    Electronic thermometer: Leave in place until you hear a tone or see a flashing or steady light.

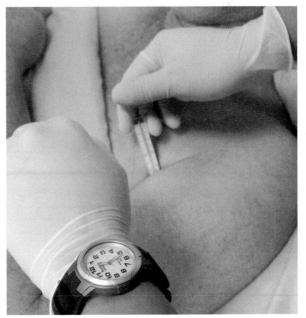

Fig. 13-14. *After inserting the thermometer, fold the resident's arm over her chest and hold it in place for the required time.*

11. *Mercury-free thermometer*: Gently remove the thermometer. Wipe with tissue from stem to bulb or remove sheath. Dispose of tissue or sheath. Read temperature. Remember the temperature reading.

   Digital thermometer: Remove the thermometer. Read temperature on display screen. Remember the temperature reading.

   Electronic thermometer: Read the temperature on the display screen. Remember the temperature reading. Remove the probe.

12. *Mercury-free thermometer*: Clean thermometer according to facility policy. Return it to plastic case or container.

   Digital thermometer: Using a tissue, remove and dispose of sheath. Clean thermometer according to facility policy. Replace the thermometer in case.

   Electronic thermometer: Press the eject button to discard the cover. Return the probe to the holder.

13. Remove and discard gloves. Wash your hands.

14. Put resident's arm back into sleeve of gown. Make resident comfortable.

15. Return bed to lowest position. Remove privacy measures.

16. Leave call light within resident's reach.

17. Wash your hands.

18. Be courteous and respectful at all times.

19. Report any changes in the resident to the nurse. Document procedure using facility guidelines. Immediately record the resident's name, temperature, date, time and method used (axillary).

5. Explain pulse and respirations

When the left ventricle of the heart contracts, it causes a wave of blood to move through an ar-

tery. This "pulse" is what you feel at the wrist or other pulse site. The pulse count is the number of times the heart beats per minute. Sometimes the abbreviation **BPM** (beats per minute) is used after a pulse count. The heartbeat or pulse is measured with the fingers or by electronic devices that automatically measure the pulse. There are many areas on the body where a pulse can be felt. Common pulse sites are shown in Figure 13-15.

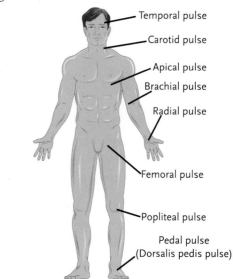

Fig. 13-15. *Common pulse sites.*

For adults, the normal pulse rate is 60 to 100 beats per minute. When a pulse is too high, a person has **tachycardia**. If it is too low, a person has **bradycardia**.

The pulse rate is affected by different factors, including the following:

- **Age**: Pulse rate decreases with advanced age.

- **Sex**: Males may have a slightly lower pulse rate than females.

- **Exercise**: Pulse rate increases with exercise. However, someone who has exercised regularly for years may have a lower pulse, which can be normal for that person.

- **Stress**: Fear, anxiety, and pain cause the pulse to increase.

- **Hemorrhage**: The pulse rate increases when blood is first lost due to the heart trying to work harder to circulate the blood.

- **Medications**: Medications can increase or decrease the heart rate.

- **Fever and illness**: When a person is ill and has a fever, blood vessels may **dilate**, or widen, due to the rise in temperature. A decrease in blood pressure then occurs due to the dilated blood vessels. The heart responds by working harder and increasing the pulse rate.

Respiration is the process of **inspiration** (inhaling air into the lungs) and **expiration** (exhaling air out of the lungs). One respiration consists of an inspiration and an expiration. The chest rises during inspiration and falls during expiration. The normal respiration rate for adults ranges from 12 to 20 breaths per minute.

Different types of respirations are:

- **Apnea**: the absence of breathing; may be temporary

- **Dyspnea**: difficulty breathing

- **Eupnea**: normal respirations

- **Orthopnea**: shortness of breath when lying down that is relieved by sitting up

- **Tachypnea**: rapid respirations

- **Cheyne-Stokes respiration**: type of respiration with periods of apnea lasting at least ten seconds, along with alternating periods of slow, irregular respirations and rapid, shallow respirations (see Chapter 27 for more information)

6. List guidelines for taking pulse and respirations

The **radial pulse** is the most common site for counting pulse beats. This pulse is found on the inside of the wrist on the thumb-side of the body. A pulse may be regular, having the same amount of time between the beats, or irregular, having varying amounts of time between the beats.

You will sometimes use a stethoscope to measure pulse rate. A **stethoscope** is an instrument used for listening to sounds within the body, such as the heartbeat or air in the lungs. Clean the earpieces and diaphragm of the stethoscope with alcohol wipes before and after each use. The diaphragm is the larger, round side of the stethoscope; you will use this side to hear a pulse (Fig. 13-16). The smaller round side of the stethoscope is called the bell side.

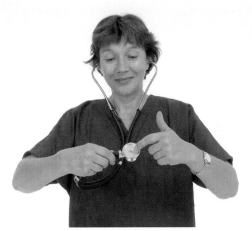

Fig. 13-16. *Use the diaphragm side of the stethoscope to hear a pulse and to take blood pressure. The diaphragm is the larger side of the stethoscope.*

When checking a resident's pulse, observe for the following:

- The pulse rate (the number of beats in one minute—normal range is 60 to 100 beats per minute)

- The overall pattern of the pulse: is the pulse regular or irregular?

- The quality or type of pulse: is the pulse strong or weak?

The respiratory rate is usually counted directly after taking the pulse because people tend to breathe more quickly if they know they are being observed. Keep your fingers on the resident's wrist or on the stethoscope over the heart to avoid making it obvious that you are watching her breathing (Fig. 13-17).

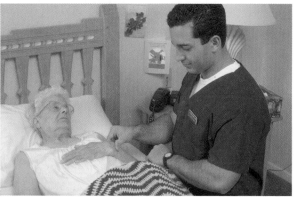

Fig. 13-17. Count the respiratory rate directly after taking the radial pulse. Keep your fingers on the resident's wrist to avoid making it obvious that you are watching her breathing.

When counting respirations, observe for the following:

- The respiratory rate (the number of times the resident breathes in one minute—normal range is 12 to 20)

- The overall pattern of respirations: is breathing regular or irregular?

- The quality or type of breathing: is shortness of breath or difficulty breathing (dyspnea) noted? Does the resident have noisy breathing? Normal breathing is quiet. Is the breathing deep or shallow?

Measuring and recording radial pulse and counting and recording respirations

Equipment: watch with second hand, pen and paper

1. Identify yourself by name. Identify the resident. Greet the resident by name.

2. Wash your hands.

3. Explain procedure to resident. Speak clearly, slowly, and directly. Maintain face-to-face contact whenever possible.

4. Provide for the resident's privacy with a curtain, screen, or door.

5. Place the fingertips of your index finger and middle finger on the thumb side of resident's wrist to locate radial pulse (Fig. 13-18). Do not use your thumb.

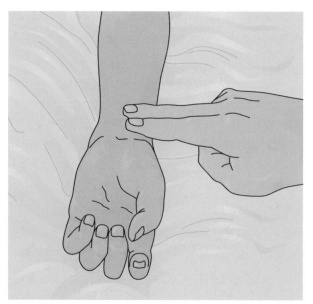

Fig. 13-18. Measure the radial pulse by placing the fingertips of your index finger and middle finger on the thumb side of the wrist.

6. Count beats for one full minute.

7. Keep your fingertips on the resident's wrist. Count respirations for one full minute. Observe for the pattern and character of the resident's breathing. Normal breathing is smooth and quiet.

8. Remove privacy measures. Make resident comfortable.

9. Leave call light within resident's reach.

10. Wash your hands.

11. Be courteous and respectful at all times.

12. Report any changes in the resident to the nurse. Document procedure using facility guidelines. Record pulse rate, date, time and method used (radial). Record the respiratory rate and the pattern or character of breathing.

The **apical pulse** is heard by listening directly over the heart with a stethoscope. The apical pulse is on the left side of the chest, just below the nipple. This type of pulse is checked on residents who have a weak radial pulse or an irregular pulse. It may also be taken on infants and people with heart disease.

Measuring and recording apical pulse

Equipment: stethoscope, watch with second hand, alcohol wipes, pen and paper

1. Identify yourself by name. Identify the resident. Greet the resident by name.

2. Wash your hands.

3. Explain procedure to resident. Speak clearly, slowly, and directly. Maintain face-to-face contact whenever possible.

4. Provide for the resident's privacy with a curtain, screen, or door.

5. Before using stethoscope, wipe diaphragm and earpieces with alcohol wipes.

6. Fit the earpieces of the stethoscope snugly in your ears. Place the flat metal diaphragm on the left side of the chest, just below the nipple. Listen for the heartbeat.

7. Use the second hand of your watch. Count beats for one full minute (Fig. 13-19). Each "lub dub" you hear is counted as one beat. A normal heartbeat is rhythmical. Leave the stethoscope in place to count respirations.

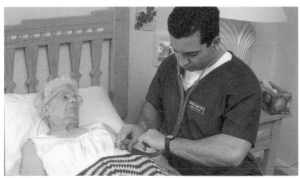

Fig. 13-19. Count the heartbeats for one full minute to measure the apical pulse.

8. Clean earpieces and diaphragm of stethoscope with alcohol wipes. Store stethoscope.

9. Make resident comfortable. Remove privacy measures.

10. Leave call light within resident's reach.

11. Wash your hands.

12. Be courteous and respectful at all times.

13. Report any changes in the resident to the nurse. Document procedure using facility guidelines. Record pulse rate, date, time, and method used (apical). Note any differences in the rhythm.

An apical pulse is also taken to compare the apical pulse to a pulse somewhere else in the body, such as the wrist (radial). In some cases, the apical and radial pulse counts differ. This is significant when evaluating circulation or a heart problem.

An apical pulse is normally about the same as a radial pulse. When the radial pulse is less than the apical pulse, it may indicate poor circulation to an extremity. The apical pulse will always be the same or higher than any other pulse on the body. It will never be lower than another pulse.

The pulse deficit is the difference between an apical pulse and another pulse. For example, if the apical pulse is 80 beats in one minute, and the radial pulse is 68 beats in one minute, the pulse deficit is 12 (80 - 68 = 12).

Measuring and recording apical-radial pulse

Equipment: stethoscope, watch with second hand, alcohol wipes, pen and paper

Find a co-worker to assist you.

1. Identify yourself by name. Identify the resident. Greet the resident by name.

2. Wash your hands.

3. Explain procedure to resident. Speak clearly, slowly, and directly. Maintain face-to-face contact whenever possible.

4. Provide for the resident's privacy with a curtain, screen, or door.

5. Before using stethoscope, wipe diaphragm and earpieces with alcohol wipes.

6. Fit the earpieces of the stethoscope snugly in your ears. Place the flat metal diaphragm on the left side of the chest, just below the nipple. Listen for the heartbeat.

7. Your co-worker should place her fingertips on the thumb side of resident's wrist to locate the radial pulse.

8. After both pulses have been located, look at the second hand of your watch. When the second hand reaches the "12" or "6," say, "Start," and both people will count beats for one full minute. Say, "Stop" after one minute (Fig. 13-20).

9. Clean earpieces and diaphragm of stethoscope with alcohol wipes. Store stethoscope.

10. Make resident comfortable. Remove privacy measures.

11. Leave call light within resident's reach.

12. Wash your hands.

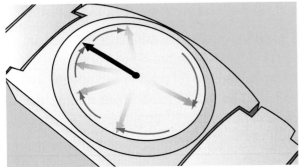

Fig. 13-20. Use the second hand on your watch to count the beats for one full minute.

13. Be courteous and respectful at all times.

14. Report any changes in the resident to the nurse. Document procedure using facility guidelines. Record both pulse rates, date, time, and method used (apical-radial). Record pulse deficit if the pulse rates are not the same (subtract radial pulse measurement from apical pulse to get pulse deficit). Note any differences in the rhythm.

7. Identify factors that affect blood pressure

Blood pressure is the measurement of the force of the blood against the walls of certain blood vessels, called arteries. Arteries carry blood away from the heart. The left ventricle of the heart causes the blood to surge out of the heart and travel through the body. The force of this movement of blood is the blood pressure. Blood pressure is measured in millimeters of mercury (mm Hg). A blood pressure reading is recorded as a fraction—for example, 120/80.

The top number in a blood pressure reading is called the **systolic** blood pressure. This is the pressure of the blood on the walls of the arteries. This occurs when the heart is contracting to pump blood out from the left ventricle into the body. The normal range for systolic blood pressure for an adult is 100–119 mm Hg.

The bottom number is the **diastolic** blood pressure. The lower reading is the pressure of the blood when the heart is relaxed. This relaxation happens when the heart is not contracting, between the heartbeats. The normal range for diastolic blood pressure for an adult is 60–79 mm Hg. The diastolic measurement is always lower than the systolic measurement.

When blood pressure is too high (140/90 or higher), it is called **hypertension**. People with hypertension have elevated systolic and/or diastolic blood pressures.

When blood pressure is too low (100/60 or lower) it is called **hypotension**. Loss of blood or slowed blood flow can cause hypotension, which can be life-threatening. More information on these disorders can be found in Chapter 19. **Orthostatic hypotension**, which is also called postural hypotension, is a sudden drop in blood pressure that occurs when a person stands or sits up. Dizziness, lightheadedness or fainting may accompany orthostatic hypotension.

More aggressive high blood pressure guidelines from the Seventh Report of the Joint National Committee (JNC 7) were released in 2003. Under the new guidelines, a definition for prehypertension was added. **Prehypertension** is defined as having a systolic measurement of 120–139 mm Hg and a diastolic measurement of 80–89 mm Hg. Prehypertension means that a person does not have high blood pressure now, but is likely to have it in the future. Nursing assistants must report any abnormal blood pressure readings, as directed.

Blood pressure is affected by different factors, including:

- **Age**: Elderly people with circulatory disorders (Chapter 19) may have higher blood pressure readings.

- **Exercise**: Regular exercise and being active decreases blood pressure.

- **Stress**: Long-term, chronic stress can raise blood pressure.

- **Race**: African-Americans are more likely to have high blood pressure than Caucasians.

- **Heredity**: People whose parents have or have had high blood pressure are more likely to develop it than others.

- **Obesity/unhealthy diet**: Being overweight and eating unhealthy diets increase blood pressure.

- **Alcohol**: Regular, high alcohol intake can raise blood pressure.

- **Tobacco products**: Smoking or chewing tobacco products are contributing factors in high blood pressure.

- **Time of day**: Blood pressure may be lower in the morning and higher later in the day.

- **Illness**: People who have certain diseases, such as diabetes and kidney disease, have a higher frequency of high blood pressure.

8. List guidelines for taking blood pressure

Blood pressure is measured with a device called a **sphygmomanometer**. You will need to gather alcohol wipes, a stethoscope, a blood pressure cuff, and a sphygmomanometer when preparing to take a blood pressure. Some facilities do not allow nursing assistants to take blood pressure readings. Follow facility policy and the care plan.

It is important to choose the correct size cuff to take a blood pressure reading. Available sizes include standard, pediatric, and large. Check with the nurse if you have questions about the size of the blood pressure cuff. The cuff must be the proper size and put on the arm correctly so the amount of pressure on the artery is correct. If not, the reading will be falsely high or low.

Types of sphygmomanometers include:

- **Aneroid sphygmomanometer**. This device has a round gauge that is portable or is attached to the wall (Fig. 13-21). It may also hook onto clothing.

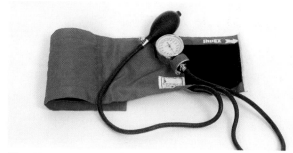

Fig. 13-21. An aneroid sphygmomanometer.

- **Electronic sphygmomanometer**. This device automatically inflates and deflates to measure blood pressure (Fig. 13-22). The readings are displayed digitally. The use of a stethoscope is not required with electronic sphygmomanometers. Ask for instructions on use if you have not been trained to use this equipment.

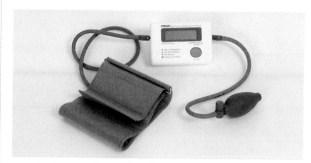

Fig. 13-22. An electronic sphygmomanometer.

- **Non-invasive blood pressure monitoring (NIBP)**. These monitoring devices measure blood pressure faster than other methods. They may also measure other vital signs, as well as perform other measurements. For example, some machines measure the temperature, pulse, and respiration, and have the ability to measure blood oxygen levels. You will receive training for these devices if they are used at your facility. Follow facility policy on the use of these machines.

The **brachial pulse** is used to take a blood pressure reading. This is the pulse inside of the elbow, about one to one and a half inches above the elbow (Fig. 13-23). Both the radial and brachial pulse are used in taking blood pressure.

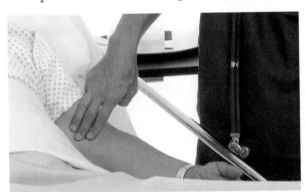

Fig. 13-23. *The brachial pulse is located on the inside of the elbow, about one to one and a half inches above the elbow.*

Do not take blood pressure on an arm or a side of the body when these situations exist:

- An intravenous line (IV) is present
- An amputation has been performed
- The cuff does not fit the arm properly
- The arm has a cast
- Burns or injuries are present
- The arm is being used for dialysis
- The arm or side has had recent trauma
- The arm or side is paralyzed due to stroke
- The side has had a mastectomy (or any breast surgery)

When taking blood pressure, observe for the following:

- The blood pressure reading: A normal reading should be from 100/60 to 119/79 (140/90 or above is high and needs to be reported).

- The quality or type of sounds: Are the sounds you hear when listening with your stethoscope strong or weak?

Different Methods for Taking Blood Pressure

This textbook includes two methods for taking blood pressure: the one-step method and the two-step method. In the two-step method, you will get an estimate of the systolic blood pressure before you start. After getting an estimated systolic reading, you will deflate the cuff and begin again. With the one-step method, you will not get an estimated systolic reading before obtaining the blood pressure reading. Your state may require that you know one or both of these methods. Follow your facility's policy on which method to use.

Measuring and recording blood pressure (one-step method)

Equipment: sphygmomanometer, stethoscope, watch with second hand, alcohol wipes, pen and paper

1. Identify yourself by name. Identify the resident. Greet the resident by name.

2. Wash your hands.

3. Explain procedure to resident. Speak clearly, slowly, and directly. Maintain face-to-face contact whenever possible.

4. Provide for the resident's privacy with a curtain, screen, or door.

5. Ask the resident to roll up his or her sleeve, approximately five inches above the elbow. Do not measure blood pressure over clothing.

6. Position resident's arm with palm up. The arm should be level with the heart.

7. With the valve open, squeeze the cuff. Make sure it is completely deflated.

8. Place blood pressure cuff snugly on resident's upper arm. The center of the cuff with sensor/arrow is placed over the brachial artery (1-1½ inches above the elbow toward inside of elbow) (Fig. 13-24).

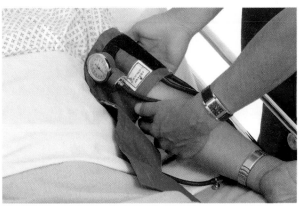

Fig. 13-24. *Place the center of the cuff over the brachial artery.*

9. Before using the stethoscope, wipe diaphragm and earpieces with alcohol wipes.

10. Locate brachial pulse with fingertips.

11. Place diaphragm of the stethoscope over brachial artery.

12. Place earpieces of the stethoscope in ears.

13. Close the valve (clockwise) until it stops. Do not over-tighten it (Fig. 13-25).

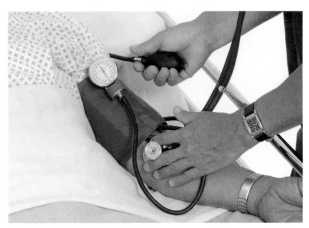

Fig. 13-25. *Close the valve by turning it clockwise until it stops.*

14. Inflate cuff to 30 mm Hg above the point at which the pulse is last heard or felt.

15. Open the valve slightly with thumb and index finger. Deflate cuff slowly.

16. Watch gauge. Listen for sound of pulse.

17. Remember the reading at which the first clear pulse sound is heard. This is the systolic pressure.

18. Continue listening for a change or muffling of pulse sound. The point of a change or the point the sound disappears is the diastolic pressure. Remember this reading.

19. Open the valve. Deflate cuff completely. Remove cuff.

20. Wipe diaphragm and earpieces of the stethoscope with alcohol. Store equipment.

21. Make resident comfortable. Remove privacy measures.

22. Leave call light within resident's reach.

23. Wash your hands.

24. Be courteous and respectful at all times.

25. Report any changes in the resident to the nurse. Document procedure using facility guidelines. Record both the systolic and diastolic pressures. Write the numbers like a fraction, with the systolic reading on top and the diastolic reading on the bottom (for example: 120/80). Note which arm was used. Write "RA" for right arm and "LA" for left arm.

Measuring and recording blood pressure (two-step method)

Equipment: sphygmomanometer, stethoscope, watch with second hand, alcohol wipes, pen and paper

1. Identify yourself by name. Identify the resident. Greet the resident by name.

2. Wash your hands.

3. Explain procedure to resident. Speak clearly, slowly, and directly. Maintain face-to-face contact whenever possible.

4. Provide for the resident's privacy with a curtain, screen, or door.

5. Ask the resident to roll up his or her sleeve, approximately five inches above the elbow. Do not measure blood pressure over clothing.

6. Position resident's arm with palm up. The arm should be level with the heart.

7. With the valve open, squeeze the cuff. Make sure it is completely deflated.

8. Place blood pressure cuff snugly on resident's upper arm. The center of the cuff with sensor/arrow is placed over the brachial artery (1-1½ inches above the elbow toward inside of elbow).

9. Locate the radial (wrist) pulse with fingertips.

10. Close the valve (clockwise) until it stops. Inflate cuff slowly, watching gauge.

11. Stop inflating when you can no longer feel the pulse. Note the reading. The number is an estimate of the systolic pressure.

12. Open the valve. Deflate cuff completely.

13. Write down estimated systolic reading.

14. Before using the stethoscope, wipe diaphragm and earpieces of stethoscope with alcohol wipes.

15. Locate brachial pulse with fingertips.

16. Place diaphragm of the stethoscope over brachial artery.

17. Place earpieces of the stethoscope in ears.

18. Close the valve (clockwise) until it stops. Do not over-tighten it (Fig. 13-26).

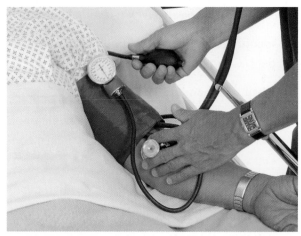

Fig. 13-26. *Close the valve, but do not over-tighten it. Tight valves are difficult to release.*

19. Inflate cuff to 30 mm Hg above your estimated systolic pressure.

20. Open the valve slightly with thumb and index finger. Deflate cuff slowly.

21. Watch gauge. Listen for sound of pulse.

22. Remember the reading at which the first clear pulse sound is heard. This is the systolic pressure.

23. Continue listening for a change or muffling of pulse sound. The point of a change or the point the sound disappears is the diastolic pressure. Remember this reading.

24. Open the valve. Deflate cuff completely. Remove cuff.

25. Wipe diaphragm and earpieces of the stethoscope with alcohol. Store equipment.

26. Make resident comfortable. Remove privacy measures.

27. Leave call light within resident's reach.

28. Wash your hands.

29. Be courteous and respectful at all times.

30. Report any changes in the resident to the nurse. Document procedure using facility guidelines. Record both the systolic and diastolic pressures. Write the numbers like a fraction, with the systolic reading on top and the diastolic reading on the bottom (for example: 120/80). Note which arm was used. Write "RA" for right arm and "LA" for left arm.

Tip

Orthostatic Hypotension

Some people have a decrease in blood pressure when they move from a lying to a sitting or a standing position. A resident who has orthostatic hypotension may need to have his blood pressure measured three times. The first measurement will be taken while the resident is lying down. The second will be taken while the resident is sitting up, and the third will be taken when the resident is standing. You will document and report all three readings. An example is Lying down=130/80, Sitting=110/76, and Standing=90/66.

9. Describe guidelines for pain management

It is important to observe and report residents' pain. Pain is sometimes referred to as the "fifth vital sign," because it is as important to monitor pain as it is to monitor the other vital signs.

It can be very difficult to cope with pain. It is uncomfortable and can greatly affect residents' daily lives and their ability to perform ADLs. Pain can swiftly drain energy and hope.

Pain is different for each person; what bothers one person may not bother another. All caregivers are responsible for recognizing pain and taking appropriate action to provide pain management. As the person who is with residents the most, you play a significant role in pain monitoring, management, and prevention. Care plans are made and adjusted based on your reports.

Treat residents' complaints of pain seriously and take action to help them (Fig. 13-27). Ask appropriate questions to help manage the pain, such as the following:

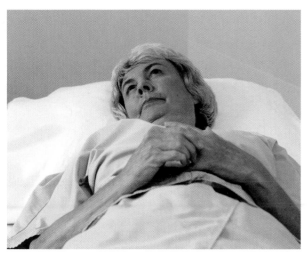

Fig. 13-27. Believe residents when they say they are in pain and take quick action to help them. Being in pain is unpleasant. Be empathetic.

- Where is the pain? Please point to the exact site or area to show me.

- When did the pain start?

- How long does the pain last? Minutes? Seconds? Ask how often it occurs.

- How severe is the pain? To help find out, use available pain scales at your facility. Pain scales are tools that help measure the level of a person's pain. One type is a numerical pain scale. You ask the resident to rate the pain on a scale of 1 to 10, with 10 being the worst. Another is a visual pain scale, which includes drawings of faces with different expressions. Ask the resident to pick the face that most closely resembles the intensity of pain he is experiencing.

- Does the pain come and go?

- Have you experienced this pain before? If so, has anything helped to relieve it?

- What medicine, if any, do you take for the pain?

- Do you remember what you were doing when the pain started?

Ask the resident to describe the pain and, using the resident's words, report to the nurse. Take notes if you need to remember the exact words.

Notice signs of pain specific to each resident. Culture plays a role in determining whether or not a resident will be able to express his pain. Some residents will state freely when they are in pain. Others will not feel comfortable reacting in some way to pain or saying that they are in pain.

Some residents will not express pain due to a fear of addiction to pain medication or worrying about constipation or fatigue from the pain medication. Residents may believe that pain is a normal part of aging, although it is not. Other residents may think that staff members are too busy to deal with their pain.

If a resident is not likely to tell staff that he is in pain, watch for body language or other signs that the person is in pain. Signs of pain to observe and report to the nurse include the following:

Observing and Reporting: Pain

- O/R Increased pulse, respirations, blood pressure
- O/R Sweating
- O/R Nausea
- O/R Vomiting
- O/R Tightening the jaw
- O/R Squeezing eyes shut
- O/R Holding or guarding a body part
- O/R Frowning
- O/R Grinding teeth
- O/R Increased restlessness
- O/R Agitation or tension
- O/R Change in behavior
- O/R Crying
- O/R Sighing
- O/R Groaning
- O/R Breathing heavily
- O/R Difficulty moving or walking

Guidelines: Measures to Reduce Pain

- G Report complaints of pain or unrelieved pain promptly to the nurse.

- G Check on the resident often and ask if the pain has been relieved.

- G Offer back rubs frequently (Fig. 13-28).

- G Assist in frequent changes of position. Be careful when moving, lifting, or transferring a resident in pain. Make sure to have enough help to transfer a resident in pain.

- G Offer warm baths or showers.

- G Encourage slow, deep breaths if the resident has difficulty breathing.

- G Always be patient, caring, gentle, and empathetic.

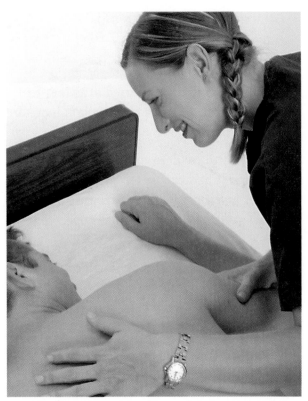

Fig. 13-28. *Back rubs can help reduce pain. Be gentle, kind, and caring when residents are in pain.*

Chapter Review

1. What are the five vital signs that are regularly monitored (LO 2)?

2. List two reasons a nursing assistant should never document a guess of a resident's vital signs (LO 2).

3. List six factors that affect body temperature (LO 3).

4. What are four symptoms of a fever (LO 3)?

5. List the four main sites on the body for measuring temperature (LO 4).

6. Which site is generally considered to be the most accurate for obtaining temperatures (LO 4)?

7. What color are rectal thermometers usually coded (LO 4)?

8. List ten conditions under which a nursing assistant should not take an oral temperature (LO 4).

9. If a resident has recently eaten or had something to drink, how long must a nursing assistant wait before she can measure his oral temperature (LO 4)?

10. When taking a rectal temperature, how long does a nursing assistant need to hold onto the thermometer while it is in the rectum (LO 4)?

11. Generally, how far should the tip of a tympanic thermometer be inserted into the ear (LO 4)?

12. What is the normal pulse rate for adults (LO 5)?

13. What is the normal respiration rate for adults (LO 5)?

14. What is the most common site for taking the pulse (LO 6)?

15. Why is the respiratory rate usually counted directly after taking the pulse, while the fingers are still on the person's wrist (LO 6)?

16. Where is the apical pulse located (LO 6)?

17. Define the pulse deficit (LO 6).

18. List the two parts of measuring blood pressure and list normal ranges for both (LO 7).

19. What reading is considered to be high blood pressure (LO 7)?

20. List seven factors that affect blood pressure (LO 7).

21. Why must a blood pressure cuff be the proper size and put on the arm correctly (LO 8)?

22. In addition to the radial pulse, what other pulse is involved in taking blood pressure measurements (LO 8)?

23. List six conditions under which a nursing assistant should not take blood pressure on an arm or one side of the body (LO 8).

24. List three reasons why some residents might not express pain openly (LO 9).

25. List 15 signs of pain to observe and report to the nurse (LO 9).

26. What are five ways a nursing assistant can help reduce a resident's pain (LO 9)?

14
Nutrition and Fluid Balance

Pernicious Anemia

A Nobel Prize was awarded to George R. Minot, William P. Murphy, and George H. Whipple for discovering that a serious and fatal disease called pernicious anemia could actually be cured. Minot worked for many years and finally discovered that with a simple change in diet, adding large amounts of liver, the disease could be cured. The three men eventually proved the disease was caused by a lack of vitamin B12. Today many people live long lives with this disease by simply getting periodic vitamin B12 shots.

"In general, mankind, since the improvement of cookery, eats twice as much as it requires."
Benjamin Franklin, 1706-1790

"Every tooth in a man's head is more valuable than a diamond."
Miguel de Cervantes, 1547-1616

1. Define important words in this chapter

apathy: a lack of interest.

diet cards: cards that list residents' names and information about special diets, allergies, likes and dislikes, and any other dietary instructions.

diuretics: medications that reduce fluid volume in the body.

fasting: a period of time during which food is given up voluntarily.

fluid balance: taking in and eliminating equal amounts of fluid.

fluid overload: a condition in which the body cannot eliminate the fluid consumed.

force fluids: a medical order for a person to drink more fluids.

glucose: natural sugar.

graduate: a measuring container for measuring fluid volume.

input: the fluid a person consumes; also called intake.

intake: the fluid a person consumes; also called input.

lactose intolerance: inability of the body to digest lactose, a type of sugar found in milk and other dairy products.

metabolism: the process of breaking down and transforming all nutrients that enter the body to provide energy, growth, and maintenance.

nutrient: substance in food that enables the body to use energy for metabolism.

nutrition: the taking in and using of food by the body to maintain health.

output: fluid that is eliminated each day through urine, feces, and vomitus, as well as perspiration; also includes suction material and wound drainage.

puree: to chop, blend, or grind food into a thick paste of baby food consistency.

restrict fluids: a medical order that limits the amount of fluids a person takes in.

special diet: a diet for people who have certain illnesses or conditions; also called therapeutic or modified diet.

vegans: vegetarians who do not eat any animal products, including milk, cheese, other dairy items, or eggs; vegans may also not use or wear any animal products, including wool, silk, and leather.

vegetarians: people who do not eat meat, fish, or poultry for religious, moral, personal, or health reasons; they may or may not eat eggs and dairy products.

2. Describe common nutritional problems of the elderly and the chronically ill

Aging and illness affect **nutrition**, or the taking in and using of food by the body to maintain health. Malnutrition, unhealthy weight loss, and dehydration are serious problems among the elderly. Malnutrition is the lack of proper nutrition that results from insufficient food intake or an improper diet. Difficulty swallowing, called dysphagia, and the inability to chew contribute to a lack of appetite. Fatigue, nausea, and pain often accompany certain illnesses, which decrease appetite. Other problems that affect nutritional intake include the following:

- Older people produce less saliva, which affects eating and swallowing. Swallowing problems put people at a high risk for aspiration, which is the inhalation of food, fluid, or foreign material into the lungs. You will learn more about aspiration later in the chapter.

- Medications can have side effects for the digestive system, such as diarrhea and constipation, both of which can interfere with appetite.

- A decrease in physical activity and mobility can cause a lack of appetite and constipation.

- The ability to smell and taste food and drink is lessened as people age. Medication can also interfere with the sense of smell and

taste. This affects the appetite and the ability to eat (Fig. 14-1).

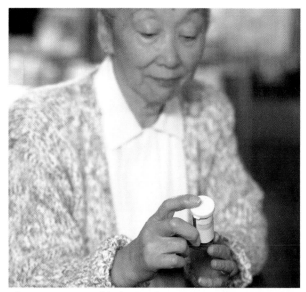

Fig. 14-1. *Many elderly people are on a variety of medications, which can affect the way food smells and tastes.*

- The inability to see well can affect the way food looks, decreasing interest in food.

- Problems with teeth, dentures, or poor oral hygiene make chewing difficult.

- Depression and lack of social interaction can decrease appetite.

- Older people may be on special diets that restrict certain foods and drinks, which can lead to poor food and fluid intake. You will learn more about special diets later in the chapter.

Some specific illnesses make eating and swallowing difficult, such as stroke, which can result in paralysis; cancers of the head, neck, or mouth; Parkinson's disease; multiple sclerosis; and Alzheimer's disease. More information on these diseases is found later in the chapter and in Chapters 22 and 24 of the textbook.

3. Describe cultural factors that influence food preferences

A resident's cultural and ethnic background has great impact on his or her food preferences. Traditions in families and cultures influence food choices (Fig. 14-2). The country or the area of the country that a person is from affects his or her food choices. For example, people from the southwestern U.S. are more apt to like spicy foods. People from Asia may prefer rice with their meals, rather than potatoes or bread.

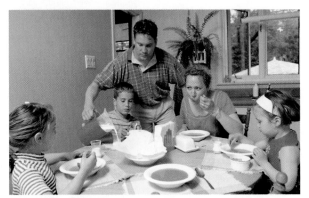

Fig. 14-2. Family traditions influence food likes and dislikes.

Certain people have foods they cannot eat due to religious reasons. For example, many Jewish people do not eat pork or shellfish, and do not eat meat products at the same meal with dairy products. Some Catholics do not eat meat on Fridays. Muslims may not drink alcohol, and people from many religious traditions may occasionally fast. **Fasting** is a practice during which food is voluntarily given up for a period of time.

Some people are vegetarians or vegans. **Vegetarians** do not eat meat, fish, or poultry. They may or may not eat eggs and dairy products. **Vegans** are vegetarians who do not eat any animal products, including milk, cheese, other dairy items, or eggs. Vegans may also not use or wear any animal products, including wool, silk, and leather.

A resident's food preferences are first discussed upon admission to a facility. Periodically these evaluations may need to be redone as a resident's likes and dislikes, as well as nutritional needs, change.

Honoring food preferences is a legal responsibility of the facility. Nursing assistants must report requests for diet substitutions to the nurse right away.

4. Identify six basic nutrients

The human body cannot survive without food and water. Good health requires a daily amount of each of the main nutrients for cells, tissues, organs, and systems to continue to function properly. A **nutrient** is something in food that enables the body to use energy for metabolism. **Metabolism** is the process of breaking down and transforming all nutrients that enter the body in order to provide energy, growth, and maintenance. There are six main nutrients required by the body for healthy growth and development:

1. **Water** is the most essential nutrient for life; it is needed by every cell in the body. Water helps move oxygen and other nutrients into the cells and remove the waste products from each of the cells. Without water, a person can only live a few days. Water helps with digestion and absorption of food. It helps to maintain a normal body temperature through perspiration. Keeping enough fluid in the body is necessary for good health (Fig. 14-3).

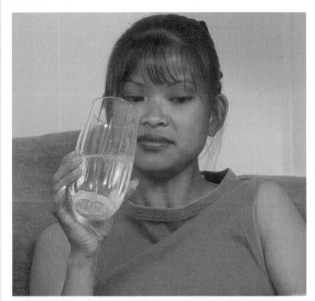

Fig. 14-3. Water is the most essential nutrient for life. Drinking plenty of water promotes good health.

2. **Fats** are a good source of energy. Fat also gives flavor to foods (Fig. 14-4). Fat falls into four categories: saturated, trans fat, monounsaturated, and polyunsaturated. Saturated and trans

fats can increase cholesterol levels and the risk of some diseases, like cardiovascular disease. Monounsaturated and polyunsaturated fats can be helpful in the diet, and can decrease the risk of cardiovascular disease and type 2 diabetes.

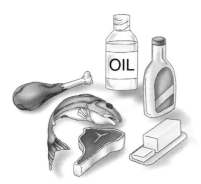

Fig. 14-4. Sources of fat.

3. **Carbohydrates** supply the body with energy and help the body use fat efficiently. Carbohydrates also add needed fiber to diets, which helps with solid waste elimination (Fig. 14-5).

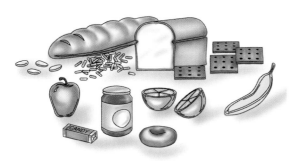

Fig. 14-5. Sources of carbohydrates.

4. **Proteins** are needed by every cell in the body. They help the body grow new tissue, enable tissue repair, and provide additional energy (Fig. 14-6).

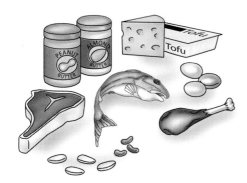

Fig. 14-6. Sources of protein.

5. **Vitamins** are substances that are needed by the body to function. The body does not make most vitamins; they can only be obtained by eating certain foods. Some vitamins are fat-soluble, meaning they are carried and stored in body fat. Vitamins A, D, E, and K are examples. Others are water-soluble vitamins, meaning they are broken down by water in the body and cannot be stored. They are eliminated through urine and feces. Vitamins B and C are examples of water-soluble vitamins.

6. **Minerals** help the body function normally. Many minerals are needed daily by the body. Some minerals keep bones and teeth strong, while others help maintain fluid balance. Minerals give the body energy and control body processes. They are found in many foods.

5. Explain the USDA's MyPlate

In 2011, in response to increasing rates of people who are overweight or obese, the United States Department of Agriculture (USDA) developed MyPlate to help people build a healthy plate at meal times (Fig. 14-7). The MyPlate icon emphasizes vegetables, fruits, grains, protein, and low-fat dairy. It replaces the USDA's MyPyramid icon, which was introduced in 2005.

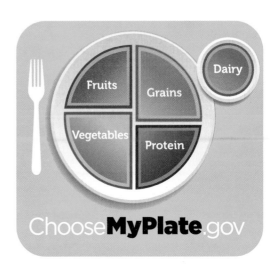

Fig. 14-7. The MyPlate icon and web address were developed by the U.S. Department of Agriculture in 2011 to help promote healthy eating practices.

The goal of MyPlate is to give people an easier way to make healthy food choices. The new visual is based on scientific information about nutrition and health. It shows the amounts of each food group that should be on a person's plate.

MyPlate's message of adopting healthy eating habits supports the *2010 Dietary Guidelines for Americans*. The *Dietary Guidelines for Americans* issues recommendations for improving health by promoting healthy eating and physical activity. It is reviewed, revised (if necessary), and published every five years.

MyPlate gives suggestions and tools for making healthy choices; however, it does not provide specific messages about what a person should eat. The MyPlate icon includes the following food groups:

Vegetables and fruits: Make half your plate fruits and vegetables. Vegetables include all fresh, frozen, canned, and dried vegetables, and vegetable juices. There are five subgroups within the vegetable group, organized by their nutritional content. These are dark green vegetables, red and orange vegetables, dry beans and peas, starchy vegetables, and other vegetables. A variety of vegetables from these subgroups should be eaten every day. Dark green, red, and orange vegetables have the best nutritional content (Fig. 14-8).

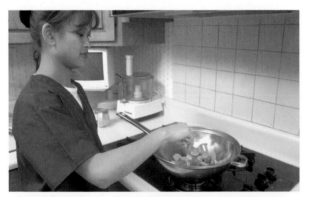

Fig. 14-8. Eating a variety of vegetables, especially dark green, red, and orange vegetables, every day helps promote good health.

Vegetables are low in fat and calories and have no cholesterol (although sauces and seasonings may add fat, calories, and cholesterol). They are

good sources of dietary fiber, potassium, vitamin A, vitamin E, and vitamin C.

Fruits include all fresh, frozen, canned, and dried fruits, and 100% fruit juices. Most choices should be whole, cut-up, or pureed fruit, rather than juice, for the additional dietary fiber provided. Fruit can be added as a main dish, side dish, or as a dessert.

Fruits, like vegetables, are naturally low in fat, sodium, and calories and have no cholesterol. They are important sources of dietary fiber and many nutrients, including folic acid, potassium, and vitamin C. Foods containing dietary fiber help provide a feeling of fullness with fewer calories. Folic acid helps the body form red blood cells. Vitamin C is important for growth and repair of body tissues.

Grains: Make half your grains whole grains. Grains include all foods made from wheat, rice, oats, cornmeal, or barley, such as bread, pasta, oatmeal, breakfast cereals, tortillas, and grits. Grains can be divided into two groups: whole grains and refined grains. Whole grains contain bran and germ, as well as the endosperm. Refined grains retain only the endosperm. Examples of whole grains include brown rice, wild rice, bulgur, oatmeal, whole-grain corn, whole oats, whole wheat, and whole rye. Consuming foods rich in fiber reduces the risk of heart disease and other diseases, and may reduce constipation.

Protein: MyPlate guidelines emphasize the importance of eating a variety of protein foods every week. Meat, poultry, seafood, and eggs are animal sources of proteins. Beans, peas, soy products, nuts, and seeds are plant sources of proteins.

Eat seafood twice a week in place of meat or poultry (Fig. 14-9). Consider seafood higher in oils and low in mercury, such as salmon or trout. Choose lean meat and poultry. Include eggs and egg whites on a regular basis. Eat plant-based protein foods more often. Beans and peas, soy products (tofu, tempeh, veggie burgers), nuts, and seeds are low in saturated fat and high in fiber. Some nuts and seeds (flax, walnuts) are excellent sources of essential fatty acids. These acids may reduce the risk of cardiovascular disease. Sunflower seeds and almonds are good sources of vitamin E.

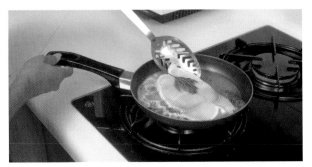

Fig. 14-9. *Fish contains healthy oils and is a good source of protein.*

Dairy: All milk products and foods made from milk that retain their calcium content, such as yogurt and cheese, are part of the dairy category. Most dairy group choices should be fat-free or low-fat (1%). Choose fat-free or low-fat milk or yogurt more often than cheese. Milk and yogurt contain less sodium than most cheeses.

Milk provides nutrients that are vital for the health and maintenance of your body. These nutrients include calcium, potassium, vitamin D, and protein. Fat-free or low-fat milk provides these nutrients without the extra calories and saturated fat (Fig. 14-10). Soy products enriched with calcium are an alternative to dairy foods.

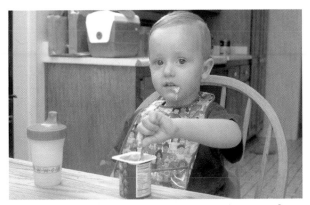

Fig. 14-10. *Low-fat milk or yogurt is a good source of calcium without the added saturated fat.*

Additional tips for making healthy food choices include the following:

Balance calories. Calorie balance is the relationship between the calories obtained from food and fluids consumed and the calories used during normal body functions and physical activity. Proper calorie intake varies from person to person. To find the proper calorie intake, the USDA suggests visiting ChooseMyPlate.gov.

Enjoy your food, but eat less. Eating too fast or eating without paying attention to your food can lead to overeating. Recognize when you feel hungry and when you are full. Notice what you are eating. Stop eating when you feel satisfied.

Avoid oversized portions. Choose smaller-sized portions when eating. Portion out food before you eat it, and use smaller bowls and plates for meals. When eating out, split food with others or take part of your meal home.

Foods to eat more often are vegetables, fruits, whole grains, and fat-free or 1% milk and low-fat dairy products. These foods have better nutrients for health.

Foods to eat less often are foods high in solid fats, added sugars, and salt. These foods include fatty meats, like bacon and hot dogs, cheese, fried foods, ice cream, and cookies.

Compare sodium in foods. Read product labels to determine if they contain salt or sodium. Foods high in sodium include the following:

- Cured meats, including ham, bacon, lunch meat, sausage, salt pork, and hot dogs

- Salty or smoked fish, including herring, salted cod, sardines, anchovies, caviar, smoked salmon, or lox

- Processed cheese and some other cheeses

- Salted foods, including nuts, pretzels, potato chips, dips, and spreads, such as salted butter and margarine

- Vegetables preserved in brine, such as

pickles, sauerkraut, pickled vegetables, olives, and relishes

- Sauces with high concentrations of salt, including Worcestershire, chili, steak, and soy sauces; ketchup, mustard, and mayonnaise

- Commercially-prepared foods such as breads, canned soups and vegetables, and certain breakfast cereals

Select canned foods that are labeled "sodium free," "very low sodium," "low sodium," or "reduced sodium."

Drink water instead of sugary drinks. Drinking water or unsweetened beverages reduces sugar and calorie intake. Sweetened beverages, such as soda, fruit punch, and sports drinks, are a major source of sugar and calories in diets.

If you would like more information about the USDA's MyPlate, visit ChooseMyPlate.gov.

6. Explain the role of the dietary department

The dietary department is responsible for providing nutritious meals and snacks to all residents. Each resident is evaluated upon admission in order to create his or her diet plan. The dietary department creates food to match the diet ordered by the doctor, while also taking into consideration the resident's likes and dislikes and nutritional needs.

In addition to planning and making meals, the dietary department prepares food so that residents are able to manage it. The food must also look appetizing. The dietary department also prepares diet cards. **Diet cards** list the resident's name and information about special diets, allergies, likes and dislikes, as well as any other dietary instructions (Fig. 14-11).

For residents who are unable to eat in the dining room, meals arrive on a floor in a warming unit. Each meal comes with a diet card. You must verify that each resident has received the correct

meal by checking the resident's identification against the diet card.

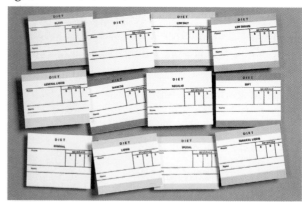

Fig. 14-11. *Sample diet cards.* (REPRINTED WITH PERMISSION OF BRIGGS CORPORATION, 800-247-2343, WWW.BRIGGSCORP.COM)

Dietary staff must follow strict infection prevention guidelines in food preparation. Surveys are done by health departments to check for cleanliness and infection prevention practices.

Menus

Menus are prepared for different diets and are completed each day at some facilities. If menus are used at your facility, you may be asked to read them to residents and to help to complete the menus. Make sure you have the correct diet order menu for each resident. Speak slowly and clearly and answer any questions or concerns the resident may have. Make the selections sound appetizing. Encourage nutritious choices, but allow the resident to make the final decisions. Make sure to check one or more items from every category, as well as a beverage. Fill out menus and turn them in promptly. When food arrives, check to see that the resident has received what he or she ordered.

7. Explain the importance of following diet orders and identify special diets

Special diets are often ordered for residents who have certain illnesses or conditions (Fig. 14-12). Sometimes they are ordered to help a resident gain or lose weight. Some diets are ordered for a short time before a medical test or surgery. Doctors prescribe the special diet, also called a "therapeutic" or "modified" diet, and then the dietician plans the diet, along with input from the resident.

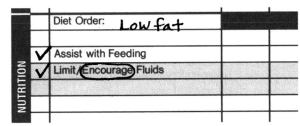

Fig. 14-12. *The care plan specifies the special diet ordered, as well as additional dietary instructions.*

Residents who have orders for specific diets require additional care and supervision. Special diets may restrict or eliminate certain foods or fluids. As stated earlier, it is very important to check resident identification against the diet card before serving meal trays. Also check the food on the tray to see if it matches the diet ordered. Serving a resident the wrong food can cause serious problems, such as allergic reactions and possibly death.

The following information identifies many types of therapeutic diets and abbreviations you are likely to see for these diets on a diet card:

Liquid Diet. Liquid diets are made up of foods that are liquid at room temperature. Liquid diets are usually ordered as "clear" or "full." A clear liquid diet consists of fluids that you can see through, such as clear soups and juices. A full liquid diet includes clear liquids with the addition of cream soups, milk, and ice cream. This diet may be ordered for a short time due to a medical condition or ordered before surgery or a diagnostic test.

Soft Diet and Mechanical Soft Diet. The soft diet is soft in texture. This diet restricts or eliminates foods that are hard to chew and swallow, such as raw fruits and vegetables and some meats. High-fiber foods, fried foods, and spicy foods may also be limited to help with digestion. The soft diet is often used for people who are making the transition from a liquid diet to a regular diet. It is also used for people who are recovering from surgery or a long illness, have dental problems, or extreme weakness.

The mechanical soft diet gets its name from how foods are prepared, such as with blenders, food processors, or cutting utensils. These items are used to chop or blend foods to make them easier to chew and swallow. In contrast to the soft diet, the mechanical soft diet does not limit spices, fat, and fiber. Only the texture of foods is changed. For example, meats can be ground and moistened with sauces or water to ease swallowing. This diet is used for people recovering from surgery, who have difficulty swallowing, or who suffer from dental problems.

Pureed Diet. To **puree** food means to chop, blend, or grind it into a thick paste of baby food consistency. This consistency means the food should be thick enough to hold its form in the mouth, but does not need to be chewed. The pureed diet is used for people who have trouble chewing and swallowing and who cannot tolerate regular or mechanical soft diets.

Bland Diet. In the bland diet, foods that irritate the stomach and digestive tract are eliminated. These include spicy foods and citrus juices. Some people must also avoid dairy products. This diet is used for people who have intestinal problems or conditions, such as Crohn's disease or irritable bowel syndrome (IBS) (Chapter 15).

Lactose-Free Diet. **Lactose intolerance** is the inability of the body to digest lactose, a type of sugar found in milk and other dairy products. A lactose-free diet means that all products with lactose must be eliminated. These include milk and all foods or beverages made with milk. Other types of milk may be allowed, such as lactose-free milk or soy milk, among others.

High-Residue or High-Fiber Diet. High-residue or high-fiber diets increase the intake of fiber and whole grains, such as whole grain cereals, bread and raw fruits and vegetables (Fig. 14-13). This diet helps with problems such as bowel disorders, constipation, and other gastrointestinal illnesses (Chapter 15).

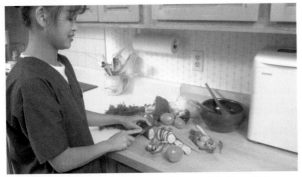

Fig. 14-13. Intake of raw vegetables and fruits will be ordered for a high-residue or high-fiber diet.

Low-Residue or Low-Fiber Diet. This diet decreases the intake of fiber, grains, seeds, and other foods, such as dairy and coffee. The low-residue diet is used for people with bowel disorders such as diverticulitis (Chapter 15).

Modified Calorie Diets. A high-calorie diet increases the amount of calories to help a person gain weight. This may be necessary due to malnutrition, surgery, or illness. In order to lose weight or to maintain weight, a person is put on a low-calorie diet, which decreases calorie intake. Common abbreviations for these diets are "High-Cal" or "Low-Cal."

Residents' Rights

Obesity and Bias

Residents, their families and friends, and staff members may be overweight or obese. Studies have shown that prejudice often exists toward people who are obese. Refrain from making judgments about people who are overweight or obese. Do not make negative comments or show disgust or distaste. Be compassionate and supportive.

Low-Sodium Diet. People with heart disease or kidney disease are put on low-sodium diets. When a resident is on a low-sodium diet, salt will be restricted. No salt shakers or salt packets should be on a meal tray. Condiments with high concentrations of salt, including Worcestershire, barbecue, chili, steak, and soy sauces, ketchup, mustard, and mayonnaise may be restricted as well. The abbreviations for this diet are "Low Na," which means low sodium, or "NAS," which stands for "No Added Salt."

High-Protein Diet. A high-protein diet is used for people recovering from surgery and for healing serious wounds, such as burns. High-protein foods, such as meat, fish, and cheese or those foods with added protein, such as protein milkshakes, are encouraged.

Low-Protein Diet. This diet is often used for people who have kidney or liver disease. Protein is restricted because the body cannot use the protein properly and it may lead to further damage of these organs. Protein is never completely eliminated from the diet, though, because the body needs protein to function. Vegetables and starches, such as breads, cereals, and pasta, are encouraged.

Low-Fat/Low-Cholesterol Diet. People who have heart disease and artery problems are often placed on this diet. The low-fat/low-cholesterol diet is also used for people who have gallbladder or liver disease. Low-fat and low-cholesterol foods, such as skim milk, low-fat cottage cheese, and white meats of turkey and chicken, and fish are usually permitted. A common abbreviation for this diet is "Low-Fat/Low-Chol."

High-Potassium Diet. This diet is used for people who take diuretics or for people who take blood pressure medications. **Diuretics** are medications that reduce fluid volume in the body. Because diuretics increase urine output, a person's body may be low in potassium. Foods high in potassium include bananas, grapefruit, oranges, orange juice, prune juice, prunes, dried apricots, figs, raisins, dates, cantaloupes, tomatoes, potatoes with skins, sweet potatoes and yams, winter squash, legumes, avocados, and unsalted nuts.

Fluid-Restricted Diet. People with severe heart disease and kidney disease may have trouble processing fluid and may be on a fluid-restricted diet. You will need to measure and document the amount of fluid consumed and eliminated. The fluid a person consumes is called **intake**, or **input**. You will learn more about fluid restrictions and documenting intake later in the chapter. Additional fluids or foods that count as fluids, such as soups, ice cream, etc., cannot be offered to a resident on a fluid-restricted diet. The abbreviation for this diet is "RF," which stands for "Restrict Fluids."

Diabetic Diet. Diabetes is a condition in which the pancreas does not produce enough insulin. Insulin converts **glucose**, or natural sugar, into energy for the body. Without insulin to process glucose, these sugars collect in the blood. This causes problems with circulation and can damage vital organs.

People with diabetes must be very careful about what they eat (Fig. 14-14). A registered dietician and the resident will make up a meal plan, including snacks, that must be followed exactly. Calories and carbohydrates are carefully controlled, and protein and fats are also regulated. The foods and the amounts are determined by nutritional and energy needs. Diabetic residents must eat the right amount of the right type of food at the right time, and they must eat everything that is served. This is necessary to maintain blood sugar. Encourage them to eat all of their meals and snacks. Do not offer other foods without the nurse's approval. If a resident will not finish meals and snacks, or throws food away, notify the nurse immediately.

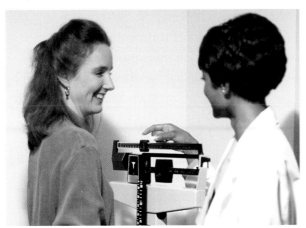

Fig. 14-14. *Diabetics must be very careful about what they eat and must keep their weight in a healthy range.*

A diabetic's meal tray may have artificial sweeteners and low-calorie jelly and maple syrup.

When serving coffee or tea to a diabetic resident, use artificial sweeteners rather than sugar. The common abbreviations for this diet on a diet card are "NCS," which stands for "No Concentrated Sweets" or "LCS," which stands for "Low Concentrated Sweets." For more information on diabetic diets, visit the American Diabetes Association's (ADA) website at diabetes.org. For more information on diabetes, see Chapter 23.

Gluten-Free Diet. This diet is free of a protein called gluten, which is found in wheat, rye, and barley. It is used for people with celiac disease. This is a disorder that can cause damage to the intestines if gluten is consumed. Foods containing wheat flour are eliminated from the diet. Examples of food that normally contains wheat include tortillas, crackers, breads, cakes, pasta, and cereals. Some sauces and dressings also have wheat in them. Other items that may contain gluten include beer, hot dogs, candy, broths, and medications. In addition, vitamins, lipsticks, and lip balms may have gluten in them.

Gluten intolerance is a condition that causes uncomfortable symptoms, such as abdominal pain, gas, and diarrhea, when a person eats products containing gluten. However, unlike with celiac disease, there is no damage to the intestines when gluten is consumed. Eliminating gluten from the diet is usually enough to manage symptoms.

Vegetarian Diet. A vegetarian diet may be needed due to a medical condition or health problem, such as diabetes or obesity, or it simply may be a person's choice not to eat meat due to cultural, ethical, personal, or religious reasons. Different types of vegetarian diets are:

- A lacto-ovo vegetarian diet excludes all meats, fish and poultry, but allows eggs and dairy products.

- A lacto-vegetarian diet eliminates poultry, meats, fish, and eggs, but allows dairy products.

- An ovo-vegetarian diet omits all meats, fish, poultry, and dairy products, but allows eggs.

- A vegan diet eliminates all poultry, meats, fish, eggs and dairy products, along with foods that contain these products.

Tip

NPO

The abbreviation "NPO" stands for "nothing by mouth." It comes from the Latin *nil per os*. This means that a resident is not allowed to have anything to eat or drink. Some residents have a serious problem with swallowing, and it is unsafe to give them anything by mouth. These residents will receive nutrition another way, either through a feeding tube or intravenously (Chapter 26). Some residents may be NPO for a short time before a medical test or surgery. If you see this abbreviation on a diet card or on the resident's care plan, do not offer the resident any food or drink, including water or ice chips.

8. Explain thickened liquids and identify three basic thickening consistencies

Residents with dysphagia, or difficulty swallowing, are evaluated by speech-language pathologists or speech therapists to determine if they should consume thickened liquids to ease swallowing. Thickened liquids have a thickening powder or agent added to them, which improves the ability to control fluid in the mouth and throat. Residents with swallowing problems may require thickened fluids to reduce the risk of choking on fluids. They tend to choke on thinner fluids, such as water or tea. Thickened liquids move down the throat more slowly, reducing coughing and limiting the risk for choking.

After the speech-language pathologist assesses a resident, the doctor writes the order for the type of thickening the resident needs. The dietary department then prepares the liquids or the thickening agent is added on the nursing unit before serving. If you have any responsibilities for thickening liquids, you will be properly trained in performing this task.

Follow instructions carefully for residents who have orders for thickened liquids. These residents are unable to drink any fluid that is not thickened. This means fluids such as soda, water, tea, and coffee are not allowed with their diets. Check with the nurse before serving any fluids to residents with these restrictions.

These are three types of thickened consistencies generally used by facilities:

1. **Nectar Thick**. This consistency is similar to a fruit nectar or other thicker juices, such as tomato juice. A resident can drink this from a cup with or without a straw.

2. **Honey Thick**. This consistency is similar to that of honey. It will pour very slowly, and spoons are usually used to consume these types of liquids.

3. **Pudding Thick**. This consistency is semi-solid, much like the consistency of pudding. A spoon will stand up straight when put into this thickened liquid. Spoons are used to consume these liquids.

9. List ways to identify and prevent unintended weight loss

Sometimes residents unintentionally lose weight, which is a serious problem for the elderly. The unintended weight loss may be due to a medical condition, such as cancer, HIV, diabetes, or other diseases. It can also be due to an unappetizing diet. Unintended weight loss puts a person at a greater risk for malnutrition. This is why it is important to report any weight loss you notice, no matter how small.

When weight loss occurs, staff will look for causes and may re-evaluate special diet orders. This will help them decide whether to modify the diet to encourage the resident to eat more. The resident may be better off eating a less strict diet. If you notice food going uneaten or if a resident complains to you or others about the food, report this to the nurse.

Warning signs for unintended weight loss include the following:

Observing and Reporting: Unintended Weight Loss and Malnourishment

O/R Resident needs help eating or drinking

O/R Resident eats less than 70% of meals/snacks

O/R Resident has mouth pain

O/R Resident has dentures that do not fit properly

O/R Resident has difficulty chewing or swallowing

O/R Resident coughs or chokes while eating

O/R Resident is sad, cries, or withdraws from others

O/R Resident is confused, wanders, or paces

If you notice any of these signs, report it immediately to the nurse. Also report if the resident has any of the following signs or symptoms, which could indicate malnourishment:

O/R Feeling of coldness throughout body

O/R Weight loss

O/R Abdominal distention

O/R Abdominal pain

O/R Constipation

O/R Edema (swelling in body tissues caused by excess fluid)

O/R Cracks or splits at the corners of the mouth

O/R Inflammation of the mucous membranes of the mouth

O/R Dry or peeling skin

O/R Brittle, easily-cracked nails

O/R Rapidly thinning hair that breaks off easily; hair that changes or loses color

O/R Frequent infections

O/R Muscle weakness

O/R Fainting

O/R Fatigue

O/R Withdrawal or **apathy** (lack of interest)

O/R Anxiety and irritability

O/R Problems with sleeping

O/R Low body temperature

O/R Slow pulse

O/R Low blood pressure

In addition, follow these guidelines to help prevent unintended weight loss:

Guidelines: Preventing Unintended Weight Loss

G Report observations and warning signs to the nurse immediately.

G Report any decrease in appetite to the nurse. If a resident has a loss of appetite, ask him or her about it.

G Encourage residents to eat by talking about eating and the food being served in a positive way (Fig. 14-15).

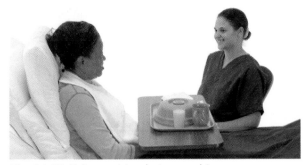

Fig. 14-15. *Being positive during mealtime can encourage residents to eat. It helps prevent unintended weight loss.*

G Check diet cards and meal trays to make sure residents are receiving the correct food.

G Respond promptly to resident complaints about foods. Serve favorite foods.

G Season food to the resident's preferences.

G   Use special adaptive equipment, as needed, to increase independence with eating.

G   Record the meal/snack intake as ordered.

G   Ask for a dietician, occupational therapist, or speech-language pathologist consultation if necessary.

Tip

Making the Most of Snacks and Nourishments

Residents are usually fed three meals a day, along with additional snacks or nourishments. Supplemental snacks or nourishments include liquids such as milk, juice, and specially-formulated nutritional drinks that may contain added protein, vitamins, or other ingredients. Solid snacks include foods like cheese and crackers, peanut butter, sherbet, gelatin, or small sandwiches. These items may be served once or twice or more often per day.

Sometimes snacks or nourishments are required by special diets. For example, a diabetic needs all of her snacks to maintain her blood sugar while on insulin injections. Another resident who is losing too much weight will need to drink all of his nutritional supplements to maintain a healthy weight. Due to illness and the problem of unintended weight loss, encourage residents to eat all of their snacks or supplements. If a resident does not finish a snack, a family member eats it, or you find it in the trash, notify the nurse.

---

10. Describe how to make dining enjoyable for residents

Often the most anticipated times of the day for residents are breakfast, lunch, and dinner. Meals provide time to see friends and socialize. Mealtimes are also the time for getting proper nourishment. Due to serious problems of weight loss and dehydration, nursing assistants are responsible for encouraging eating and promoting healthy appetites. To make mealtimes enjoyable and pleasant, follow these guidelines:

Guidelines: Dining

G   Follow a routine for dining. This encourages structure in residents' days.

G   Residents may want to look their best. Assist them with their grooming requests. All residents should be neat and clean for meals. Dress residents appropriately for dining.

G   Make sure that residents have their eyeglasses, hearing aids, dentures, and any other equipment required for eating comfortably.

G   Help to give oral care before meals, if requested.

G   Assist them as necessary with washing hands before eating.

G   Help with toileting or help them to the bathroom before eating.

G   Honor requests to seat residents by their friends. Seat residents with common interests together. Encourage conversation.

G   Position residents properly for eating. This position is usually upright at a 90-degree angle, which helps prevent swallowing and choking problems.

G   Place residents in appropriate chairs. Wheelchairs should be positioned at the right height for the table. Many tables at facilities are adjustable. These tables should be adjusted to the right height for wheelchairs. Make sure special seats, such as geriatric chairs (geri-chairs, see Chapter 11), are available if needed for a particular resident. Residents who use geri-chairs must be sitting upright, not reclining, while eating.

G   Serve food promptly to maintain the correct temperature of the food.

G   Give residents the proper eating tools they will need for their meals. If they need assistive devices, such as special utensils or cups, make sure they are available (Fig. 14-16).

G   Cut food into small portions when necessary. Do this before bringing food to the table, if possible. This promotes dignity.

G   Allow enough time for eating. Do not rush residents through their meals.

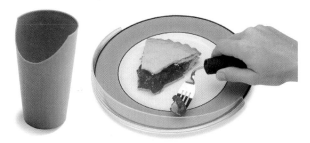

Fig. 14-16. *Examples of assistive devices that can help with eating.* (PHOTOS COURTESY OF NORTH COAST MEDICAL, INC., 800-821-9319, WWW.NCMEDICAL.COM)

G   Keep the noise level low. Do not shout or bang trays or plates. Soft music may accompany the meal (Fig. 14-17).

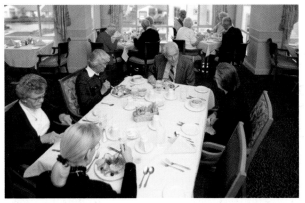

Fig. 14-17. *An appealing environment is important for promoting appetites. Keep the noise level low.*

G   Remain cheerful and positive during mealtime. Make conversation when residents wish to talk.

G   Honor requests regarding food. Residents have the legal right to ask for and receive different food. They also may be able to have additional food when requested. Check diet orders first before getting any extra food or additive, such as sugar or salt.

11. Describe how to serve meal trays and assist with eating

Meals are usually served on trays or are brought from the kitchen. Nursing assistants must work quickly to make sure food is served at the proper temperature and that residents do not have to wait long for their meals. Follow these guidelines for serving meals to residents:

Guidelines: Serving Meal Trays

G   Wash your hands before serving any meal trays. Wear gloves, if required.

G   Check the diet card for special diet orders, and identify each resident before serving a meal tray. Make sure the food looks correct for each person. As you learned earlier, serving a resident the wrong food can cause serious health problems, even death.

G   Serve all residents sitting at one table before serving other tables, so the residents will be able to eat together.

G   If a resident needs your help to eat, leave the tray on the cart until you are able to do this task. Keep the door to the food cart closed after removing each tray. Maintaining the proper temperature of food helps prevent foodborne illnesses.

G   Prepare the food before helping residents eat. Only do what residents cannot do for themselves.

G   Open juice or milk cartons, if residents need help. If a resident is able to use a straw and wants one, place it in the container using the wrapper; do not touch straws with your fingers. Pour beverages into cups if residents do not want to use cartons. Get coffee, tea, or other drinks when residents request them.

G   Butter rolls, bread, and vegetables as residents prefer.

G   Season food according to what the resident wants, even pureed food. Remember not to season food with salt if a resident is on a low-sodium diet.

G   When serving additional snacks or nourishments to residents, follow the same guidelines as for serving regular meal trays. Provide any necessary assistance with snacks and nourishments. Report to the nurse if residents do not finish their supplemental snacks or nourishments.

You may be required to serve meal trays to residents in isolation. Carefully follow Isolation Precautions, in addition to Standard Precautions, ordered for each resident. Apply PPE as needed, and make sure dietary department staff puts on proper PPE as well.

For residents in isolation, food trays may be served using regular dishes and standard utensils. These items are then washed and, in some cases, disinfected.

Food inside an isolation room must never be shared with visitors, other residents, or staff. Discard uneaten food in the proper container in the isolation room. Apply PPE before entering the room to remove a meal tray.

Residents differ in the amount of assistance they need with eating. Good organization on your part will help make the dining experience run smoothly. Prepare residents who require the least assistance first. Make sure everything is ready, such as opening cartons and cutting and seasoning food. When the resident is ready to feed himself, you can move on to the next resident. Continue this process until all residents who can eat on their own are set up and eating.

Check back with these residents from time to time to see if they need anything else.

Some residents will be completely unable to feed themselves. When assisting residents with feeding, promote independence by encouraging them to do whatever they can for themselves. For example, if a resident can hold and use a napkin, she should. If she can hold and eat finger foods, offer them. As mentioned earlier, special assistive devices for eating can be helpful, too.

Promoting independence with eating positively affects self-esteem. It is very difficult when a person has to depend on another person for assistance with a basic need such as eating. Empathize with residents and be sensitive to this. Provide privacy as needed when eating.

Eating is a social time, and even residents who must be fed or who get their nutrition via tubes (Chapter 26) may still enjoy being social with others. While assisting with eating, make conversation if the resident wishes, using appropriate topics, such as the news and weather (Fig. 14-18). Pay attention to the person you are helping; do not talk to other staff members while assisting residents with eating. Say positive things about the food being served. For example, "This smells really good," and, "This looks really fresh." Meal time should be a pleasant experience, and cheerful company can actually increase how much a resident eats and drinks. Do not rush residents through their meals.

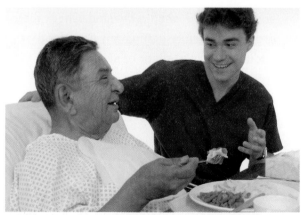

Fig. 14-18. *Be friendly and social while helping residents with eating. Encourage them to do whatever they can for themselves.*

In addition, follow these guidelines for helping residents at meal time:

- Offer a clothing protector to the resident before assisting with eating. Do not refer to the clothing protector as a "bib." If he refuses to wear one, respect his wishes. Residents have the right to choose whether or not to use a clothing protector (Fig. 14-19).

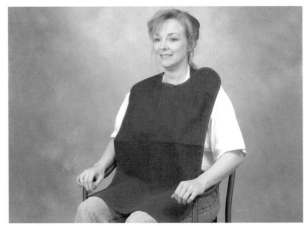

Fig. 14-19. Residents have the right to choose whether or not to use a clothing protector. Respect each resident's decision. (REPRINTED WITH PERMISSION OF BRIGGS CORPORATION, 800-247-2343, WWW.BRIGGSCORP.COM)

- Treat the resident with respect. Do not make fun of or judge any food choices.

- Follow all infection prevention precautions.

- Sit at the resident's eye level and make eye contact. Give the resident your full attention.

- Identify foods and fluids in front of the resident. Call pureed foods and soft foods by their correct names. For example, ask, "Would you like some steak?" rather than asking if they want "some of this brown stuff."

- Ask the resident which foods he wants to eat first and honor his choices.

- Do not mix foods unless the resident requests it.

- If you are concerned that food is too hot, do not touch it to test its temperature. Put your hand over the food to sense the heat. Do not blow on it to cool it if it feels too hot. Offer other foods first while you wait for it to cool down.

- Alternate between food and drink. Offer fluids to the resident throughout the meal.

- If a resident wants different food than what is being served, tell the dietician or the nurse right away.

- If a resident refuses to eat, respect this. Do not insist that he eat the food, but report it to the nurse immediately.

Feeding a resident who cannot feed self

Equipment: meal tray, clothing protector, 2-3 washcloths or wipes

1. Identify yourself by name. Identify the resident. Greet the resident by name.

2. Wash your hands.

3. Explain procedure to resident. Speak clearly, slowly, and directly. Maintain face-to-face contact whenever possible.

4. Provide for the resident's privacy with a curtain, screen, or door.

5. Pick up diet card. Ask resident to state his or her name. Verify that resident has received the right tray.

6. Raise the head of the bed. Make sure resident is in an upright sitting position (at a 90-degree angle).

7. Adjust bed height so you will be able to sit at resident's eye level. Lock bed wheels.

8. Place meal tray where it can be easily seen by the resident, such as on the overbed table.

9. Help resident to clean hands with hand wipes if resident cannot do it on her own.

10. Help resident to put on clothing protector, if desired.

11. Sit facing resident. Sit at resident's eye level (Fig. 14-20). Sit on the stronger side if resident has one-sided weakness.

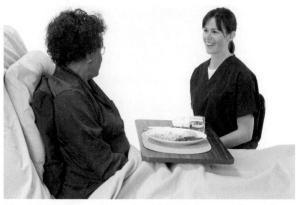

Fig. 14-20. *The resident should be sitting upright and you should be sitting at her eye level.*

12. Tell the resident what foods are on tray. Offer a drink of beverage and ask what resident would like to eat first.

13. Offer the food in bite-sized pieces, telling the resident the content of each bite of food offered (Fig. 14-21). Alternate types of food, allowing for resident's preferences. Do not feed all of one type before offering another type. Report any swallowing problems to the nurse immediately. If resident has one-sided weakness, direct food to the unaffected, or stronger, side.

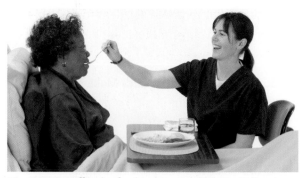

Fig. 14-21. *Offer the food in bite-sized pieces. Tell resident the content of each bite of food.*

14. Offer sips of beverage to resident throughout the meal.

15. Make sure resident's mouth is empty before next bite or sip.

16. Talk with the resident during the meal (Fig. 14-22).

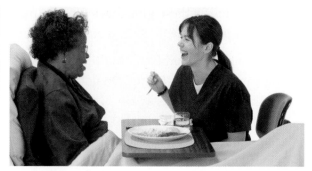

Fig. 14-22. *Cheerful company makes mealtime more enjoyable and may increase how much the resident eats and drinks.*

17. Use washcloths or wipes to wipe food from resident's mouth and hands as needed during the meal. Wipe again at the end of the meal (Fig. 14-23).

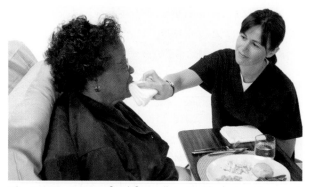

Fig. 14-23. *Wiping food from the mouth during the meal helps to maintain the resident's dignity.*

18. Remove clothing protector if used. Dispose of in proper container.

19. Remove food tray. Check for eyeglasses, dentures, hearing aids, or any personal items before removing tray. Place tray in proper area to be picked up.

20. Make resident comfortable. Make sure the bed is free from crumbs.

21. Return bed to lowest position. Remove privacy measures.

22. Leave call light within resident's reach.

23. Wash your hands.

24. Be courteous and respectful at all times.

25. Report any changes in the resident to the nurse. Document procedure using facility guidelines. Record intake of solid food and fluids properly (see Learning Objective 14 for more information).

Residents' Rights and Eating

Residents have the right to refuse food and drink. Residents also have the right to ask for and receive different kinds of food. Report any refusals of food or requests for different food right away.

12. Describe how to assist residents with special needs

Residents with certain diseases or conditions, such as Parkinson's disease, stroke, dementia, head trauma, blindness, and confusion may need additional help with eating. For example, a resident who has Parkinson's disease may have tremors or shaking and stiffness, which make it very difficult to eat without help. Follow these guidelines for special dining techniques.

Guidelines: Dining Techniques

G Use assistive or adaptive devices for eating when necessary. They help people feed themselves. Utensils with padded handles and plates with high edges to prevent food from sliding off are two examples of assistive devices for eating.

G To help maintain independence with eating, use physical and verbal cues. The hand-over-hand approach is an example of a physical cue. The resident lifts a utensil if he is able, and you put your hand over his to help with eating (Fig. 14-24). With your hand placed over the resident's hand, assist in getting food on the utensil. Steer the utensil from the plate to the mouth and back. Repeat this until the resident is finished with his meal.

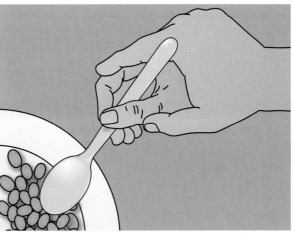

Fig. 14-24. The hand-over-hand approach is used when a resident can help by lifting utensils. It helps promote independence.

G Verbal cues must be short and clear so that they are easily understood. After each task is done, give additional prompts one at a time, for example, "Pick up your spoon." "Put some potatoes on your spoon." "Lift the spoon to your mouth." These types of phrases are repeated until the resident has finished eating.

G For residents who have had a stroke and have a weaker side, always put food into the stronger, or unaffected, side of the mouth. This helps prevent choking. Make sure food is swallowed before offering more bites.

G For residents who have Parkinson's disease, dementia, confusion, or trauma, use physical and verbal cues if needed. Allow enough time to chew and swallow. Place food and drinks within the resident's reach.

G For residents who are visually impaired or blind, read menus to them if needed. Allow enough time for decision-making on menu items. When assisting with eating, face them when speaking and use a normal tone of voice. Place plate or tray directly in front of residents. Use the face of an imaginary clock to explain the position of what is in front of them (Fig. 14-25). If necessary, let residents know when to open their mouths and what food they are eating.

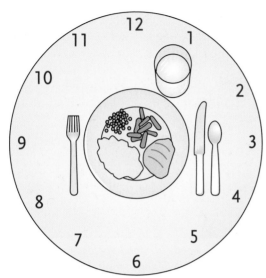

Fig. 14-25. *Use the face of an imaginary clock to explain the position of food to visually-impaired residents.*

G   If the resident eats too quickly, remind him to chew, and set the utensils down between bites. Use smaller cups and plates and put less food on plates.

G   If the resident bites down on utensils, ask the resident to open his mouth. Wait until the jaw relaxes to pull the utensil out of the mouth. Offer finger foods instead. Use smaller utensils, but do not use plastic utensils. Avoid using forks.

G   If the resident cannot or will not chew, lightly press on the edge of the lips or on the chin to stimulate chewing. You can also show him how to chew by doing it yourself. Serve softer foods that require less chewing; dip meats and other foods in sauce or gravy.

G   If the resident will not stop chewing, ask him to stop chewing. Offer smaller bites of food and feed softer foods that do not need as much chewing.

G   If the resident holds food in his mouth or will not swallow, remind him to swallow after every bite. After feeding a bite of food, lightly press an empty teaspoon against the lips to encourage the person to swallow the food. This may help stimulate saliva production, along with the swallowing reflex.

G   If the resident pockets food in his cheek, ask him to chew and swallow the food. Touch the outside of the cheek and ask him to use his tongue to get the food. Using your fingers on the cheek near the lower jaw, gently push food toward teeth. Avoid offering food such as rice that can stick inside the mouth or on dentures. Give sips of fluids often. Check the mouth for food often before offering more food, but do not place your fingers inside the mouth. Ask the resident to open his mouth so that you can check for food. Ask residents not to stand up with food in their mouths.

G   If the resident has poor lip closure, remind him to close his lips. Show him how to close his lips if necessary. A speech-language pathologist or a nurse may teach this resident to practice blowing a whistle to help him close his lips.

G   If the resident has no teeth or is missing teeth, a dentist will do an assessment of oral health. Thickened liquids or soft or pureed diets may be ordered.

G   If the resident has dentures that do not fit properly, report it to the nurse immediately. A dentist will evaluate the resident as soon as possible for denture replacement. Thickened liquids or soft or pureed diets may be ordered until dentures are replaced.

G   If the resident has a change in vision, it can cause problems with seeing food clearly, which may reduce appetite. Make sure resident wears eyeglasses and that they are clean. Report to the nurse if eyeglasses are damaged or broken. Read menus out loud and describe food in front of the resident using the imaginary clock if necessary.

G   If the resident has a protruding tongue or tongue thrust, use special straws and cups to help. A tongue thrust is a forceful protrusion of the tongue, often during eating and drinking. The jaw will need to be encouraged to move upward so that the tongue will retract and the lips will close on the eating utensil. A speech-language pathologist or a nurse may teach this resident to practice blowing a whistle to help him close his lips.

G If the resident will not open his mouth, touch his lower lip to encourage him to open the mouth. Identify each bite of food you offer. Do not feed sticky food such as peanut butter.

G If the resident falls asleep while eating, seat him with residents who talk a lot and are very social. Make appropriate conversation while he is eating.

G If the resident chokes when drinking, remind him to lift his chin before taking a sip of fluid. Offer fluids when he has no food in his mouth. Do not distract the resident by talking while he is eating. The resident should be seated, not standing, while drinking.

G If the resident is susceptible to choking when eating, avoid foods like cake, hot dogs, peanut butter, nuts, popcorn, raw vegetables and small, shiny fruits, like grapes.

G If the resident forgets to eat, remind him to take another bite. Offer praise and encouragement. Do not rush the person.

G If the resident drools excessively, make sure he is in an upright eating position, using good posture. A consultation with a speech-language pathologist may be ordered to help the resident learn better swallowing techniques. If drooling interferes with basic safety, medications may be ordered to decrease the drooling. Clothing protectors, towels, or pads may be used to protect clothing.

G If the resident has poor sitting balance, seat him in a regular dining room chair with armrests, rather than a wheelchair. Position him upright at a 90-degree angle. Knees should be flexed, and feet and arms should be fully supported. Push the chair under the table and place his forearms on the table.

G If the resident tends to lean to one side, ask him to keep his elbows on the table. Using a wheelchair wedge cushion may help.

G If the resident tends to fall forward, using a geriatric chair may help. A wheelchair wedge cushion may also help.

G If the resident has poor neck control, a soft neck brace may stabilize the head. A wedge cushion behind the head and shoulders can help a resident in a geriatric chair.

For tips on feeding residents who are cognitively impaired, see Chapter 22.

13. Discuss dysphagia and list guidelines for preventing aspiration

Difficulty in swallowing, or dysphagia, can be a serious problem for elderly residents. Causes of dysphagia include: illness (stroke is one example), certain medications, problems with the mouth and throat muscles, weakness, and food choices. Problems with teeth or dentures also put a person at risk for swallowing problems. The need for proper oral care can affect the ability to eat or drink safely.

Signs and symptoms of swallowing problems must be reported to the nurse immediately. Nurses, doctors, and care team members, such as the speech-language pathologist, will determine what steps to take to reduce dysphagia. The following are signs and symptoms of dysphagia to report to the nurse:

Observing and Reporting: Dysphagia

O/R Eating very slowly

O/R Avoidance of eating

O/R Spitting out pieces of food

O/R Difficulty chewing food

O/R Difficulty swallowing small bites of food or pills

°/ʀ Swallowing several times when eating a single bite

°/ʀ Dribbling saliva, food or fluid from the mouth

°/ʀ Keeping food inside the mouth or cheeks during and after meals

°/ʀ Vomiting while eating or drinking

°/ʀ Frequent throat clearing

°/ʀ Food or fluid coming up into or out of the nose

°/ʀ Coughing during or after meals

°/ʀ Choking during meals or while drinking

°/ʀ Gurgling sound in voice during or after meals

°/ʀ Problems breathing when eating or drinking

°/ʀ Visible effort to swallow

°/ʀ Watering eyes when eating or drinking

In addition, observing and reporting the following may help the care team assess a resident who has dysphagia:

°/ʀ Type of food or drink that caused the problem

°/ʀ Time of day the problem occurred

°/ʀ Whether or not the resident had dentures in place when the problem happened

°/ʀ Whether or not the resident was talking or laughing when the choking occurred

°/ʀ How the resident was positioned while eating or drinking

°/ʀ Whether or not the resident was ambulating (walking) while eating or drinking

As you have learned, swallowing problems cause a high risk for choking on food or drink. When a person chokes, mucus, food or fluids, or emesis (vomitus) may move into the lungs. Inhaling food, drink, or foreign material into the lungs is called aspiration, which can cause pneumonia or death. To ensure residents' safety, follow these guidelines to prevent aspiration:

Guidelines: Preventing Aspiration

G Place residents in proper position for eating and drinking. They must sit upright at a 90-degree angle (Fig. 14-26). Do not feed residents in a reclining position.

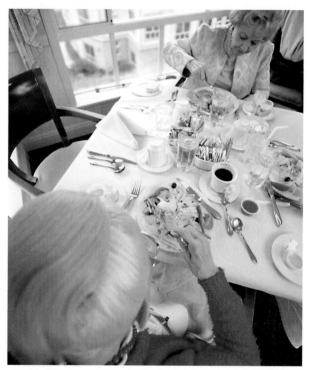

Fig. 14-26. *Sitting as upright as possible when eating and drinking helps prevent aspiration.*

G Feed residents slowly.

G Avoid distractions while eating.

G Offer small pieces of food or small spoonfuls of pureed food.

G Offer a bite of food, then a liquid. Repeat this.

G Place food in the non-paralyzed, or unaffected, side of the mouth, if one side is paralyzed.

G Make sure food is actually swallowed after each bite before offering more food or fluids. However, do not put your fingers inside a resident's mouth.

G Keep residents sitting upright for at least 30 minutes after eating and drinking.

G Provide quality mouth care after eating.

G   Closely observe residents who choke easily during eating and drinking. Report signs of aspiration, such as gagging, vomiting, clutching throat, cyanosis (bluish skin color), darkening skin, unconsciousness, shortness of breath, difficulty breathing, or resident complaints of chest pain or tightness in the chest to the nurse immediately.

More information on swallowing difficulties and alternative methods of feeding is in Chapter 26.

14. Describe intake and output (I&O)

As you learned earlier, the fluid a person consumes is called intake, or input. **Output** is the fluid that is eliminated each day that cannot stay in the body. Output includes urine, feces, and vomitus, as well as perspiration and moisture in the air that a person exhales. It also includes suction material and wound drainage. When a person maintains equal intake and output, or consumes and eliminates equal amounts of fluid, it is called **fluid balance**.

Most people maintain fluid balance naturally. However, residents on special diets or who have certain illnesses may need to have their intake and output (I&O) measured. Measuring I&O means that staff record and add together all of the amounts of food and fluids the resident takes in and eliminates within 24 hours. This is recorded on an Intake/Output (I&O) sheet (Fig. 14-27).

Fluids are usually measured in milliliters (mL). Milliliters are units of measurement in the metric system. One milliliter is 1/1000 of a liter and is equal to one cubic centimeter (cc). Ounces (oz) are converted to milliliters. One ounce equals 30 milliliters, so to convert ounces to milliliters, multiply by 30. **Graduates** are containers that measure fluid in milliliters and may also measure in ounces (Fig. 14-28). It is important to know how to convert ounces to milliliters, as well as other common conversions. See the box below for information on conversions.

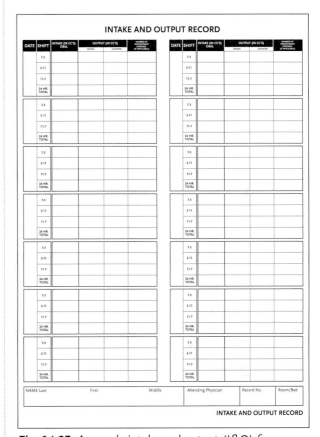

Fig. 14-27. A sample intake and output (I&O) form.

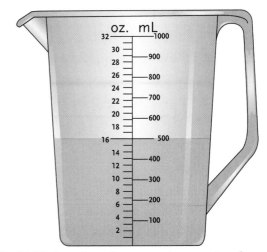

Fig. 14-28. A graduate is a measuring container for measuring fluid volume.

Conversions

One milliliter (mL) is a unit of measure equal to one cubic centimeter (cc). Follow your facility's policies on whether to document using "mL" or "cc."

1 oz. = 30 mL or 30 cc
2 oz. = 60 mL
3 oz. = 90 mL
4 oz. = 120 mL
5 oz. = 150 mL
6 oz. = 180 mL
7 oz. = 210 mL
8 oz. = 240 mL
¼ cup = 2 oz. = 60 mL
½ cup = 4 oz. = 120 mL
¾ cup = 6 oz. = 180 mL
1 cup = 8 oz. = 240 mL
2 cups = 16 oz. = 480 mL
4 cups = 32 oz. = 960 mL

For example, a resident has an eight-ounce glass of juice. She consumes about half of the juice, or four ounces. To determine her intake, convert ounces to milliliters. Multiply four ounces by 30; the answer is 120 mL, which is what you document on the intake sheet.

Measuring and recording intake and output

Equipment: I&O sheet, graduate (measuring container), pen and paper

Measure intake first.

1. Identify yourself by name. Identify the resident. Greet the resident by name.

2. Wash your hands.

3. Explain procedure to resident. Speak clearly, slowly, and directly. Maintain face-to-face contact whenever possible.

4. Provide for the resident's privacy with a curtain, screen, or door.

5. A list of container sizes should be available to help with measuring. For example, a water cup equals 240 mL, a cereal bowl equals 150 mL, and a milk carton equals 240 mL. If amounts are not available, use a graduate to measure how much fluid a resident is served. Note the amount of fluid the resident is served on paper.

6. When the resident has finished a meal or snack, measure any leftover fluids. Note this amount on paper.

7. Subtract the leftover amount from the amount served. If you have measured in ounces, convert to milliliters (mL) by multiplying by 30.

8. Record amount of fluid consumed (in mL) in input column on I&O sheet. Record the time and what fluid was consumed.

9. Wash your hands.

Measuring output is the other half of monitoring fluid balance.

Equipment: I&O sheet, graduate, gloves, additional PPE if required, pen and paper

1. Wash your hands.

2. Put on gloves before handling bedpan/urinal.

3. Pour the contents of the bedpan or urinal into measuring container. Do not spill or splash any of the urine.

4. Place container on flat surface. Measure amount of urine at eye level. Keep container level (Fig. 14-29).

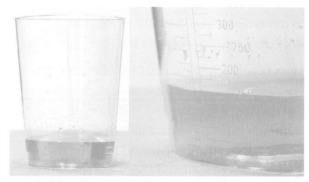

Fig. 14-29. *Keep container level while measuring output.*

5. After measuring urine, empty contents of measuring container into toilet. Do not splash. Flush toilet.

6. Place container and bedpan in area for cleaning or clean and store according to policy.

7. Remove and discard gloves.

8. Wash hands before recording output.

9. Record contents of container in output column on sheet. Report any changes to the nurse.

To record food intake, the percentage method is often used. Menus that list the percentage of total calories of each item served may be used. A dietician calculates these percentages. It is important to accurately record how much of the meal the resident has eaten. To do this, observe how much of each item was consumed. Then adjust the percentage of total calories the item provided. Finally, add the adjusted percentages for a total percentage consumed.

For example, egg, toast, and milk is on a resident's breakfast tray. The egg is worth 20% of calories needed for her breakfast. If she finishes half of the egg, you would document that she consumed 10% of that food. If the toast is worth 15%, and she eats all of the toast, you would record the full 15% toward the total calories consumed. This is one example of how to document intake using the percentage method. Facilities may document intake in other ways. Follow your facility's policy. Document food and drink intake carefully. Accuracy is important. Report if a resident eats less than 70% of his or her meal.

15. List ways to identify and prevent dehydration

Water is one of the most important nutrients for life. Drinking at least 64 ounces (eight 8-ounce glasses) of water or other fluids per day can help prevent constipation, urinary incontinence, and dehydration. Dehydration is a serious condition that occurs when a person does not have enough fluid in the body. Proper fluid intake also helps to dilute wastes and flush out the urinary system, which lessens the risk of infection (Fig. 14-30).

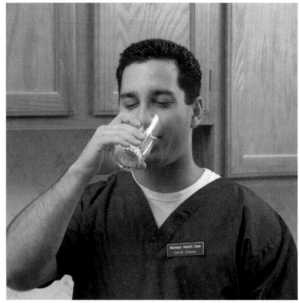

Fig. 14-30. *Remember, drinking plenty of water is good for you, too!*

Because the sense of thirst lessens as people age, fluids should be offered to residents often. A "force fluids" (FF) order may be written for a resident who is at risk of being dehydrated. **Force fluids** means to encourage the resident to drink more fluids.

Warning signs of dehydration include the following:

Observing and Reporting: Dehydration

If you notice any of these signs, report them immediately to the nurse.

O/R Resident drinks less than six 8-ounce glasses of liquids per day

O/R Resident drinks little or no fluids at meals

O/R Resident needs help drinking from a cup or glass

O/R Resident has trouble swallowing liquids

O/R Resident has frequent vomiting, diarrhea, or fever

O/R Resident is easily confused or tired

O/R Resident is thirsty

^O/R   Resident has a dry mouth

^O/R   Resident has a decrease in urinary output

Also report if the resident has any of these signs or symptoms:

^O/R   Severe thirst

^O/R   Dry mouth and mucous membranes

^O/R   Cracked lips

^O/R   Dry, warm, wrinkled, or clammy skin

^O/R   Sunken eyes

^O/R   Flushed face

^O/R   Dark urine

^O/R   Strong-smelling urine

^O/R   Constipation or weight loss

^O/R   Weakness, dizziness, lightheadedness, or confusion

^O/R   Headache

^O/R   Irritability

^O/R   Rapid or weakened pulse

^O/R   Irregular heartbeat

^O/R   Low blood pressure

Preventing dehydration is an important nursing assistant responsibility. Follow these guidelines to help prevent dehydration:

Guidelines: Preventing Dehydration

G   Observe residents carefully for signs and symptoms of dehydration. Report observations and warning signs to the nurse immediately.

G   Encourage residents to drink fluids every time you see them, if allowed. Offer fresh water or other fluids often (Fig. 14-31).

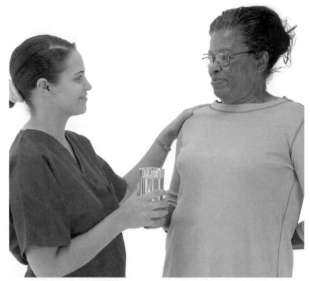

Fig. 14-31. *Encouraging residents to drink every time you see them can help prevent dehydration.*

G   Offer fluids that residents prefer, such as water, juice, or milk. Some residents will prefer fluids without ice. Honor this preference. If the resident wants ice in his drink, use and store the ice scoop properly. Do not let ice touch your hand and then fall back into the container. Place the ice scoop in the proper receptacle after each use. Report if the resident complains about the fluids being offered.

G   Make sure water pitcher and cup are close enough to the resident and light enough for the resident to lift, approximately half-full.

G   Offer assistance if the resident cannot drink without help. Use assistive devices as needed.

G   Offer ice chips, flavored ice sticks, and gelatin often. These items are considered liquids. Do not offer ice chips or sticks if resident has a swallowing problem.

G   Keep accurate I&O records.

G   Follow posted schedules for offering fluids.

One method of encouraging fluids is outlined in the acronym on the next page:

POURR

Post a regular schedule for offering fluids to residents.

Observe residents carefully for signs and symptoms of dehydration.

Use other kinds of fluids, such as flavored frozen ice sticks, to improve fluid balance and increase fluid intake.

Remind all staff, visitors, and volunteers as necessary of the importance of following the schedule.

Report changes in fluid balance or any signs and symptoms of dehydration promptly.

Residents' Rights

A request for a drink must be honored.

When residents are thirsty, they may ask for water, juice, or some other beverage. Respond promptly to these requests. Residents have a legal right to have their basic needs, like eating and drinking, met. The only time you should not honor this request is when a resident has a fluid restriction or has an "NPO" order. NPO is an abbreviation for "nothing by mouth." In this situation, explain why a drink cannot be given. Report the request to the nurse.

16. List signs and symptoms of fluid overload and describe conditions that may require fluid restrictions

Fluid overload is a condition that occurs when more fluid enters the body than is eliminated from the body. The body cannot eliminate the additional fluid, and fluid gathers in certain areas of the body, such as the ankles. Fluid overload can occur when the heart, kidneys, or lungs are not working properly. People can also have this problem after having surgery.

Observing and Reporting: Fluid Overload

O/R Weight gain (daily weight gain of one to two pounds)

O/R Fatigue

O/R Difficulty breathing or shortness of breath, especially if lying down

O/R Swelling of the ankles, feet, fingers, or hands

O/R Coughing

O/R Decreased urine output

O/R Increased heart rate

O/R Skin that appears tight, smooth, and shiny

O/R Swollen abdomen due to excess fluid, called ascites

Treating fluid overload usually consists of a reduction in activity, medicine to eliminate the excessive fluid, increasing the number of pillows used for sleep, and careful monitoring of weight gain and edema.

Fluid restrictions are ordered when the amount of fluid must be carefully measured and limited due to certain disorders. Examples are congestive heart failure (CHF) (Chapter 19), or chronic renal failure (Chapter 16). Some residents will have a **restrict fluids** (RF) order, which means the person is allowed to drink, but must limit the daily amount to a level set by the doctor. When a resident has a restrict fluids order, do not give that resident extra fluids or a water pitcher unless the nurse approves it. Other reasons for fluid restrictions include:

- Recent surgery

- Illness, such as a gastrointestinal (GI) illness

- Special medical test ordered

- Feeding done through a special tube (See Chapter 26 for more information.)

Chapter Review

1. List five common nutritional problems that elderly people may experience (LO 2).

2. List two factors that influence food choices (LO 3).

3. List the six basic nutrients and identify which nutrient is the most essential for life (LO 4).

4. According to MyPlate's suggestions, what should half of your plate be made up of (LO 5)?

5. List some examples of plant sources of protein foods (LO 5).

6. According to MyPlate, what should most dairy group choices be (LO 5)?

7. List the information contained on diet cards (LO 6).

8. Why is it very important to check resident identification against the diet card before serving meal trays (LO 7)?

9. How is the mechanical soft diet different from the soft diet (LO 7)?

10. What is one common abbreviation for a low-sodium diet (LO 7)?

11. What is the difference between a clear liquid diet and a full liquid diet (LO 7)?

12. Why must diabetic residents eat the right amount of the right type of food at the right time, and eat everything that is served (LO 7)?

13. What does the abbreviation "NPO" stand for (LO 7)?

14. Explain three basic thickening consistencies (LO 8).

15. What is the benefit of thickening liquids (LO 8)?

16. List six warning signs for unintended weight loss that should be reported (LO 9).

17. What is the proper position in which to place a resident for eating (LO 10)?

18. Look at the guidelines for dining in Learning Objective 10. List four that promote residents' dignity (LO 10).

19. When serving meal trays, why should nursing assistants only do what residents cannot do for themselves? Why should residents be encouraged to do whatever they can for themselves (LO 11)?

20. Give two examples, other than those listed in Learning Objective 11, of positive things to say about food being served (LO 11).

21. If a resident refuses to wear a clothing protector, what should the nursing assistant do (LO 11)?

22. How should a nursing assistant properly test the temperature of food if she feels it might be too hot (LO 11)?

23. To which side of the mouth should food be directed if a resident has a weaker side—the weaker (affected) or stronger (unaffected) side (LO 12)?

24. When assisting a resident who is visually impaired, how should the nursing assistant explain the position of food and objects in front of the resident (LO 12)?

25. For each of the following conditions, list a technique that would help with eating (LO 12):

The resident bites down on utensils

The resident will not chew

The resident pockets food in his cheek

The resident has poor sitting balance

The resident has poor neck control

26. List 11 signs and symptoms of dysphagia (LO 13).

27. List eight guidelines for preventing aspiration (LO 13).

28. List four examples of output (LO 14).

29. Define "fluid balance" (LO 14).

30. How many milliliters (mL) equal one ounce (oz.) (LO 14)?

31. How many ounces of water or other liquids should a healthy resident be encouraged to drink every day (LO 15)?

32. List four warning signs of dehydration that should be reported (LO 15).

33. List six ways to prevent dehydration (LO 15).

34. List seven symptoms of fluid overload (LO 16).

35. What is a "restrict fluids (RF)" order (LO 16)?

15
The Gastrointestinal System

Privies Over the Centuries

"Sewage disposal was not unprovided for in the 14th century, though far from adequate. Privies . . . and public latrines existed, though they did not replace open street sewers. Castles and wealthy townhouses had privies built . . . with a hole in the bottom allowing the deposit to fall into a river or a ditch. . . . Town houses away from the riverbank had cesspools in the backyard . . . they frequently seeped into wells and other water sources. . . . the 15th and later centuries preferred to ignore human elimination."

Barbara Tuchman, from *A Distant Mirror*, Random House, Inc.

"One should eat to live, not live to eat."

Moliere, 1622-1673

". . . Give no more to every guest Than he's able to digest."

Jonathan Swift, 1667-1745

1. Define important words in this chapter

absorption: the digestive process in which digestive juices and enzymes break down food into materials the body can use.

anatomy: the study of body structure.

biology: the study of all life forms.

body systems: groups of organs that perform specific functions in the human body.

bowel elimination: the physical process of releasing or emptying the colon or large intestine of solid waste, called stool or feces.

cells: the basic structural unit of all organisms.

chyme: semi-liquid substance made as a result of the chemical breakdown of food in the stomach.

colon: the large intestine.

colostomy: surgically-created opening through the abdominal wall into the large intestine to allow feces to be expelled.

constipation: the inability to eliminate stool, or the infrequent, difficult and often painful elimination of a hard, dry stool.

Crohn's disease: a disease that causes the wall of the intestines (large or small) to become inflamed (red, sore, and swollen).

defecation: the process of eliminating feces from the rectum through the anus.

diarrhea: frequent elimination of liquid or semi-liquid feces.

digestion: the process of breaking down food so that it can be absorbed into the cells.

diverticulitis: inflammation of sacs that develop in the wall of the large intestine due to diverticulosis.

diverticulosis: a disorder in which sac-like pouchings develop in weakened areas of the wall of the large intestine (colon).

duodenum: the first part of the small intestine, where the common bile duct enters the small intestine.

electrolytes: chemical substances that are essential to maintaining fluid balance and homeostasis in the body.

elimination: the process of expelling wastes.

enema: a specific amount of water, with or without an additive, introduced into the colon to eliminate stool.

fecal impaction: a mass of dry, hard stool that remains packed in the rectum and cannot be expelled.

fecal incontinence: an inability to control the muscles of the bowels, which leads to an involuntary passage of stool or gas; also called anal incontinence.

feces: solid body waste excreted through the anus from the large intestine; also called stool.

flatulence: air in the intestine that is passed through the rectum; also called gas or flatus.

fracture pan: a bedpan that is flatter than a regular bedpan; used for small or thin people or those who cannot lift their buttocks onto a standard bedpan.

gastroesophageal reflux disease (GERD): a chronic condition in which the liquid contents of the stomach back up into the esophagus.

gastrointestinal tract: a continuous tube from the opening of the mouth all the way to the anus, where solid wastes are eliminated from the body.

heartburn: a condition that results from a weakening of the sphincter muscle which joins the esophagus and the stomach; also known as acid reflux.

hemorrhoids: enlarged veins in the rectum that can cause itching, burning, pain, and bleeding.

homeostasis: the condition in which all of the body's systems are balanced and are working at their best.

ileostomy: surgically-created opening into the end of the small intestine, the ileum, to allow feces to be expelled.

ingestion: the process of taking food or fluids into the body.

irritable bowel syndrome (IBS): a chronic condition of the gastrointestinal tract that is worsened by stress.

malabsorption: a condition in which the body cannot absorb or digest a particular nutrient properly.

occult: hidden.

organ: a structural unit in the human body that performs a specific function.

ostomy: surgical creation of an opening from an area inside the body to the outside.

pathophysiology: the study of the disorders that occur in the body.

peristalsis: muscular contractions that push food through the gastrointestinal tract.

physiology: the study of how body parts function.

portable commode: a chair with a toilet seat and a removable container underneath; used for elimination; also called a bedside commode.

specimen: a sample, such as tissue, blood, urine, stool, or sputum, used for analysis and diagnosis.

stoma: an artificial opening in the body.

suppository: a medication given rectally to cause a bowel movement.

tissues: a group of cells that performs similar tasks.

ulcerative colitis: a chronic inflammatory disease of the large intestine.

ureterostomy: a type of urostomy in which a surgical creation of an opening from the ureter through the abdomen is made for urine to be eliminated.

urostomy: the general term used for any surgical procedure that diverts the passage of urine by redirecting the ureters.

2. Explain key terms related to the body

Biology is the study of all life forms. Anatomy and physiology are a part of the science of biology. **Anatomy** is the study of body structure, while **physiology** looks at how body parts function.

The human body is made up of many different kinds of cells. **Cells** are the basic structural unit of all organisms. Living cells divide, grow, and die, renewing the tissues and organs of the body. There are different types of cells, but most are made up of the same components. Examples of cells are blood, nerve, and muscle cells.

Tissues are made up of groups of cells. Together, these groups of cells perform specific body functions. Examples of tissues are epithelial, connective, muscle, and nervous.

Groups of tissues come together to form **organs**. Each organ has a specific function to perform to keep the body healthy. The heart is an example of an organ.

Organs in the human body are organized into body systems. **Body systems** are made up of different organs that perform specific functions in the body. Each system in the body has its own unique function. Two examples are the circulatory system, consisting of the heart, blood vessels, and blood, and the urinary system, consisting of the kidneys, ureters, bladder, and urethra. Chapters 15 through 24 discuss body systems and related care. This textbook has organized the human body into these ten systems:

1. Gastrointestinal or Digestive
2. Urinary
3. Reproductive
4. Integumentary, or Skin
5. Circulatory or Cardiovascular
6. Respiratory
7. Musculoskeletal
8. Nervous
9. Endocrine
10. Immune and Lymphatic

Staying healthy and functioning normally is very important. In order to do this, the body must keep certain internal conditions stable, regardless of external factors. This is called homeostasis. **Homeostasis** is the condition in which all of the body's systems are balanced and are working at their best. Keeping body temperature around 98.6° Fahrenheit, regardless of how cold or hot it is outside, is an example of homeostasis.

Pathophysiology is the study of the disorders (conditions or diseases) that occur in the body. You will learn about diseases, along with normal, age-related changes for each body system listed above. Knowing what normal changes of aging are for each body system will help you better recognize any abnormal changes in your residents.

3. Explain the structure and function of the gastrointestinal system

The gastrointestinal (GI) system, also called the digestive system, is made up of two sections: the gastrointestinal tract and the accessory organs (Fig. 15-1). The **gastrointestinal tract** is a continuous tube from the opening of the mouth all the way to the anus, where solid wastes are eliminated from the body.

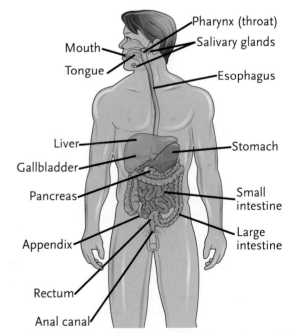

Fig. 15-1. *The GI system consists of all the organs needed to digest food and process waste.*

Food enters the mouth as a person eats. The tongue moves food around in the mouth. The salivary glands secrete a fluid called saliva, which begins lubricating and dissolving the food. The teeth break up food during a process called mastication (chewing). Food forms into a bolus, a mass of food that is easier to swallow. The bolus moves into the pharynx or throat, where it travels down to the esophagus, a tube about ten inches in length. This occurs as part of the swallowing reflex. Breathing pauses during swallowing because breathing and swallowing cannot occur at the same time. The epiglottis acts like a lid, shutting off the larynx during the swallowing process. This blocks food from entering the trachea and causing choking. Food moves into the stomach from the esophagus because of muscular contractions, called **peristalsis**, that push it toward the stomach.

When the food reaches the stomach, it mixes with gastric juice. This fluid is capable of killing most microorganisms that enter the stomach. The stomach changes the food into a substance called **chyme**. Food usually stays in the stomach for about two to six hours after eating. From there, the chyme passes into the first part of the small intestine, called the **duodenum**. The small intestine is about 20 feet long and is approximately one inch in diameter.

The small intestine receives secretions from the liver and the pancreas. The small intestine also secretes intestinal digestive juice from its walls. The liver produces bile, which is stored in the gallbladder. Bile is a substance that breaks down fats. When needed, the gallbladder sends the bile to the small intestine through the common bile duct. The pancreas produces juices that digest carbohydrates, proteins, and fats. These juices are sent to the small intestine through the pancreatic duct, which joins the common bile duct.

The small intestine is lined with villi, tiny finger-like projections that absorb food and fluids. **Absorption** takes place because nutrients from food are broken down into tiny molecules that move into the blood. Approximately 90% of food and fluids is absorbed in the small intestine.

The rest of absorption occurs in the large intestine. It is about two and one-half inches in diameter and about five feet long. The large intestine helps regulate water balance by absorbing water and electrolytes and eliminating solid waste products as **feces**. **Electrolytes** are chemical substances that are essential to maintaining fluid balance and homeostasis within the body.

The first part of the large intestine, the cecum, has a valve that prevents the feces from moving backward into the small intestine. The appendix is attached to the cecum. The exact function of the appendix is not known. The rest of the large intestine consists of the ascending, transverse, descending, and sigmoid **colon**, along with the rectum and anus. The chyme takes three to ten hours to become feces within the colon. Feces is made up of water, solid waste material, bacteria, and mucus. Feces is eliminated from the body by peristalsis through the anus, the rectal opening. This process is called **defecation**.

The functions of the gastrointestinal system are:

- **Ingestion** of food (taking food or fluids into the body)

- **Digestion** of food (breaking down food so that it can be absorbed into the cells)

- Absorption of nutrients

- **Elimination** of waste products from food/fluids

Destination: Homeostasis

Fluid balance is a vital part of the body's ability to maintain homeostasis. A person becomes dehydrated when his output is greater than his intake. The body reacts quickly to try to correct dehydration. One of the primary responses is to stimulate thirst. If the intake of water and other fluids is not increased, the body responds by decreasing sweating and urination. If fluid balance is not restored, other more severe symptoms occur. Eliminating dehydration can be as simple as drinking a glass of water. When fluids are re-introduced into the body, fluid balance and homeostasis are restored.

Process of Digestion

Lazzaro Spallanzani (1729-1799), an Italian scientist, studied digestion. He performed experiments with birds called kites. In his studies with these birds, he found that gastric juice works to dissolve food in the stomach.

4. Discuss changes in the gastrointestinal system due to aging

For each system in the body, there are normal changes of aging. Knowing these normal changes for each body system will help you better recognize and understand what is abnormal for the body as a person ages.

Normal age-related changes for the gastrointestinal system include the following:

- Ability to taste decreases.
- Process of digestion takes longer and is less efficient.
- Body waste moves more slowly through the intestines, causing more frequent constipation.
- Difficulty chewing and swallowing may occur.
- Absorption of vitamins and minerals decreases.
- Production of saliva and digestive fluids decreases.

For each body system, there are signs and symptoms that need to be reported to the nurse if observed. You will learn more about these observations in Learning Objectives 5 and 7.

5. List normal qualities of stool and identify signs and symptoms to report about stool

Bowel elimination is the physical process of releasing or emptying the colon or large intestine of stool or feces. Feces, or stool, are solid waste products eliminated by the colon. The frequency of bowel movements varies; they can occur as often as one to three times per day or as infre-

quently as several times a week. Regular bowel movements help keep the gastrointestinal system healthy. It is especially important for elderly people to have regular bowel movements because they help prevent serious problems, such as fecal impactions, from occurring.

Stool is normally brown in color, and its consistency is soft, moist, and formed (not loose). Certain foods can change its color. For example, red gelatin or beets can make stool appear red. Green, leafy vegetables can make stool look green. Iron supplements can cause stool to turn black. Stool is tubular in shape, which is due to its passage through the colon. The amount of stool produced per day depends upon the food eaten.

Normal bowel elimination means not having any pain with passing stool. A change in stool's appearance, such as blood, pus, mucus, or worms in stool, can signal a health problem. Report any of the following to the nurse:

Observing and Reporting: Stool

- O/R Bloody or abnormally-colored stool (whitish, black [tarry])
- O/R Hard, dry stools
- O/R Liquid stools (diarrhea)
- O/R Constipation (inability to have a bowel movement)
- O/R Pain when having a bowel movement
- O/R Blood, pus, mucus, or discharge in stool
- O/R Fecal incontinence (involuntary loss of stool)

6. List factors affecting bowel elimination and describe how to promote normal bowel elimination

There are many things that may affect normal bowel elimination:

Growth and Development: Aging affects the regularity of bowel elimination. Peristalsis slows due to a decrease in muscle tone. Tooth loss and less saliva may make eating less appealing and more challenging. Nutrients are not absorbed as well, making digestion more difficult.

To promote normal elimination, encourage fluids and nutritious meals. Supplements may be ordered. Encourage regular exercise and activity as allowed. Provide good oral care and make sure dentures are clean, in place, and fit properly.

Psychological Factors: The lack of privacy may affect bowel elimination. Having a roommate for the first time, being in a place that is not home, and needing help with elimination can disrupt normal elimination patterns. Anxiety, stress, fear, or anger can increase the frequency of bowel movements, causing watery, loose stools, and may even cause incontinence. Depression can decrease the frequency of elimination.

To promote normal elimination, always provide privacy and allow plenty of time for elimination. Leave the call light within reach. Respond to call lights and requests for help with toileting immediately. If residents want to talk about their concerns, take the time to listen to them. Report their concerns to the nurse.

Diet: A diet low in fiber may decrease elimination and cause constipation. Foods high in animal fats, such as dairy products, red meat, and eggs may also cause constipation. Products containing caffeine may cause or aggravate diarrhea. Other foods are gas-causing, which can increase elimination but may also cause discomfort. Beans, whole grains, apples, cabbage, onions, dairy products, and carbonated drinks are examples of foods that can cause gas.

To promote normal elimination, encourage nutritious meals. Increase fiber intake and decrease fatty, sugary foods if constipation is a problem.

Fluid Intake: The sense of thirst decreases as a person ages. A decrease in fluids may cause constipation. A lack of strength or coordination can also lower fluid intake. Some beverages, such as orange or prune juice, can cause an increase in bowel elimination.

To promote normal elimination, encourage fluid intake. Generally, a healthy person needs at least 64 ounces of fluid each day. Remind residents to drink often if they do not have a fluid restriction. Make sure pitcher and water are within reach and are light enough for residents to lift. Assist with fluid intake as needed.

Physical Activity and Exercise: A lack of exercise and mobility can weaken muscles and slow elimination. Regular physical activity helps bowel elimination by strengthening abdominal and pelvic muscles (Fig. 15-2). This helps peristalsis.

To promote normal elimination, increase daily exercise. Encourage regular walks and other types of activities that are allowed.

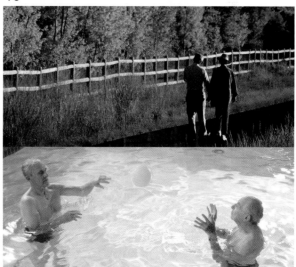

Fig. 15-2. *Regular exercise is important. Encourage walks and other types of approved exercise.*

Personal Habits: Certain times of day may be more common for having bowel movements. Drinking warm fluids can increase bowel movements by stimulating peristalsis. Elimination usually occurs after meals. Familiar places, such as the resident's own bathroom, may encourage bowel elimination. Positioning in bed also affects elimination. A resident who is lying flat on his back (supine) will have difficulty with elimination because it is difficult to contract the muscles in this position.

To promote normal elimination, make sure residents are helped to the bathroom at the time of day that is best for each person. Use the bathroom the resident prefers or get a portable commode if the resident cannot make it to the bathroom. Raise the head of the bed for residents who use a bedpan. The best position for elimination is squatting and leaning forward.

Medications: Some medications affect bowel elimination. Antibiotics can cause diarrhea; pain relievers may cause constipation.

To promote normal elimination, laxatives may be ordered. Laxatives can help with elimination, but may cause diarrhea. Report diarrhea or constipation to the nurse promptly.

Assisting with Elimination

A bedpan is used by residents who cannot get out of bed to go to the bathroom. Women use bedpans for urination and bowel movements. Men generally use urinals for urination and bedpans for bowel movements. There are two kinds of bedpans: standard bedpans and fracture bedpans (Fig. 15-3). A **fracture pan** is flatter than the regular bedpan and is used for small or thin people or those who cannot lift their buttocks onto a standard bedpan.

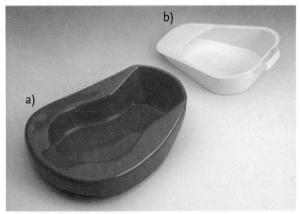

Fig. 15-3. a) Standard bedpan and b) fracture pan.

Feces and urine are considered infectious wastes. Wear gloves when handling bedpans, urinals, or basins that contain wastes. Wear ad-ditional PPE as needed. Use caution when removing bedpans or waste containers from beds; avoid spilling the contents. Do not place this equipment on an overbed table or on top of a side table. Use a bedpan cover or disposable pad to transfer bedpans to the bathroom. Dispose of wastes in the toilet, unless a nurse needs to check the contents. Immediately after use, place these containers in the proper area for cleaning or clean and store them according to policy. Cleaning them right away helps to avoid odors.

When placing a bedpan, position a standard bedpan so that the wider end is aligned with a resident's buttocks. Position a fracture pan with the handle toward the foot of the bed. You may need to warm the bedpan with warm water if it is cold to the touch. Dry it completely before placing it under a resident.

Assisting a resident with use of a bedpan

Equipment: bedpan, bedpan cover, disposable bed protector, bath blanket, toilet paper, disposable washcloths or wipes, soap, towel, 2 pairs of gloves

1. Identify yourself by name. Identify the resident. Greet the resident by name.

2. Wash your hands.

3. Explain procedure to resident. Speak clearly, slowly, and directly. Maintain face-to-face contact whenever possible.

4. Provide for the resident's privacy with a curtain, screen, or door.

5. Adjust bed to safe level, usually waist high. Before placing bedpan, lower head of bed. Lock bed wheels.

6. Put on gloves.

7. Cover the resident with a bath blanket. Ask him to hold it while you pull down the top covers underneath. Do not expose more of the resident than is needed.

8. Place the bed protector under the resident's buttocks and hips. To do this, have the resident roll away from you. If the resident cannot do this, you must turn him away from you (see Chapter 11). Be sure resident cannot roll off the bed. Move to empty side of bed. Place bed protector on the area where the resident will lie on his back. The side of the protector nearest the resident should be fanfolded (folded several times into pleats) and tucked under the resident (Fig. 15-4).

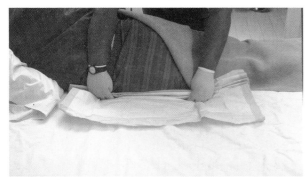

Fig. 15-4. *Fanfold the bed protector near the resident's back.*

Ask resident to roll onto his back, or roll him back as you did before, if he is unable. Unfold rest of bed protector so it completely covers area under and around the resident's hips (Fig. 15-5).

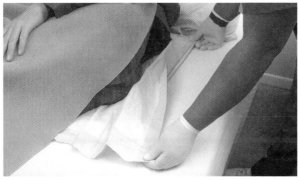

Fig. 15-5. *Unfold the rest of the bed protector so it completely covers area under and around the resident's hips.*

9. Ask resident to remove undergarments or help him do so.

10. Place bedpan near his hips in correct position. **Standard bedpan** should be positioned with the wider end aligned with resident's

buttocks. **Fracture pan** should be positioned with handle toward foot of bed.

11. If resident is able, ask him to raise hips by pushing with feet and hands at the count of three (Fig. 15-6). Slide the bedpan under his hips.

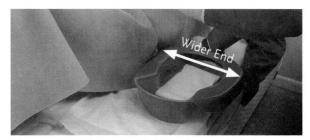

Fig. 15-6. *On the count of three, slide the bedpan under the resident's hips. The wider end of bedpan should be aligned with resident's buttocks.*

If a resident cannot help you in any way, keep the bed flat and roll the resident away from you. Slip the bedpan under the hips and gently roll him back onto the bedpan. Keep the bedpan centered underneath.

12. Remove and discard gloves. Wash your hands.

13. Raise the head of the bed until the resident is in a sitting position. Prop the resident into a semi-sitting position using pillows.

14. Place toilet tissue and washcloths or wipes within resident's reach. Ask resident to clean his hands with a hand wipe when finished, if he is able.

15. Leave call light within resident's reach. Wash your hands. Ask resident to signal when finished. Leave the room.

16. When called by the resident, return and wash your hands. Put on clean gloves.

17. Lower the head of the bed. Make sure resident is still covered. Do not overexpose the resident.

18. Remove bedpan carefully and gently. Cover bedpan. Remove the bed protector.

19. Give perineal care if help is needed. Wipe from front to back. Dry the perineal area with a towel. Help the resident put on undergarment. Place the towel in a hamper or bag, and discard disposable supplies.

20. Take bedpan to the bathroom. Note color, odor, amount, and consistency of contents. Empty contents into toilet unless the nurse needs to check the contents. If you notice anything unusual about the stool or urine (for example, the presence of blood), do not discard it. You will need to inform the nurse.

21. Flush toilet. Place bedpan in area for cleaning or clean and store it according to policy.

22. Remove and discard gloves. Wash your hands.

23. Make resident comfortable.

24. Return bed to lowest position. Remove privacy measures.

25. Leave call light within resident's reach.

26. Wash your hands.

27. Be courteous and respectful at all times.

28. Report any changes in the resident to the nurse. Document procedure using facility guidelines.

Bedpans and urinals are usually kept in the bathroom when they are not being used. If the bathroom is shared, this equipment may need to be labeled. Follow facility policy for storage. Men generally use a urinal for urinating (Fig. 15-7).

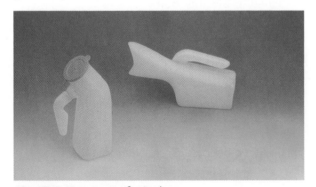

Fig. 15-7. *Two types of urinals.*

Assisting a male resident with a urinal

Equipment: urinal, disposable bed protector, disposable washcloths or wipes, 2 pairs of gloves

1. Identify yourself by name. Identify the resident. Greet the resident by name.

2. Wash your hands.

3. Explain procedure to resident. Speak clearly, slowly, and directly. Maintain face-to-face contact whenever possible.

4. Provide for the resident's privacy with a curtain, screen, or door.

5. Adjust bed to a safe level, usually waist high. Lock bed wheels.

6. Put on gloves.

7. Place the bed protector under the resident's buttocks and hips.

8. Hand the urinal to the resident. If the resident cannot do so himself, place urinal between his legs and position penis inside the urinal (Fig. 15-8). Replace bed covers.

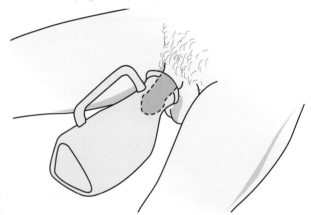

Fig. 15-8. *Position the penis inside the urinal if the resident cannot do it himself.*

9. Remove and discard gloves. Wash your hands.

10. Place wipes within resident's reach. Ask the resident to clean his hands with a hand wipe when finished, if he is able. Leave call light within reach. Wash your hands. Ask resident to signal when done. Leave the room.

11. When called by the resident, return and wash your hands. Put on clean gloves.

12. Have resident hand urinal to you, or gently remove urinal. Remove the bed protector. Discard disposable supplies.

13. Take urinal to the bathroom. Note color, odor, amount, and qualities (for example, cloudiness) of contents before flushing. Empty contents into toilet unless the nurse needs to check the contents.

14. Flush toilet. Place urinal in proper area for cleaning or clean and store it according to policy.

15. Remove and discard gloves. Wash your hands.

16. Return bed to lowest position. Remove privacy measures.

17. Make resident comfortable.

18. Leave call light within resident's reach.

19. Wash your hands.

20. Be courteous and respectful at all times.

21. Report any changes in the resident to the nurse. Document procedure using facility guidelines.

Portable, or bedside, commodes are used for people who can get out of bed but who find it difficult to walk to the bathroom. A **portable commode** is a chair with a toilet seat and a removable container underneath (Fig. 15-9). The removable container must be cleaned after each use. Commodes may have wheels. The wheels must be locked before helping residents onto commodes. Once seated, leave the resident alone to use the commode, if it is safe to do so.

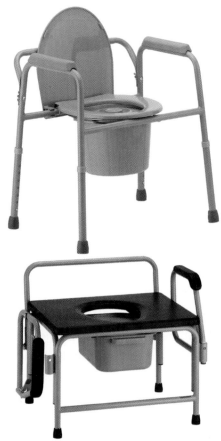

Fig. 15-9. *The top photo shows a regular portable commode and the bottom photo shows a bariatric portable commode, which can be used for people who are overweight or obese.* (PHOTO COURTESY OF NOVA MEDICAL PRODUCTS, WWW.NOVAMEDICALPRODUCTS.COM)

Helping a resident use a portable commode

Equipment: portable commode with basin, toilet paper, disposable washcloths or wipes, non-skid footwear, towel, bath blanket, 3 pairs of gloves

1. Identify yourself by name. Identify the resident. Greet the resident by name.

2. Wash your hands.

3. Explain procedure to resident. Speak clearly, slowly, and directly. Maintain face-to-face contact whenever possible.

4. Provide for the resident's privacy with a curtain, screen, or door.

5. Lock commode wheels. Adjust bed to lowest position. Lock bed wheels.

6. Put on gloves.

7. Help resident out of bed and to portable commode. Make sure resident is wearing non-skid shoes and that the laces are tied.

8. If needed, help resident remove clothing and sit comfortably on toilet seat. Place toilet tissue and washcloths or wipes within resident's reach. Ask resident to clean his hands with a hand wipe when finished, if he is able.

9. Place bath blanket over resident's legs. Leave call light within resident's reach. Remove and discard gloves. Wash your hands. Ask resident to signal when finished. Leave the room.

10. When called by the resident, return and wash your hands. Put on clean gloves.

11. Give perineal care if help is needed. Wipe from front to back. Dry the perineal area with a towel. Help the resident put on undergarment. Place the towel in a hamper or bag. Discard disposable supplies.

12. Remove and discard gloves. Wash your hands.

13. Help resident back to bed. Leave bed in lowest position. Remove privacy measures.

14. Make resident comfortable.

15. Put on clean gloves.

16. Remove waste basin. Note color, odor, amount, and consistency of contents. Empty contents into toilet unless the nurse needs to check the contents.

17. Flush toilet. Place container in proper area for cleaning or clean it according to facility policy.

18. Remove and discard gloves. Wash your hands.

19. Leave call light within resident's reach.

20. Wash your hands.

21. Be courteous and respectful at all times.

22. Report any changes in the resident to the nurse. Document procedure using facility guidelines.

Tip

Be careful when cleaning bedpans and commodes.

Cleaning bedpans can be tricky. If you are using a spray nozzle to clean a bedpan, the contents can spray on you. Be very careful not to splash or spray waste while you are disposing of it. Urine and stool are considered infectious waste. Wear appropriate PPE when cleaning bedpans and commodes. After cleaning, properly remove PPE and wash your hands.

7. Discuss common disorders of the gastrointestinal system

Heartburn

Heartburn, also known as acid reflux, occurs when the sphincter muscle that joins the esophagus and the stomach weakens. Normally this muscle tries to prevent return, or reflux, of stomach contents back into the esophagus. If this is not done, stomach juices will move into the esophagus and cause burning and pain. The esophagus has a delicate lining that can be damaged by these stomach juices. Symptoms include a burning feeling in the esophagus and pain in the chest, around the breastbone (sternum) or the rib area. The pain may also move into the neck area. Pain usually occurs directly after a eating a meal. Heartburn often causes a bitter taste in the mouth or the feeling of food coming back up into the throat or the mouth. This may worsen when a person is lying down. Treatment includes medication—antacids are one example—as well as a change in diet and/or sleep position.

Gastroesophageal Reflux Disease (GERD)

Gastroesophageal reflux disease (GERD) is a chronic condition in which the liquid contents of the stomach back up into the esophagus. The liquid can inflame and damage the lining of the esophagus, which can cause bleeding, ulcers, or difficulty swallowing. Frequent heartburn is a common symptom of GERD. Other symptoms are chest pain, hoarseness in the morning, difficulty swallowing, or a tightness in the throat. Coughing and foul-smelling breath can also occur with GERD. Possible causes of GERD are hiatal hernia, a weak lower esophageal sphincter, and slow digestion. Other causes are diets high in acidic and spicy foods, obesity, smoking, and alcohol use.

Treatment includes stopping smoking and not drinking alcohol, avoiding spicy and acidic foods, and losing weight. Wearing loose-fitting clothing may help. Bending over to lift objects can push acid up into the esophagus and make GERD worse. It should be avoided. Serving frequent, small meals throughout the day is advised, as well as serving the last meal of the day three to four hours before bedtime. Sitting up for at least two to three hours after eating may help. Elevation of the head of the bed and using extra pillows to keep the body upright help reduce acid reflux while in bed (Fig. 15-10).

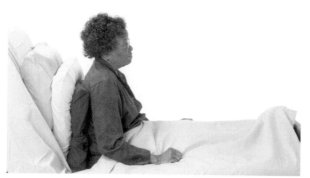

Fig. 15-10. *Sitting upright, elevating the head of the bed, and using extra pillows help reduce acid reflux.*

Ulcers

Ulcers are raw sores in the stomach (peptic or gastric ulcers) and the small intestine (duodenal ulcers). Dull or burning pain occurs one to three or more hours after eating, accompanied by belching or vomiting. Peptic ulcers may cause bleeding, and stool may appear black (tarry). Ulcers are caused by excessive acid secretion. Infection of the stomach by a bacteria called Helicobacter pylori may also cause ulcers. Excessive aspirin use may be a factor in the development of ulcers. Treatment includes antacids and other

medications, as well as a change in diet. Alcohol, caffeine, and cigarette use should be avoided, as they increase the production of gastric acid.

Ulcerative Colitis and Crohn's Disease

Ulcerative colitis is a disorder that causes inflammation of and sores in the lining of the large intestine (colon). It is a form of inflammatory bowel disease (IBD). Symptoms include diarrhea (which may be bloody), abdominal pain, cramping, rectal bleeding, poor appetite, fever, and weight loss. Ulcerative colitis can cause intestinal bleeding and death if not treated.

Crohn's disease is a disease that causes the wall of the intestines (large or small) to become inflamed (red, sore and swollen). Crohn's disease is also a form of inflammatory bowel disease (IBD). Symptoms include diarrhea, abdominal pain, fever, weight loss, and joint pain.

There is no known cause of ulcerative colitis or Crohn's disease. Research has shown that they tend to run in families. The immune system may overreact to normal bacteria present in the intestines and cause inflammation. Bacteria and viruses also may cause the diseases.

Treatment includes medications to stop inflammation; however, medication does not cure ulcerative colitis or Crohn's disease. Surgery may be performed if medications do not help these disorders. Surgical treatment may include an ileostomy or colostomy. More information on these types of ostomies can be found in Learning Objective 11 of this chapter.

Diverticulosis and Diverticulitis

Diverticulosis is a disorder of the intestinal wall of the large intestine (colon). Sac-like pouchings of the intestinal wall develop in weakened areas of this wall. A small percentage of people with diverticulosis develop inflammation inside the pouchings called **diverticulitis**. With diverticulitis, stool and bacteria become trapped inside the sacs, causing pain and fever. If the condition worsens, the intestine can tear, causing stool to enter the abdominal cavity and cause peritonitis (inflammation of the lining of the abdominal cavity due to microorganisms). One cause of diverticulitis is a low-fiber diet. The lack of fiber may cause the weakening of the intestinal wall.

Treatment for diverticulitis includes rest, medications to reduce inflammation and treat infection, and special diets. Surgery is sometimes necessary.

Flatulence

Flatulence, also called gas or flatus, is the presence of excessive air in the digestive tract. It is passed through the rectum and may cause cramping or abdominal pain. High fiber foods can cause gas. It can also be caused by eating foods that a person cannot tolerate, such as lactose in dairy products. The inability to digest lactose, a type of sugar in milk and other dairy products, is called lactose intolerance. Other causes of flatulence, or gas, are:

- Swallowing air when eating

- Antibiotics

- **Malabsorption**, which means that nutrients from the intestinal tract are not properly absorbed; can also be accompanied by diarrhea.

- **Irritable bowel syndrome (IBS)**, which is a chronic condition of the GI tract that is worsened by stress. IBS causes abdominal pain and discomfort, bloating, and constipation. No exact cause has been identified.

For the relief of flatulence, two positions are used to help reduce gas: the left-side-lying, or left-lateral, position, and the supine (flat on the back) position. Lying on the left side allows gas to escape due to gravity. Placing a resident in this position for at least 20 minutes usually assists in the elimination of gas. The supine position can be used with residents who are recovering from surgery. This position allows gas inside the abdomen due to surgery to escape more quickly. A rectal tube may also be placed in the rectum to reduce gas.

Constipation

Constipation is the inability to eliminate stool, or the infrequent, difficult and often painful elimination of a hard, dry stool. It occurs when body waste moves slowly through the intestines. As you have learned, constipation is a common problem for elderly people. As people age, digestion takes longer and is less efficient. It can also result from poor diet, lack of exercise, a decrease in fluid intake, medications, disease, or ignoring the urge to eliminate. Signs of constipation include abdominal swelling, gas, and irritability. The resident's medical chart may also show no recent bowel movement.

Treating constipation often involves increasing fiber in the diet, as well as physical activity, if possible. Medications may be ordered, such as laxatives, enemas, or suppositories. An **enema** is a specific amount of water or other fluid, with or without an additive, introduced into the colon to help eliminate stool. You will learn more about enemas later in this chapter. A **suppository** is a medication given rectally to cause a bowel movement. Some states allow nursing assistants to give a rectal suppository. A procedure on how to give a suppository is included in your instructor's material.

Diarrhea

Diarrhea is the frequent elimination of liquid or semi-liquid feces. Abdominal cramps, urgency, nausea, and vomiting can accompany diarrhea, depending on the cause. Infections, microorganisms, irritating foods, and medications can cause diarrhea. Treatment is usually medication and a change of diet. A diet of bananas, rice, applesauce, and tea/toast (BRAT diet) is often suggested.

Fecal Incontinence

Fecal incontinence (also called "anal incontinence") is an inability to control the muscles of the bowels, which leads to an involuntary passage of stool or gas. Causes of fecal incontinence include muscle and nerve damage, disorders of the spinal cord or anus, injuries to the anal muscles during childbirth, injuries due to anal operations, trauma, fecal impaction, constipation, and tumors. Treatment often includes changes in diet, medication, bowel training, and surgery. You will learn more about bowel training in Learning Objective 12 of the chapter.

Fecal Impaction

A **fecal impaction** is a build-up of dry, hardened feces in the rectum that results from unrelieved constipation. A person cannot remove an impaction naturally. Signs and symptoms of a fecal impaction include no stool for several days, cramping, abdominal or rectal pain, abdominal swelling (distention), nausea, and vomiting. Another sign is the seeping or oozing of liquid stool, which can be mistaken for diarrhea. Other signs are an increase in urination or the inability to urinate, fever, confusion, or disorientation. When an impaction occurs, the nurse or doctor will insert one or two gloved fingers into the rectum to break the mass into fragments. Usually the stool can then be passed. A fecal impaction can be a serious, even fatal, condition if a complete bowel obstruction occurs and is not immediately treated. Report signs and symptoms promptly to the nurse. Ways to prevent fecal impactions include drinking plenty of fluids, eating a high-fiber diet, following a toileting schedule, and exercising regularly.

Hemorrhoids

Hemorrhoids are enlarged veins in the rectum. They may also be visible outside the anus. Untreated constipation, obesity, pregnancy, chronic diarrhea, overuse of enemas or laxatives, and straining during bowel movements are common causes of hemorrhoids. Rectal itching, burning, pain, and bleeding during bowel elimination are symptoms of hemorrhoids. Treatment includes changing the person's diet, such as adding more fiber and increasing water intake, medications, compresses, and sitz baths (Chapter 18). Surgery may be necessary. Excessive cleaning and wiping of the area should be avoided. When cleaning the anus, be very gentle. Avoid using scented soaps, as these may further irritate the anal area.

Information on hepatitis, a gastrointestinal system disorder, is found in Chapter 6.

8. Discuss how enemas are given

An enema is given when help eliminating stool from the colon is needed. A specific amount of water flows inside of the colon in order to help remove stool. Some facilities allow nursing assistants to give enemas. If your facility allows this, follow facility policies, and make sure you are trained to give enemas. Talk to the nurse if you have any questions or concerns.

Enemas are ordered for these reasons:

- Preparation for a diagnostic test
- Preparation for surgery
- To remove stool that a resident cannot eliminate on his or her own

Doctors will write an enema order. There are four different types of enemas:

- Tap water enema (TWE): 500-1000 mL water from a faucet (nothing added to the water)
- Soapsuds enema (SSE): 500-1000 mL water with 5 mL of mild castile soap added
- Saline enema: 500-1000 mL water with two teaspoons of salt added
- Commercial enema (also called "pre-packaged" enema): 120 mL solution; may have oil or other additive

Tap water, soapsuds, and saline enemas are all considered cleansing enemas. Cleansing enemas require more fluid than commercial enemas do. Equipment needed for cleansing enemas includes an IV pole, the enema solution, and tubing and a clamp. Encourage residents to hold in the enema solution as long as possible—at least 10 to 20 minutes for the best results.

When giving a cleansing enema, remove the air from the enema tubing before inserting the tube into the rectum. Allowing a small amount of water to flow into a bedpan will allow the air to escape.

Provide plenty of privacy for the resident with this procedure. Make sure others cannot see the resident and that he is not unnecessarily exposed in any way.

During an enema, the resident must be in the Sims' position (Fig. 15-11). If the person is positioned on the left side, the water does not have to flow against gravity. Water temperature should not be over 105°F to avoid internal burning. Water that is too cold can cause intense cramping.

Give the enema slowly, holding the enema tubing in place. Enemas are given gradually to avoid causing cramping. Stop immediately if the resident has pain or if you feel resistance. Be reassuring and gentle during the procedure. Observe for cramping, pain or discomfort, bleeding, the ability to retain the fluid, and any change in the resident's condition during and following the enema.

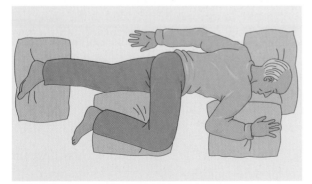

Fig. 15-11. *Place the resident in the Sims' position for an enema, which is a left side-lying position.*

Tip

Enemas and Vital Signs

Stimulation of the rectal area by any type of tube may temporarily increase the heartbeat and blood pressure. Residents with heart disease may not be able to have enemas. Follow the nurse's instructions regarding the use of enemas.

Giving a cleansing enema

Equipment: 2 pairs of gloves, bath blanket, IV pole, enema solution, additive (if needed), tubing and clamp, disposable bed protector, bedpan, bedpan cover, lubricating jelly, bath thermometer, tape measure, toilet paper, disposable washcloths or wipes, towel, robe, non-skid footwear

1. Identify yourself by name. Identify the resident. Greet the resident by name.

2. Wash your hands.

3. Explain procedure to resident. Speak clearly, slowly, and directly. Maintain face-to-face contact whenever possible.

4. Provide for the resident's privacy with a curtain, screen, or door.

5. Adjust bed to safe working level, usually waist high. Lock bed wheels.

6. Help resident into left-sided Sims' position. Cover with a bath blanket.

7. Place the IV pole beside the bed. Raise the side rail.

8. Clamp the enema tube. Prepare the enema solution. Add specific additive, if ordered. Fill bag with 500-1000 mL of warm water (105°F) and swish fluid to mix well. Check water temperature with bath thermometer.

9. Unclamp the tube. Let a small amount of solution run through the tubing to release the air. Re-clamp the tube.

10. Hang bag on IV pole. Using the tape measure, make sure bottom of enema bag is not more than 12 inches above the resident's anus (Fig. 15-12).

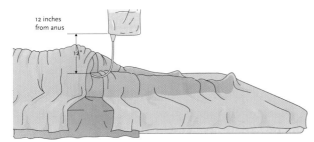

Fig. 15-12. Bottom of the bag should not be more than 12 inches above the anus.

11. Put on gloves.

12. Place bed protector under resident. Ask resident to remove undergarments or help him do so. Place bedpan close to resident's body.

13. Lubricate two to four inches of the tip of the tubing with lubricating jelly.

14. Ask resident to breathe deeply. This relieves cramps during procedure.

15. Place one hand on the upper buttock. Lift to expose the anus. Ask the resident to take a deep breath and exhale (Fig. 15-13). Using other hand, gently insert the tip of the tubing two to four inches into the rectum. Stop immediately if you feel resistance or if the resident complains of pain. If this happens, clamp the tubing. Tell the nurse immediately.

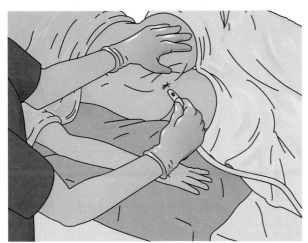

Fig. 15-13. Lift the upper buttock to expose the anus. Ask the resident to take a deep breath before inserting the tubing.

16. Unclamp the tubing. Allow the solution to flow slowly into the rectum. Ask resident to take slow, deep breaths. If resident complains of cramping, clamp the tubing and stop for a couple of minutes. Encourage him or her to take as much of the solution as possible. Resident should let you know when he cannot accept any more fluid.

17. Clamp the tubing before the bag is empty when the solution is almost gone. Gently remove the tip from the rectum. Place the tip into the enema bag. Do not contaminate yourself, resident, or bed linens.

18. Ask the resident to hold the solution inside as long as possible.

19. Help resident to use bedpan, commode, or get to the bathroom. Raise the head of the bed, if resident is using bedpan. If the resident uses a commode or bathroom, put on robe and non-skid footwear. Lower the bed to its lowest position before the resident gets up.

20. Remove and discard gloves. Wash your hands.

21. Place toilet paper and washcloths or wipes within resident's reach. Ask the resident to clean his hands with a hand wipe when finished, if he is able. If the resident is using the bathroom, ask him not to flush the toilet when finished.

22. Place the call light within resident's reach. Wash your hands. Ask resident to signal when finished. Leave the room.

23. When called by the resident, return and wash your hands. Put on clean gloves.

24. Lower the head of the bed, if raised. Make sure resident is still covered. Do not overexpose the resident.

25. Remove bedpan carefully and gently. Cover bedpan. Remove the bed protector.

26. Give perineal care if help is needed. Wipe from front to back. Dry the perineal area with

a towel. Help the resident put on undergarment. Place the towel in a hamper or bag, and discard disposable supplies.

27. Take bedpan to the bathroom. Call the nurse to observe enema results, whether in bedpan or in toilet. Consistency, color, and amount will be observed. Empty contents into toilet.

28. Flush toilet. Place bedpan in proper area for cleaning or clean and store it according to policy.

29. Remove and discard gloves. Wash your hands.

30. Make resident comfortable.

31. Return bed to lowest position. Remove privacy measures.

32. Leave call light within resident's reach.

33. Wash your hands.

34. Be courteous and respectful at all times.

35. Report any changes in the resident to the nurse. Document procedure using facility guidelines.

Commercial enemas may contain oil, such as mineral oil, or other additives. The goals of using an oil-retention enema include the following: lubricating the intestine to make stool pass more easily; softening stool for ease of elimination; encouraging gentle bowel movements; reducing straining with bowel movements; and eliminating a fecal impaction.

With commercial enemas, no IV pole, tubing, or clamp are needed. They come in a prepackaged kit; no mixing is usually required. The tip of a commercially-prepared enema is usually pre-lubricated and should only be inserted about one-and-a-half inches into the rectum. Commercial enemas generally take longer to work than cleansing enemas. Encourage residents to hold in the enema solution as long as possible. For best results, fluid should be retained for at least

20 minutes. Oil-retention enemas should be retained for 30 to 60 minutes.

Giving a commercial enema

Equipment: 2 pairs of gloves, bath blanket, standard or oil retention commercial enema kit, disposable bed protector, bedpan, bedpan cover, lubricating jelly, toilet paper, disposable washcloths or wipes, towel, robe, non-skid footwear

1. Identify yourself by name. Identify the resident. Greet the resident by name.

2. Wash your hands.

3. Explain procedure to resident. Speak clearly, slowly, and directly. Maintain face-to-face contact whenever possible.

4. Provide for the resident's privacy with a curtain, screen, or door.

5. Adjust bed to safe working level, usually waist high. Lock bed wheels.

6. Help resident into left-sided Sims' position. Cover with a bath blanket.

7. Put on gloves.

8. Place bed protector under resident. Ask resident to remove undergarments or help him do so. Place bedpan close to resident's body.

9. Uncover resident enough to expose anus only.

10. Add extra lubricating jelly to the tip of bottle if needed.

11. Ask resident to breathe deeply to relieve cramps during procedure.

12. Place one hand on the upper buttock. Lift to expose the anus. Ask the resident to take a deep breath and exhale. Using other hand, gently insert the tip of the tubing about one and a half inches into the rectum. Stop immediately if you feel resistance or if the resident complains of pain.

13. Slowly squeeze and roll the enema container so that the solution runs inside the resident. Stop when the container is almost empty.

14. Gently remove tip from the rectum, continuing to keep pressure on the container until you place bottle inside the box upside down (Fig. 15-14).

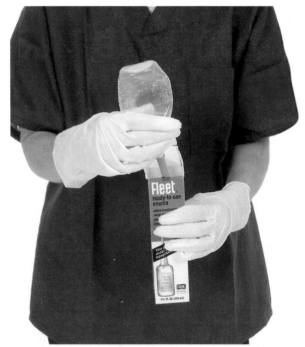

Fig. 15-14. *Place enema bottle upside-down in the box.*

15. Ask the resident to hold the solution inside as long as possible.

16. Help resident to use bedpan, commode, or go to the bathroom. Raise the head of the bed, if resident is using bedpan. If the resident uses a commode or bathroom, put on robe and non-skid footwear. Lower the bed to its lowest position before the resident gets up.

17. Remove and discard gloves. Wash your hands.

18. Place toilet paper and washcloths or wipes within resident's reach. Ask the resident to clean his hands with a hand wipe when finished, if he is able. If the resident is using the bathroom, ask him not to flush the toilet when finished.

19. Place the call light within resident's reach. Wash your hands. Ask resident to signal when finished. Leave the room.

20. When called by the resident, return and wash your hands. Put on clean gloves.

21. Lower the head of the bed, if raised. Make sure resident is still covered. Do not overexpose the resident.

22. Remove bedpan carefully and gently. Cover bedpan. Remove the bed protector.

23. Give perineal care if help is needed. Wipe from front to back. Dry the perineal area with a towel. Help the resident put on undergarment. Place the towel in a hamper or bag, and discard disposable supplies.

24. Take bedpan to the bathroom. Call the nurse to observe enema results, whether in bedpan or in toilet. Consistency, color, and amount will be observed. Empty contents into toilet.

25. Flush toilet. Place bedpan in proper area for cleaning or clean and store it according to policy.

26. Remove and discard gloves. Wash your hands.

27. Make resident comfortable.

28. Return bed to lowest position. Remove privacy measures.

29. Leave call light within resident's reach.

30. Wash your hands.

31. Be courteous and respectful at all times.

32. Report any changes in the resident to the nurse. Document procedure using facility guidelines.

A follow-up cleansing enema may be ordered after using an oil-retention enema. This helps clean the bowels more thoroughly and eliminate remaining oil in the intestine. The resident may want to bathe after this procedure and the bowel movements that follow. Assist as needed.

9. Demonstrate how to collect a stool specimen

You may be asked to collect a stool specimen from a resident. A **specimen** is a sample, such as tissue, blood, urine, stool, or sputum, used for analysis and diagnosis. Specimens are used for different types of tests. A stool sample may be needed to test for blood, pathogens, and other things. Stool may be collected and tested for ova and parasites (O&P) to detect worms or amoebas. If testing stool for ova and parasites, deliver the specimen to the lab immediately. These tests must be done while the stool is still warm. Stool that cannot be sent to the lab immediately may need to be placed in a special refrigerator used strictly for specimens. Never place a specimen in a refrigerator that is used for food or drinks. Follow instructions for transporting or storing stool specimens collected for testing.

When collecting a stool specimen, first show the resident the correct container to use. Ask the resident not to get urine or toilet paper in the sample because they can ruin the sample and create the need for a new specimen.

A plastic collection container called a "hat" is sometimes inserted into a toilet to collect and measure urine or stool (Fig. 15-15). Hats should be labeled with the resident's name and room number and must be cleaned after each use.

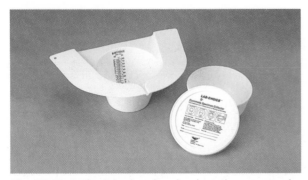

Fig. 15-15. A "hat" is placed under the toilet seat to collect a specimen.

Ask the resident to let you know when he or she can have a bowel movement. Be ready to collect the specimen.

Collecting a stool specimen

Equipment: specimen container and lid, completed label (labeled with resident's name, date of birth, room number, date, and time), 2 tongue blades, 2 pairs of gloves, bedpan (if resident cannot use portable commode or toilet), "hat" for toilet (if resident uses toilet or commode), 2 plastic bags, toilet paper, laboratory slip, disposable washcloths or wipes, supplies for perineal care, pen

1. Identify yourself by name. Identify the resident. Greet the resident by name.

2. Wash your hands.

3. Explain procedure to resident. Speak clearly, slowly, and directly. Maintain face-to-face contact whenever possible.

4. Provide for the resident's privacy with a curtain, screen, or door.

5. Put on gloves.

6. When the resident is ready to move bowels, ask him not to urinate at the same time. Ask him not to put toilet paper in with the sample. Provide a plastic bag for toilet paper.

7. Fit hat to toilet or commode, or provide resident with bedpan. Place toilet paper and washcloths or wipes within resident's reach. Ask the resident to clean his hands with a hand wipe when finished, if he is able.

8. Ask the resident to signal when he is finished with the bowel movement. Make sure call light is within reach.

9. Remove and discard gloves. Wash your hands. Leave the room.

10. When called by the resident, return and wash your hands. Put on clean gloves.

11. Give perineal care if help is needed.

12. Using the two tongue blades, take about two tablespoons of stool and put it in the container. Cover it tightly, apply label, and place specimen in a clean plastic bag.

13. Wrap the tongue blades in toilet paper and place them in plastic bag with used toilet paper. Discard bag in the proper container. Empty the bedpan or container into the toilet. Flush the toilet. Place in proper area for cleaning or clean it according to facility policy.

14. Remove and discard gloves. Wash your hands.

15. Make resident comfortable.

16. Return bed to lowest position. Remove privacy measures.

17. Leave call light within resident's reach.

18. Wash your hands.

19. Be courteous and respectful at all times.

20. Report any changes in the resident to the nurse. Document procedure using facility guidelines. Take specimen and lab slip to designated place promptly.

Collecting a specimen from a resident in isolation requires special handling. Some steps are done outside the isolation room. Two labels are completed, leaving one label outside on a biohazard bag. Proper PPE must be put on before entering the room. After collecting the specimen and covering the container, place one completed label on the container. When you are ready to leave the isolation room, complete all actions to safely leave the room. Remove and discard gloves, and wash your hands last.

Using a clean paper towel, carefully pick up the specimen container and leave the room. Immediately put the specimen container into the biohazard bag on the isolation cart. Discard the paper towel in the appropriate container. Seal the bag properly and take the specimen to the proper site. Wash your hands again.

10. Explain occult blood testing

Hidden, or **occult**, blood is found inside stool with a microscope or a special chemical test. This may be a sign of a serious physical problem, such as cancer. The Hemoccult® test checks for occult blood in stool. The collecting and testing of stool to check for occult blood is a common procedure. In some facilities, staff members do not perform this test; the staff at laboratories do it instead. Follow the care plan and your facility's policy. Specific dietary orders or medications may be necessary prior to occult blood testing. Check the expiration date on testing cards before using.

Testing a stool specimen for occult blood

Equipment: labeled stool specimen, Hemoccult® test kit (Fig. 15-16) or other ordered test kit, 1 or 2 tongue blades, plastic bag, gloves

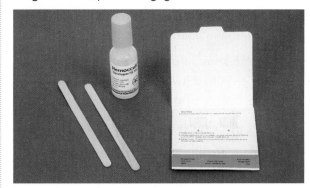

Fig. 15-16. *A Hemoccult® test kit.*

1. Wash your hands.

2. Put on gloves.

3. Open the test card.

4. Pick up a tongue blade. Get small amount of stool from specimen container.

5. Using a tongue blade, smear a small amount of stool onto Box A of test card (Fig. 15-17).

6. Flip tongue blade (or use new tongue blade). Get some stool from another part of specimen. Smear small amount of stool onto Box B of test card.

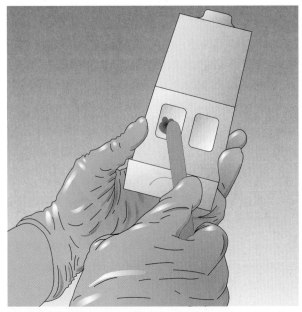

Fig. 15-17. *Smear a small amount of stool onto Box A.*

7. Close the test card. Turn over to other side.

8. Open the flap.

9. Open developer. Apply developer to each box. Follow manufacturer's instructions.

10. Wait the amount of time listed in instructions, usually between 10 and 60 seconds.

11. Watch the squares for any color changes. Record color changes. Follow instructions.

12. Place tongue blade(s) and test packet in plastic bag.

13. Dispose of plastic bag properly in biohazard container.

14. Remove and discard gloves.

15. Wash your hands.

16. Document procedure using facility guidelines. Report results to the nurse.

11. Define the term "ostomy" and identify the difference between colostomy and ileostomy

An **ostomy** is the surgical creation of an opening from an area inside the body to the outside. The terms "colostomy" and "ileostomy" refer to

the surgical removal of a portion of the intestines. In a resident with one of these ostomies, the end of the intestine is brought to the outside of the body through an artificial opening in the abdomen. This opening is called a **stoma**. Stool, or feces, is eliminated through the ostomy rather than through the anus.

An ostomy may be necessary due to bowel disease, such as diverticulitis, Crohn's disease, or colon cancer. An ostomy can be either permanent or temporary; a temporary ostomy allows the intestines to heal from a specific condition.

The terms "colostomy" and "ileostomy" tell what section of the intestine was removed and the type of stool that will be eliminated (Fig. 15-18). A **colostomy** is a surgically-created opening into the large intestine to allow feces to be expelled. With a colostomy, stool may be semi-solid. An **ileostomy** is a surgically-created opening into the end of the small intestine, the ileum, to allow feces to be expelled. Stool will be liquid and may be irritating to the skin.

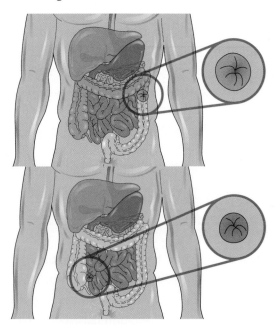

Fig. 15-18. *An illustration of a colostomy on the top and an ileostomy on the bottom.*

Residents who have had an ostomy wear a disposable drainage bag, or appliance, that fits over the stoma to collect the feces. The bag is custom-fitted over the stoma to collect the stool (Fig. 15-19). The bag is attached to the skin by adhesive, and a belt may be used to secure it.

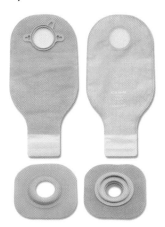

Fig. 15-19. *The top of this photo shows the front and back of one type of drainage bag for an ostomy. An example of a skin barrier is at the bottom of the photo.* (PHOTOS COURTESY OF HOLLISTER INCORPORATED, LIBERTYVILLE, ILLINOIS)

Many people with ostomies feel embarrassed or angry. They often feel they have lost control of a basic bodily function. Ostomies can cause odor, discomfort, and fear of the bag falling off. You can do a great deal to help residents with ostomies feel better about themselves. Be sensitive and supportive and always provide privacy for ostomy care. Do not act uncomfortable with ostomy care, especially with the odor or the changing of the bag. Follow these guidelines when giving ostomy care:

Guidelines: Ostomy Care

G   Follow Standard and/or Transmission-Based Precautions, including wearing gloves and any additional PPE needed, when caring for ostomies. Wash your hands carefully.

G   Make sure residents with ostomies receive good skin care and proper hygiene.

G   Remove ostomy bags carefully to avoid tearing the resident's skin.

G   Before removing the drainage bag, allow a little air out of the bag to remove any built-up pressure. This can prevent the bag from exploding.

G   Observe contents of ostomy bag before disposing of used bag. If anything unusual is noted, such as blood or a change in the stool quality or amount, notify the nurse.

G   Empty, clean, and replace the ostomy bag whenever stool is eliminated.

G   Assist residents with ostomies to wash their hands properly.

G   During ostomy care, observe for signs of skin irritation, rashes, swelling, or bleeding around stoma. Report these signs, along with complaints of pain or discomfort, immediately.

G   Use skin barriers, such as creams and pastes, as ordered.

G   Make sure the bottom of drainage bag is securely clamped before applying it to the stoma.

G   Make sure bag is attached securely to the resident before completing ostomy care.

G   Make sure the bag is secure before the resident goes to activities or appointments or receives visitors.

G   Be supportive, empathetic, and caring. Your support will help the resident to handle this important change in lifestyle.

Caring for an ostomy

Equipment: disposable bed protector, bath blanket, clean ostomy drainage bag and belt, toilet paper or gauze squares, basin of warm water, mild soap or cleanser, washcloth, skin barrier as ordered, 2 towels, plastic disposable bag, gloves, special deodorant, if used

1.   Identify yourself by name. Identify the resident. Greet the resident by name.

2.   Wash your hands.

3.   Explain procedure to resident. Speak clearly, slowly, and directly. Maintain face-to-face contact whenever possible.

4. Provide for the resident's privacy with a curtain, screen, or door.

5. Adjust bed to safe working level, usually waist high. Lock bed wheels. Raise head of bed.

6. Put on gloves.

7. Place bed protector under resident. Cover resident with a bath blanket. Pull down the top sheet and blankets. Expose only the ostomy site. Offer resident a towel to keep clothing dry.

8. Undo the ostomy belt if used. Pull gently on one edge of ostomy appliance to release air.

9. Remove ostomy bag carefully. Place it in plastic bag. Note the color, odor, consistency, and amount of stool in the bag.

10. Wipe area around stoma with toilet paper or gauze squares. Discard paper/gauze in plastic bag.

11. Add small amount of mild soap or cleanser to the warm water. Using a washcloth, wash the area gently in one direction, away from the stoma (Fig. 15-20). Rinse. Pat dry with another towel. Apply skin barrier as ordered. Temporarily cover stoma opening with gauze squares.

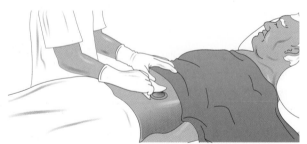

Fig. 15-20. *Wash the area gently, moving in one direction, away from the stoma.*

12. Apply deodorant to bag if used. Remove gauze squares, and place in plastic bag. Put the clean ostomy drainage bag on resident. Hold in place and seal securely. Make sure the bottom of the bag is clamped. Attach to ostomy belt if used.

13. Remove bed protector and discard. Place soiled linens in proper container.

14. Remove bag and gauze squares. Discard bag and squares in the proper container.

15. Remove and discard gloves. Wash your hands.

16. Make resident comfortable.

17. Return bed to lowest position. Remove privacy measures.

18. Leave call light within resident's reach.

19. Wash your hands.

20. Be courteous and respectful at all times.

21. Report any changes in the resident to the nurse. Document procedure using facility guidelines.

Other Types of Ostomies

A **urostomy** is the general term used for any surgical procedure that diverts the passage of urine by re-directing the ureters. A **ureterostomy** is a type of urostomy in which an opening from a ureter is brought through the abdomen for urine to be eliminated.

12. Explain guidelines for assisting with bowel retraining

Residents who have had an illness, injury, or a period of inactivity may need assistance in re-establishing a regular routine and normal bowel function. Retraining is the process of assisting residents to regain control of their bowels.

Taking regular trips to the bathroom at specific times each day will help with bowel retraining. Doctors may order suppositories, enemas, laxatives, or stool softeners to assist. Most care team members will be involved with charting and implementing bowel retraining. Understand and follow the care plan for each resident.

Guidelines: Bowel Retraining

G   Follow the care plan consistently. Explain the training schedule to the resident. Direct any questions the resident has to the nurse.

G   Follow Standard Precautions. Wear gloves when handling body wastes. For residents in isolation, additional PPE may be needed. Follow the care plan.

G   Observe the resident's elimination habits. This helps predict when a trip to the bathroom or a bedpan will be necessary.

G   Keep a record of elimination, including episodes of incontinence. Keeping accurate records will help establish a routine.

G   Offer a bedpan or a trip to the bathroom at specific times each day.

G   Answer call lights promptly.

G   Provide privacy for elimination, and do not rush the resident.

G   Help with perineal care as needed. This promotes proper hygiene. Watch for skin changes and report them.

G   Encourage fluids throughout the day, if allowed.

G   Encourage the proper diet.

G   Dispose of wastes promptly and properly.

G   Praise attempts and successes in controlling the bowels.

G   Never show frustration or anger toward residents who are incontinent. That is abusive behavior, and negative reactions will only make the problem worse. Be positive and patient with the retraining efforts.

Handling Incontinence

Always act professionally when handling bowel incontinence or helping to re-establish routines. Bowel incontinence is difficult enough for residents without them having to worry about your reactions. Be patient when setbacks occur.

Chapter Review

1.   Define these terms: anatomy, physiology, cells, tissues, organs, body systems, and homeostasis (LO 2).

2.   How does peristalsis aid in elimination (LO 3)?

3.   What is feces (LO 3)?

4.   What are four functions of the gastrointestinal system (LO 3)?

5.   List five normal age-related changes of the gastrointestinal system (LO 4).

6.   List three normal qualities of stool (LO 5).

7.   List seven things to observe and report about stool (LO 5).

8.   For each of the seven factors that affect bowel elimination listed in Learning Objective 6, describe one way nursing assistants can promote normal elimination (LO 6).

9.   When is a fracture pan used for elimination rather than a standard bedpan (LO 6)?

10.   How should a standard bedpan be positioned? How should a fracture pan be positioned (LO 6)?

11.   When are portable commodes used (LO 6)?

12.   How should a resident who has GERD be positioned after eating (LO 7)?

13.   List two types of treatments for ulcerative colitis or Crohn's disease (LO 7).

14.   What are five causes of flatulence (LO 7)?

15.   List three possible treatments for constipation (LO 7).

16.   What are five causes of fecal incontinence (LO 7)?

17.   List six signs and symptoms of a fecal impaction (LO 7).

18.   What should be avoided when caring for a resident who has hemorrhoids (LO 7)?

19.   Describe four types of enemas (LO 8).

20. What position must the resident be in for an enema (LO 8)?

21. If a resident feels pain while receiving an enema, what should the nursing assistant do (LO 8)?

22. When giving a cleansing enema, how far above a resident's anus should the bottom of the enema bag be placed (LO 8)?

23. Why does a stool specimen need to be delivered to the lab immediately when testing for ova and parasites (LO 9)?

24. What items should not be included in a stool specimen (LO 9)?

25. What is the term for a plastic collection container that is inserted into a toilet to collect and measure urine or stool (LO 9)?

26. How is occult blood found in stool (LO 10)?

27. Define the term "ostomy" (LO 11).

28. When may an ostomy be necessary (LO 11)?

29. How do colostomies and ileostomies differ (LO 11)?

30. List ten guidelines for bowel retraining (LO 12).

16
The Urinary System

1. Define important words in this chapter

24-hour urine specimen: a urine specimen consisting of all urine voided in a 24-hour period.

calculi: kidney stones.

chronic renal failure (CRF): progressive condition in which the kidneys cannot filter certain waste products; also called chronic kidney failure.

clean-catch specimen: a urine specimen that does not include the first and last urine that is voided; also called mid-stream.

condom catheter: a catheter that has an attachment on the end that fits onto the penis; also called an external or Texas catheter.

dialysis: a process that cleans the body of wastes that the kidneys cannot remove due to kidney failure.

end-stage renal disease (ESRD): condition in which kidneys have failed and dialysis or transplantation is required to sustain life.

indwelling catheter: a catheter that stays inside the bladder for a period of time; urine drains into a bag.

ketones: chemical substances that the body produces when it does not have enough insulin in the blood.

micturition: the process of emptying the bladder of urine; also called urination or voiding.

routine urine specimen: a urine specimen that can be collected any time a person voids.

specific gravity: a test performed to measure the density of urine.

sphincter: a ring-like muscle that opens and closes an opening in the body.

straight catheter: a catheter that does not stay inside the person; it is removed immediately after urine is drained or collected.

urinary incontinence: the inability to control the bladder, which leads to an involuntary loss of urine.

urinary tract infection (UTI): a disorder that causes inflammation of the bladder; also called cystitis.

voiding: the process of emptying the bladder of urine; also called urination or micturition.

2. Explain the structure and function of the urinary system

The urinary system consists of two kidneys, two ureters, the urinary bladder, the urethra, and the meatus (Fig. 16-1). The kidneys are bean-shaped organs. They lie slightly above the waist against the rear wall of the abdominal cavity and on either side of the spine. Each kidney is about four to five inches in length, one inch thick, and weighs between four and six ounces. The kidneys are partially protected by the back muscles and the lower ribs. The kidneys clean and filter waste products and toxic materials from the blood. They regulate the amount of electrolytes within the body. They also help to regulate blood pressure and water balance.

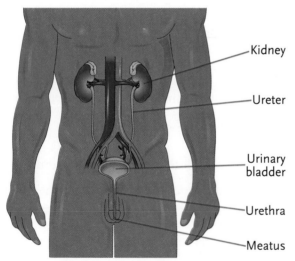

Fig. 16-1. The urinary system consists of two kidneys and two ureters, the bladder, the urethra, and the meatus.

Substances needed by the body are reabsorbed; the substances not needed—toxins and waste products—stay in the kidney and form urine. The urine is then transferred to the bladder through tubes called the ureters. The ureters are narrow tubes about one foot in length. When

a person urinates, the ureters also prevent the backflow of urine into the kidneys.

The urinary bladder temporarily stores the urine. When the bladder has collected about 200 to 400 mL of urine, nerve impulses are transferred to the lower portion of the spinal cord. The spinal cord sends nerve impulses back, causing the muscles of the bladder to contract. This relaxes the internal sphincter. The urine moves into the urethra, the tube that carries the urine out of the body. In males, the urethra is approximately seven to eight inches long. In females, it is approximately three to four inches long (Fig. 16-2).

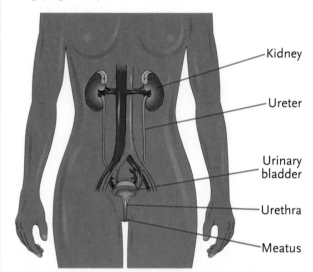

Fig. 16-2. The female urethra is shorter than the male urethra. Because of this, the female bladder is more likely to become infected by bacteria traveling up the urethra.

There is an external sphincter in the body that needs to voluntarily relax in order to pass urine. A **sphincter** is a ring-like muscle that opens and closes an opening in the body. Urine then passes out of the body through the meatus, the opening at the end of the urethra. This is the process of urinating, which is also called **micturition** or **voiding**. When this sphincter is damaged, weakened, or loses contact with the nervous system, it can cause urinary incontinence. **Urinary incontinence** is the inability to control the bladder, which leads to an involuntary loss of urine. You will learn more about urinary incontinence later in this chapter.

The functions of the urinary system are to:

- Eliminate waste products from the blood
- Maintain water balance in the body
- Regulate the levels of electrolytes in the body
- Assist in regulation of blood pressure

Destination: Homeostasis

When the body's fluid balance is disturbed, the kidneys work hard to try to continue to remove waste products from the blood. When water intake decreases, the body adjusts by retaining or saving more water. To do this, the kidneys increase the amount of water returned to the bloodstream. This causes less water to be moved into the urine, which temporarily produces a more concentrated form of urine. In this way, the body's water balance remains stable, maintaining homeostasis.

Tip

Tiny stones can be a big pain.

A kidney stone is a hard mass developed from crystals that separate from the urine and build up on the inner surfaces of the kidney. The stones are also called renal calculi. They can block a ureter, which causes extreme pain. Urine production is decreased during a blockage. This is due to a reflex that causes tiny vessels in the kidney to constrict, or become smaller. Report symptoms, such as blood in the urine, painful urination, a frequent urge to urinate, back pain, or flank pain, that may indicate kidney stones.

3. Discuss changes in the urinary system due to aging

Normal age-related changes for the urinary system include the following:

- The kidneys do not filter the blood as efficiently.
- Bladder muscle tone weakens.
- Bladder holds less urine, which causes more frequent urination.
- Bladder may not empty completely, causing an increased chance of infection.

4. List normal qualities of urine and identify signs and symptoms to report about urine

Urination is the physical process of releasing or emptying the bladder of urine. Urine consists of waste products removed from the blood. Humans must urinate several times daily in order to remain healthy. Regular urination is vital to keep the urinary system healthy.

Urine is normally light, pale yellow, or amber in color (Fig. 16-3). Certain medications and some foods change the color of urine. For example, beets, berries, and some food dyes can make urine appear pink or red. Urine should be clear or transparent and have a faint smell. Urine can become cloudy as it stands, but if it is cloudy when freshly voided, it can be a sign of infection. Normal urine output varies with age and the amount and type of liquids consumed. Adults usually produce approximately 1200 to 1500 mL of urine per day. Elderly adults may produce less urine.

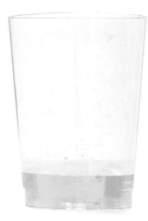

Fig. 16-3. *Urine is normally light or pale yellow in color. It should be clear, not cloudy.*

Normal urine elimination means there is no pain during urination. There should be no blood, pus, mucus, protein, bacteria, glucose or other abnormal matter in urine. You will learn more about glucose later in the chapter. A change in the appearance of urine can signal a health problem. Report any of the following signs or symptoms to the nurse:

Observing and Reporting: Urine

O/R Cloudy urine

O/R Dark or rust-colored urine

O/R Strong-, offensive-, or fruity-smelling urine

O/R Pain, burning, or pressure when urinating

O/R Blood, pus, mucus, or discharge in urine

O/R Episodes of incontinence

5. List factors affecting urination and describe how to promote normal urination

There are many things that may affect normal urination:

Growth and Development: Aging affects the bladder's ability to hold urine. The bladder is not able to hold the same amount of urine as it did when a person was younger. Older people may have to urinate more often. Urination during the night occurs more frequently with the elderly. The bladder may not empty completely, causing a higher risk of infection. In males, an inability to urinate properly may be due to an enlargement of the prostate gland.

To promote normal urination, encourage the intake of fluids. Provide water and other beverages often for residents who do not have a fluid restriction. Offer frequent trips to the bathroom. Follow a schedule, if possible. Respond to call lights and bathroom requests promptly. The best position for women to urinate is sitting; for men, it is standing. Avoid the flat-on-back (supine) position if possible, as it does not put pressure on the bladder and works against gravity. Promote exercise and activity, as ordered in the care plan. Help with perineal care as needed, wiping from front to back. Good perineal care will help reduce the risk of infection. Assist residents in washing hands.

Encourage Kegel exercises; these exercises use the pelvic floor muscles to strengthen muscle tone. To find your Kegel muscles, stop the flow of urine once or twice while urinating. To do Kegel exercises, squeeze the muscles for five to ten seconds and relax for ten seconds. These can be done many times per day and can be done anywhere in any position.

Psychological Factors: A lack of privacy can affect urination. Having a roommate for the first time, being in a place that is not home, and needing help with elimination can disrupt normal elimination patterns. Stress and fear can affect urination. They can cause a person to void frequent, small amounts of urine. Depression can alter urination patterns. A person may not be motivated to change exercise habits and increase fluid intake. This can make urinary elimination more difficult.

To promote normal urination, always provide plenty of privacy and allow time for urination. Do not rush the resident. Leave the call light within reach. Respond to call lights and requests for help with toileting immediately. If residents want to talk about their concerns, take the time to listen to them. Report their concerns to the nurse.

Fluid Intake: The sense of thirst generally decreases as a person ages. Reduced fluid intake decreases urine production. The body's ability to remove wastes in the urine may be affected. When wastes build up, infections and other problems can occur. Drinking alcoholic beverages and caffeinated beverages increases urine production. Fluids high in sodium decrease urine output.

To promote normal urination, encourage fluid intake. Generally, a healthy person needs 64 ounces (1920 mL) of fluid each day. Remind residents to drink often. Be aware of excessive caffeine, sodium, alcohol, or sugar in the resident's diet. Make sure pitcher and water are within reach and are light enough for each resident to lift. Offer a straw if the resident prefers using one. Assist with fluid intake as needed.

Physical Activity and Exercise: A lack of exercise lessens sphincter control, which can increase episodes of incontinence. Childbirth can affect a woman's muscle tone. Indwelling catheters (Learning Objective 8) and trauma can affect muscle tone, and increase the risk of infection.

To promote normal urination, increase daily exercise. Encourage regular walks and other types of activities that are allowed.

Personal Habits: If a resident is confined to bed, urination may be more difficult due to his position. As stated before, the sitting position for women and standing position for men are the best positions for urination. Complete emptying of the bladder may be difficult when having to use a bedpan or urinal.

To promote normal urination, raise the head of the bed. Try running water in the bathroom sink to encourage urination.

Medications: Some medications affect urination. Residents who have high blood pressure may be taking diuretics, which are medications that reduce fluid in the body by increasing urine output.

To promote normal urination, offer a trip to the bathroom or bedpan or urinal often. Encourage fluids if allowed, even if this causes more frequent urination.

Disorders: Certain disorders affect urination. Fevers cause increased sweating and may decrease urine production. Diabetes, diseases of the bladder or urethra, infection, and congestive heart failure (CHF) can affect urination. You will learn more about these diseases later in this chapter and in Chapters 19 and 23 of the textbook.

Residents' Rights

Help residents promptly.

Do your residents wait too long to void? This is unhealthy for their urinary systems. Residents should be taken to the bathroom as soon as they need to urinate. They should never have to wait. Accidents are not the only problem with waiting. Holding urine in the bladder for too long can cause bacteria to grow. This leads to infection.

See Chapter 15 for procedures on how to assist residents with bedpans and urinals.

6. Discuss common disorders of the urinary system

Urinary Tract Infection (UTI)

A **urinary tract infection (UTI)**, or cystitis, causes inflammation of the bladder. This occurs when bacteria enter the urinary tract through the urethra and then begin to multiply in the bladder. The most common cause of this bacterial infection is from *E. coli* bacteria, which is a form of bacteria commonly found in the gastrointestinal tract. It moves from the anus into the urethra and then the bladder, causing a urinary tract infection.

Women are more susceptible to UTIs than men. This is due to the female urethra being shorter than the male urethra. Bacteria can reach a woman's bladder more easily. Women often develop urinary tract infections after having sexual intercourse. Urinating immediately after sexual intercourse helps prevent these infections.

Symptoms of UTIs include burning or pain with urination, blood in the urine, and frequency of and urgency with urination.

Drinking plenty of water and other fluids can help prevent UTIs. Cranberry, orange, and blueberry juices, which are rich in vitamin C, help to acidify urine, which can prevent infection. Wiping from front to back after elimination helps to prevent infection (Fig. 16-4). Taking showers, rather than baths, can help prevent UTIs. Antibiotics are usually prescribed to treat UTIs. Report to the nurse if a resident has cloudy, dark, or foul-smelling urine. Report complaints of burning or discomfort during urination, or if a resident urinates often and in small amounts.

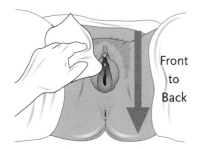

Fig. 16-4. *After elimination, wipe from front to back to prevent infection.*

Chronic Renal Failure

Chronic renal failure (CRF), also called chronic kidney failure, is a condition in which the kidneys cannot effectively filter waste products from the blood. The kidneys are also unable to perform other life-sustaining duties. Chronic renal failure worsens over time. With this disorder, the kidneys slowly become damaged. Waste products and fluid accumulate in the body.

This disease can result from diabetes, high blood pressure (hypertension), chronic urinary tract infections, inflammation of the kidneys (nephritis), or some medications, especially certain analgesics. Symptoms may appear only after damage to the kidneys has been done. Initial signs and symptoms of this disorder are:

- Unintended weight loss

- Nausea and vomiting

- Fatigue

- Headache

- Frequent hiccups

- Itching

If kidney function is seriously impaired, dialysis may be necessary. Kidney **dialysis** is an artifi-

cial means of removing the body's waste products. It is done when the person's kidneys are no longer able to perform their responsibilities. It can improve and extend life for several years. Dialysis is done regularly and continuously until a kidney transplant is performed or until the person dies. Residents will have fluid restrictions of different degrees when on dialysis.

End-stage renal disease (ESRD) occurs when the kidneys have failed and dialysis or transplantation is required to sustain life. Diabetes is the most common cause of ESRD. Dialysis must be performed for people who have ESRD.

Urine Retention

Urine retention is an inability to adequately or completely empty the bladder. Retention can be short-term or long-term. Surgical procedures, obstruction, infection, and some disorders, such as multiple sclerosis and diabetes, are common causes of urine retention. You will learn more about these diseases in Chapters 22 and 23 of the textbook. In men, the most common cause of urine retention is enlargement of the prostate gland. Symptoms include the following:

- Lower abdominal pain

- A painful urge, but inability, to urinate

- Swollen (distended) bladder

- Abdominal swelling

- Frequent urge to urinate

- Difficulty in starting to urinate

- Weak flow of urine

- Dribbling at the end of urinating and in between urinating

Report to the nurse if you note any of the symptoms listed above. If the condition is not treated, it can lead to a UTI or damage to the urinary tract and kidneys. Urine retention is usually treated with medications and catheterization (use of a tube to drain urine from the bladder).

7. Discuss reasons for incontinence

Urinary incontinence is the inability to control the muscles of the bladder, which leads to an involuntary loss of urine. Incontinence can occur in residents who are confined to bed, ill, or paralyzed. Other physical reasons for incontinence include the following:

- Circulatory or nervous system diseases or injuries, such as stroke, dementia, or multiple sclerosis

- Prostate problems

- Childbirth

Incontinence is not a normal part of aging. Whatever the reason for incontinence, it is important for nursing assistants to act professionally when handling this problem. Never show anger or frustration toward residents who are incontinent. Residents who are incontinent need reassurance and understanding.

There are different types of incontinence:

- Stress incontinence is a loss of urine due to an increase in intra-abdominal pressure; it may be caused by sneezing, laughing, or coughing

- Urge incontinence is involuntary voiding due to an abrupt urge to void.

- Mixed incontinence means symptoms of both urge and stress incontinence are present.

- Functional incontinence is urine loss caused by environmental, cognitive, or physical reasons.

- Overflow incontinence is due to overflow or over-distention of the bladder.

Incontinence can be very difficult for residents to handle emotionally. Residents may avoid discussing the problem due to embarrassment. It may cause frustration and anger. Family and friends may share these feelings as well. Nursing assistants can help by always being professional and positive when dealing with episodes of incontinence. In addition, follow these guidelines:

Guidelines: Urinary Incontinence

G Know residents' routines and urinary habits. Know their physical signs, such as holding the lower abdomen, which might indicate the need to urinate.

G Follow toileting schedules and the care plan carefully.

G Leave call lights within reach. Answer call lights promptly to prevent accidents.

G Offer a bedpan or take residents to the bathroom often.

G Encourage plenty of fluids, unless residents have a fluid restriction.

G Walking can stimulate the circulation and the need to go to the bathroom. Take daily walks close to a bathroom.

G Disposable incontinence pads or briefs for adults help keep wastes away from the skin (Fig. 16-5). Change wet or soiled briefs immediately. Always refer to incontinence products as briefs or pads; never call them diapers. Residents are not infants, and this is disrespectful.

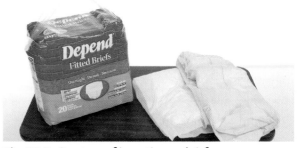

Fig. 16-5. One type of incontinence brief.

G Change bed linens any time they are wet or soiled. Leaving residents in wet linens puts them at risk for pressure ulcers (Chapter 18). It is also abusive or neglectful behavior.

G   Use bed protectors or plastic or disposable sheets for residents who are incontinent.

G   When residents wear incontinence briefs, check them at least every two hours. Change briefs whenever they are wet or soiled. Observe and report any signs of skin irritation. Tell the nurse if the brief does not appear to fit properly.

G   Change wet or soiled clothing immediately.

G   Give good skin care and good perineal care. This helps prevent skin breakdown. Urine is irritating to the skin. Bathe residents often.

G   Provide privacy for episodes of incontinence. Keep your voice low to keep incontinence a private matter. Never expose more of the resident than is necessary.

G   Be calm, patient, and professional.

G   Family and friends may watch how you behave to see how they should react to the problem. Be reassuring and remain positive.

Residents' Rights

No shortcuts with resident care.

Residents are sometimes incontinent in bed. Do not take shortcuts when changing bed linen after episodes of incontinence. If you replace a disposable pad without changing the wet linen, it can irritate the skin and put residents at risk for pressure ulcers. Remove all wet linen and disposable pads as soon as possible. Replace them with clean ones. Promote your residents' health and dignity.

8. Describe catheters and related care

Residents who are unable to pass urine normally may need a urinary catheter. A catheter is a tube used to add or drain fluid that is inserted through the skin or into a body opening. Some residents will need straight catheterization. A **straight catheter** is a type of catheter that is inserted to drain urine present in the bladder, and is removed after urine is drained or collected. This catheter does not stay inside the person.

Other residents may require that a catheter remain inside the bladder for a period of time.

This type of a catheter is called an **indwelling catheter** (Fig. 16-6). This catheter is held in place by a balloon filled with sterile water and the urine drains into a bag.

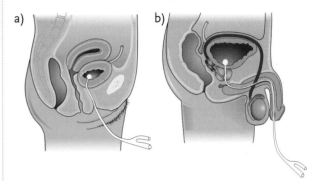

Fig. 16-6. a) An indwelling catheter (female). b) An indwelling catheter (male).

Another type of catheter that is used for males is called an external, or **condom catheter** (sometimes called a "Texas catheter"). It has an attachment on the end that fits onto the penis and is fastened with special tape. The urine drains through the condom catheter into the tubing, then into the drainage bag. Smaller bags, called "leg bags" collect the urine. They attach to the resident's leg (Fig. 16-7). A condom catheter is changed daily or as needed.

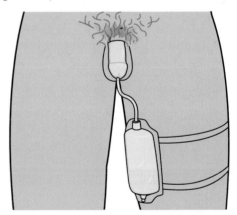

Fig. 16-7. A condom catheter with a leg bag.

Catheters are inserted by nurses or doctors. Nursing assistants usually do not insert, irrigate, or remove catheters. However, you may be asked to give daily catheter care, clean the area around the urethral opening, and empty the drainage bag. The bag is emptied into a measuring container, called a graduate. You learned about measuring urinary output in Chapter 14.

Serious complications, such as infections, can occur from poor catheter care. These infections can be life-threatening. Follow these care guidelines for working with catheters:

Guidelines: Catheters

G Wear gloves when emptying catheter drainage bags.

G When draining the bag, open and close the tubing clamp without touching the tip of the clamp to any other object. If the tip touches other objects, it can transfer pathogens to the inside of the tubing, which can move up into the bladder and cause infection.

G Do not let the catheter drainage spout touch the graduate when draining the catheter bag.

G Make sure the drainage bag always hangs lower than the level of the hips or bladder, including when the resident is ambulating or in a wheelchair. Urine must never flow back into the bladder from the tubing or bag, as it can cause infection.

G Do not hang the drainage bag from the bedrail; the drainage bag should be secured to a non-movable part of the bed frame. When in a wheelchair, the bag may fit into a special pouch located on the side of or at the back of the wheelchair.

G Keep the drainage bag off the floor. Make sure the catheter tubing does not touch the floor.

G Keep tubing as straight as possible. Make sure there are no kinks in the tube and that the resident is not lying on the tubing. The tubing should be over the leg, not underneath it. This can prevent urine from draining properly. Do not hang tubing over side rails.

G Keep the genital area clean to prevent infection. Pathogens can enter the bladder more easily with catheters. Daily careful care of the genital area is important.

G When cleaning the urinary meatus, move in one direction, away from the meatus. Use a clean area of the cloth for each stroke.

G Report to the nurse if you notice any of the following: blood in the urine, urine leaking from the catheter, catheter bag filling suddenly or not filling for several hours. Also report complaints of pain or pressure, or odor.

G Secure the tubing properly to the leg with a catheter strap.

G Be careful not to disconnect the catheter when positioning or transferring residents with catheters. Do not try to re-attach a catheter tube that has disconnected. Inform the nurse immediately so that he or she can re-attach the tube. This is a sterile procedure.

Providing catheter care

Equipment: bath blanket, disposable bed protector, bath basin with warm water, soap, bath thermometer, 2-4 washcloths or wipes, towel, gloves

1. Identify yourself by name. Identify the resident. Greet the resident by name.

2. Wash your hands.

3. Explain procedure to resident. Speak clearly, slowly, and directly. Maintain face-to-face contact whenever possible.

4. Provide for the resident's privacy with a curtain, screen, or door.

5. Adjust bed to safe working level, usually waist high. Lock bed wheels.

6. Lower head of bed. Position resident lying flat on her back.

7. Remove or fold back top bedding. Keep resident covered with bath blanket.

8. Test water temperature with thermometer or your wrist and ensure it is safe. Water temperature should be 105° F. Have the resident check water temperature. Adjust if necessary.

9. Put on gloves.

10. Avoid contact with clothing and soiled pads or soiled linens throughout procedure.

11. Ask the resident to flex her knees and raise the buttocks off the bed by pushing against the mattress with her feet. Place clean bed protector under her buttocks.

12. Expose only the area necessary to clean the catheter.

13. Place towel or pad under catheter tubing before washing.

14. Apply soap to wet washcloth. If a male resident is uncircumcised, pull back the foreskin first. Clean area around meatus. Use a clean area of the washcloth for each stroke.

15. Hold catheter near meatus. Avoid tugging the catheter.

16. Clean at least four inches of catheter nearest meatus. Move in only one direction, away from meatus (Fig. 16-8). Use a clean area of the cloth for each stroke.

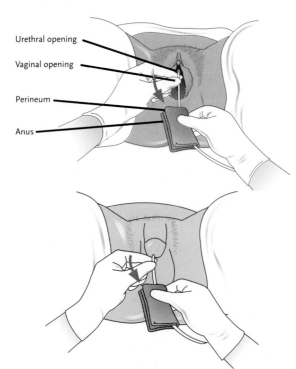

Urethral opening

Vaginal opening

Perineum

Anus

Fig. 16-8. Hold the catheter near the meatus, so that you do not tug on it. Moving in only one direction, away from meatus, helps prevent infection.

17. Rinse area around meatus, using a clean area of washcloth for each stroke. Pat dry with clean cloth.

18. Rinse at least four inches of catheter nearest meatus. Move in only one direction, away from meatus. Use a clean area of the cloth for each stroke.

19. Remove bed protector and discard. Remove towel or pad from under catheter tubing and place in proper containers.

20. Empty basin in toilet and flush toilet. Place in proper area for cleaning or return to storage.

21. Remove gloves and discard. Wash your hands.

22. Replace top covers. Remove bath blanket. Make resident comfortable.

23. Return bed to lowest position. Remove privacy measures.

24. Leave call light within resident's reach.

25. Wash your hands.

26. Be courteous and respectful at all times.

27. Report any changes in the resident to the nurse. Document procedure using facility guidelines.

Emptying a catheter drainage bag

Equipment: graduate (measuring container), alcohol wipes, paper towels, gloves

1. Identify yourself by name. Identify the resident. Greet the resident by name.

2. Wash your hands.

3. Explain procedure to resident. Speak clearly, slowly, and directly. Maintain face-to-face contact whenever possible.

4. Provide for the resident's privacy with a curtain, screen, or door.

5. Put on gloves.

6. Place graduate on paper towel on the floor.

7. Open the drain or clamp on the bag. Allow urine to flow out of the bag into the graduate. Do not let spout or clamp touch the graduate (Fig. 16-9).

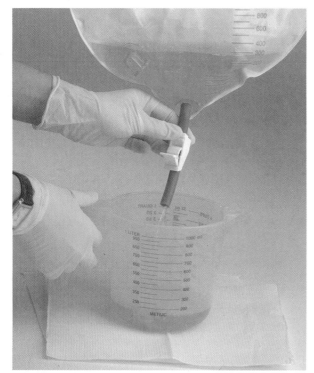

Fig. 16-9. Keep the spout and clamp from touching the graduate while draining urine.

8. When urine has drained, close clamp. Using alcohol wipe, clean the drain clamp. Replace the drain in its holder on the bag.

9. Go into the bathroom. Place graduate on a flat surface and measure at eye level. Note the amount and the appearance of the urine. Empty urine into toilet and flush toilet.

10. Place container in area for cleaning or clean and store it according to policy. Discard paper towel.

11. Remove and discard gloves. Wash your hands.

12. Leave call light within resident's reach.

13. Wash your hands.

14. Be courteous and respectful at all times.

15. Report any changes in the resident to the nurse. Document procedure and amount of urine (output) using facility guidelines.

Changing a condom catheter

Equipment: condom catheter and collection bag, catheter tape (if not a self-adhesive catheter), gloves, plastic bag, bath blanket, disposable bed protector, supplies for perineal care

1. Identify yourself by name. Identify the resident. Greet the resident by name.

2. Wash your hands.

3. Explain procedure to resident. Speak clearly, slowly, and directly. Maintain face-to-face contact whenever possible.

4. Provide for the resident's privacy with a curtain, screen, or door.

5. Adjust bed to safe working level, usually waist high. Lock bed wheels.

6. Lower head of bed. Position resident lying flat on his back.

7. Remove or fold back top bedding. Keep resident covered with bath blanket.

8. Put on gloves.

9. Place clean bed protector under his buttocks.

10. Adjust bath blanket to expose only genital area.

11. Gently remove condom catheter. Disconnect condom from tube and immediately cap tube. Do not allow tube to touch anything. Place condom and tape in the plastic bag.

12. Help as necessary with perineal care.

13. Move pubic hair away from the penis so it does not get rolled into the condom.

14. Hold penis firmly. Place condom at tip of penis. Roll towards base of penis. Leave at

least one inch of space between the drainage tip and glans of penis to prevent irritation. If resident is not circumcised, be sure that foreskin is in normal position.

15. Gently secure condom to penis with special tape provided or use self-adhesive (Fig. 16-10). Apply in a spiral. Never wrap tape all the way around penis because it can impair circulation.

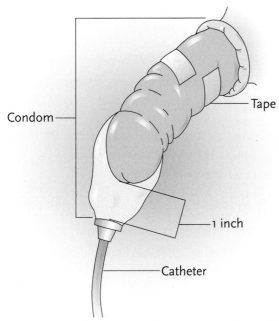

Fig. 16-10. *Gently secure condom to penis with provided tape.*

16. Connect catheter tip to drainage tubing. Do not touch tip to any object but drainage tubing. Make sure tubing is not twisted or kinked.

17. Check to see if collection bag is secured to leg. Make sure drain is closed.

18. Remove bed protector and discard. Dispose of plastic bag properly. Place soiled clothing and linens in proper containers.

19. Clean and store supplies.

20. Remove and discard gloves. Wash your hands.

21. Replace top covers. Remove bath blanket. Make resident comfortable.

22. Return bed to lowest position. Remove privacy measures.

23. Leave call light within resident's reach.

24. Wash your hands.

25. Be courteous and respectful at all times.

26. Report any changes in the resident to the nurse. Document procedure using facility guidelines.

After a condom catheter is applied, check on it often to make sure urine is draining freely. Reapply condom catheter if it falls off. Report to the nurse if you notice signs that the catheter is interfering with circulation in the penis, such as pale, gray, or blue-tinged skin or if the resident complains of numbness, tingling, or pain.

Continuous Bladder Irrigation (CBI)

Some residents who have an indwelling catheter have an order for continuous bladder irrigation (CBI). This may be needed after surgery on the urinary tract or when a resident has had a catheter for some time and needs to flush out the catheter. The goal of this procedure is to keep the catheter system open and clear of blockage.

When a CBI is ordered, a special type of catheter tubing is needed. A 3-in-1 style is used (Fig. 16-11):

- Tube 1 drains the urine.

- Tube 2 allows fluid to be injected to inflate a tiny balloon inside the bladder. This keeps the catheter in place and prevents it from slipping out of the bladder.

- Tube 3 allows the irrigation fluid to flow inside the bladder to flush out the system.

The nurse performs the irrigation procedure. To calculate urine output for a resident with CBI, use this example:

Irrigation fluid used during shift: 750 mL

Fluid output in the catheter drainage bag when emptied: 1250 mL

1250 mL - 750 mL = 500 mL total urine output

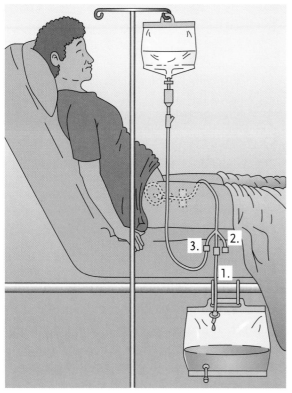

Fig. 16-11. *Bladder irrigation using a three-way catheter.*

9. Explain how to collect different types of urine specimens

Urine specimens are collected for different types of tests (Fig. 16-12). When collecting a urine specimen, make sure that you have the correct resident. The specimen must be put in the proper container and labeled with the resident's name, date of birth, room number, date, and time. Some urine specimens require special containers.

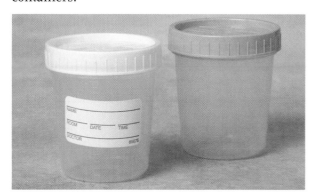

Fig. 16-12. *Specimens must always be labeled with the resident's name, date of birth, room number, the date, and time, before being taken to the lab.* (REPRINTED WITH PERMISSION OF BRIGGS CORPORATION, 800-247-2343, WWW.BRIGGSCORP.COM)

Urine that cannot be sent to the lab immediately may need to be placed in a special refrigerator used strictly for specimens. Never place a specimen in a refrigerator that is used for food.

When collecting a urine specimen, show the resident the correct container to use. The resident should be prepared to give a specimen the next time he or she has to urinate. Urine specimens must be collected properly in order to obtain accurate results. Ask the resident not to get toilet paper or stool in the sample because they can ruin the sample. After obtaining the specimen, take it to the lab or proper place promptly.

There are many tests that can be performed on urine. A **routine urine specimen** can be collected any time the resident voids. The resident will void into a bedpan, urinal, commode, or hat.

Collecting a routine urine specimen

Equipment: specimen container and lid, completed label (labeled with resident's name, date of birth, room number, date, and time), 2 pairs of gloves, bedpan or urinal (if resident cannot use portable commode or toilet), "hat" for toilet (if resident can get to the bathroom), 2 plastic bags, disposable washcloths or wipes, toilet paper, paper towel, supplies for perineal care, pen, laboratory slip

1. Identify yourself by name. Identify the resident. Greet the resident by name.

2. Wash your hands.

3. Explain procedure to resident. Speak clearly, slowly, and directly. Maintain face-to-face contact whenever possible.

4. Provide for the resident's privacy with a curtain, screen, or door.

5. Put on gloves.

6. Help the resident to the bathroom or commode, or offer the bedpan or urinal.

7. Have resident void into "hat," urinal, or bedpan. Ask the resident not to put toilet paper

or stool in with the sample. Provide a plastic bag to discard toilet paper.

8. Place toilet paper and washcloths or wipes within resident's reach. Ask the resident to clean his hands with a hand wipe when finished, if he is able.

9. Ask the resident to signal when he is finished. Make sure call light is within reach.

10. Remove and discard gloves. Wash your hands. Leave the room.

11. When called, return and wash your hands. Put on clean gloves.

12. Give perineal care if help is needed.

13. Take bedpan, urinal, or commode pail to the bathroom.

14. Pour urine into the specimen container. Specimen container should be at least half full.

15. Cover the urine container with its lid. Do not touch the inside of container. Wipe off the outside with a paper towel and discard. Apply label, and place in clean plastic bag.

16. If using a bedpan or urinal, discard extra urine in the toilet. Flush toilet. Place in proper area for cleaning or clean it according to policy.

17. Remove and discard gloves. Wash your hands.

18. Make resident comfortable.

19. Return bed to lowest position. Remove privacy measures.

20. Leave call light within resident's reach.

21. Wash your hands.

22. Be courteous and respectful at all times.

23. Report any changes in the resident to the nurse. Document procedure using facility guidelines. Take specimen and lab slip to designated place promptly.

Urine Straining

Urine is strained to detect the presence of **calculi**, or kidney stones, that can develop in the urinary tract. Urine straining is the process of pouring all urine through a fine filter to catch any particles. Kidney stones can be as small as grains of sand or as large as golf balls. If any stones are found, they are saved and then sent to a laboratory for examination. To strain urine, you will collect a routine urine specimen. In the bathroom, pour it through a strainer or a 4x4-inch piece of gauze into a specimen container. Any stones are trapped in the filter. The filter is placed in the specimen container and then into a plastic bag for transport to the lab.

A **clean-catch**, or mid-stream (CCMS), **specimen** is collected by first cleaning the perineal area, and then urinating a small amount into the toilet to clear the urethra. After urinating a small amount into the toilet, the sample is then collected mid-stream in a clean or sterile container. The resident stops urinating, if possible, and the container is removed from the stream. Then the resident finishes voiding into the toilet. The specimen is called mid-stream because the first and last urine that is voided are not included in the sample. This specimen is often collected to detect bacteria in the urine.

Collecting a clean-catch (mid-stream) urine specimen

Equipment: specimen kit with container, completed label (labeled with resident's name, date of birth, room number, date and time), cleaning solution, gauze or towelettes, gloves, bedpan or urinal (if resident cannot use portable commode or toilet), plastic bag, washcloth, toilet paper, disposable washcloths or wipes, paper towel, supplies for perineal care, pen, laboratory slip

1. Identify yourself by name. Identify the resident. Greet the resident by name.

2. Wash your hands.

3. Explain procedure to resident. Speak clearly, slowly, and directly. Maintain face-to-face contact whenever possible.

4. Provide for the resident's privacy with a curtain, screen, or door.

5. Put on gloves.

6. Open the specimen kit. Do not touch the inside of the container or lid.

7. If the resident cannot clean his or her perineal area, you will do it. See bed bath procedure in Chapter 12 for reminder on how to give perineal care.

8. Ask the resident to urinate a small amount into the bedpan, urinal, or toilet, and to stop before urination is complete.

9. Place the container under the urine stream. Do not touch the resident's body with the container. Have the resident start urinating again. Fill the container at least half full. Have resident stop urinating and remove container if possible. Have the resident finish urinating in bedpan, urinal, or toilet.

10. After urination, give perineal care if help is needed. Ask the resident to clean his hands with the hand wipes, if he is able.

11. Cover the urine container with its lid. Do not touch the inside of the container. Wipe off the outside with a paper towel and discard. Apply label, and place in clean plastic bag.

12. If using a bedpan or urinal, discard extra urine in the toilet. Flush toilet. Place in proper area for cleaning or clean it according to policy.

13. Remove and discard gloves. Wash your hands.

14. Make resident comfortable.

15. Return bed to lowest position. Remove privacy measures.

16. Leave call light within resident's reach.

17. Wash your hands.

18. Be courteous and respectful at all times.

19. Report any changes in the resident to the nurse. Document procedure using facility

guidelines. Take specimen and lab slip to designated place promptly.

A **24-hour urine specimen** tests for certain chemicals and hormones. This specimen collects all the urine voided by a resident in a 24-hour period. Usually the collection begins at 7 a.m. and runs until 7 a.m. the next day. When beginning a 24-hour urine specimen collection, the resident must void and discard the first urine. The collection begins with an empty bladder. All urine must be collected and stored properly. If any is thrown away, spilled, or improperly stored, the collection will need to be restarted.

Collecting a 24-hour urine specimen

Equipment: 24-hour specimen container with lid, completed label (labeled with resident's name, date of birth, room number, date, and time), bedpan or urinal for residents confined to bed, "hat" for toilet (if resident can get to the bathroom), gloves, toilet paper, disposable washcloths or wipes, supplies for perineal care, sign to alert other team members that a 24-hour urine specimen is being collected, laboratory slip with date and time of first void

1. Identify yourself by name. Identify the resident. Greet the resident by name.

2. Wash your hands.

3. Explain procedure to resident. Speak clearly, slowly, and directly. Maintain face-to-face contact whenever possible. Emphasize that all urine must be saved. Ask the resident not to put toilet paper or stool in with the sample.

4. Provide for the resident's privacy with a curtain, screen, or door.

5. Place a sign near the resident's bed to let all care team members know that a 24-hour specimen is being collected. Sign may read "Save all urine for 24-hour specimen."

6. When starting the collection, have the resident completely empty the bladder. Discard the urine. Note the exact time of this voiding. The collection will run until the same time the next day (Fig. 16-13).

7. Wash hands and put on gloves each time the resident voids. Measure I&O each time if needed.

INTAKE-OUTPUT RECORD

Resident/Patient Name		Room No.	
	FLUID INTAKE	URINE	EMESIS or DRAINAGE
7:00 A.M. to 3:00 P.M.			
	8-Hour Total		
3:00 P.M. to 11:00 P.M.			
	8-Hour Total		
11:00 P.M. to 7 A.M.			
	8-Hour Total		

Form 3039 © Briggs, Des Moines, IA 50306 PRINTED IN U.S.A. R404

DON'T BREAK THE LAW   (Save   1-800-247-2343
MAKE THE CALL   13¾*   www.BriggsCorp.com
*savings on buying vs. copying

Fig. 16-13. *One type of form to record urine output over 24 hours.* (REPRINTED WITH PERMISSION OF BRIGGS CORPORATION, 800-247-2343, WWW.BRIGGSCORP.COM)

8. Pour urine from bedpan, urinal, or hat into the container. Container may be stored on ice or in a special refrigerator when not used. The ice keeps the specimen cool. It also prevents components and chemicals in the urine from breaking down, which can prevent proper analysis. Follow facility policy.

9. After each voiding, give perineal care if help is needed. Ask the resident to clean his hands with a hand wipe, if he is able.

10. Clean equipment after each voiding.

11. Remove and discard gloves.

12. Wash your hands.

13. After the last void of the 24-hour period, add the urine to the specimen container. Remove the sign.

14. Make resident comfortable.

15. Return bed to lowest position. Remove privacy measures.

16. Leave call light within resident's reach.

17. Wash your hands.

18. Be courteous and respectful at all times.

19. Report any changes in the resident to the nurse. Document procedure using facility guidelines. Take specimen containers and lab slip to designated place promptly.

A catheterized urine specimen is obtained when a person cannot urinate on his or her own, when an infection in the urinary tract may be present, or if the person is retaining urine. A nurse will collect this type of specimen. To collect this urine specimen, the nurse will insert a straight catheter through the urethra into the bladder using sterile technique. The urine is obtained this way to avoid contamination.

A specimen may have to be collected from a resident who has a urostomy. The nurse will remove the urostomy appliance and collect this specimen directly from the stoma. The appliance is then re-sealed over the stoma.

Five "Rights" of Specimen Collection

Knowing and remembering the five "rights" of specimen collection will help prevent mistakes and ensure that specimens are collected properly:

1. The Right Resident
2. The Right Specimen
3. The Right Container
4. The Right Date/Time
5. The Right Storage/Delivery

Properly collecting specimens helps avoid resident discomfort and embarrassment, as well as saving time and money.

10. Explain types of tests that are performed on urine

Facilities use different methods to test urine. Your facility may use a dip strip that can test for such things as pH level, glucose, ketones, blood, and specific gravity. These strips, called reagent strips, have different sections that change color when they react with urine (Fig. 16-14).

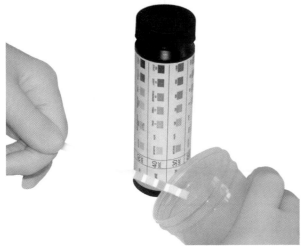

Fig. 16-14. *Reagent strips change color when they react with urine. The color is then compared to a color chart to determine levels of each chemical factor.* (PHOTO COURTESY OF LW SCIENTIFIC, INC., WWW.LWSCIENTIFIC.COM, 800-726-7345)

Testing pH levels: The pH scale ranges from 0 to 14. The lower the number, the more acidic the fluid. The higher the number, the more alkaline the fluid. Normal pH range for urine is 4.6–8.0. A pH imbalance may be due to medication, food, or illness.

Testing for glucose and ketones: In diabetes mellitus, commonly called diabetes, the pancreas does not produce enough insulin or does not produce any insulin (see Chapter 23). Insulin is the substance the body needs to convert glucose, or natural sugar, into energy. Without insulin to process glucose, these sugars collect in the blood. Some sugar appears in the urine.

Diabetics may also have ketones in the urine. **Ketones** are chemical substances produced when the body burns fat for energy or fuel. They are produced when there is not enough insulin to help the body use sugar for energy. Without enough insulin, glucose builds up in the blood. Since the body cannot use glucose for energy, it breaks down fat instead. When this occurs, ketones build up in the blood and spill into the urine.

Testing for blood: In normal urine, blood should not be present. Illness and disease can cause blood to appear in urine. Some blood is hidden, or occult. This blood can be detected by testing the urine.

Specific gravity: A **specific gravity** test is done to test urine density. It can be ordered to make sure the kidneys are functioning properly. Density is how much a substance weighs compared to another substance, which in this case is water. Urine can be very dilute, or close to water. It can also be very dense, or concentrated. This test is done to see how the urine compares to water. Normal values are between 1.002 to 1.028.

When you perform urine testing with testing strips, check the expiration date to make sure that the strips have not expired. Testing strips that have expired may give inaccurate results. This can prolong the resident's discomfort or problem. Inform the nurse and get a new bottle if the strips have expired. Testing strips are usually stored in a light-resistant bottle. Remove strips one at a time when testing a urine specimen. Cap tightly before storing.

The doctor will order the specific type of specimen to be collected and how often urine tests should be done. Follow the care plan and the nurse's instructions.

Testing urine with reagent strips

Equipment: urine specimen as ordered, reagent strip, gloves, paper towel

1. Wash your hands.

2. Put on gloves.

3. Place paper towel on surface before setting urine specimen down.

4. Take a strip from the bottle and recap bottle. Close it tightly.

5. Dip the strip into the specimen.

6. Follow manufacturer's instructions for when to remove strip. Remove strip at correct time.

7. Follow manufacturer's instructions for how long to wait after removing strip. After proper time has passed, compare strip with color chart on bottle. Do not touch bottle with strip.

8. Read results.

9. Discard used items. Discard specimen in the toilet. Flush toilet.

10. Remove and discard gloves.

11. Wash your hands.

12. Record and report results. Document procedure using facility guidelines.

11. Explain guidelines for assisting with bladder retraining

Illness, injury, or inactivity can cause a loss of normal bladder function. Residents may need help in re-establishing a regular routine and normal bladder function. Incontinence may be a problem when retraining the bladder. Be professional when episodes of incontinence occur. As you have learned, problems with incontinence can be embarrassing or difficult to discuss. Be sensitive to this situation. Be empathetic and maintain a positive attitude.

Most care team members will be involved with charting and implementing bladder retraining. Accurate charting is very important. Follow the care plan for each resident.

Guidelines: Bladder Retraining

G   Follow the plan consistently. Explain the training schedule to the resident. Direct any questions the resident has to the nurse.

G   Follow Standard Precautions. Wear gloves when handling body wastes. For residents in isolation, additional PPE may be needed. Follow the care plan.

G   Observe your residents' elimination habits. This helps predict when a trip to the bathroom or a bedpan or urinal will be necessary.

G   Keep a record of elimination, including episodes of incontinence. Keeping accurate records will help establish a routine.

G   Offer a bedpan or urinal or a trip to the bathroom before beginning long procedures and after the procedures have been completed (Fig. 16-15).

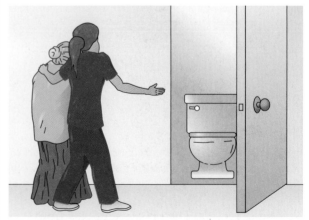

Fig. 16-15. Offer regular trips to the bathroom, especially before and after performing care.

G Answer call lights promptly. Residents should never have to wait to go to the bathroom.

G Provide privacy with elimination and do not rush the resident.

G Help the resident with good perineal care as needed. This promotes proper hygiene and helps prevent skin breakdown. Watch for skin changes and report them.

G Encourage plenty of fluids throughout the day if allowed, even if incontinence is a problem. About 30 minutes after fluids are consumed, offer a bedpan, urinal, or trip to the bathroom.

G Have the resident lean forward slightly to put pressure on the bladder. If he or she is having trouble urinating, try running water in the sink.

G Dispose of wastes properly.

G Keep accurate intake and output (I&O) records. Output includes episodes of incontinence.

G Offer praise and positive words for attempts and successes in controlling the bladder.

G Never show frustration or anger toward residents who are incontinent. The problem is out of their control. Be positive and patient with the retraining efforts.

Residents' Rights

Bladder Retraining

Residents have the right to assistance with their elimination needs as often as necessary. It is important that they not feel intimidated by the frequency of their requests for help. Take time to let residents know that you are willing to help as often as needed.

Chapter Review

1. What is the name of the tube that carries the urine out of the body (LO 2)?

2. Is a woman's urethra longer or shorter than a man's (LO 2)?

3. List four functions of the urinary system (LO 2).

4. List four normal age-related changes of the urinary system (LO 3).

5. List three normal qualities of urine (LO 4).

6. List six things to observe and report about urine (LO 4).

7. For each of the six factors (not including disorders) that affect urination listed in Learning Objective 5, describe one way nursing assistants can promote normal urination (LO 5).

8. What is the best position for women to urinate? What is the best position for men (LO 5)?

9. Why are women more susceptible to UTIs than men (LO 6)?

10. List three signs and symptoms of UTIs (LO 6).

11. How should residents wipe after elimination in order to prevent infection (LO 6)?

12. What is dialysis (LO 6)?

13. List eight signs and symptoms of urine retention (LO 6).

14. List five physical reasons for incontinence (LO 7).

15. Define five different types of incontinence (LO 7).

16. List eight guidelines for dealing with incontinence (LO 7).

17. What is the difference between a straight catheter and an indwelling catheter (LO 8)?

18. List ten care guidelines for catheters (LO 8).

19. Why should a drainage bag for a catheter always hang lower than the level of the hips or bladder (LO 8)?

20. What items should not be included in a urine specimen (LO 9)?

21. Explain how a clean-catch urine specimen is obtained (LO 9).

22. What is a 24-hour urine specimen (LO 9)?

23. When is a catheterized urine specimen needed (LO 9)?

24. List four things reagent strips can test for in urine (LO 10).

25. About how long after fluids are taken should residents be offered a trip to the bathroom (LO 11)?

26. Why might problems with urinary incontinence be difficult to discuss (LO 11)?

17
The Reproductive System

An Amazing Recovery!

Ephraim McDowell, 1771-1830, a doctor of the Kentucky frontier, was visited in 1809 by a patient with a large ovarian cyst. He asked her to travel 60 miles to his office for an operation from which she would probably not survive. She decided to travel the distance on horseback. The physician opened her abdomen without anesthesia while she read from the Bible. He cut out an ovary weighing nearly 20 pounds. After a 25-day recovery, she left the area and returned home. The woman lived another 31 years. McDowell gained international fame for his removal of cysts.

"In the dark womb where I began
My mother's life made me . . .
Through all the months of human birth
Her beauty fed my common earth."

John Masefield, 1878-1967

"Little creature, formed of joy and mirth,
Go, love without the help of any thing on earth."

William Blake, 1757-1827

1. Define important words in this chapter

benign prostatic hypertrophy: a disorder that can occur in men as they age, in which the prostate becomes enlarged and causes problems with urination and/or emptying the bladder.

cervical cancer: a form of female reproductive cancer that begins in the cervix; can occur at any age and has few symptoms.

chlamydia: a sexually-transmitted infection caused by bacteria.

endometrial cancer: a form of female reproductive cancer that begins in the uterus; symptoms include vaginal bleeding and pelvic pain.

genital herpes: a sexually-transmitted, incurable infection caused by herpes simplex viruses type 1 (HSV-1) or type 2 (HSV-2).

genital HPV infection: a sexually-transmitted infection caused by human papillomavirus.

glands: structures in the body that produce substances.

gonads: the male and female sexual reproductive glands.

gonorrhea: a sexually-transmitted infection caused by bacteria.

hormones: chemical substances produced by the body that control numerous body functions.

impotence: the inability to have or maintain a penile erection.

menopause: the end of menstruation.

menstruation: the shedding of the lining of the uterus that occurs approximately every 28 days; also known as the menstrual cycle or period.

ovarian cancer: a form of female reproductive cancer that begins in the ovaries; can occur at any age and has few symptoms.

ovum: female sex cell or egg.

prostate cancer: a form of male reproductive cancer that begins in the prostate gland; usually occurs in older men, and symptoms include urinating during the night, a weak flow of urine, painful urination, blood in urine, and problems with maintaining an erection.

sexually-transmitted infections (STIs): infections caused by sexual contact with infected people; signs and symptoms are not always apparent.

sperm: male sex cells.

syphilis: a sexually-transmitted infection caused by bacteria.

testicular cancer: a form of male reproductive cancer that begins in the testes.

trichomoniasis: a sexually-transmitted infection caused by protozoa (single-celled animals).

vaginal irrigation: a rinsing of the vagina in order to clean the vaginal tract or to introduce medication into the vagina; also called a douche.

vaginitis: an inflammation of the vagina; symptoms include vaginal discharge, itching and pain.

2. Explain the structure and function of the reproductive system

The reproductive system consists of the reproductive organs, which are different in men and women. This system allows human beings to reproduce, or create new human life. Reproduction begins when male and female sex cells, **sperm** and **ovum**, join. These sex cells are formed in the male and female sexual reproductive glands, called the **gonads**. **Glands** are structures in the body that produce substances. **Hormones** are chemical substances produced by the body that control numerous body functions, including the body's ability to reproduce. You will learn more about glands and hormones in Chapter 23.

The Male Reproductive System

The male reproductive system consists of the penis, testes, scrotum, epididymis, vas deferens,

erectile tissue, seminal vesicle, ejaculatory duct, and prostate gland (Fig. 17-1). The testes are found within the sac of skin known as the scrotum. The scrotum supports the testes and regulates the temperature of the testes. The testes produce testosterone, the male hormone needed for the reproductive organs to function properly, and sperm.

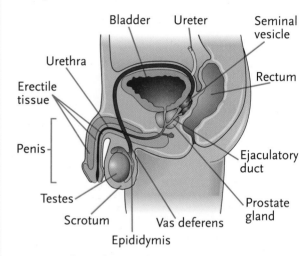

Fig. 17-1. *The male reproductive system.*

Sperm travel from the testes to the epididymis, a coiled tube that can be as long as 20 feet. The epididymis receives and stores sperm. After maturing in the epididymis, sperm move into the vas deferens, the tube that sperm travel through in order to reach the ejaculatory duct. During their trip, the sperm mix with fluid produced in three glands, the seminal vesicles, the prostate gland, and Cowper's glands.

From the ejaculatory duct, sperm empty into the urethra, where they are released from the body through the penis. The penis is the sex organ located outside the body, in front of the scrotum. The penis is composed of erectile tissue that becomes filled with blood during sexual excitement. As the penis fills with blood, it becomes enlarged and erect and is able to release semen. Semen is released in small amounts during ejaculation, from about two to five mL at a time. Every milliliter of semen contains 50 to 150 million sperm.

The Female Reproductive System

The female reproductive system is made up of the ovaries, fallopian tubes, uterus, vagina, the external genitals—the vulva—and the mammary glands or breasts (Fig. 17-2). The ovaries produce the female sex cells or eggs (ova) and they produce the female hormones, estrogen and progesterone. Each month from puberty to menopause, ova are released from ovaries (usually alternating ovaries) during the process called ovulation. This monthly cycle is maintained by estrogen and progesterone. The ovum or egg cell then travels into the respective fallopian tube, one of two tubes that open into the uterus.

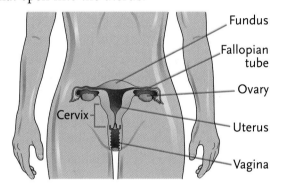

Fig. 17-2. The female reproductive system.

Fundus
Fallopian tube
Ovary
Uterus
Vagina
Cervix

As the ovum reaches the fallopian tube, it may be fertilized by a sperm that will swim its way up into the tube. If it is not fertilized, the ovum will die within about 24 to 48 hours. Sperm usually die within two days. If an ovum is fertilized, it moves into the uterus, or womb. The uterus is a hollow, pear-shaped, muscular organ located within the pelvis. It lies behind the bladder and in front of the rectum.

A fertilized ovum will implant into the lining of the uterus, or the endometrium. This is where the fetus develops. If an ovum is not fertilized, the secretion of female hormones decreases. The endometrium then breaks up and is expelled in a process called **menstruation**.

The vagina is the muscular canal that opens to the outside of the body. It serves as the outlet for the blood during a woman's menstrual cycle. It acts as the receiver of sperm during sexual intercourse and is the birth canal.

The breasts or mammary glands are the glands that nourish a baby. They are responsible for the production of milk within the alveolar glands inside the breast. These glands send the milk into milk ducts that come together at the nipple in the area called the areola. This process is called lactation.

The functions of the reproductive system are:

Male

- To manufacture sperm and the male hormone testosterone

Female

- To manufacture ova (eggs) and female hormones, estrogen and progesterone

- To provide an environment for the development of a fetus

- To produce milk (lactation) for the nourishment of a baby after birth

Destination: Homeostasis

Homeostasis can be affected by changes in the reproductive system. For example, a male's testosterone level can increase due to stressors. This increase in the hormone level causes the brain to send a message to the male reproductive glands to decrease the production of testosterone. The testosterone level then returns to normal, and the body returns to homeostasis.

3. Discuss changes in the reproductive system due to aging

Normal age-related changes for the reproductive system include the following:

Male

- The prostate gland enlarges.

- The number and capability of sperm decreases.

- Sexual response slows; it may take longer to achieve an erection and to reach orgasm.

Female

- **Menopause** occurs when menstruation ends, usually between the ages of 45 and 55, and ends the female's ability to reproduce.

- Decrease in production of estrogen and progesterone leads to a loss of calcium, causing brittle bones and, potentially, osteoporosis. Decrease in estrogen also makes females more prone to urinary tract infections.

- Vaginal walls become drier and thinner; this may cause discomfort during sexual intercourse.

4. Discuss common disorders of the reproductive system

Sexually-Transmitted Infections (STIs)

Sexually-transmitted infections (STIs), formerly referred to as "sexually-transmitted diseases (STDs)," are caused by sexual contact with infected persons. STIs do not always have visible signs and symptoms.

STIs are transmitted through sexual contact, such as sexual intercourse (vaginal and anal), contact of the mouth with the genitals or anus, and contact of the hands with the genital area. Some STIs can also be transmitted via needles used in IV drug use, as well as through childbirth or breastfeeding.

The transmission of some STIs can be reduced or stopped by using latex condoms. The human immunodeficiency virus (HIV) can be transmitted sexually, as well. HIV and AIDS are discussed in depth in Chapter 24.

Chlamydia infection is caused by bacteria. Symptoms of chlamydia include burning with urination, yellow or white discharge from the penis or vagina, swelling of the testes, painful intercourse, and abdominal and low back pain. In many cases, no symptoms are apparent. This disorder may cause an eye infection (conjunctivitis, or "pink eye") or pneumonia in babies born

to infected mothers. It may also cause infertility and pelvic inflammatory disease (PID) if not promptly and properly treated. Treatment includes the use of antibiotics.

Genital herpes is caused by herpes simplex viruses type 1 (HSV-1) or type 2 (HSV-2). Usually genital herpes is caused by HSV-2. It cannot be treated with antibiotics, nor can it be cured. Once infected with genital herpes, a person may have repeated outbreaks of the disease for the rest of his or her life. Symptoms include itching and painful, red blisters or open sores. Herpes may also cause a burning sensation while urinating or during intercourse, low-grade fever, headache, and muscle aches. Herpes sores are infectious, and may appear quickly after sexual contact with an infected partner. However, a person can also spread genital herpes when sores are not present. Treatment consists of anti-viral medications. The medication does not cure the disease, but it can help lessen the frequency, duration, and intensity of the episodes.

Genital HPV infection is a sexually-transmitted infection caused by human papillomavirus (HPV). These viruses are spread primarily through genital contact and can infect the genital area of both men and women. This includes the penis, vulva, lining of the vagina, cervix, rectum, or anus. Many people have no signs or symptoms of HPV. Some HPV infections cause women to have an abnormal pap test. Genital warts may appear. They may also lead to the development of cervical cancer. Treatment to remove warts is done in a doctor's office or through the use of medications. Treatment for HPV also consists of methods used by doctors to treat changes in the cervix that occur with infection. There is no cure for HPV. However, an HPV vaccine, licensed by the Food and Drug Administration (FDA), is available.

Gonorrhea is a sexually-transmitted infection caused by bacteria. It is easier to detect in men because many women with gonorrhea show no early symptoms. Symptoms in men include painful or burning urination, a white, yellow, or green cloudy pus-like discharge from the penis, and painful or swollen testes. Symptoms in women include cloudy vaginal discharge, along with vaginal bleeding between periods. Rectal symptoms, such as itching, soreness, bleeding, or painful elimination of stool, can occur in both sexes. This disorder can cause blindness, joint infection, or a serious blood infection in babies born to infected mothers. It can also cause sterility and pelvic inflammatory disease (PID) if not treated. Treatment consists of antibiotics.

Syphilis is caused by bacteria. Syphilis is generally easier to detect in men than in women. The first stage is marked by small, painless sores called chancres that form on the penis soon after infection. In women, these sores may form inside the vagina. If left untreated, the infection progresses to the second stage, in which rashes appear on one or more areas of the body. These rashes do not usually cause itching. A headache and a fever may occur, along with sore throat, weight loss, and muscle aches. The third stage usually takes years to develop. During this stage, the symptoms from the second stage disappear. The person will still have the disease, and if not treated with penicillin or other antibiotics, the infection spreads to the heart, brain, and other vital organs. Untreated syphilis will eventually be fatal. The sooner it is treated, the better the chance is of preventing long-term damage and avoiding infection of others.

Trichomoniasis is a sexually-transmitted infection caused by protozoa (single-celled animals). Men may have no symptoms. However, mild discharge, irritation or a burning sensation after urination or ejaculation sometimes occurs. Symptoms of infection in women include a green-yellow vaginal discharge with a strong odor, irritation, or itching. The infection may cause discomfort during intercourse or urination. Treatment consists of the administration of the prescription drug metronidazole.

Other Sexually-Transmitted Diseases

Other diseases that may be sexually transmitted include scabies and pubic lice. For information on these diseases and others, visit the CDC's website, cdc.gov.

Hepatitis B is a liver disease transmitted by sexual contact with an infected person. It is also transmitted by sharing infected needles, contact with infected blood, or to a baby from an infected mother during childbirth. For more information on hepatitis, see Chapter 6.

Trivia

The Scourge of Syphilis

The first epidemic of syphilis affected sailors who returned from Columbus' first voyage to The Americas. At that time it was called "Naples Disease" and the "French Disease."

Paul Ehrlich, 1854-1915, a doctor and medical scientist, developed a substance called salvarsan that was effective in treating syphilis. It was used as a primary drug to treat syphilis until antibiotics became the treatment of choice during the 1940s. Ehrlich won the Nobel Prize for Medicine in 1908.

Vaginitis

Vaginitis is an inflammation of the vagina; symptoms include vaginal discharge, itching, and pain. There are many different types of vaginitis. Bacterial vaginosis occurs when there is an overgrowth of normal bacteria inside the vagina. Yeast infections are caused by an overproduction of a fungus called *Candida albicans*. Vaginal atrophy is caused by lower estrogen levels that can occur in women after menopause. Non-infectious vaginitis is caused by irritation or an allergic reaction to a product, such as bubble bath, soaps, and fabric softeners.

Creams, suppositories, antibiotics, and estrogen supplements are treatments for vaginitis. For non-infectious vaginitis, treatment consists of eliminating the product(s) suspected of causing the vaginitis.

Female Reproductive Cancers

Ovarian cancer begins in the ovaries. It can occur in women at any age. Symptoms are not always apparent, which is why it may not be discovered until it is in a late stage. Some symptoms may occur, including abdominal pressure, indigestion, low back pain, and constipation. There is no definitive screening test for ovarian cancer. Pelvic examinations and ultrasound testing may be performed to help diagnose this type of cancer. Treatment includes surgery, radiation, and chemotherapy.

Endometrial cancer begins in the uterus. Symptoms of this type of cancer include vaginal bleeding and pelvic pain. Pelvic examinations and ultrasounds are used to diagnose this type of cancer. If detected early, endometrial cancer is highly curable by removing the uterus.

Cervical cancer begins in the cervix. It can occur at any age. Symptoms are not always apparent, but include vaginal bleeding, change in menstrual cycles, painful intercourse, and blood-tinged vaginal discharge. Pap tests, scopes, and biopsies are tests that check for cervical cancer. A vaccine for cervical cancer is available for younger women. If detected early, cervical cancer is curable.

Benign Prostatic Hypertrophy (BPH)

Benign prostatic hypertrophy is a disorder that is quite common in men over the age of 60. Studies show that one-third to one-half of all men over this age show signs of this disorder. When a man has BPH, the prostate becomes enlarged, which causes pressure on the urethra. When the urethra becomes compressed, urination becomes difficult. Other symptoms of BPH are a feeling of incomplete urination, frequent urination, and a weak stream of urine. Dribbling of urine right after urinating, the need to urinate often during the night, and incontinence are symptoms, too. The cause of BPH is unknown. Medications and/or surgery are generally used to treat BPH.

Prostate enlargement is not a cancerous condition. However, as men age, they are at increased risk for prostate cancer.

Male Reproductive Cancers

Prostate cancer is a type of cancer that forms in the prostate gland, normally in older men. Certain men have a higher risk of prostate cancer. Risk factors include having a family history of prostate cancer and being 60 years of age or older. Regular prostate checks are often a part of annual exams, and a screening test is available. Symptoms of prostate cancer are urinating during the night, a weak flow of urine, painful urination, blood in urine, and problems with maintaining an erection. This type of cancer tends to be slow-growing and treatable, if caught early. Treatment includes removal of the prostate, hormone therapy, and chemotherapy.

Testicular cancer occurs in the testes, the male reproductive glands. It is the most common form of cancer in younger men, from ages 15 to 39, but can also occur in older men. Men older than 40 can have a higher risk of death from the disease. Regular self-examinations and doctor examinations can diagnose this form of cancer. Symptoms include a noticeable lump in the testes, pain in the testicles, breast tenderness, and an ache in the groin. Testicular cancer is highly curable. Treatment includes surgical removal of the testes, chemotherapy, and radiation therapy.

5. Describe sexual needs of the elderly

Sexual needs continue throughout a person's life. All people, regardless of age, have sexual needs and desires (Fig. 17-3). The ability to engage in sexual activities, such as intercourse and masturbation, continues unless a disease or injury occurs. You can help by providing privacy whenever necessary for sexual activity and respecting your residents' sexual needs.

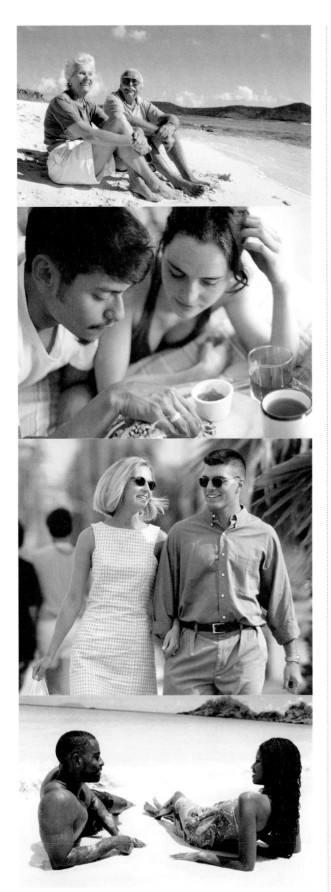

Fig. 17-3. Sexual needs, behavior, and desires are present in all age groups.

Some things that can affect sexual activity in the elderly include the following:

- Illness affecting the ability of men and women to perform sexually

- Erectile dysfunction (ED) (impotence) in males

- Vaginal atrophy (weakening or wasting of muscles), pain, and dryness in females

- Fear of inadequate sexual performance

- Depression

- A lack of privacy

- Medications

In the past, male impotence was often viewed as a normal response to aging. **Impotence** is the inability to have or maintain an erection. However, it is not a normal change of aging. Medications can help this problem. Report any resident complaints about impotence to the nurse.

For women, special creams and medications can help with vaginal dryness. Report complaints about dryness or pain to the nurse.

You learned about sexually-transmitted infections in Learning Objective 4 of this chapter. Nurses and doctors can educate sexually-active older adults about how to reduce the risk of contracting these infections. Nursing assistants can help by reporting any signs or symptoms of STIs to the nurse immediately.

Remember that older adults are sexual beings like all humans, and they have the right to choose how they express their sexuality. In all age groups, there is a wide variety of sexual behavior. This is also true of residents in long-term care facilities. An attitude that any expression of sexuality by the elderly is cute, funny, or disgusting deprives residents of their right to dignity and respect. All residents have a right to be treated with dignity and to have their privacy respected.

If you encounter any sexual situation, such as a resident masturbating or two consenting adult residents engaged in sexual activity, provide privacy and leave the area. Do not judge any sexual behavior you see.

6. Describe vaginal irrigation

Vaginal irrigation, or a vaginal douche, is a rinsing of the vagina in order to clean the vaginal tract prior to surgical procedures or examinations or due to vaginal drainage. It is also performed to introduce medication into the vagina to treat disorders or to reduce discomfort, such as itching or redness. These irrigations are only performed with a doctor's order.

Disposable irrigation kits or bags with tubing may be used for this procedure. The solution will run into the vagina through a special irrigation kit. The solution will run back out of the vagina into a bedpan or toilet, or in the shower due to gravity. Irrigations may be ordered with water and can include any of the following additives:

- Vinegar
- Baking soda
- Medication

Commercial irrigation kits are also available. The additives are usually already mixed in with the solution. The tip is approximately two to three inches long and may be pre-lubricated. If using a commercial vaginal irrigation, attach the tip securely onto the bottle. If the fluid needs to be mixed more thoroughly, turn the bottle back and forth gently. Do not shake the bottle.

Guidelines: Vaginal Irrigation

G Always provide privacy during this procedure. Keep the resident covered with a blanket.

G Place the woman in the dorsal recumbent position (flat on her back with knees flexed and slightly separated; feet are flat on bed) (Fig. 17-4).

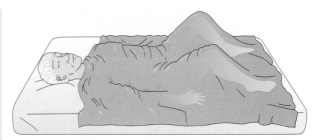

Fig. 17-4. *The dorsal recumbent position.*

G First have fluid flow over the external vulva. Then insert the tip into the vagina.

G Do not force the tip into the vagina. If you are unable to insert the tip, stop, and use the call light to call the nurse.

G When giving a vaginal irrigation, observe and report any of the following:

- Pain or discomfort
- Increase or decrease in vaginal discharge
- Bleeding
- Itching or burning
- Abdominal swelling

Many facilities do not allow nursing assistants to perform this procedure. Follow your facility's policy regarding vaginal irrigations. If assisting with this procedure, make sure the resident urinates before beginning the procedure.

Giving a vaginal irrigation

Equipment: vaginal irrigation kit, including bag, tubing and tip, lubricating jelly, gloves, bed protector, bath blanket, towel, bedpan and bedpan cover

1. Identify yourself by name. Identify the resident. Greet the resident by name.

2. Wash your hands.

3. Explain procedure to resident. Speak clearly, slowly, and directly. Maintain face-to-face contact whenever possible.

4. Provide for the resident's privacy with a curtain, screen, or door.

5. Adjust bed to safe working level, usually waist high. Lock bed wheels.

6. Lower head of bed. Position resident lying flat on her back.

7. Put on gloves.

8. Cover the resident with a bath blanket. Ask her to hold it while you pull down the top covers underneath. Do not expose more of her than is necessary.

9. Place a bed protector under the resident's buttocks and hips.

10. Hang prepared vaginal irrigation bag on IV pole and lower pole so that bag is 12 inches above resident's perineal area.

11. Remove resident's underpants, exposing only as much of the resident's body as necessary.

12. Place the bedpan under the resident and make sure she is in the dorsal recumbent position.

13. Open the clamp and allow a little water to run from the tubing into the bedpan to clear air from the tubing.

14. Lubricate tip of tubing, if not already lubricated.

15. Insert nozzle slowly and gently into vagina about two to three inches (Fig. 17-5).

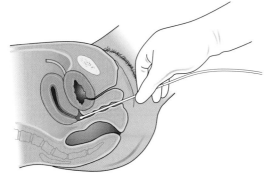

Fig. 17-5. *Insert nozzle slowly and gently into vagina about two to three inches.*

16. Begin slow flow of water or fluid by releasing clamp. Before vaginal irrigation bag is empty, clamp tubing.

17. Remove tubing slowly and gently and place tubing tip inside top of bag.

18. Raise the head of the bed so that the resident is in a semi-sitting position on the bedpan so that the solution can drain.

19. After solution has drained into bedpan, remove bedpan and cover it. Remove the bed protector and discard.

20. Bring bedpan to bathroom and check contents for anything unusual. Empty bedpan unless nurse needs to check the contents.

21. Flush toilet. Place bedpan in area for cleaning or clean and store it according to policy.

22. Place soiled linens and clothing in proper containers.

23. Remove and discard gloves. Wash your hands.

24. Put clothing back on. Remove bath blanket and replace top covers. Make resident comfortable.

25. Return bed to lowest position. Remove privacy measures.

26. Leave call light within resident's reach.

27. Wash your hands.

28. Be courteous and respectful at all times.

29. Report any changes in the resident to the nurse. Document procedure using facility guidelines.

Residents' Rights

Gynecological Exams

A gynecological examination may be done in the resident's room or in a special examination room. It can also be performed in an emergency room or an urgent care center. When these exams are done, it is important to be sensitive to the resident's feelings and concerns. Gynecological examinations may be embarrassing, uncomfortable, and frightening. Listen to residents who want to talk, and answer any questions that are within your scope of practice. Refer any questions that you cannot answer to the nurse or doctor. Make sure to provide privacy throughout the exam.

Chapter Review

1. List the functions of the male and female reproductive systems (LO 2).

2. What is the name of the male hormone needed for the reproductive organs to function properly (LO 2)?

3. What two female hormones help maintain the monthly cycle of menstruation (LO 2)?

4. What are the names of the male sex cells and the female sex cells (LO 2)?

5. List all normal age-related changes of the reproductive system for males and females (LO 3).

6. How are sexually-transmitted infections (STIs) transmitted from one person to another (LO 4)?

7. Which two STIs listed are caused by a virus and cannot be cured (LO 4)?

8. Why does urination become more difficult for men who have BPH (LO 4)?

9. When encountering a sexual situation between consenting residents, what should a nursing assistant do (LO 5)?

10. List seven factors that can affect sexual activity in the elderly (LO 5).

11. Why is it important not to judge residents' sexual behavior (LO 5)?

12. List three reasons that vaginal irrigations are given (LO 6).

13. List five signs and symptoms about vaginal irrigation that must be reported to the nurse (LO 6).

18 The Integumentary System

The Field of Dermatology in its Infancy

Ferdinand Hebra (1816-1880) was one of the first doctors to specialize in the diseases of the skin. He founded a division of dermatology. One of the discoveries he made concerned scabies, a disorder that causes intense itching. Hebra noted that when the itch-mite parasite was destroyed, scabies was cured. He also made the important discovery that scabies was contagious and that it could be transmitted from one person to another.

"'Tis not a lip or eye we beauty call/But the joint force and full result of all."

Alexander Pope, 1688-1744

"Men should be judged, not by their tint of skin . . . But by the quality of thought they think."

Adela Florence Cory Nicolson, 1865-1904

1. Define important words in this chapter

bony prominences: areas of the body where the bone lies close to the skin.

bruise: a purple, black, or blue discoloration on the skin caused by the leakage of blood from broken blood vessels into the surrounding tissues; also called a contusion.

closed wound: a type of wound in which the skin's surface is not broken.

dermis: the inner layer of the two main layers of tissue that make up the skin.

eczema: a temporary or chronic skin disorder that results in redness, itching, burning, swelling, cracking, weeping, and lesions; also called dermatitis.

epidermis: the outer layer of the two main layers of tissue that make up the skin.

gangrene: death of tissue caused by infection or lack of blood flow.

integument: natural protective covering.

lesion: an area of abnormal tissue or an injury or wound.

melanin: the pigment that gives skin its color.

melanocyte: cell in the skin that produces and contains the pigment called melanin.

necrosis: the death of living cells or tissues caused by disease or injury.

open wound: a type of wound in which the skin's surface is not intact.

pressure points: areas of the body that bear much of its weight.

pressure ulcer: a serious wound resulting from skin breakdown; also known as pressure sore, decubitus ulcer, or bed sore.

psoriasis: a chronic skin condition caused by skin cells growing too quickly which results in red, white, or silver patches, itching and discomfort.

scabies: a contagious skin infection caused by mites burrowing into the skin that results in pimple-like irritations, rashes, intense itching, and sores.

shingles: a viral infection caused by the same virus that causes chickenpox; results in pain, itching, rashes, and possibly fever and chills.

sitz bath: a warm soak of the perineal area to clean perineal wounds and reduce inflammation and pain.

skin cancer: the growth of abnormal skin cells; symptoms include changes in mole, wart, or spot on the skin, sores that do not heal, itching, pain, and skin that is oozing or bleeding.

tinea: a fungal infection that causes red, scaly patches to appear in a ring shape, generally on the upper body, or the hands and feet.

wart: contagious hard bump caused by a virus.

2. Explain the structure and function of the integumentary system

The integumentary system consists of the following parts: the skin, hair, nails, oil glands, sweat glands, subcutaneous tissue, and nerve endings (Fig. 18-1). The skin is a natural protective covering, or **integument**. The skin is an organ, and it is the largest organ in the human body. It is considered an organ because it has different types of tissues that together function to perform activities of the body. The skin covers and protects the body, provides sensation through nerves, regulates body temperature, and prevents the loss of too much water.

The two basic layers of the skin are the epidermis and the dermis. The **epidermis** is the outer layer of the skin, which is composed of dead cells. These cells are continuously shed as new cells move up from the dermis. The epidermis does not contain blood vessels. Keratin is a substance found in the dead skin cells of the epidermis. Keratin has waterproof qualities that protect the inside of the body when it gets wet. Beneath the very top of the epidermis lie other types of cells. One is the **melanocyte**, which contains **melanin**, the substance that gives skin its color. The more melanin your skin produces, the darker your skin color.

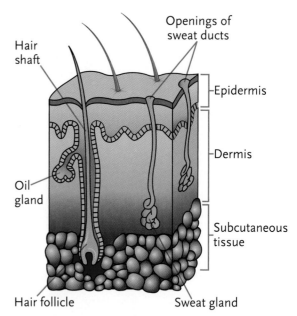

Fig. 18-1. *Cross-section showing the integumentary system.*

The skin is a sense organ. Receptors are found in the skin that give us the ability to feel and touch. One type of receptor is found near the surface of the skin and the other is found within the dermis.

The **dermis** is the inner layer of the skin. Within the dermis lie the structures responsible for unique fingerprints. These ridges are called the dermal-papillae and form before birth. Fingerprints and footprints, which grow as a child becomes an adult, will always have the same pattern and can identify people throughout their lives. Hair and nail follicles, sweat and oil glands, blood vessels, and receptors for touch, temperature, pressure, and pain are also housed in the dermis.

Hair grows from roots located in the dermis. Every hair consists primarily of dead cells, made up of protein called keratin and the pigment that gives hair its color. Hair protects the body. The hair inside the nose protects against inhaling irritants in the air. Hair on the head, underarms, and genitals protect sensitive areas from injuries. Eyebrows and eyelashes help keep objects from getting into the eyes.

Collagen fibers, which make skin tough, are found within the dermis. Elastic fibers are also found in the dermis. They give the skin its elasticity, or ability to stretch.

The subcutaneous layer is positioned immediately underneath the dermis. This is the area of the body where fat, or adipose tissue, lies. This adipose tissue also serves as a cushion over bone and provides some protection as it insulates the body from cold weather. Humans' fat layer is thinner than the fat layer in other mammals.

The functions of the integumentary system are to:

- Protect internal organs from injury
- Protect the body against bacteria
- Prevent the loss of too much water
- Regulate body temperature
- Respond to heat, cold, pain, pressure, and touch
- Excrete waste products in sweat
- Help with production of vitamin D

Destination: Homeostasis

When cells die or become damaged, homeostasis is disturbed. When the surface of the skin is opened, such as by a cut, the inflammatory response begins. Blood flow increases to the area. Signs of inflammation, such as redness, swelling, heat and pain, occur. Platelets, along with a substance called fibrin, form a clot. White blood cells, called phagocytes, travel to the area and start cleaning the wound of bacteria. A scab, which is a hard, protective structure, forms over the area. Normal tissue eventually develops and, over time, the scab is pushed off of the area, leaving new skin. When normal tissue repair is complete, the injured area returns to homeostasis.

Tip

Observing residents' skin is a daily duty!

Every time you help residents bathe and/or dress, carefully and closely observe their skin. This helps identify any changes in the skin, which need to be reported immediately. Pressure ulcers, skin cancer, and contagious skin diseases can pose serious health risks if not caught early and treated. You will be the person who sees residents most often on a daily basis. Your careful observations can help prevent serious illnesses.

3. Discuss changes in the integumentary system due to aging

Normal age-related changes for the integumentary system include the following:

- Amount of fat and collagen decreases, causing skin to sag.
- Elastic fibers lose elasticity, causing wrinkles.
- Hair and nail growth slows.
- Skin becomes drier due to decreased production of perspiration and oil.
- Skin becomes thinner and more fragile, causing more frequent skin injuries, tearing, and infections.
- Protective fatty tissue layer thins, so person feels colder.
- Hair thins and turns gray, due to a decrease in the melanocyte activity (Fig. 18-2).
- Brown spots on the skin may appear due to an increase in the production of certain melanocytes in areas exposed to the sun.

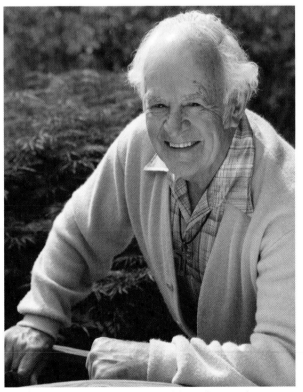

Fig. 18-2. *Hair growth slows, and hair thins and turns gray as a person ages.*

4. Discuss common disorders of the integumentary system

Pressure ulcers, a major disorder of the integumentary system, are discussed in Learning Objective 5 of this chapter.

Burns

You first learned about how to prevent burns and scalds in Chapter 8. Burns can be caused by fire, hot liquids, warm water applications, such as warm moist compresses, electrical equipment, such as hair dryers and heaters, hot objects, or certain chemicals.

When a burn occurs, there may be a varying degree of skin damage (Fig. 18-3). The different degrees or classifications of burns are:

Degree	Layer of Skin	Damage Involved
First-degree (superficial)	Epidermis (outer layer)	Redness and pain
Second-degree (partial-thickness)	Dermis (deeper layer)	Some skin damage; redness, pain, swelling, and blistering
Third-degree (full-thickness)	Epidermis, dermis, and underlying tissue	Serious scarring; muscle and bone may be affected; white or charred skin; pain; swelling; and peeling skin

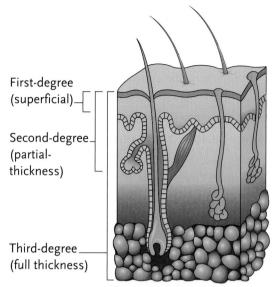

Fig. 18-3. *Different degrees of burns.*

First-degree (superficial)

Second-degree (partial-thickness)

Third-degree (full thickness)

Burns and scalds are very painful and can require surgery. They can cause a resident's condition to deteriorate quickly. When caring for a resident who has burns, be careful not to cause additional pain. Before giving care, it may be necessary to arrange with the nurse to have the resident's pain medication given. That way it takes effect before you begin the care. Be gentle when moving and positioning residents in order to reduce pain and the chance of damaging dressings. Use special protective devices, such as pads or draw sheets, as ordered. Encourage fluids and follow diet instructions closely. Measure intake and output (I&O) carefully (Chapter 14).

Report to the nurse if you notice pus or other fluids around burn areas or if the resident complains of pain. Report any decrease in appetite or intake and output.

You may be asked to assist the nurse with dressing care, which you will learn more about later in the chapter.

Scabies

Scabies is a skin infection that causes pimple-like irritations to form on the skin. These irritations are caused by tiny mites that burrow into the skin to lay eggs. A rash, intense itching, and sores can occur, and the sores may become infected. The symptoms may take a month or more to appear.

Scabies is contagious and is usually transmitted by direct person-to-person contact. Using an infected person's towel, washcloth, clothing, or bedding can also spread scabies. The elderly and others with weakened immune systems are at a higher risk of acquiring scabies.

Treatment consists of the use of special lotions. Follow instructions for handling and washing clothing and linens. Use proper PPE when touching areas that have been treated.

Even after treatment, the itching may continue for a while. Anyone who may have been infected with scabies should be treated at the same time, such as residents, their families and friends, and their roommates.

Shingles

Shingles is a viral infection that causes a painful rash. Shingles is also called "herpes zoster" or "zoster." It is caused by the same virus that causes chickenpox. This virus is called varicella-zoster virus (VZV). The disease can occur in anyone who has had chickenpox. The infection begins with pain or itching at the site where the rash will appear. The person may have fever or chills. Severe pain can occur after the rash is gone; this happens in about 20% of the people and is more commonly seen in the elderly. The pain may last for many years.

Shingles cannot be transmitted through person-to-person contact. However, the VZV virus can spread to someone who has not had chickenpox, and that person may then develop chickenpox. The virus is spread when the disease is in its blister form (Fig. 18-4). When the blisters have crusts, the disease is no longer contagious.

A shingles rash must remain covered at all times. Infected people should wash their hands

often and should not touch or scratch the rash. Medication is used to treat shingles. If the medication is started immediately, it can reduce the severity of the disease and shorten the length of the illness. A doctor should be contacted when shingles first appears. Waiting to treat this infection reduces the effectiveness of the medication.

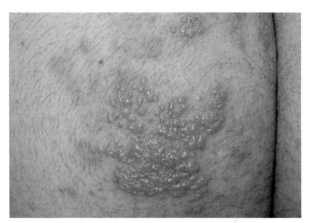

Fig. 18-4. *Shingles in blister form.* (PHOTO COURTESY OF DR. JERE MAMMINO, DO)

There is a vaccine for shingles that is often recommended for people over the age of 60. The vaccine may reduce the risk of getting shingles or reduce the pain associated with the disease.

Wounds

Wounds fall into two categories: open and closed. Skin that is not intact is considered an **open wound**. A **closed wound** is a wound where the skin's surface is not broken, such as a bruise or internal bleeding. Types of open wounds include the following:

- An abrasion is a tearing or wearing away of the surface skin due to friction. Another word for abrasion is "scrape" or "excoriation." Abrasions usually bleed very little, but the area must be kept clean to help prevent infection.

- An avulsion is a tearing away of tissues during a violent act or accident, such as a gunshot wound or an explosion. A dog bite is another example. Bleeding in this type of wound is usually heavy.

- An incision is a cut caused by a sharp-edged object, such as glass, a knife, or a razor. Bleeding in this type of wound is generally rapid and heavy; however, when an incision is made during surgery, the bleeding is usually controlled.

- A laceration is an irregular or jagged wound that is caused by blunt tearing of soft tissue. For example, it can result from the tearing of skin that occurs during childbirth. A laceration may cause rapid and extensive bleeding.

- A puncture wound is a wound from a sharp object that causes a small hole in the tissues. For example, a needle or a nail can cause a puncture wound. Bleeding may be slight or heavy.

A contusion, also called a **bruise**, is a common type of a closed wound. Trauma to the outside of the body can cause a contusion. The skin's surface generally remains intact, but internal damage and bleeding can occur.

Symptoms of wounds are pain, tissue damage, discoloration, and light or heavy bleeding. Fever, chills, or trouble breathing may occur. If any of these symptoms are observed, report to the nurse immediately. New wounds require immediate medical attention and assessment and monitoring by a nurse.

Treatment includes stopping bleeding and cleaning the wound. A dressing will need to be applied to the wound. Stitches or special bandages may be needed. In some cases, a tetanus shot is required. A bite from an animal may require rabies shots.

Skin Lesions

There are different types of lesions that can occur on the skin. A **lesion** is an area of abnormal tissue or an injury or wound.

Macules are the most simple skin lesion. Macules are flat spots that can be seen but not felt. They are visible because they change the color of the skin. Freckles are an example.

Papules are skin lesions that are raised, little round bumps on the skin. Papules can be felt. They do not contain pus. Contact dermatitis is an example.

Pustules are raised spots filled with pus, such as acne or infected boils.

Vesicles are small blisters that contain fluid. They can occur on the skin or inside the mouth. Chickenpox is an example.

Wheals are large raised, irregular areas, that are usually itchy (Fig. 18-5). Hives from an allergic reaction are an example.

Hematoma is a collection of blood in one area. The spot can be visible as a bruise, but may also occur on internal organs. Hematomas can become larger over time. They may also change color.

Purpura are small, purplish spots caused by bleeding under the skin. In elderly people, these spots are called senile purpura. Senile purpura occurs because blood vessels become more fragile with age.

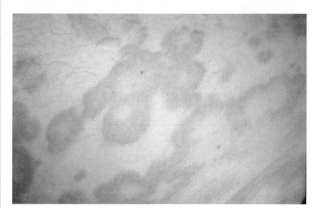

Fig. 18-5. *An example of wheals.* (PHOTO COURTESY OF DR. JERE MAMMINO, DO)

Gangrene

Gangrene means death of tissue. It is caused by a lack of blood flow due to factors such as burns, diabetes, injuries, circulatory disorders, a weakened immune system, and complications from surgery. Gangrene must be treated immediately.

Symptoms of gangrene include discoloration of the skin (usually black or blue), sores that do not heal, pain, loss of feeling, and foul-smelling discharge. The person may experience chills or have a change in vital signs.

Be familiar with residents' normal ranges for vital signs. Report elevated temperature, pulse or respiration rate, change in blood pressure, or difficulty breathing.

Treatments depend on the extent of the spread of the gangrene and may include antibiotics, surgery, amputation, or hospitalization.

Eczema (Dermatitis)

Eczema, or dermatitis, is a general term for a variety of skin problems. Dermatitis means inflammation of the skin. Eczema can be a temporary or chronic skin disorder in which redness, itching, burning, swelling, cracking, or weeping (oozing fluid) of the skin, and lesions can occur.

Causes of eczema include stress, allergies, family history, and irritating agents in the environment. Some people who have eczema also have asthma or other allergies.

Treatment of eczema includes protecting the skin surfaces from worsening. Topical steroid creams and soothing or drying lotions prescribed by a dermatologist (a doctor specializing in conditions of the skin) may help treat the problem.

Discouraging residents from scratching the skin can help healing. Certain types of oral medications can reduce the itching. With contact eczema (contact dermatitis), avoiding the irritating agent can help prevent the problem from occurring again. Follow orders for limiting harsh soaps and other products. Monitor vital signs, especially temperature. If eczema worsens, severe itching or pain develops, or if signs of infection occur, notify the nurse. Signs of infection are warmth, redness, swelling in the affected area, or a change in vital signs, especially fever.

Psoriasis

Psoriasis is a chronic skin condition in which cells of the skin grow too fast, causing red, white or silver patches to form. The patches can be small or large and usually occur on the arms, elbows, lower back, knees, or feet. Psoriasis can

be mild or severe. Larger patches can cause itching and discomfort, along with embarrassment. People with psoriasis can also have arthritis and pain.

Psoriasis is usually inherited. It may also be caused or aggravated by a dry climate, cold weather, stress, and a weakened immune system.

Treatment includes topical creams, shampoos, and lotions. Oral medication may also help. Phototherapy, which is special ultraviolet light treatments for the skin, may be performed. Some people with psoriasis make dietary changes and use sun therapy to treat the disorder.

Fungal Infections

Fungal and yeast (one type of fungus) infections can occur anywhere on the body. However, they most commonly occur in moist areas, such as the toes, under the breasts, and the groin area. Red, scaly patches appear, accompanied by itching, rawness, and pain. Jock itch, vaginal yeast infections, and athlete's foot are all examples of fungal infections. **Tinea** is a fungal infection that causes red scaly patches to appear in a ring shape, generally on the upper body, or the hands and feet (Fig. 18-6).

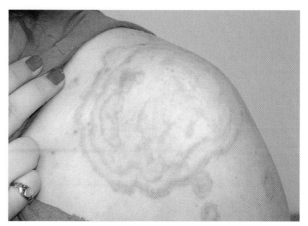

Fig. 18-6. *Tinea is a fungal infection that causes red scaly patches to appear in a ring-like shape.* (PHOTO COURTESY OF DR. JERE MAMMINO, DO)

Perspiration usually causes fungal infections. These infections often worsen in the summer, when perspiration increases. Tight-fitting clothing may also cause fungal infections. Treatment includes topical antifungal creams and medications. The earlier the treatment begins, the faster the infection heals. Report any skin changes, skin abrasions, flaking, redness, sores, and scratching to the nurse.

Warts

A **wart** is a rough, hard bump (Fig. 18-7). The bump or bumps may be spongy-looking with red, yellow, brown, or black spots. Warts are contagious, and are caused by a virus that invades the skin, usually through a cut or tear. They may spread to other areas of the body if not treated. People are more prone to developing warts if they have a weakened immune system.

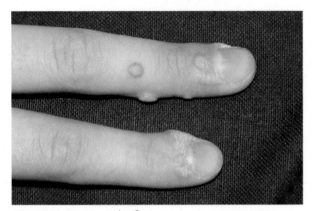

Fig. 18-7. Warts on the fingers. *(PHOTO COURTESY OF DR. JERE MAM-MINO, DO)*

Treatment includes medication and/or removal with a laser or a special instrument. Wash your hands frequently to help prevent the spread of warts to other parts of the body.

Skin Cancer

Skin cancer is the growth of abnormal skin cells. There are different types of skin cancer. The most serious form is malignant melanoma. If the cancer is caught in its early stages, it is normally treatable. If the skin cancer spreads, it can be fatal. Signs and symptoms of skin cancer include changes in a mole, wart, or spot on the skin, sores that do not heal, itching, pain, and skin that is oozing or bleeding. Dark-skinned

people have a higher risk of skin cancer on their palms, soles of their feet, and under their nails.

Treatment of skin cancer involves removing the cancerous area and sometimes the surrounding tissue. Advanced melanoma may be treated with interferon, a protein. To reduce the risk of getting skin cancer, reduce sun exposure, wear sunscreen, and wear hats and protective clothing. Have skin checked regularly by a dermatologist.

Report any changes in residents' skin to the nurse, including the following:

- **A**symmetry: one-half of a mole, spot, or birthmark does not match the other half.

- **B**order: the edges of a mole are irregular or blurred.

- **C**olor: the color of a mole varies with red, pink, black, brown, white, or blue areas.

- **D**iameter: a mole is over six millimeters in size (the size of a pencil eraser). Some melanomas are smaller than this, so report any spot you notice.

5. Discuss pressure ulcers and identify guidelines for preventing pressure ulcers

When a person is confined to bed for long periods of time, the amount of blood that circulates to the skin is reduced. The risk of skin breakdown increases. This breakdown usually occurs at the points of the body that bear much of the body's weight. These points are called **pressure points**, and there are many on the human body. They are mainly located at **bony prominences**, which are areas of the body where the bone lies close to the skin. These areas include the elbows, shoulder blades, sacrum (tailbone), hips and knees (inner and outer parts), ankles, heels, toes, and the back of the neck and the head. Other areas at risk for skin breakdown include the ears, the area under the breasts or scrotum, the area between the folds of the buttocks or abdomen, and skin between the legs (Fig. 18-8).

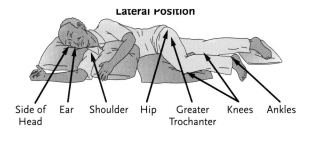

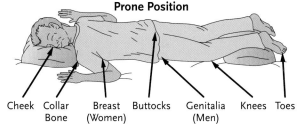

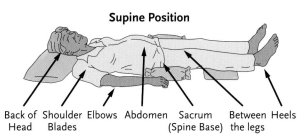

Fig. 18-8. *Pressure ulcer danger zones.*

When skin breaks down due to poor circulation, the amount of oxygen the cells receive is reduced and necrosis results. **Necrosis** is the death of living cells or tissues. This is due to prolonged pressure on an area or any other cause that interferes with circulation. Moisture and warmth also contribute to skin breakdown. Once skin has broken down and is weakened, sores can occur and may become infected, causing damage to the underlying tissue. The sores or wounds that result from skin deterioration and shearing are called **pressure ulcers**. Shearing is rubbing or friction resulting from the skin moving one way and the bone underneath it remaining fixed or moving in the opposite direction. Pressure ulcers are also called pressure sores, decubitus ulcers, or bed sores.

The first signs of skin breakdown include pale, white, or reddened skin. Darker skin may look purple. The skin may be dry, cracked, or torn. Blisters, bruises, or rashes may be visible.

Pressure ulcers are a common, serious problem in long-term care. If caught early, a break or tear in the skin can heal fairly quickly without other complications. However, once a pressure ulcer forms, it can become bigger, deeper, and infected. Pressure ulcers are painful and difficult to heal, and can lead to life-threatening infections. Pressure ulcers are much easier to prevent than to cure. Prevention is very important.

There are four stages of pressures ulcers (Fig. 18-9):

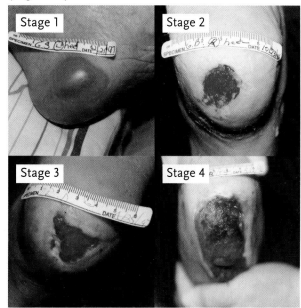

Fig. 18-9. *Pressure ulcers are categorized by four stages.*
(PHOTOS COURTESY OF DR. TAMARA D. FISHMAN AND THE WOUND CARE INSTITUTE, INC.)

Stage 1: Skin is intact, but reddens or appears blue or gray. In darker-skinned people, the area may appear purple or darker than the skin surrounding the area. People with darker skin may also have skin that is swollen or feels warm or firm. In this stage, redness or discoloration is not relieved within 15 to 30 minutes after removing pressure. Stage 1 can be reversed if discovered promptly and treated. If not treated promptly, the pressure ulcer will worsen and progress into other stages.

Stage 2: There is partial-thickness skin loss involving the epidermis and the dermis. The ulcer is superficial and looks like a blister or shallow crater. It is accompanied by pain, and the skin around the pressure ulcer may be discolored. There is no dead (necrotic) tissue in the site at this stage.

Stage 3: There is full thickness skin loss (both the epidermis and dermis will be gone), and the ulcer looks like a deep crater. The bottom of the wound may have yellow, dead tissue. The damage may extend to the muscle. Stage 3 pressure ulcers require weeks or months to fully heal.

Stage 4: There is full thickness skin loss extending through all layers of the skin, tissue, and possibly, muscle, bone, and other structures, such as joints or tendons. The ulcer will look like a deep crater and will have some necrotic tissue. The healing process extends over months. Serious infections can result. Stage 4 pressure ulcers may require a skin graft.

Nursing assistants are in the best position to observe for signs of pressure ulcers since they see residents' skin on a daily basis. Inspect each resident's skin every time you provide care. Notify the nurse if you observe any of these signs:

Observing and Reporting: Pressure Ulcers

O/R Pale, white, reddened, gray, or purple skin

O/R Dry, cracked, or flaking skin

O/R Torn skin

O/R Blisters, bruises, or wounds on the skin

O/R Rashes or any skin discoloration

O/R Tingling, warmth, or burning of the skin

O/R Itching or scratching

O/R Swelling of the skin

O/R Wet skin

O/R Broken skin anywhere on the body, including between the toes or around the toenails

O/R Changes in existing wounds or ulcers, including size, depth, drainage, color, odor

In addition to immobility, there are other risk factors for pressures ulcers. Wrinkled linens that

do not lie flat under residents, as well as crumbs or other irritating objects in the bed, can increase the risk for pressure ulcers. Malnutrition and dehydration increase the risk, too. Urinary incontinence is also a major risk factor for pressure ulcers. Follow these guidelines to help prevent pressure ulcers from occurring:

Guidelines: Preventing Pressure Ulcers

G Report any changes in a resident's skin.

G Perform regular skin care and closely observe residents' skin each time it is performed. Check areas that can be irritated by an IV, oxygen delivery device, or bandages.

G Keep skin clean and dry. Give skin care immediately after episodes of incontinence. Change clothing and bed linens as needed.

G Assist immobile residents to change position as ordered, but at least every two hours.

G Ask every resident in a wheelchair or any other chair to change position frequently. Follow facility policy on frequency of this practice.

G Be careful during transfers. Avoid rubbing skin against linen or other surfaces. Be gentle so that you do not tear fragile skin.

G Keep linens dry, clean, and wrinkle-free.

G Perform range of motion exercises as ordered.

G Massage the skin often if allowed. This increases circulation. Do not massage any white, red, or purple areas or put any pressure on them. Massage healthy skin around the areas.

G Use special positioning devices (Chapter 25) to help reduce pressure as ordered (Fig. 18-10).

G Use pillows to separate skin surfaces.

G Follow diet and fluid orders carefully; encourage fluids and good nutrition.

G Use moisturizers as ordered on unbroken skin. Follow the care plan. Do not use
creams, lotions, soaps, or other products on
non-intact skin.

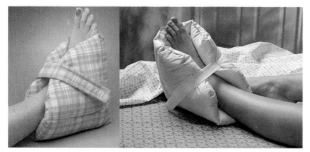

*Fig. 18-10. Padded heel protectors help keep feet properly
aligned and prevent pressure ulcers.* (REPRINTED WITH PERMISSION OF
BRIGGS CORPORATION, 800-247-2343, WWW.BRIGGSCORP.COM)

Tip

Urinary Incontinence and Pressure Ulcers
The Minimum Data Set (MDS) guidelines state to
count any time that a resident's skin, pad, brief, or
underwear is wet from urine as an episode of incontinence. This is true even if it is a small amount of
urine. Document this carefully, following facility policy. This is important to help prevent pressure ulcers.

6. Explain the benefits of warm and cold applications

Applications of heat or cold can have beneficial
effects on injuries, infections, fevers, and other
conditions. The body responds to heat and cold
in different ways.

Heat helps relieve pain and muscular tension
and decreases swelling. It elevates the temperature in the tissues, increases waste removal from
the area, and increases blood flow due to dilated
blood vessels. Increased blood flow brings more
oxygen and nutrients to the tissues for healing.
However, there are risks associated with warm
applications, too. Heat can cause burns, make
bleeding worse, and cause confusion, dizziness, or fainting due to a reduction of blood to
the brain. The elderly are at an increased risk
for burns and other complications because they
have thinner, more fragile skin.

With cold applications, blood flow decreases
due to the constriction of the vessels. The movement of oxygen and nutrients into the tissues
decreases. Cold applications help stop bleeding,
minimize swelling, and reduce pain. Cold helps
bring down high temperatures. Risks of cold applications include cyanosis or pale skin, chills,
and shivering. Lack of blood flow to the application area and the cold temperature may damage
tissue.

Warm or cold applications can be either moist
or dry. Moisture strengthens the effect of heat
and cold, which means that moist applications
are more likely to cause injury. Be careful when
using these applications. Know how long they
should be performed, and use the correct temperature listed in the care plan. Check on the
applications often.

Types of moist applications include:

• Compresses (warm or cold)

• Soaks (warm or cold)

• Tub baths (warm)

• Sponge bath (warm or cold)

• Sitz bath (warm)

• Ice packs (cold)

Types of dry applications include:

• Aquamatic K-pad® (warm or cold)

• Disposable warm pack (warm)

• Ice bag (cold)

• Disposable cold pack (cold)

• Warming blankets (warm)

• Cooling blankets (cold)

Some facilities do not allow nursing assistants to
prepare and apply warm and cold applications.
Only perform procedures that are assigned to
you and that you are trained to do. If your facility does allow you to perform this care, carefully
follow the procedure manuals and the care plan.

Provide privacy when giving warm and cold applications. If you note any of the following, stop the application and report to the nurse immediately. These signs may indicate that the application is causing tissue damage:

- Excessive redness
- Pain
- Blisters
- Numbness

Remember, if the resident has non-intact skin or open sores, wear gloves when applying warm or cold applications. You should always wear gloves when assisting with a sitz bath. A **sitz bath** is a warm soak of the perineal area to clean perineal wounds and reduce inflammation and pain.

> **Tip**
>
> **Hot opens; cold closes.**
>
> When using warm and cold applications, it helps to remember what happens with each kind of application. The following tip may help you remember the body's response to heat and cold:
>
> Hot opens, or dilates, (blood vessels). Cold closes, or constricts (blood vessels).

> **Tip**
>
> **The 20-minute rule**
>
> When warm and cold applications are applied for too long, the opposite effect of what is intended occurs. This means that if you leave an ice bag on an affected area for longer than 20 minutes, the blood vessels may start to open again. This can increase bleeding and swelling at the injury site. Remember to limit warm or cold applications to 20 minutes at a time.

Applying warm moist compresses

Equipment: washcloth or compress, plastic wrap, towel, basin, bath thermometer

1. Identify yourself by name. Identify the resident. Greet the resident by name.

2. Wash your hands.

3. Explain procedure to resident. Speak clearly, slowly, and directly. Maintain face-to-face contact whenever possible.

4. Provide for the resident's privacy with a curtain, screen, or door.

5. Fill basin one-half to two-thirds with warm water. Test water temperature with thermometer or your wrist. Ensure it is safe. Water temperature should be no more than 105°F. Have resident check water temperature. Adjust if necessary.

6. Soak the washcloth in the water. Wring it out. Immediately apply it to the area needing a warm compress. Note the time. Quickly cover the washcloth with plastic wrap and the towel to keep it warm (Fig. 18-11).

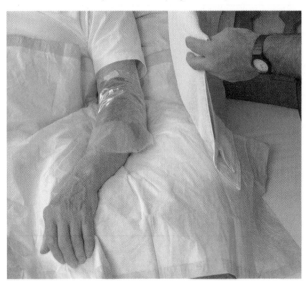

Fig. 18-11. *Cover warm compresses to keep them warm.*

7. Check the area every five minutes. Remove the compress if the area is red or numb or if the resident has pain or discomfort. Change the compress if cooling occurs. Remove the compress after 20 minutes.

8. Commercial warm compresses are also available. If you are using these, follow the package directions and the nurse's instructions.

9. Remove privacy measures. Make resident comfortable.

10. Empty, rinse, and wipe basin. Return to proper storage. Discard plastic wrap.

11. Place soiled clothing and linens in appropriate containers.

12. Leave call light within resident's reach.

13. Wash your hands.

14. Be courteous and respectful at all times.

15. Report any changes in the resident to the nurse. Document procedure using facility guidelines.

Administering warm soaks

Equipment: towel, basin, bath thermometer, bath blanket

1. Identify yourself by name. Identify the resident. Greet the resident by name.

2. Wash your hands.

3. Explain procedure to resident. Speak clearly, slowly, and directly. Maintain face-to-face contact whenever possible.

4. Provide for the resident's privacy with a curtain, screen, or door.

5. Fill the basin half full of warm water. Test water temperature with thermometer or your wrist, and ensure it is safe. Water temperature should be no more than 105°F. Have resident check water temperature. Adjust if necessary.

6. Immerse the body part in the basin. Pad the edge of the basin with a towel if needed (Fig. 18-12). Use a bath blanket to cover the resident if needed for extra warmth.

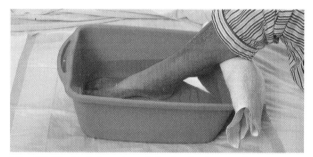

Fig. 18-12. *Pad the edge of the basin for comfort.*

7. Check water temperature every five minutes. Add warm water as needed to maintain the temperature. Never add water warmer than 105°F. To prevent burns, tell the resident not to add warm water. Observe the area for redness. Discontinue the soak if the resident has pain or discomfort.

8. Soak for 15-20 minutes, or as ordered.

9. Remove basin. Use the towel to dry the resident.

10. Remove privacy measures. Make resident comfortable.

11. Empty, rinse, and wipe basin. Return to proper storage.

12. Place soiled clothing and linens in appropriate containers.

13. Leave call light within resident's reach.

14. Wash your hands.

15. Be courteous and respectful at all times.

16. Report any changes in the resident to the nurse. Document procedure using facility guidelines.

Applying an Aquamatic K-Pad®

Equipment: K-Pad® and control unit (Fig. 18-13), covering for pad, distilled water

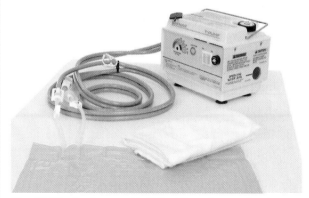

Fig. 18-13. *An Aquamatic K-Pad® and control unit.*

1. Identify yourself by name. Identify the resident. Greet the resident by name.

2. Wash your hands.

3. Explain procedure to resident. Speak clearly, slowly, and directly. Maintain face-to-face contact whenever possible.

4. Provide for the resident's privacy with a curtain, screen, or door.

5. Make sure the surface on the bedside table is dry. Place the control unit on the bedside table. Make sure cords are not frayed or damaged. Check that tubing between pad and unit is intact.

6. Remove cover of control unit to check level of water. If it is low, fill it with distilled water to the fill line.

7. Put the cover of control unit back in place.

8. Plug unit in. Turn unit on. Temperature should have been pre-set. If it was not, check with the nurse for proper temperature. If you need to set the temperature, you must remove the key after doing so. Place key in proper place.

9. Place the pad in the cover. Do not pin the pad to the cover.

10. Uncover area to be treated. Place the covered pad. Note the time. Make sure the tubing is not hanging below the bed. It should be coiled on the bed. Make sure tubing has no kinks.

11. Return and check area every five minutes. Remove the pad if the area is red or numb or if the resident reports pain or discomfort.

12. Check water level. Refill with distilled water to the fill line when necessary.

13. Turn off unit and remove pad after 20 minutes.

14. Remove privacy measures. Make resident comfortable.

15. Clean K-pad® according to instructions and return to storage.

16. Place used linen in appropriate container.

17. Leave call light within resident's reach.

18. Wash your hands.

19. Be courteous and respectful at all times.

20. Report any changes in the resident to the nurse. Document procedure using facility guidelines.

Sitz baths cause circulation to be increased to the pelvic area. Residents with perineal swelling (such as hemorrhoids) may have sitz baths ordered. During sitz baths, blood flow to other parts of the body decreases. This is because the bath causes increased blood flow to the pelvic area. Residents may feel weak, faint, or dizzy after a sitz bath. Stop the bath if the resident complains of feeling dizzy or faint. Sitz baths may cause the need or urge to void. Always wear gloves when helping with a sitz bath.

A disposable sitz bath fits on the toilet seat. It is attached to a plastic bag containing warm water (Fig. 18-14).

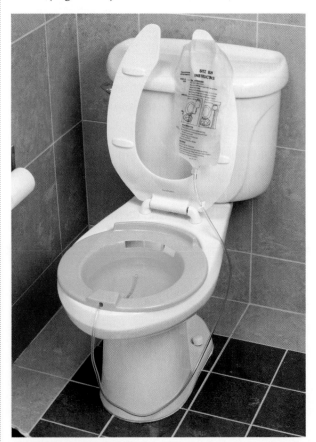

Fig. 18-14. *A disposable sitz bath.* (REPRINTED WITH PERMISSION OF BRIGGS CORPORATION, 800-247-2343, WWW.BRIGGSCORP.COM)

Assisting with a sitz bath

Equipment: disposable sitz bath, bath thermometer, towels, gloves

1. Identify yourself by name. Identify the resident. Greet the resident by name.

2. Wash your hands.

3. Explain procedure to resident. Speak clearly, slowly, and directly. Maintain face-to-face contact whenever possible.

4. Provide for the resident's privacy with a curtain, screen, or door.

5. Put on gloves.

6. Fill the sitz bath container two-thirds full with warm water. Place the sitz bath on the toilet seat. Water temperature should generally be no more than 105°F. Check the water temperature using the bath thermometer. If the sitz bath is ordered for pain and to stimulate circulation, the water temperature may need to be higher. Follow the care plan.

7. Help the resident undress and get seated on the sitz bath. A valve on the tubing connected to the bag allows the resident or you to fill the sitz bath again with warm water.

8. You may be required to stay with the resident during the bath for safety reasons. If you leave the room, check on the resident every five minutes to make sure he or she is not dizzy or weak. Make sure resident knows how to use the emergency pull cord in the bathroom if it is needed.

9. Help the resident off of the sitz bath after 20 minutes. Provide towels. Help with dressing if needed.

10. Empty, rinse, and wipe sitz bath container. Return to proper storage.

11. Place soiled clothing and linens in appropriate containers.

12. Remove and discard gloves. Wash your hands.

13. Make resident comfortable. Remove privacy measures.

14. Leave call light within resident's reach.

15. Wash your hands.

16. Be courteous and respectful at all times.

17. Report any changes in the resident to the nurse. Document procedure using facility guidelines.

Commercial warm or cold packs may be used. There are different types of commercial packs. Follow the manufacturer's instructions and the procedure manual when using these packs. Some packs are used once and disposed of, while others are cleaned and re-used. To activate the warm or cold pack, you may need to squeeze the package. Apply a cover before applying the pack to the skin. Follow instructions on cleaning non-disposable packs. Check the site every five minutes and remove the pack after 20 minutes or as ordered. Report to the nurse if you note any of the following: pale skin, burning, numbness and tingling, or pain.

This procedure teaches you how to apply a non-commercial ice pack.

Applying ice packs

Equipment: ice pack or sealable plastic bag and crushed ice, towels or cover for pack or bag

1. Identify yourself by name. Identify the resident. Greet the resident by name.

2. Wash your hands.

3. Explain procedure to resident. Speak clearly, slowly, and directly. Maintain face-to-face contact whenever possible.

4. Provide for the resident's privacy with a curtain, screen, or door.

5. Fill plastic bag or ice pack one-half to two-thirds full with crushed ice. Seal bag. Remove excess air. Cover bag or ice pack with towel or cover (Fig. 18-15).

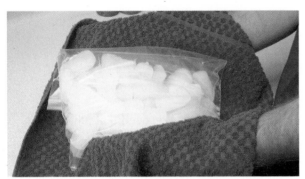

Fig. 18-15. *Seal the bag filled with ice and cover it with a towel.*

6. Apply pack or bag to the area as ordered. Note the time. Use another towel to cover bag if it is too cold.

7. Check the area after five minutes for blisters or pale, white, or gray skin. Stop treatment if resident reports numbness or pain.

8. Remove ice pack or bag after 20 minutes or as ordered.

9. Remove privacy measures. Make resident comfortable.

10. Empty and store ice pack.

11. Place used linen in appropriate container.

12. Leave call light within resident's reach.

13. Wash your hands.

14. Be courteous and respectful at all times.

15. Report any changes in the resident to the nurse. Document procedure using facility guidelines.

Residents with high temperatures may need to have a cooling or tepid sponge bath. Sponge baths can reduce body temperature. High fevers can have serious side effects, such as convulsions and confusion.

Prior to the bath, vital signs, including temperature, will need to be taken. During the procedure, vital signs will need to be taken at specific intervals. Follow your facility's procedure to perform the sponge bath. Possible complications of sponge baths are chills, shivering, a sudden change in vital signs, or breathing problems. If any of these occur, stop the bath, cover the resident completely, and immediately call for the nurse.

Warming and Cooling Blankets

Warming blankets, also called hypothermia blankets, may be used when a resident has severe sub-normal body temperature. Cooling blankets, also called hyperthermia blankets, may be used when a resident has a high fever.

Warming or cooling blankets are plugged into an electrical socket, and then the resident is placed on the blanket to try to raise or lower his body temperature. Ice bags or commercial ice packs may be used along with a cooling blanket.

The nurse is responsible for this procedure. He or she will apply it, adjust the setting, and monitor the procedure. Cover the blanket with a sheet before the resident lies down on it if needed. You may be asked to take vital signs before, during, and after the warming/cooling blanket procedure.

Notify the nurse if you observe pale or cyanotic skin or nailbeds, sudden changes in vital signs, breathing difficulties, numbness or tingling, or pain. If you note any damage to the blanket, leakage, or sparking, turn the blanket off and get the nurse.

7. Discuss non-sterile and sterile dressings

Open wounds increase the risk of infection because breaks in the skin are a way for bacteria and other microorganisms to enter the body. In order to protect wounds from bacteria, dressings are applied. Dressings can be either non-sterile or sterile. Non-sterile dressings are applied to dry wounds that have less chance of infection. Sterile dressings are required when the wound is new, open, or draining. They are also required when there is a higher risk of infection.

Nursing assistants may help with non-sterile and sterile dressing changes. It is important to know the correct method to perform each procedure. When giving any type of dressing care, it is important not to further damage the wound area or damage the dressing or tape. Be careful not to cause pain to the resident. Ask the nurse if pain medication is needed prior to changing the dressing. Notify the nurse if the resident tells you that he is allergic to latex.

Assisting the nurse with changing a non-sterile dressing

Equipment: package of square gauze dressings, adhesive tape, scissors, 2 pairs of gloves, plastic bag

1. Identify yourself by name. Identify the resident. Greet the resident by name.

2. Wash your hands.

3. Explain procedure to resident. Speak clearly, slowly, and directly. Maintain face-to-face contact whenever possible.

4. Provide for the resident's privacy with a curtain, screen, or door.

5. The nurse will prepare a clean, flat, dry surface for the dressing materials. Keep the plastic bag close by for immediate disposal of old dressing materials.

6. You may be asked to open packages for the nurse or cut strips of tape. Cut pieces of tape long enough to secure the dressing. Open gauze square packages without touching the insides or the gauze. If asked to set package down, place the opened package on a clean, flat surface.

7. Put on gloves.

8. Only expose the area where the dressing will be changed. The nurse will remove soiled dressing. Dispose of used dressing in proper container.

9. Remove and discard gloves in plastic bag.

10. Wash your hands.

11. Put on new gloves. The nurse will observe the wound and then apply the fresh gauze over

the wound and tape it in place (Fig. 18-16). Assist as directed.

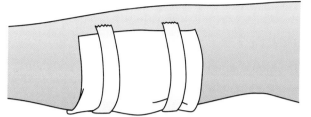

Fig. 18-16. *The nurse will apply and secure the dressing.*

12. Remove and discard gloves. Wash your hands.

13. Make resident comfortable. Remove privacy measures.

14. Leave call light within resident's reach.

15. Wash your hands.

16. Be courteous and respectful at all times.

17. Report any changes in the resident to the nurse. Document procedure using facility guidelines.

Sterile gloves will be used for sterile dressing care. A sterile field—the area that is kept sterile—is created with sterile dressing care. You may need to assist the nurse with sterile dressing care. Examples of supplies that are considered sterile are sterile dressings, sterile drapes or pads, and tubing and catheters. Packages are generally marked in some way to indicate whether the supply is sterile or non-sterile. Check expiration dates on packages to make sure gloves can still be used.

Make sure not to contaminate the sterile field or the sterile gloves. If any part of the sterile field becomes contaminated, the entire process must be re-started.

Applying sterile gloves

Equipment: 2 pairs of sterile gloves in correct size

1. Wash your hands.

2. Using a clean, flat, dry surface, remove outer wrapper from gloves. Place inner wrapper on the clean surface. The word "Left" should be on your left side, and the word "Right" should be on your right side.

3. Slowly open the inner wrapper, only touching the small flaps of the wrapper.

4. The gloves will have been placed palm-side up with cuffs in place. Pick up the first glove by the bottom end of the cuff. Slip your fingers into the glove without touching the outside of the glove (Fig. 18-17). If you touch the outside of the glove, it will be contaminated. You will have to start over with a new pair of gloves. Wait to adjust the glove until the second glove is on your other hand.

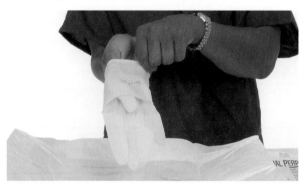

Fig. 18-17. Touching the bottom end of the cuff, slip your fingers into the glove, without touching the outside of the glove.

5. Slip your gloved hand into the second glove in the area under the cuff.

6. Slowly slip the fingers of your ungloved hand into the second glove, and pull it completely over your hand and wrist (Fig. 18-18).

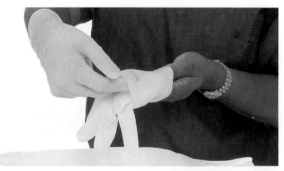

Fig. 18-18. Touching the area under the cuff of the second glove, slip the fingers of your ungloved hand inside.

7. With your gloved second hand, finish pulling the first glove up and over the wrist. Adjust the fingers now if any adjustment is necessary.

8. If either glove has a tear in it, stop and start again with the second set of sterile gloves.

9. Keep your gloved hands in front of you and above the level of your waist at all times during the procedure.

10. Assist the nurse with sterile procedure.

___

Trivia

The History of the Rubber Glove

In the early 20th century, William Halsted developed rubber gloves to protect his nurse's (and future wife's) hands. A student suggested that surgeons adopt them. The gloves were very thick, though, and many surgeons would not wear them. Some surgeons wore cloth gloves over the rubber ones. Over the years, rubber gloves became thinner and easier to wear. Today's gloves are made of different materials, such as nitrile or latex.

Chapter Review

1. What are the two basic layers of the skin (LO 2)?

2. List four functions of the integumentary system (LO 2).

3. List eight normal age-related changes of the integumentary system (LO 3).

4. Briefly describe the damage and/or symptoms caused by first-, second-, and third-degree burns (LO 4).

5. How is scabies usually transmitted (LO 4)?

6. What causes shingles (LO 4)?

7. Give one example each of an open and a closed wound (LO 4).

8. Where does skin breakdown most often occur (LO 5)?

9. List the first signs of skin breakdown (LO 5).

10. Why is prevention of pressure ulcers so important (LO 5)?

11. List four risk factors for pressure ulcers (LO 5).

12. How often should immobile residents be helped to change position (LO 5)?

13. What are some benefits of applying heat to the body? What are some benefits of applying cold to the body (LO 6)?

14. What signs may indicate that a warm or cold application is causing tissue damage (LO 6)?

15. Generally speaking, for how long should warm or cold applications be applied (LO 6)?

16. Under what circumstances are non-sterile dressings usually used? When are sterile dressings used (LO 7)?

19
The Circulatory or Cardiovascular System

Discovering the Pathways of the Blood

William Harvey (1578-1657), an English physician, wrote *On the Movement of the Heart and Blood in Animals*, which was published in 1628. He noted that blood moves throughout the body in a closed system. He came to the conclusion that the blood recycles itself and moves inside the body in a single direction, not back and forth.

Harvey also identified that the heart is a pump and that it works by using the force of muscle. He found the heart has two phases: systole, when the heart contracts and empties itself of blood, and diastole, when the chambers of the heart are filled with blood.

" . . . It ennobled our hearts and enriched our blood . . ."

Richard Leveridge, 1670-1758

" . . . So in my veins red life might stream again . . ."

John Keats, 1795-1821

1. Define important words in this chapter

anemia: a condition in which the amount of red blood cells or hemoglobin in the body is less than normal.

angina pectoris: chest pain, pressure, or discomfort.

anti-embolic stockings: special stockings used to help prevent swelling and blood clots and aid circulation; also called elastic stockings.

artery: vessel that carries blood away from the heart.

atria: the upper two chambers of the heart.

capillaries: tiny blood vessels in which the exchange of gases, nutrients, and waste products occurs between blood and cells.

cardiomyopathy: a weakening of the heart muscle due to enlargement or thickening, which reduces the heart's ability to pump blood effectively.

congestive heart failure (CHF): a condition in which the heart muscle is damaged and fails to pump effectively.

coronary artery disease (CAD): a condition in which the coronary arteries become damaged and narrow over time, causing chest pain and other symptoms.

diastole: phase when the heart muscle relaxes.

heart: four-chambered pump that is responsible for the flow of blood in the body.

hypoxia: a condition in which the body does not receive enough oxygen.

ischemia: a lack of blood supply to an area.

myocardial ischemia: a condition in which the heart muscle does not receive enough blood and lacks oxygen; can cause angina pectoris.

nitroglycerin: medication that relaxes the walls of the coronary arteries.

occlusion: a complete obstruction of a blood vessel.

orthopnea: shortness of breath when lying down that is relieved by sitting up.

peripheral vascular disease (PVD): a condition in which the legs, feet, arms, or hands do not have enough blood circulation.

phlebitis: inflammation of the veins in the lower extremities.

pulmonary edema: a condition in which there is an accumulation of fluid in the lungs; usually due to heart failure.

sequential compression device (SCD): a machine used to help improve circulation, reduce fluid build-up, and prevent blood clots; compression sleeves are placed around the legs and are inflated and deflated regularly.

stable angina: chest pain that occurs when a person is active or under severe stress.

systole: phase where the heart is at work, contracting and pushing blood out of the left ventricle.

unstable angina: chest pain that occurs while a person is at rest and not exerting himself.

vein: vessel that carries blood to the heart.

ventricles: the lower two chambers of the heart.

2. Explain the structure and function of the circulatory system

The circulatory, or cardiovascular, system is made up of the heart, blood vessels, and blood (Fig. 19-1). The **heart** is the pump of the circulatory system. It is positioned between the lungs, slightly to the left of the middle of the chest. The heart muscle is made up of three layers: the pericardium, the myocardium and the endocardium.

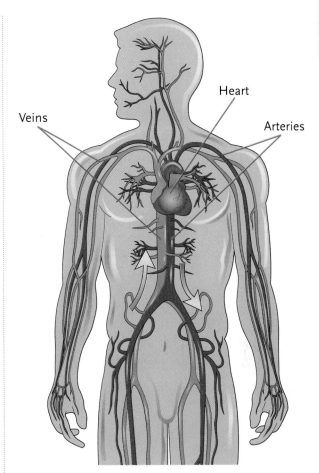

Veins   Heart   Arteries

Fig. 19-1. The heart, blood vessels, and blood are the main parts of the circulatory system.

The heart is composed of four main chambers: the **atria** (the upper left and right chambers) and the **ventricles** (the lower left and right chambers). The right atrium receives de-oxygenated blood from the body. It is delivered via the superior vena cava from the head and upper extremities and the inferior vena cava, which delivers blood from the rest of the body (Fig. 19-2).

The heart functions in two phases: systole and diastole. During **systole**, the lower chambers of the heart, the ventricles, contract. This contraction causes blood to move out of the ventricles of the heart and into the arteries. The ventricles relax after contraction and fill up with blood again. This part of heart function is known as **diastole**. This is the relaxation phase of the heart, or when the heart rests.

Blood is pumped from the right atrium to the right ventricle. The right ventricle pumps the de-oxygenated blood into the lungs via the pulmonary arteries. These are the only arteries in the body that carry de-oxygenated blood; the other arteries carry oxygen-rich blood. The exchange of carbon dioxide for oxygen is made during this process. The blood then travels back into the heart through the pulmonary veins. These are the only veins in the body that carry oxygen-rich blood.

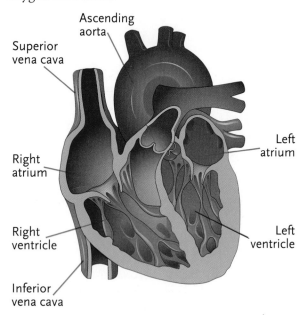

Fig. 19-2. *The four chambers of the heart connect to the body's largest blood vessels.*

While in the lungs, carbon dioxide is removed when we exhale, or breathe out, and oxygen is added when we inhale, or take a breath. This exchange of gases returns oxygen-rich blood to the left ventricle. The left ventricle then pumps the oxygen-rich blood out of the heart via the largest **artery** in the body, the aorta. The blood is delivered to all of the arteries in the body through the arterial system (Fig. 19-3).

With the exception of the pulmonary arteries, the arteries carry oxygen-rich blood away from the heart to deliver the oxygen to the cells. When blood arrives at the cell level, it moves into arterioles, the tiniest of the arterial vessels. The arterioles deliver the blood to the tiny blood vessels called **capillaries**. Gas, nutrient, and waste exchanges happen within capillaries. Capillaries have very thin walls, allowing blood to move

in and out of the tiny vessels. During capillary exchange, oxygen and nutrients move from the blood into the tissues, and tissue fluid and waste products move from the tissues into the blood.

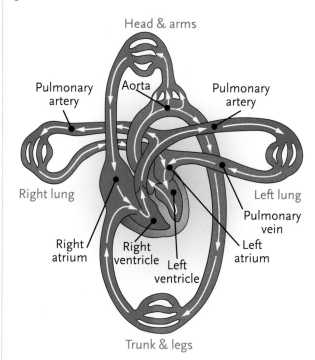

Fig. 19-3. *The flow of blood through the heart.*

Capillaries connect to the venules, small veins. The venules collect the de-oxygenated blood from the capillaries and then drain this blood into the veins. The **veins** carry the de-oxygenated blood back to the heart, and the whole process begins again.

Blood is made up of solids and liquids: cells and plasma. Plasma makes up about 55% of blood; blood cells make up the remaining 45%. Blood is composed of three different types of blood cells: red blood cells, or erythrocytes; white blood cells, or leukocytes; and platelets, or thrombocytes.

Red blood cells (erythrocytes) contain hemoglobin, which carries oxygen through the blood vessels. Red blood cells also transport carbon dioxide from the cells through the heart to the lungs. The lungs are responsible for the elimination of carbon dioxide from the body via exhaling. Red blood cells are produced by bone marrow, a substance found inside hollow bones.

Iron, found in bone marrow and red blood cells, is essential to blood. It gives blood its red color. Iron in the diet allows the body to produce new red blood cells. Red blood cells function for a short time, and then they die. They are filtered out of the blood by the liver and spleen.

White blood cells (leukocytes) protect the body from bacteria and viruses and other foreign substances. When the body becomes aware of these invaders, white blood cells rush to the site of infection and multiply rapidly. The bone marrow, spleen, and thymus gland produce white blood cells.

Platelets (thrombocytes) cause the blood to clot, which prevents excess bleeding. Platelets are also produced by the bone marrow.

Plasma, the liquid portion of the blood, is made up mostly of water. The plasma carries oxygen, nutrients, waste products, hormones, salts, antibodies, and the substance necessary for the blood to clot.

The functions of the circulatory system are:

The heart:
- Pumps blood through blood vessels to every cell in the human body

The blood:
- Transports oxygen, nutrients, hormones, salts, and antibodies to cells
- Removes carbon dioxide and other waste products from the cells
- Controls pH level and body temperature
- Clots the blood and fights pathogens and poisons

Destination: Homeostasis

A sudden decrease in blood pressure, as in the case of shock (decrease in amount of blood to organs and tissues) or a severe hemorrhage (loss of blood), causes an imbalance in homeostasis. One of the body's responses to this change is to trigger the sympathetic nervous system to increase the heart rate, along with the force of the contraction of the heart. This increases the output of blood from the heart. The change in the output of blood increases blood pressure. The heart tries to restore an adequate volume of blood to all body tissues. When blood volume is back to normal levels, the body has returned to homeostasis.

3. Discuss changes in the circulatory system due to aging

Normal age-related changes for the circulatory system include the following:
- Heart pumps less efficiently.
- Blood vessels narrow.
- Blood vessels become less elastic.
- Blood flow decreases.

4. Discuss common disorders of the circulatory system

Hypertension (HTN) or High Blood Pressure

When blood pressure consistently measures 140/90 or higher, a person is diagnosed as having hypertension, or high blood pressure. The major cause of hypertension is the hardening and narrowing of the blood vessels. It can also result from kidney disease, tumors of the adrenal glands, pregnancy, extreme stress or pain, and certain medications. Arteries may become hardened, or narrower, because of a build-up of plaque on the walls of the blood vessels, and this can also cause hypertension (Fig. 19-4).

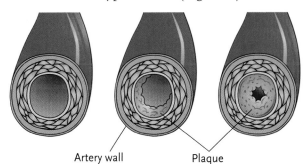

Artery wall   Plaque

Fig. 19-4. *Arteries may harden or narrow because of a build-up of plaque. Hardened arteries cause high blood pressure.*

Prehypertension is a condition in which a person's systolic blood pressure measurement is between 120–139 mm Hg and diastolic measurement is between 80–89 mm Hg. Prehypertension means that a person does not have hypertension now, but is likely to have it in the future.

Hypertension can develop in persons of any age. Signs and symptoms of hypertension are not always obvious, especially in the early stages of the disease. Often the illness is only discovered when a blood pressure measurement is taken by a healthcare provider. Persons with the disease may complain of headache, blurred vision, and dizziness.

Hypertension can lead to a myocardial infarction (heart attack). This is often caused by fatty deposits completely blocking off a coronary artery. This is called an occlusion or a coronary occlusion. An **occlusion** is an obstruction of a blood vessel. Occlusions cause damage to a part of the heart muscle from the lack of blood supply. **Ischemia** is a lack of blood supply to an area. If hypertension is not treated promptly, it can also result in a cerebrovascular accident (CVA), or stroke. Hypertension can also lead to kidney disease or blindness.

Medication is usually ordered to treat hypertension. This helps lower blood pressure and can prevent the complications listed above. Diuretics may also be prescribed. Diuretics are medications that reduce fluid in the body. Extra fluid can increase blood volume and weight, which increases the workload on the heart. Residents may have prescribed exercise programs and special diets, such as low-fat or low-sodium diets. Reducing the intake of sodium (salt) in the diet helps reduce extra fluid in the body. Stopping smoking can increase the size of the blood vessels, increasing the flow of blood. Nicotine constricts (closes) blood vessels. Lowering stress levels can also help people with hypertension.

Nursing assistants may be asked to measure blood pressure often. You can also assist by encouraging residents to follow their prescribed diets and exercise programs.

The Silent Killer

Signs of hypertension include nosebleeds, eye hemorrhages (blood showing up in the white of an eye), dizziness, trembling, shortness of breath, and headaches. Hypertension puts a person at high risk for a heart attack or stroke. If you notice any of these signs and symptoms, report them to the nurse.

Coronary Artery Disease (CAD)

The coronary arteries supply blood to the heart. **Coronary artery disease (CAD)** occurs when the coronary arteries become damaged. Over time, a build-up of arterial plaque forms and the arteries narrow. This plaque can partially or completely block the arteries.

When the blood supply to the heart is reduced, myocardial ischemia occurs. **Myocardial ischemia** is a condition in which the heart muscle does not get enough blood, and therefore lacks enough oxygen. When the heart is deprived of oxygen, chest pain can occur. However, myocardial ischemia can occur without causing pain or discomfort. Chest pain, pressure, or discomfort due to CAD is known as **angina pectoris** (Fig. 19-5). Angina pectoris is a symptom of myocardial ischemia.

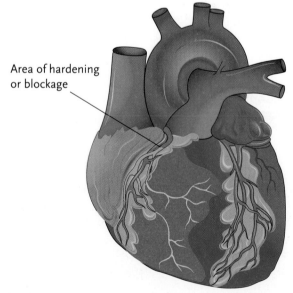

Area of hardening or blockage

Fig. 19-5. Angina pectoris is chest pain that results from the heart not getting enough oxygen.

Angina pectoris is classified as stable or unstable. **Stable angina** is chest pain that occurs when a person is active or under severe stress. **Unstable angina** is chest pain that occurs while a person is at rest and not exerting himself.

The pain of angina can be mild or severe. Angina is usually described as intense pressure in the chest, a tightness in the chest, or pain in the back, neck, jaw, or shoulder. Some people have pain that radiates down the inside of the left arm. The person may sweat or look pale and have trouble breathing. Cyanosis of the lips, nailbeds and mucous membranes may develop. Dizziness may occur. To help residents with angina, follow these guidelines:

Guidelines: Angina

G   Reduce emotional distress as much as possible. Stress can cause or worsen angina.

G   Residents will need to take their medication as ordered. Nitroglycerin is usually ordered for angina. **Nitroglycerin** is medication that relaxes the walls of the coronary arteries. This medication comes in various forms, such as pills, patches, or sprays. If pills are used, the resident places a pill under his tongue as soon as chest pain occurs. Nitroglycerin pills must be kept nearby at all times, even when residents leave the facility. Notify the nurse immediately if the resident needs help taking this medication. Nursing assistants are not allowed to give medication. Notify the nurse if a nitroglycerin patch falls off. Nitroglycerin may also come in the form of a spray that the person sprays onto or under the tongue. Side effects of nitroglycerin include headache, dizziness, fainting, slow or rapid pulse rate, and a drop in blood pressure. Report these side effects to the nurse.

G   Make sure residents get enough rest. Rest is very important for people suffering from angina pectoris. It reduces the heart's need for extra oxygen. However, rest may not help

people who are suffering from unstable angina.

G   Residents will need to avoid big meals, especially right before bedtime. People with angina should not overeat.

G   Encourage residents to follow their exercise plan as ordered by the doctor. During exercise, observe for chest pain. Report to the nurse if a resident has pain or difficulty during exercising.

G   Climate can affect symptoms of coronary artery disease. Humid weather can cause breathing problems. Residents may need to avoid hot and humid weather.

G   Be encouraging if residents have quit or are trying to quit smoking.

Cardiomyopathy

Extensive CAD can cause **cardiomyopathy**, or a heart muscle that no longer pumps effectively. Cardiomyopathy can also be caused by a virus, diabetes, thyroid problems, drug and alcohol use, a birth defect, or unknown causes. The prognosis for cardiomyopathy is not good. This condition is the most common reason for heart transplants.

Tip

Laughter—The Best Medicine?

Studies have shown that laughing relaxes the arteries, which in turn, can help people with CAD or other illnesses. Be positive with residents and share appropriate humor when the situation is right. It may be "just what the doctor ordered!"

Tip

Healthy Gums and CAD

There may be a link between heart disease, strokes, and diabetes and poor gum health. Make sure your residents receive regular, careful oral care.

Myocardial Infarction (MI) or Heart Attack

When all or part of the blood flow to the heart muscle is blocked, oxygen and nutrients fail to reach the cells in that area. Waste products are not removed and muscle cells die. This is called a myocardial infarction (MI) or a heart attack (Fig. 19-6). When a clot (thrombosis) causes an MI by blocking the blood supply to an area of the heart, it is called a coronary thrombosis.

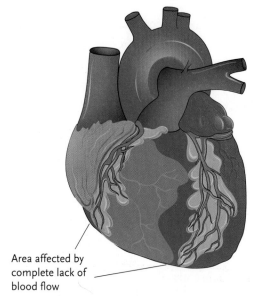

Area affected by complete lack of blood flow

Fig. 19-6. *A heart attack occurs when all or part of the blood flow to the heart is blocked.*

After a myocardial infarction, the area of the heart that has been damaged can no longer function and usually turns into scar tissue. The undamaged part of the heart muscle must then compensate (take over) for the part of the heart that has died. This can increase the workload on the part of the heart that is still able to function. See Chapter 8 for warning signs of an MI.

After a myocardial infarction, cardiac rehabilitation is usually ordered. Cardiac rehabilitation may continue for a period of a few months up to six months or more. This comprehensive program consists of a variety of components, including the following:

- A low-cholesterol, low-fat, and low-sodium diet may be ordered. A dietician or nutritionist helps plan the diet.

- Most residents will be placed on a regular exercise program. The exercise program usually starts slowly, advancing to a higher level of exercise. The person's cardiac system, including the pulse and blood pressure, will be closely monitored during these exercise sessions. In some cases, the person's heart will have to be monitored during the exercise sessions.

- Medications to regulate the heart rate and blood pressure may be prescribed.

- Stopping smoking will be encouraged.

- A stress management program may be initiated to help reduce stress levels.

- Residents recovering from MIs may be told to avoid cold temperatures.

> **Tip**
>
> **Do not ignore shortness of breath or chest pain.**
>
> If a resident complains of shortness of breath or chest pain, report these signs to the nurse immediately. See Chapter 8 for more warning signs of a myocardial infarction.

Peripheral Vascular Disease (PVD)

Peripheral vascular disease (PVD) is a condition in which the blood supply to the legs, feet, arms, or hands is decreased due to poor circulation. This is primarily due to a build-up of arterial plaque over time. Peripheral vascular disease refers to disease of the blood vessels; it does not include the vessels of the heart and brain. Other causes of PVD are a reduction in cardiac output (amount of blood being pumped out of the heart with each contraction), trauma, and inflammation of the veins in the lower extremities, called **phlebitis**. When the blood supply is reduced, the oxygen supply is reduced, causing damage to tissues.

The most common type of PVD is peripheral arterial disease (PAD). It is similar to coronary artery disease. A blockage is created by arterial plaques that build up in the artery walls. Blood circulation decreases, mostly in the arteries leading to the kidneys, stomach, arms, legs, and feet. The pain associated with PAD occurs because there is not enough blood supply to the muscles during exercise. This decreased blood flow causes the pain or cramping in the legs that is the most common symptom of PAD.

Signs and symptoms of PVD include:

- Painful cramping in the hips, thighs, or calves when walking, climbing stairs or doing other exercise
- Painful cramping in the legs that does not go away when exercise stops
- Cyanotic (blue or gray-tinged) hands or feet
- Bluish nailbeds
- Arms and/or legs that feel cold or cool to the touch
- Edema (swelling) in the hands or feet
- Ulcers on the legs or feet, especially sores that do not heal
- Gangrene (see Chapter 18)

Identifying and managing the cause of peripheral vascular disease is done to improve circulation to the peripheral blood vessels. For example, if the cause is arterial plaque, a low-cholesterol diet may be ordered to try to prevent further plaque from forming. Many people do not show symptoms of PAD.

Nursing assistants can help by carefully observing residents for signs and symptoms or changes that might signal poor circulation. Following orders for weighing residents daily and measuring intake and output (I&O) is important. Residents must be encouraged to follow any ordered fluid restrictions and/or special diets. Be positive if the resident has quit smoking.

Observing and Reporting: Peripheral Vascular Disease

Report any of the following signs and symptoms to the nurse:

- O/R Resident complaints of pain or discomfort in his hands, legs, or feet
- O/R Any change in the hands, legs, or feet
- O/R Change in any vital sign, especially in pulse or blood pressure
- O/R Increase in edema
- O/R Weight gain
- O/R Intake or output change
- O/R Headache or any pain in the head or neck area
- O/R Complaints about the inability to see clearly
- O/R Any type of chest, back, jaw, or shoulder pain or discomfort
- O/R Disorientation, dizziness, or confusion

For some cases of poor circulation, special stockings are ordered to help prevent swelling and blood clots. These stockings increase blood circulation and help reduce fluid retention. They are called **anti-embolic** or elastic **stockings**. They should only be used with a doctor's order. Some residents should not use these stockings.

Anti-embolic stockings increase blood circulation by causing smooth, even compression of the legs so that the blood moves better through the vessels. Measurements are taken for these stockings so that the person is given the correct size. There are two styles: thigh-high and knee-high.

Each stocking has a seamed hole in the fabric around the toe or underneath the foot. This allows the skin color of the feet and toes to be observed. Cyanosis can be seen without taking the stockings all the way off. Carefully observe the toes for cyanosis throughout the day.

Using these stockings poses some risks. If the stocking is turned over at the top, the compression can double, causing the blood flow in the leg to be blocked. These stockings should be applied in the morning when legs are at their smallest size. It is more difficult to apply them later in the day. These stockings should be put on while feet are still elevated, before the resident gets out of bed. Follow the manufacturer's instructions for putting them on. Avoid causing pain throughout the procedure.

Putting knee-high elastic stockings on a resident

Equipment: elastic stockings

1. Identify yourself by name. Identify the resident. Greet the resident by name.

2. Wash your hands.

3. Explain procedure to resident. Speak clearly, slowly, and directly. Maintain face-to-face contact whenever possible.

4. Provide for the resident's privacy with a curtain, screen, or door.

5. Adjust bed to safe working level, usually waist high. Lock bed wheels.

6. The resident should be in the supine position (on his back) in bed. With resident lying down, remove his or her socks, shoes, or slippers, and expose one leg. Expose no more than one leg at a time.

7. Take one stocking and turn it inside-out at least to the heel area (Fig. 19-7).

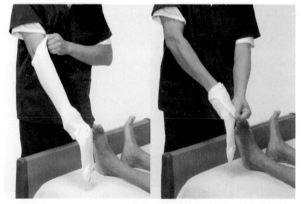

Fig. 19-7. *Turning the stocking inside-out allows stocking to roll on gently.*

8. Gently place foot of stocking over toes, foot, and heel (Fig. 19-8). Make sure the heel is in the right place (heel should be in heel of stocking).

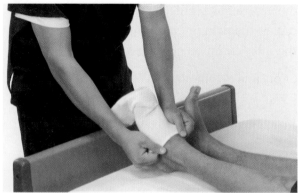

Fig. 19-8. *Place the foot of the stocking over the toes, foot, and heel. Promote the resident's comfort and safety. Avoid force and over-extension of joints.*

9. Gently pull top of stocking over foot, heel, and leg.

10. Make sure there are no twists or wrinkles in stocking after it is on the leg. It must fit smoothly (Fig. 19-9). The opening in the stocking that allows observation of skin color should be either on the top or the bottom of the toe area, depending upon the manufacturer. Check toes for possible pressure from stocking and adjust as needed.

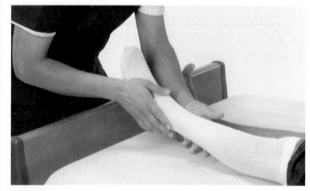

Fig. 19-9. *Make stocking smooth and twist- and wrinkle-free. Twists or wrinkles cause the stocking to be too tight, which reduces circulation.*

11. Repeat steps 7 through 10 for the other leg.

12. Make resident comfortable.

13. Return bed to lowest position. Remove privacy measures.

14. Leave call light within resident's reach.

15. Wash your hands.

16. Be courteous and respectful at all times.

17. Report any changes in the resident to the nurse. Document procedure using facility guidelines.

A **sequential compression device (SCD)** is a machine used to reduce fluid build-up, improve circulation, and prevent blood clots. A plastic, air-filled sleeve is applied to the legs and hooked up to the machine, which has an on/off switch. The machine inflates and deflates the sleeves on its own, causing alternating compression of the legs. It acts in the same way that the muscles do during normal activity (Fig. 19-10).

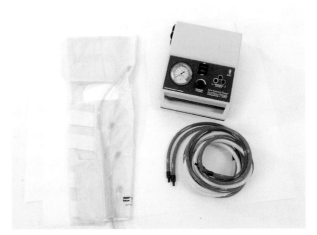

Fig. 19-10. A sequential compression device.

This method of therapy is sometimes used with anti-embolic stockings. A measurement is needed to order the correct size of sequential compression stockings. As with any electrical equipment, report to the nurse if you notice damage to any part of this equipment.

Congestive Heart Failure (CHF)

Coronary artery disease, myocardial infarction, hypertension, heart valve problems, or other disorders may damage the heart. When the heart muscle has been damaged, it fails to pump effectively. When the left side of the heart is affected, blood backs up into the lungs. When the right side of the heart is affected, blood backs up into the legs, feet, or abdomen. When one or both sides of the heart stop pumping blood effectively, it is called **congestive heart failure (CHF)**. CHF occurs when the normal cardiac output cannot meet the body's needs for activities of daily living (ADLs). Signs and symptoms of CHF include:

• Fatigue

• Reduction in the ability to exercise or be active

• Difficulty breathing, or dyspnea

• Shortness of breath, or **orthopnea** (shortness of breath when lying down that is relieved by sitting up)

• Increased pulse

• Irregular heartbeat

• Chest pain

• Dizziness

• Confusion

• Weight gain

• Lack of appetite

• Edema, especially in the feet or ankles

• Swelling in the abdomen (abdominal distention)

• Abdominal pain

• Increased urination, especially at night

Other symptoms may occur, depending on the side of the heart that is affected. In right-sided failure, the blood build-up causes swelling of the feet and ankles and can cause the liver and the abdomen to retain fluid. In left-sided heart failure, the build-up of fluid in the lungs causes shortness of breath. These are the symptoms of CHF associated with each side of the heart:

• Left-sided failure: fatigue, orthopnea, coughing, rapid pulse, and weight gain

• Right-sided failure: fatigue, weakness, edema of the extremities (especially the ankles), bulging neck veins, irregular heartbeat, and fainting

Congestive heart failure may be treated and controlled through medication and a care plan that encourages rest. Diuretics help reduce excess fluid build-up inside the body, thereby reducing edema. Other medications may also help the heart contract more effectively, which increases the movement of blood through the body. Certain medications improve the flow of blood, which helps reduce the workload of the heart. Nursing assistants can help residents with CHF by doing the following:

Guidelines: Congestive Heart Failure

G   Encourage rest and limited activity as ordered. Have the resident sit or lie down if dizziness or fainting (syncope) occur.

G   Measure daily weight and intake and output accurately.

G   Encourage residents to follow orders for fluid restrictions and low-sodium diets.

G   Use special stockings as ordered.

G   Provide extra pillows for residents who have trouble breathing while lying flat in bed.

G   Assist with personal care and ADLs as needed.

G   Assist with ROM exercises to improve muscle tone when activity is limited (Fig. 19-11).

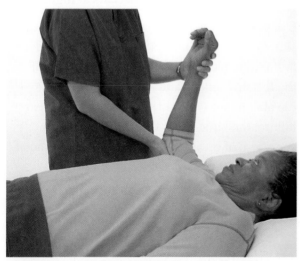

Fig. 19-11. Range of motion exercises improve muscle tone and help circulation. See Chapter 25 for more information.

G   Report any of the following signs and symptoms to the nurse:

- Dizziness, confusion, or fainting
- Fatigue
- Increased respiratory rate, pulse, or blood pressure
- Irregular heartbeat
- Palpitations
- Dyspnea
- Coughing
- Wheezing
- Chest tightness or chest pain
- Lack of appetite
- Abdominal swelling or pain
- Edema
- Weight gain from fluid retention
- Bulging neck veins
- Change in urinary output

Pulmonary Edema

In left-sided heart failure, fluid builds up in the lungs, which presses on the air sacs, causing shortness of breath. This can cause **pulmonary edema**. Pulmonary edema is a life-threatening condition; it can be caused by an infection or it can be a complication of CHF or an MI.

Symptoms of pulmonary edema include shortness of breath, wheezing, coughing, gurgling when breathing, anxiety, and restlessness. A person may feel like he is drowning. Emergency treatment is necessary with acute pulmonary edema. Oxygen will be ordered, and a ventilator may be necessary to help the person breathe. Other follow-up treatments include medication and cardiac rehabilitation.

Blood Disorders

Anemia is a condition in which the amount of red blood cells or hemoglobin in the body is less than normal. This prevents adequate oxygen from reaching the organs and tissues, a condition called **hypoxia**. Anemia is the most common blood disorder. It is diagnosed by a blood test.

Symptoms of anemia include fatigue, weakness, pale skin, problems with the tongue, brittle nails, and difficulty concentrating. A deficiency of iron (iron-deficiency anemia) is the most common form of anemia. Treatment includes a diet of foods rich in iron, vitamins, iron supplements, and methods to treat constipation that can occur with added dietary iron. If excess bleeding is the suspected cause of the anemia, other tests may be performed.

Pernicious anemia is a form of anemia caused by a lack of a substance that absorbs vitamin B12 from the digestive tract. This type of anemia is common in people over the age of 60. Symptoms include bleeding gums, problems with the tongue, rapid pulse, unsteadiness, shortness of breath, pale skin, diarrhea, and numbness and tingling in the hands and feet. Treatment includes monthly vitamin B12 injections, B12 given through the nose, or vitamin B12 pills, along with a well-balanced diet.

Tip

"The Gift of Life"

Have you ever considered donating blood to help others? The process does not take long, and this act can actually save a life. Think about calling the American Red Cross or another agency and donating blood. You'll be glad you did.

Chapter Review

1. What is the largest artery in the body (LO 2)?

2. What are the three different types of blood cells that make up blood (LO 2)?

3. What gives blood its red color (LO 2)?

4. What is the main component of plasma? (LO 2)?

5. List four functions of blood (LO 2).

6. List three normal age-related changes of the circulatory system (LO 3).

7. What four conditions can result from hypertension (LO 4)?

8. List three ways that hypertension is treated (LO 4).

9. How is the pain of angina pectoris commonly described (LO 4)?

10. List three care guidelines for a resident with angina pectoris (LO 4).

11. What are five components that may be included in a cardiac rehabilitation program after a person has had an MI (LO 4)?

12. What is the most common form of PVD (LO 4)?

13. List six signs and symptoms of PVD (LO 4).

14. List three ways nursing assistants can help a resident who has PVD (LO 4).

15. How do anti-embolic stockings help prevent swelling and blood clots (LO 4)?

16. When should anti-embolic stockings be applied (LO 4)?

17. List eight signs and symptoms of CHF that must be reported to the nurse (LO 4).

18. List six ways nursing assistants can help a resident who has CHF (LO 4).

19. List three common symptoms of anemia (LO 4).

20
The Respiratory System

Respiration and the "Vapours" of the Heart

Galen, an early physician and author of many medical works, studied the process of respiration. He formed a belief that respiration actually cooled a person's heart. Galen also thought that chest movement added air that helped get rid of certain "vapours" of the heart. Much later, William Harvey, a doctor and researcher, developed the primary theory that the lungs change venous blood to arterial blood.

". . . Full of sweet dreams, and health, and quiet breathing."

John Keats, 1795-1821

"Nothing to breathe but air.
Quick as a flash 'tis gone . . ."

Benjamin Franklin King, Jr., 1857-1894

1. Define important words in this chapter

alveoli: tiny, grape-like sacs in the lungs where the exchange of oxygen and carbon dioxide occurs.

asthma: a chronic and episodic inflammatory disease that makes it difficult to breathe and causes coughing and wheezing.

bronchi: branches of the passages of the respiratory system that lead from the trachea into the lungs.

bronchiectasis: a condition in which the bronchi become permanently dilated (widened) and damaged.

bronchitis: an irritation and inflammation of the lining of the bronchi.

chest percussion: clapping the chest to help lungs drain with the force of gravity.

chronic obstructive pulmonary disease (COPD): a chronic, progressive, and incurable lung disease that causes difficulty breathing.

emphysema: a chronic, incurable lung disease in which the alveoli in lungs become filled with trapped air; usually results from smoking and chronic bronchitis.

expiration: the process of exhaling air out of the lungs.

hemoptysis: the coughing up of blood from the respiratory tract.

inspiration: the process of breathing air into the lungs.

lungs: main organs of respiration responsible for the exchange of oxygen and carbon dioxide.

multidrug-resistant TB (MDR-TB): disease that occurs when the full course of medication is not taken for tuberculosis (TB).

oxygen therapy: the administration of oxygen to increase the supply of oxygen to the lungs.

pneumonia: acute inflammation in the lung tissue caused by a bacterial, viral, or fungal infection and/or chemical irritants.

respiration: the process of inhaling air into the lungs and exhaling air out of the lungs.

sputum: mucus coughed up from the lungs.

trachea: an air passage that goes from the throat (pharynx) to the bronchi; also called the windpipe.

tuberculosis (TB): a contagious lung disease caused by a bacterium that is transmitted through the air; causes coughing, difficulty breathing, fever, and fatigue.

2. Explain the structure and function of the respiratory system

The respiratory system is composed of the nose, nasal cavity, pharynx, larynx, trachea, bronchi, lungs, and alveoli (Fig. 20-1). The nose serves as the front line of the body's air filtration. Air enters the nose and moves through the nasal cavity. Nasal hairs are located in the nasal cavity, which has a mucous membrane lining. The hairs and mucus work to filter particles, such as bacteria and other microbes, dust, smoke, and pollen from the air as it moves through the cavity. These particles are then moved by the cilia, fine, threadlike projections that work to sweep away particles and fluid, to the pharynx, or throat, to be eliminated from the body.

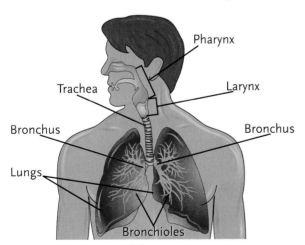

Fig. 20-1. An overview of the respiratory system.

The nasal cavity also warms and humidifies the cooler inhaled air before it continues along toward the pharynx. The pharynx allows for the passage of air and food. The air then moves through the pharynx down to the larynx, or voice box. The larynx is made up of nine pieces of cartilage, including the thyroid cartilage (often called the "Adam's apple") and the epiglottis. The epiglottis acts like a lid, shutting off the larynx during the swallowing process. This blocks food from entering the **trachea**, or windpipe, which can cause choking.

The larynx enables humans to speak. Exhaled air passes over the vocal cords and causes them to vibrate. Males have lower voices because they have thicker and longer vocal cords than females. This causes their vocal cords to vibrate more slowly, which lowers the overall pitch of their voices.

The trachea transfers air to the lungs. The trachea is lined with a mucous membrane. During the movement through the trachea, more foreign particles attach to the mucus, and the cilia there move the particles up toward the pharynx for elimination from the body.

From the trachea, the air travels into the **bronchi**, the branches of the respiratory system that enter into the lungs. The bronchi turn into the tiniest branches, called the bronchioles. These tiny branches end in the grape-like clusters called **alveoli**. These are known as the air sacs of the lungs. The exchange of oxygen and carbon dioxide occurs in the alveoli.

The **lungs** are large organs in the chest cavity. They are covered by a membrane called the pleura, which covers and protects the lungs. The pleura is made up of two layers that have a small amount of fluid in between them. This fluid allows the pleura to move easily without rubbing together as the lungs expand and contract.

The lungs expand and contract the chest cavity when we breathe in, or inhale (**inspiration**). Inspiration is an active process. Expiration is a passive process. The lungs relax and the chest cavity gets smaller when we exhale (**expiration**). The process of inspiration uses more energy than the process of expiration. **Respiration**, the body taking in oxygen and removing carbon dioxide, involves inspiration (breathing in) and expiration (breathing out).

Oxygen is a colorless, odorless, and tasteless gas that makes up about 21% of the atmosphere. Oxygen nourishes cells, aids in respiration, and provides energy for cell metabolism. Carbon dioxide is a colorless, odorless, and tasteless gas that makes up about 1% of the atmosphere. Carbon dioxide is a waste product produced by the cells.

There are two oxygen and carbon dioxide gas exchanges that occur in the lungs and in the cells. The exchange in the lungs is called external respiration. During external respiration, oxygen moves into the blood, and carbon dioxide moves into the alveoli. The carbon dioxide is transported from the alveoli when we exhale out through the nose and the mouth.

The second exchange of gases inside the cells is called internal respiration. During internal respiration, oxygen moves into the cells and carbon dioxide moves into the blood. The second exchange is now complete. The cells have oxygen, and carbon dioxide is headed to the lungs to be exhaled. This process of breathing air in and out is continuous; it never stops. Cells must constantly be filled with a fresh supply of oxygen.

The functions of the respiratory system are to:

- Serve as an air filter, cleaning the inhaled air
- Supply oxygen to body cells
- Remove carbon dioxide from the cells
- Produce the sounds associated with speech

Destination: Homeostasis

When the blood carbon dioxide level increases due to a stressor, the area in the brain responsible for respiratory control, the medulla, sends out nerve impulses. These impulses cause the diaphragm and the other respiratory muscles to contract more forcefully and more often. This is known as hyperventilation, or rapid and deep breathing. This increase in breathing blows off the excess carbon dioxide, thereby increasing the oxygen to meet cellular needs. When the carbon dioxide level returns to normal, homeostasis is restored.

3. Discuss changes in the respiratory system due to aging

Normal age-related changes for the respiratory system include the following:

- Lung strength decreases.
- Air sacs (the alveoli) become less elastic and decrease in number.
- Airways become stiff and less elastic.
- Lung capacity decreases.
- Rib cage changes and chest muscles become weaker.
- Cough reflex becomes less effective and cough becomes weaker.
- Oxygen in the blood decreases.
- Decreased lung capacity causes voice to weaken.

4. Discuss common disorders of the respiratory system

Chronic Obstructive Pulmonary Disease (COPD)

Chronic obstructive pulmonary disease (COPD) is a chronic, progressive disease. Progressive means that the disease gets worse. COPD leads to difficulty breathing due to the obstruction of the airways, especially during exhalation. Many people live with COPD for years. It is not a reversible condition and it cannot be cured, but treatment may slow its progression. Two chronic lung diseases are grouped under COPD: chronic bronchitis and emphysema.

Bronchitis is an inflammation of the lining of the bronchi. There are two types of bronchitis: acute and chronic. Acute bronchitis is caused by an infection. It is often associated with severe colds and usually lasts a brief period of time.

Symptoms include coughing, yellow or green **sputum** (mucus coughed up from the lungs), and trouble breathing. Acute bronchitis is generally treated with antibiotics and/or anti-inflammatory medications.

Chronic bronchitis is a condition that occurs when the lining of the bronchial tubes becomes inflamed. This later causes scarring. The irritation of these tubes continues for a long period of time, which then causes excessive mucus production. A long-lasting, mucus-producing cough occurs. Air flow may be restricted and the lungs become scarred. Lung infections can occur more easily when this happens. Chronic bronchitis is caused by cigarette smoking, second-hand smoke, and air pollution or other irritants in the air.

Treatment usually consists of reducing the triggers that cause irritation. Quitting smoking is encouraged. Medications may be ordered.

Emphysema is a chronic condition in which the walls between the alveoli (air sacs) in the lungs become over-stretched. The air sacs weaken and break. Air is trapped in the air sacs and normal breathing is impaired. Emphysema usually results from cigarette smoking and chronic bronchitis. Symptoms of emphysema include shortness of breath, coughing, and difficulty breathing.

There is no cure for emphysema. Treatment focuses on providing comfort and relieving symptoms. Quitting smoking is very important. Oxygen may be ordered to help with breathing. Medication and regular respiratory therapy, including breathing exercises, may reduce discomfort.

General symptoms of COPD include:

- Coughing or wheezing
- Dyspnea (difficulty breathing)
- Shortness of breath, especially during activity
- Cyanosis

- Chest pain or tightness
- Confusion
- Weakness
- Weight loss or loss of appetite
- Fear and anxiety

Guidelines: COPD

G COPD causes difficulty with breathing. Residents may be constantly anxious or fearful about not being able to breathe. They may fear suffocation. Be supportive and calm. Be empathetic. Not being able to breathe properly is very frightening.

G Use pillows to help residents sit upright or lean forward. This may help them breathe more comfortably (Fig. 20-2).

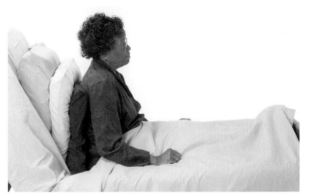

Fig. 20-2. *Using pillows to help a resident with COPD sit upright can ease breathing.*

G Be supportive of residents who are quitting smoking.

G Encourage a healthy diet.

G Offer plenty of fluids, as long as resident does not have a fluid restriction.

G Encourage periods of rest. Try to get residents to save their energy for important tasks.

G Use proper infection prevention practices. Wash your hands often and help residents do the same, if help is needed. Dispose of used tissues promptly in the nearest no-touch waste container.

G Colds can make COPD worse. Report signs and symptoms of colds or the flu immediately to the nurse.

G Medications that relax the air passages may be prescribed. These may be taken orally or inhaled directly into the lungs using sprays or inhalers. It is important for residents to take medications as ordered.

G Oxygen must be supplied to the resident exactly as ordered. Follow safety guidelines for oxygen therapy (see Chapter 7).

G Report any of the following signs and symptoms to the nurse:

- Fever
- Confusion or changes in mental state
- Refusal to take ordered medications
- Change in breathing patterns, especially shortness of breath
- Change in color or consistency of mucus or sputum
- Chest pain
- Inability to sleep due to anxiety or fear

Tip

Oxygen

When oxygen has been ordered for a resident, be alert for fire hazards, such as smoking materials, flammable liquids, and open flames, which can spark and cause fire. Remove fire hazards. Never remove an oxygen delivery system or adjust oxygen levels. That is the nurse's responsibility.

Asthma

Asthma is a chronic, episodic disorder in which irritants, allergens such as pollen or dust, infection, and cold air cause inflammation and swelling within the air passages in the lungs (Fig. 20-3). Exercise and stress can also cause or worsen asthma. When the bronchi become irritated due to any one of these conditions, they constrict, making it difficult to breathe. Thick mucus is produced by the mucous membranes, which further inhibits breathing. Air is trapped in the lungs, which causes heavy wheezing, coughing, and a tight feeling in the chest.

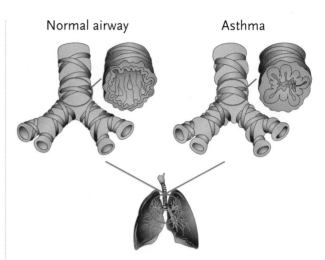

Normal airway   Asthma

Fig. 20-3. *When a person has asthma, air passages in the lungs become inflamed and swollen.*

The cause of asthma is unknown. Medications are usually ordered to treat asthma. Residents may need an inhaler with them at all times (Fig. 20-4). Encourage residents to carry their inhalers. Help them avoid the triggers that cause asthma attacks. For example, a resident with asthma should not be exposed to strong-smelling cleaning agents or heavy perfume. Smoking and second-hand smoke should be avoided as much as possible. Because stress is a trigger for asthma attacks, reducing stress levels can help. Talking with and listening to residents may help decrease stress levels.

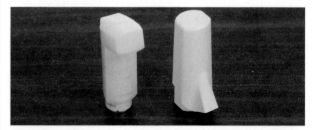

Fig. 20-4. *Encourage residents with asthma to carry their inhalers at all times.*

Observing and Reporting: Asthma

Report any of the following signs and symptoms to the nurse:

O/R Changes in vital signs, especially respiratory rate or pulse

O/R Wheezing, shortness of breath, or dyspnea

- %R Cyanosis
- %R Chest pain or tightness
- %R Refusal to use inhaler when needed

Bronchiectasis

Bronchiectasis is a condition in which the bronchi become permanently dilated (widened) and damaged. A person may be born with this disorder, or may develop it later. Bronchiectasis is caused by an infection of the airways. Cystic fibrosis is a cause of bronchiectasis. Tumors or inhaling foreign material can also cause this problem.

Bronchiectasis is a serious illness that can result in chronic coughing, shortness of breath, wheezing, weight loss, cyanosis, and coughing up blood. Respiratory infections may occur. Over time, foul-smelling sputum may cause halitosis, or bad breath.

Treatment includes proper positioning for drainage (postural drainage) and **chest percussion** (clapping the chest to help the lungs drain with the force of gravity). Recognizing infections early can reduce the severity of the condition. Report fever, chest pain, and a change in mucus or phlegm production to the nurse right away. Prompt treatment of infections will reduce the risk of complications.

Pneumonia

Pneumonia is an inflammation of the lungs caused by a viral, bacterial, or fungal infection and/or chemical irritants. The air sacs in the lungs fill with pus and other liquid.

The person usually develops a high fever, chest pain, especially when inhaling, coughing, difficulty breathing, shortness of breath, chills, and a rapid pulse. Thick secretions may be coughed up from the lungs.

People with weaker immune systems, such as young children and the elderly, are at a higher risk of developing pneumonia. Pneumonia can be a serious and potentially fatal disease, es-pecially for the elderly, who may take longer to recover. Treatment includes antibiotics and other medications, along with an inhaler. A special diet and increased fluid intake may be ordered.

Report to the nurse if a resident says he is not taking his prescribed medication. Encourage proper diet and fluid intake. Report complaints of pain promptly.

Tuberculosis (TB)

Tuberculosis, or TB, is a highly contagious lung disease caused by a bacterium that is carried on mucous droplets suspended in the air. TB is an airborne disease. People can be exposed to TB when they spend time with a person who is infected with TB. The infected person can spread the disease by coughing, breathing, singing, sneezing, or even laughing.

TB usually infects the lungs, causing coughing, difficulty breathing, fever, and fatigue. TB can be cured by taking all prescribed medication. However, if left untreated, TB may cause death.

There are two types of TB: latent TB, also called TB infection, and active TB, also called TB disease. Someone with latent TB (TB infection) carries the disease but does not show symptoms and cannot infect others. A person with active TB (TB disease) shows symptoms of the disease and can spread TB to others. Latent TB can progress to active TB. Signs and symptoms of TB include:

- Fatigue
- Loss of appetite
- Weight loss
- Slight fever and chills
- Night sweats
- Prolonged coughing
- Coughing up blood (**hemoptysis**)
- Chest pain
- Shortness of breath
- Dyspnea

Tuberculosis is more likely to be spread in areas with poor ventilation or small, confined spaces. People are more likely to get active TB (TB disease) if their immune systems are weakened by illness, malnutrition, cancer, HIV/AIDS, alcoholism, or drug abuse.

Multidrug-resistant TB (MDR-TB) is a form of tuberculosis that can develop when a person infected with TB does not take all of his prescribed medication. When the full course of proper medication is not taken, bacteria that is resistant to medication remains in the body. This means that this bacteria is less likely to be killed by medication used to treat TB. The disease then becomes more difficult to cure.

Residents who have active TB are often isolated in an airborne infection isolation room (AIIR). Air within the room is carefully controlled so that the air in the room flows directly into the outside air or is directed through special HEPA filters before being returned to the air-handling system.

Doors to an airborne infection isolation room must remain closed, except when people are entering and leaving the room. It is important to prevent contaminated room air from entering the hallways. You will be instructed on how to properly enter and exit this type of isolation room. A sign will be placed outside the room that identifies the room as an AIIR and the need for Airborne Precautions. If you believe that an AIIR system is not working properly, inform the nurse immediately.

Guidelines: Tuberculosis

G Follow Standard Precautions and Airborne Precautions.

G Wear personal protective equipment (PPE) as instructed during care. Use an N-95, PFR-95, or HEPA respirator mask to provide care (Chapter 6) (Fig. 20-5).

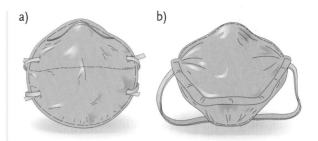

a)   b)

Fig. 20-5. a) An illustration of an N-95 respirator mask and b) an illustration of a PFR-95 respirator mask.

G Be careful when handling sputum.

G Resident must take all of the medication prescribed. Failure to take all medication is a major factor in the spread of TB.

Trivia

The History of the Mask

Masks were first regularly used when practicing medicine during the 1940s and 1950s. It is hard to believe, but many surgeons left their noses uncovered and wore masks only over their mouths. If only they had known . . .

5. Describe oxygen delivery

Every living cell in the human body needs oxygen to survive. The oxygen level in the air is adequate for most people. However, when a person has low oxygen levels, supplemental oxygen is required. **Oxygen therapy** is the administration of oxygen to increase the supply of oxygen to the lungs.

You learned about safety guidelines for oxygen use in Chapter 7. There are different ways to deliver additional oxygen to a person. Oxygen may be piped into a room at a healthcare facility from a wall outlet. Compressed oxygen comes in large cylinders or smaller, portable cylinders, which do not require electricity. Liquid oxygen in special reservoirs can be used in facilities and is also supplied in special containers for use in the home and the community. The liquid oxygen warms and becomes a gas that the person can then breathe. Oxygen concentrators are machines that run by electricity, removing oxygen from the air and storing it for use.

The doctor determines which oxygen delivery device is the best for a resident who needs additional oxygen. Oxygen is considered a drug and cannot be adjusted by nursing assistants. Common types of oxygen delivery devices include the following:

Nasal cannula: This device has a set of two prongs which are placed into the nostrils, and a plastic tube that fits behind the ears (Fig. 20-6). The tubing is attached to the oxygen delivery source, which is generally a wall outlet. A small plastic slide moves up and down on the tubing below the chin and adjusts it for comfort and stability. A nasal cannula is the simplest oxygen delivery device. It is a low-flow oxygen delivery system. This is the device you will see most often in long-term care.

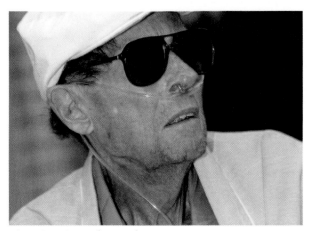

Fig. 20-6. A nasal cannula.

Simple face mask: This plastic device is shaped to fit over the nose and mouth. It is held in place with an elastic band that slides over the head and above the ears. The band can be adjusted for comfort and stability. The person breathes in through the nose and mouth, and oxygen is delivered. Plastic tubing connects the mask to the oxygen source. Simple face masks deliver low-flow oxygen. These masks can irritate the skin and may feel hot and cause claustrophobia. Masks can prevent a person from talking and eating normally.

Oxygen concentrator: An oxygen concentrator filters oxygen from normal room air. It delivers low-flow oxygen. It is generally used in conjunction with a nasal cannula. The cannula is placed on the person and is then attached to the oxygen concentrator. Oxygen concentrators are quiet and efficient. They can either be larger units that remain in a room, or smaller, portable ones that can be used when leaving the facility or the home. Oxygen concentrators plug in to electrical outlets and are generally not usable during power outages.

Guidelines: Care of the Resident using Oxygen

G   Perform frequent skin care on areas of the face where the oxygen device rests, such as by the nose, behind the ears and around the mouth.

G   Observe for redness, sores, bruising or discomfort in the ear, nose, mouth, or chin area.

G   Lubricate sensitive areas on the nose and mouth using water-based lubricants. Do not use any petroleum products on the tubing; oil-based lubricants can be a fire hazard.

G   Take vital signs as ordered.

G   Check the oxygen delivery device often for proper fit and comfort.

G   Notify the nurse if the oxygen equipment does not seem to be working. Tell the nurse if the tubing is clogged or dirty and/or if the tank level drops to the point where replacement is needed.

G   Post "No Smoking" and "Oxygen in Use" signs. These should be posted on each door and over the resident's bed. Do not allow smoking or open flames anywhere around oxygen equipment.

G   Know the location of the fire alarms and fire extinguishers.

G   Add pillows as needed to improve breathing.

G   Encourage activity as permitted so resident does not withdraw or feel isolated.

G   Provide emotional support; some oxygen delivery devices are difficult to use and can cause claustrophobic feelings.

G   If you notice any of the following, notify the nurse:

- Sores or crusts on nasal area

- Dry and/or reddened areas on the skin by the ears, nose, mouth or chin

- Complaints of discomfort or pain

- Shortness of breath

- Changes in vital signs, especially respiratory rate or pulse

- Cyanosis or any change in skin, nail, or mucous membrane color

- Chest pain or tightness

Residents who are using oxygen will need it either continuously or periodically. Continuous oxygen means the oxygen must be on at all times.

Tip

Portable Oxygen Tanks

When you are caring for anyone using an oxygen concentrator, it is important to have a portable oxygen tank available in case of a power outage. The stem of a tank must not be damaged. Portable tanks should always be kept in an upright position and in a proper oxygen cylinder holder when in use or when stored. Certain staff members are trained to use portable oxygen tanks. These devices must be quickly hooked up during emergencies. You may be trained to do this procedure only in cases of emergency.

6. Describe how to collect a sputum specimen

It is sometimes necessary to collect a specimen of mucus that comes from inside the respiratory system for testing. Sputum is not the same as saliva, which comes from the salivary glands inside the mouth. Sputum may show evidence of cancer or bacteria. The lab will study the sputum, looking for abnormal cells, microorganisms, or blood.

Some facilities allow nursing assistants to collect sputum specimens. Early morning is the best time to collect sputum. When people are flat on their backs for an entire night, mucus tends to collect inside the respiratory passages. This makes it easier to collect the sputum specimen.

The resident should rinse her mouth with water before you obtain the sputum specimen. This removes any leftover food and any excess saliva. The resident should not rinse with mouthwash before a sputum specimen collection. Mouthwash kills certain kinds of bacteria and other organisms that need to remain within the sputum for analysis.

Collecting a sputum specimen

Equipment: specimen container and lid, completed label (labeled with resident's name, room number, date, and time), tissues, plastic bag, gloves, mask, emesis basin

1. Identify yourself by name. Identify the resident. Greet the resident by name.

2. Wash your hands.

3. Explain procedure to resident. Speak clearly, slowly, and directly. Maintain face-to-face contact whenever possible.

4. Provide for the resident's privacy with a curtain, screen, or door.

5. Put on mask and gloves. If the resident has known or suspected TB or another infectious disease, wear the proper mask when collecting a sputum specimen.

6. Ask the resident to rinse her mouth with water. Assist as necessary. Have her spit rinse water in the emesis basin, if she does not use the sink.

7. Ask the resident to cough deeply, so that sputum comes up from the lungs. To prevent the spread of infectious material, give the resident tissues to cover his or her mouth. Ask the resident to spit the sputum into the container.

8. When you have obtained a good sample (about two tablespoons of sputum), cover the container tightly. Wipe any sputum off the outside of the container with tissues. Discard the tissues. Apply the label and put the container in the plastic bag and seal the bag.

9. Remove and discard gloves and mask. Wash your hands.

10. Leave call light within resident's reach.

11. Wash your hands.

12. Be courteous and respectful at all times.

13. Report any changes in the resident to the nurse. Document procedure using facility guidelines. Take specimen container and lab slip to the designated place promptly.

7. Describe the benefits of deep breathing exercises

Deep breathing exercises help expand the lungs, clearing them of mucus and preventing infections such as pneumonia. Residents who have had surgery, such as hip replacement or abdominal surgery, are instructed to do deep breathing exercises to regularly expand the lungs. The care plan may include using a deep breathing device called an incentive spirometer (Fig. 20-7). Incentive spirometry encourages the resident to take long, slow, deep breaths. The spirometer provides residents with visual or other positive feedback when they inhale. A goal volume is set, and this rate is attempted for a minimum of three seconds. Regular use can increase the capacity of the lungs and strengthen the breathing muscles. It also helps clear the lungs. Do not assist with these exercises if you have not been trained.

When assisting with an incentive spirometer, use only the resident's personal device. Do not share incentive spirometers with other residents. The spirometer should be labeled with the resident's name.

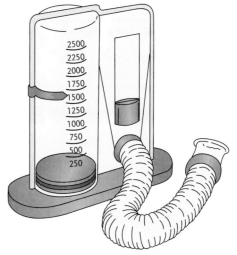

Fig. 20-7. *Incentive spirometers are used for deep breathing exercises.*

Make sure both you and the resident wash your hands prior to using the spirometer. Don gloves before assisting with this procedure. If the resident has a respiratory infection, you may need to wear additional PPE. Residents may need encouragement to use this device. Be encouraging, but do not force the resident to use the spirometer. Report to the nurse if a resident refuses to do the procedure.

Clean and store the device after each use. The unit may have its own storage bag. Follow the care plan and the nurse's instructions.

Assisting with deep breathing and coughing exercises

Equipment: gloves, pillow, tissues, emesis basin

1. Identify yourself by name. Identify the resident. Greet the resident by name.

2. Wash your hands.

3. Explain procedure to resident. Speak clearly, slowly, and directly. Maintain face-to-face contact whenever possible.

4. Provide for the resident's privacy with a curtain, screen, or door.

5. Put on gloves.

6. Position resident in the Fowler's position with a pillow over the abdomen, if needed. You may also be instructed to position the resident in a dangling position.

7. Ask her to wrap her arms around the pillow and hold the pillow tightly against her abdomen.

8. Tell the resident to take a deep breath and hold the breath for a few seconds.

9. Ask the resident to exhale for as long as possible through lips that are pursed.

10. Tell the resident to then repeat the deep breathing exercise a few more times. Ideally, the deep breathing exercise should be repeated five times in a row.

11. Make sure the tissues are nearby. Ask the resident to hold the pillow tightly, breathe in once deeply, and then cough as forcefully as possible. Collect any secretions with the tissues and dispose of tissues temporarily in the emesis basin.

12. Repeat the sequence above the designated number of times or the number of times the resident is able to perform the exercises.

13. Dispose of tissues in nearest no-touch receptacle.

14. Clean and store emesis basin.

15. Remove and discard gloves. Wash your hands.

16. Make resident comfortable. Remove privacy measures.

17. Leave call light within resident's reach.

18. Wash your hands.

19. Be courteous and respectful at all times.

20. Report any changes in the resident to the nurse. Document procedure using facility guidelines.

Chapter Review

1. What is the function of the epiglottis (LO 2)?

2. What does the larynx enable a person to do (LO 2)?

3. What is the process of breathing in and out called (LO 2)?

4. List three functions of the respiratory system (LO 2).

5. List six normal age-related changes of the respiratory system (LO 3).

6. Why might a person with COPD be fearful or anxious (LO 4)?

7. List eight care guidelines for a resident who has COPD (LO 4).

8. What are three ways a nursing assistant can help a resident with asthma (LO 4)?

9. Which populations are at a higher risk for developing pneumonia (LO 4)?

10. How is tuberculosis spread (LO 4)?

11. What is the difference between TB infection and TB disease (LO 4)?

12. List seven signs and symptoms of TB (LO 4).

13. Why is it important for a resident to take all prescribed medication if he has TB (LO 4)?

14. List ten guidelines for caring for a resident using oxygen (LO 5).

15. List five signs and symptoms that must be reported to the nurse when a resident is using oxygen (LO 5).

16. What time of day is best to collect a sputum specimen (LO 6)?

17. What conditions can require a resident to perform deep breathing exercises (LO 7)?

21
The Musculoskeletal System

Roentgen and the Discovery of the X-ray

On November 8, 1895, Wilhelm Konrad Roentgen (1845-1923) passed electric current through a tube and noted afterward that a specially-coated cardboard material nearby was glowing. He discovered that the glow came from the radiation coming out of the tube. He named the radiation "X-rays." One of his early X-rays was of his own wife's hand. The tremendous impact of this discovery was felt throughout the entire world. An amazing method to be able to see fractures and diseases of the bones had at last been found.

"And the muscular strength. . . has lasted the rest of my life."

Lewis Carroll, 1832-1898
from *Alice's Adventures in Wonderland*

"His bones ache with the day's work that earned it."

Ralph Waldo Emerson, 1803-1882

1. Define important words in this chapter

abduction: moving a body part away from the midline of the body.

adduction: moving a body part toward the midline of the body.

amputation: the surgical removal of an extremity.

arthritis: a general term that refers to inflammation of the joints.

bones: rigid connective tissues that make up the skeleton, lend support to body structures, allow the body to move, and protect the organs.

bursae: tiny sacs of fluid that are located near joints and help reduce friction.

bursitis: a condition in which the bursae become inflamed and painful.

cartilage: the protective substance that covers the ends of bones and makes up the discs that are found between vertebrae.

flexion: bending a body part.

fracture: a broken bone.

full weight-bearing (FWB): a doctor's order stating that a person has the ability to support full body weight on both legs and has no weight-bearing limitations.

joints: the points where two bones meet; provide movement and flexibility.

ligaments: strong bands of fibrous connective tissue that connect bones or cartilage and support the joints and joint movement.

muscles: groups of tissues that contract and relax, allowing motion, supporting the body, protecting organs, and creating heat.

muscular dystrophy: an inherited, progressive disease that causes a gradual wasting of muscle, weakness, and deformity.

non-weight-bearing (NWB): a doctor's order stating that a person is unable to touch the floor or support any weight on one or both legs.

osteoarthritis: a type of arthritis that usually affects weight-bearing joints, especially the hips and knees; also called degenerative joint disease.

osteoporosis: a condition in which the bones become brittle and weak; may be due to age, lack of hormones, not enough calcium in bones, or lack of exercise.

partial weight-bearing (PWB): a doctor's order stating that a person is able to support some body weight on one or both legs.

phantom limb pain: pain in a limb (or extremity) that has been amputated.

phantom sensation: warmth, itching, or tingling from a body part that has been amputated.

prosthesis: an artificial device that replaces a body part, such as an eye, hip, arm, leg, tooth, or heart valve; helps improve function and/or appearance.

rheumatoid arthritis: a type of arthritis in which joints become red, swollen, and very painful; movement is restricted and deformities of the hands are common.

sling: a bandage or piece of material that is suspended from the neck for the purpose of holding and supporting a forearm.

tendons: tough fibrous bands that connect muscle to bone.

total hip replacement (THR): a surgical replacement of the head of the femur (long bone of the leg) and the socket it fits into where it joins the hip with artificial materials.

total knee replacement (TKR): a surgical replacement of a damaged or painful knee with artificial materials.

2. Explain the structure and function of the musculoskeletal system

The musculoskeletal system is composed of muscles, bones, joints, tendons, and ligaments. The musculoskeletal system gives the body shape and structure. It allows the body to move and support itself. It also provides protection for the body and creates heat.

Muscles are made up of groups of tissues that help the body move by contracting and relaxing. They support the body, protect organs, and create heat. There are over 600 muscles in the human body. There are three types of muscles:

1. Skeletal muscles, also called voluntary muscles, control body movements by contracting and relaxing. A voluntary muscle is a muscle that can be controlled voluntarily, or at will. Skeletal muscles work together—one muscle moves the bone in one direction, and another moves it back. For example, the biceps are skeletal muscles that flex or contract when a person bends at the elbow.

2. Smooth muscles, also called involuntary muscles, make up the walls of organs, such as the bladder and uterus. Involuntary muscles are controlled automatically and are not under a person's conscious control. This type of muscle has the ability to stretch without putting a lot of stress on the muscle.

3. Cardiac muscles are involuntary muscles that are found only in the heart. The cardiac muscles contract and relax anywhere from 60 to 100 times each minute.

Bones are the rigid connective tissues that make up the skeleton, which is the framework of the human body (Fig. 21-1). Bones lend support to body structures, allow the body to move, and protect the organs. The outer layer of bone is hard or compact, while the inner layer at the end of a long bone is soft and spongy. Bone marrow lies within the spongy area of long bones. Bone marrow is responsible for the production of red and white blood cells and platelets. There are 206 bones in the human adult skeleton. There are four types of bones:

1. Long bones: the humerus (upper arm bone), the femur (upper leg or thigh bone)

2. Short bones: carpals (wrist bones), tarsals (ankle bones)

3. Flat bones: the sternum (breastbone) and scapula (shoulder blade)

4. Irregular bones: bones of the vertebrae (spine)

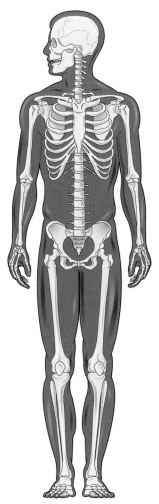

Fig. 21-1. *The skeleton is composed of 206 bones that help movement and protect organs.*

Joints are found at the places where two bones come together (articulate). The joints or articulations are structures that hold bones together and provide movement and flexibility. Joint movements depend on the way in which the joint is formed. There are three types of joints: immovable, slightly movable, and movable.

Examples of immovable joints are the bones of the cranium (skull). The joints of the skull

bones are called sutures. An example of a slightly movable joint is the joint between the pubic bones. The joint between the scapula and the humerus is an example of a freely movable joint. Other types of movable joints are the hip and shoulder joints, which are ball-and-socket joints, and the elbow and knee joints, which are types of hinge joints (Fig. 21-2).

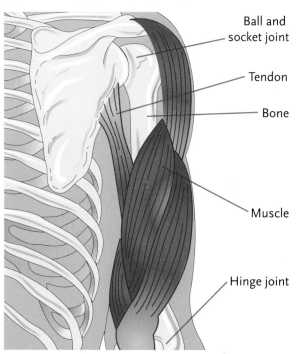

Ball and socket joint

Tendon

Bone

Muscle

Hinge joint

Fig. 21-2. *Muscles are connected to bones by tendons. Bones meet at different types of joints. Examples of the ball-and-socket joint and the hinge joint are shown here.*

Joints are found within a cavity or "capsule" that is lined with a synovial membrane. This membrane produces a fluid called synovial fluid that aids in joint lubrication. The ends of movable bones are covered with a flexible, protective substance called **cartilage** that allows free joint movement. Cartilage is also found in other parts of the body, such as the nose. **Bursae** are tiny sacs of fluid located near joints. They reduce friction during body movement.

Tendons are tough bands of connective tissue that anchor or connect muscles to bones. **Ligaments** are strong, fibrous bands that connect bones or cartilage and help support the joints and joint movement. Ligaments can become injured during sports or other strenuous activity. Torn ligaments can take a long time to heal following an injury.

The functions of the musculoskeletal system are to:

- Give shape and form to the body

- Maintain posture

- Permit movement

- Protect internal organs

- Store calcium and phosphorus

- Produce heat

- Produce some blood cells

Destination: Homeostasis

The musculoskeletal system helps to regulate the calcium levels in the blood. Bones serve as a calcium storage area. When blood calcium decreases to abnormally low levels, bones are alerted to release some of the stored calcium back into the blood. The calcium level then returns to normal range, and homeostasis is restored.

Tip

No swinging by the arms!

Pulling too hard on a person's arm can easily dislocate shoulder joints. Because of this, never jerk a resident's arm or attempt to lift or reposition a resident by pulling on the arm. Dislocations can cause extreme pain and may cause permanent damage.

3. Discuss changes in the musculoskeletal system due to aging

Normal age-related changes for the musculoskeletal system include the following:

- Muscles weaken and lose tone.

- Bones lose calcium, causing them to become porous and brittle (easily broken).

- Height is gradually lost due to shrinkage of the space between the vertebrae in the spine.

- Loss of muscle mass in the body causes weight loss.

- Joints are less flexible and are stiffer, which slows normal body movements and decreases range of motion.

4. Discuss common disorders of the musculoskeletal system

Muscular Dystrophy (MD)

Muscular dystrophy is a hereditary, progressive disease that causes various disabilities. With this disease, muscle tissue is destroyed, and the muscles atrophy. Muscle atrophy means the muscle wastes away, decreases in size, and weakens. MD causes muscle weakness, stiffness, and twitching of the hands and arms. People with this disorder may be confined to a wheelchair.

Muscular dystrophy is a genetic disorder caused by a specific gene. It generally appears at birth or during childhood. Duchenne's muscular dystrophy is a type of MD that is more common in males. Currently there is no cure for muscular dystrophy.

Guidelines: Muscular Dystrophy

G Allow enough time for the person to move about with braces or in wheelchair.

G Give frequent skin care to prevent pressure ulcers.

G Reposition resident often as ordered to help prevent pressure ulcers or contractures, which are the permanent and painful stiffening of a muscle.

G Perform range of motion exercises as directed.

G Assist with ADLs as needed. Encourage independence with ADLs so functioning muscles will not atrophy.

G If any of the following occurs, notify the nurse:

- Red skin, pale skin, or signs of the beginning of a pressure ulcer

- Stiffening of muscles
- Pain, swelling, or burning in a leg, especially the lower leg and the calf
- Symptoms of a urinary tract infection
- Signs of pneumonia, such as fever, chills, cough, and chest pains

Osteoporosis

Osteoporosis is a condition in which the bones lose mass, which causes them to be brittle and easily broken. Osteoporosis is caused by any one or a combination of the following: a lack of calcium in the diet, the loss of estrogen, a lack of regular exercise or reduced mobility, or age. Osteoporosis is more common in women, especially after menopause. Signs and symptoms of osteoporosis are low back pain, loss of height, fractures, and stooped posture (Fig. 21-3).

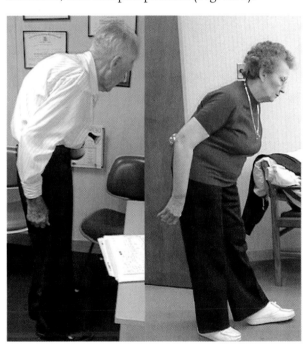

Fig. 21-3. Stooped posture, or "dowager's hump," is a common sign of osteoporosis. (PHOTOS COURTESY OF JEFFREY T. BEHR, MD)

Osteoporosis is treated with medication and exercise. Starting a doctor-approved exercise program and taking calcium supplements or other medications may help control osteoporosis. Some osteoporosis medications need to be taken weekly or monthly. The nurse may ask you to stay with the resident after she takes this medication to make sure she stays upright for the prescribed period of time.

Be patient and allow residents enough time to move. Reposition and transfer residents with osteoporosis very carefully. Follow special diet orders. Encourage ambulatory residents to walk; keep canes or walkers close by, if needed. Report to the nurse if you notice any decline in activity or movement.

> **Tip**
>
> **Fragile bones mean fragile residents!**
> When a person has osteoporosis, bones are weak and fragile. Bones can break with a simple movement. Movements that you take for granted, such as turning in bed, sitting down, or standing, can cause fragile bones to break. Be very careful when moving residents.

Arthritis

Arthritis is a general term for the inflammation of the joints that can cause pain, stiffness, and swelling. Decreased mobility may also result. Two common types of arthritis are osteoarthritis and rheumatoid arthritis.

Osteoarthritis, also called degenerative arthritis or degenerative joint disease (DJD), is a condition in which the cushiony cartilage that rests between the bones and pads the ends of the bones begins to slowly erode. The cartilage also loses its elasticity. Without the padding of the cartilage, the bones begin to rub together causing pain, redness, swelling, stiffness, and limited motion. If the condition worsens, the area may eventually become deformed. Osteoarthritis generally occurs with aging and may also be due to a joint injury. It usually affects weight-bearing joints, especially the hips and knees. Joints in the fingers, thumbs, and spine can also be affected. Cold, damp weather can increase pain and stiffness caused by osteoarthritis.

Rheumatoid arthritis is a form of arthritis that may become crippling. It affects a special membrane that lines the joint capsule, called the synovial membrane, causing stiffness, swelling, severe pain, and deformities that can be severe and disabling. Fever, fatigue, and weight loss are also symptoms of rheumatoid arthritis. The synovial membrane may eventually be completely destroyed. When this occurs, the joint becomes fixed and unable to move. It usually affects smaller joints first before progressing on to larger ones. Often rheumatoid arthritis develops early in middle age, but it can affect people of any age.

Rheumatoid arthritis is considered an autoimmune, inflammatory disease. An autoimmune illness occurs when the body's immune system attacks normal tissue in the body. A type of virus or bacteria acts as a trigger, which causes the body to turn on itself.

Treatment for arthritis includes rest and controlled exercise. Range of motion exercises may be ordered. Anti-inflammatory medications, such as ibuprofen, as well as other medications, are used to relieve pain. Weight loss can help reduce stress on the joints. Heat applications are often useful to lessen inflammation and pain. With a serious deformity, joint replacement can help.

Guidelines: Arthritis

G   Assist with the exercise program as needed. Encourage gentle activity and ambulation as ordered. Keep canes or walkers close by, if needed.

G   Perform range of motion exercises as directed.

G   Let the nurse know about 30 minutes prior to exercise if pain medication is supposed to be given beforehand.

G   Assist with ADLs as needed. Using assistive devices for bathing, dressing, and eating can promote residents' independence (Fig. 21-4).

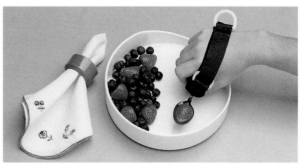

Fig. 21-4. *Special equipment can help a person with arthritis be independent.* (PHOTO COURTESY OF NORTH COAST MEDICAL, INC., WWW.NCMEDICAL.COM, 800-821-9319)

G   Encourage the use of handrails and safety bars in the bathroom.

G   Be positive and supportive. Listen to residents when they want to talk.

G   If any of the following occurs, notify the nurse:
   • Stiffness
   • Swelling
   • Pain
   • Reduced ability to perform range of motion exercises
   • Decline in activity

Bursitis

Bursitis is a condition in which the bursae (tiny sacs of fluid found near joints) become inflamed. The tissues around the joint may become painful, swollen, and tender. The shoulder, elbow, hip, and knee are joint areas that are commonly affected. Bursitis may also occur in the foot. Treatment for bursitis includes application of ice, immobilization to rest the joint, and the use of anti-inflammatory and pain medications. Removing fluid from the joint with a needle may be necessary. Cortisone injections may be administered. If the area becomes infected, antibiotics will be ordered.

Amputations

An **amputation** is the surgical removal of an extremity, such as a hand, foot, leg, or arm. Amputations are necessary due to disease, such as diabetes, which can cause severe circulatory problems. They are also performed due to cancer or injuries. Traumatic amputations are due to car accidents or an accident involving some type of machinery or equipment.

Limb amputations are performed either above or below the knee or elbow joint. The surgeon determines the extent of the removal of tissue. Some skin will be left in place to cover the residual stump. Post-operatively, the surgical site may be closed immediately or left open for a few days. A temporary prosthesis may be used until the permanent prosthesis is ready. A **prosthesis** is an artificial device that replaces a body part, such as an eye, hip, arm, leg, tooth, or heart valve (Fig. 21-5). It is used to improve function and/or appearance.

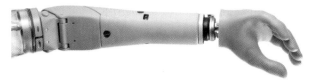

Fig. 21-5. *A type of prosthetic arm. (MOTION CONTROL UTAH ARM. PHOTO BY KEVIN TWOMEY.)*

A prosthesis is created specifically for each amputee. The prosthesis may take weeks to make and can cost tens of thousands of dollars. People who have stumps may require special, costly wheelchairs.

Prostheses for limbs are very lifelike and give greater movement and flexibility. People can walk, exercise, and do other activities, such as dancing or writing, with an artificial limb. Artificial eyes, or ocular prosthetics, dentures, and hearing aids are other types of prostheses.

Transplants of certain body parts are done on some amputees. One serious complication of transplants is rejection of the surgically-attached part. The person must take medication for the rest of his life to prevent rejection of the transplanted body part.

After an amputation, a person may feel that the amputated limb is still a part of his body. Three conditions that can occur following an amputa-

tion are phantom limb pain, phantom sensation, and stump pain. With **phantom sensation**, the person may have the feeling that the body part is still there. This involves sensations such as warmth, tingling, or itching in the area where the limb existed. **Phantom limb pain** occurs when the person feels pain in a limb (or extremity) that has been amputated. There is a variety of possible causes for phantom sensation and phantom limb pain. Causes include remaining damaged nerve endings, the level of pain the person had prior to the amputation, cold weather, surgery that was not performed correctly, scar tissue from surgery, stress, fatigue, lack of blood flow, infections, viruses, excessive pressure on the body part, swelling in the area, and inactivity. Phantom sensation and limb pain are real and should not be ignored or ridiculed. Medication or physical therapy may be used to treat these conditions.

Stump pain is pain felt in the area of the part of the limb that is still there. With stump pain, the prosthesis may need to be altered for a better fit.

Guidelines: Amputation and Prosthesis Care

G   A resident may have difficulty adjusting physically and emotionally to a new prosthesis. Residents may be depressed, sad, angry, or frustrated. Be supportive during the continuing process of adjustment.

G   Special positioning to prevent pressure ulcers is usually necessary. The doctor may order stump elevation post-operatively, which can help reduce swelling of the residual limb. The prone position may be ordered for limited time periods. Carefully follow orders for bed elevation and positioning.

G   Follow orders for positioning of the leg. Flexion, elevation of the knee, and crossing of the legs may be restricted. **Flexion** is bending a body part. Pillows cannot be used under or between the limbs.

G Assist resident as needed with ADLs. Occupational therapists may work with the resident to help with ADLs.

G Encourage activity as ordered. Check with the nurse 30 minutes prior to exercising to see if pain medication is needed.

G To prevent contractures and other complications, follow the exercise program exactly as ordered. Perform range of motion exercises as directed.

G Physical therapists will teach the resident how to bear weight on the prosthesis.

G Be very careful when handling prostheses and special wheelchairs. They are very expensive. This equipment costs tens of thousands of dollars.

G The nurse will demonstrate how to apply a prosthesis. Follow instructions to apply and remove the prosthesis. Assist the resident as needed.

G Apply special compression bandages and/or stump shrinkers as ordered to help with swelling. A stump shrinker is an elastic, compression-like bandage that fits snugly, but not too tightly, around the stump. Bandages should not be applied too tightly and should not cause pain. Stump bandages can be changed many times a day, as needed.

G Socks of different layers (for example, one-ply, two-ply, etc.), are used to cover and protect the stump before the prosthesis is applied. Change socks often and place seams on the sock to the outside to prevent abrasions, which increase the risk of infection. Make sure there are no foreign objects inside the socks before applying. Place used socks in a bag or hamper for laundering.

G Regular skin care is vital to avoid complications with the stump and the prosthesis. The residual limb can suffer complications, including trauma, allergic reactions to the materials used, and infections. Give careful skin care to the area under a prosthesis. Make sure the skin is always clean and dry. Report signs of skin problems to the nurse immediately.

G The prosthesis must be removed prior to going to bed. Bathe the stump gently. Use mild, scent-free soap and warm water (not hot). Avoid other products, such as iodine-based cleansers, because they can injure the stump. Clean the stump thoroughly and rinse completely. Use a soft, non-abrasive, towel to dry the area. If an abrasion, rash, or other problem occurs, avoid using soap. Ask resident not to use a sharp object to scratch the stump or the non-amputated limb. Apply creams to the stump area as ordered.

G Clean the socket of the prosthesis when it is removed. Use warm water and mild soap for cleaning. Use a soft cotton cloth to wipe and dry the prosthesis. Avoid using other products on the socket. Dry the prosthesis, especially the socket, completely. Leaving moisture in any area can increase the risk of infections.

G Before applying a prosthesis, make sure the area is completely dry. If you observe any complications in the stump area, report to the nurse immediately.

G Provide support for phantom pain, phantom sensation, or stump pain. The pain or sensation is real and should be treated that way.

G Do not react negatively to the stump or the prosthesis during care.

G If any of the following occur, notify the nurse:

- Redness or swelling of stump or extremity

- Drainage, bleeding, or sores of any kind on the stump or extremity

- Stump pain, burning, phantom pain, or phantom sensation

- Reduced ability to move extremity

- Cyanosis of any portion of the extremity

- Problems with the prosthesis

An Early Method of Amputation

Amputation was a very difficult procedure prior to the discovery of anesthesia. People requiring amputations experienced excruciating pain during the surgeries. Patients were often given alcohol to drink prior to the procedure to help them manage the pain. The surgical staff would hold the patient down while the amputation was being performed. The use of anesthesia allowed these surgeries to be performed without the severe pain.

Fractures

A **fracture** is a broken bone. Fractures are usually caused by some sort of trauma or accident. Fractures can occur spontaneously with diseases such as osteoporosis. Elderly people are more prone to falling, which is a common cause of fractures. Falling also contributes to other serious physical problems, including head injuries and soft tissue injuries. A fractured hip is a very serious problem that can occur with a fall.

Common signs and symptoms of fractures are pain, swelling, and bruising. The pain can be severe, and the area may be painful to touch. Pain may increase if treatment is not obtained soon after the injury. Movement may be limited. Bleeding can occur with some fractures. There are different types of fractures, including the following:

- **Closed or simple fracture**: The skin is closed. Bone is in proper position, and has not dislocated.

- **Hairline fracture**: The skin is closed. Bone has fine-line crack noted on X-ray, and has not dislocated.

- **Open or compound fracture**: The skin is open. Bone may come through the skin. The person has an increased risk of infection.

- **Greenstick fracture**: The skin is usually closed. The fracture is incomplete. Only one side of the bone is broken; the other side is bent. Greenstick fractures are more common in children.

- **Comminuted fracture**: The skin is open or closed. Bone has fractured in two or more places.

- **Compression fracture**: The fracture occurs in the spine. The skin is usually closed. Bone may break with trauma or without significant trauma. This fracture can be due to osteoporosis, tumor, or other condition. It is commonly seen in the elderly.

Preventing Falls

You first learned about fall prevention in Chapter 7. In addition to causing fractures, falls can contribute to other problems related to physical injuries, such as immobility, dehydration, and pressure ulcers. Falls can have psychological consequences as well, such as triggering fear, anxiety, and depression. If a resident is less confident, he may be unwilling to perform routine activities.

As the person who often spends the most time with residents, you play an important role in preventing falls. Make sure that pathways are clear and that there is proper lighting in rooms. Navigate stairs carefully, and point out any uneven or wet areas in walkways.

Keep hearing aids clean and encourage residents to use them. Reduce background noise when possible. Remind residents to wear eyeglasses. Encourage properly-fitting clothes (not too long) and make sure non-skid shoes or slippers are worn. Fasten straps and tie shoelaces. Assist with ambulation and encourage use of assistive devices when needed. Problems related to falls are often long-lasting and costly. Elderly residents take longer to heal from injuries. Preventing falls is very important.

Fractures are generally diagnosed with an X-ray. During the healing process, X-rays can be used to check on the success of healing. Fractures are treated by specialists. The bones must be set and allowed to heal in normal alignment. The joints above and below the fracture are immobilized.

New bone develops to heal a fractured bone. The ends of the broken bones need to be snugly set in order for them to heal properly. Bone healing can take four to eight weeks or longer. However, fractures can take even longer to heal in the elderly. When bones heal properly, there is a greater chance the area of the fracture will return to normal function.

Some fractures require a cast. Casts keep the fractured bones in place so that they may heal. Casts are generally made of fiberglass. Fiberglass casts dry very rapidly. The edges of the cast may need to be padded to reduce sharp edges. Special material may be used for this padding. The stocking under the cast can also be used to help pad the rough edges. Padding the cast helps avoid skin injury from the cast. Never put sharp objects inside a cast because they can pierce the skin. This increases the chance of infection in the area under the cast.

Guidelines: Cast Care

G Allow enough time for the person to move.

G Follow orders exactly on moving and repositioning. Tell the nurse prior to moving if pain medication is needed.

G Help with range of motion exercises as ordered.

G The extremity in a cast may need to be elevated to reduce swelling. Use pillows to assist with elevation (Fig. 21-6).

G Pad the cast edges as needed; ask the nurse for help with this.

G Assist with the use of cane, walker, or crutches as needed.

G Do not get the cast wet. Wet casts can lose their shape. If showers are allowed, tape a plastic bag around the cast before showering.

G Use bed cradles to reduce pressure from the bed linens.

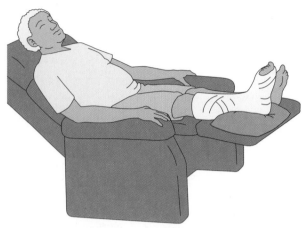

Fig. 21-6. *Elevating the extremity in a cast helps to stop swelling.*

G Keep cast clean. Protect the cast from soiling during elimination.

G If any of the following occur, notify the nurse:

- Numbness, tingling or increased swelling

- Cyanosis or pale skin

- Redness, drainage, bleeding, or sores of any kind

- Changes in temperature of the skin (hot or cold skin)

- Resident complains cast feels too tight

- Pain, burning, or pressure

- Wetness in or around a cast

- Odor around the cast

- Resident places sharp object inside the cast

A person may need physical therapy while the fracture heals and after the cast is removed because muscle atrophy and weakness can occur. Physical therapy helps return the limb to normal strength and function.

Sometimes a sling will be ordered to support an injured or broken arm in a cast. A **sling** is a bandage or piece of material that is suspended from the neck for the purpose of holding and supporting a forearm. A sling also helps reduce swelling by keeping the arm elevated. When a resident has a sling, make sure the arm is positioned comfortably and properly elevated.

Fractured Hip

Older people, especially those who have osteoporosis or a specific type of arthritis, are at risk for hip fractures. Hip fractures can result from falls or even from simple movements. If the bones are already weak, they can fracture easily.

Surgery is often performed on fractured hips. **Total hip replacement (THR)** is a surgical replacement of the head of the femur (long bone of the leg) and the socket it fits into where it joins the hip. THR may be performed due to a fractured hip that does not heal properly, a weakened hip due to age and decreased bone strength, or a hip that is painful and stiff and no longer able to bear weight. Once surgery has been performed, the resident will have a doctor's order restricting weight-bearing on that leg while the hip heals. The order will be written as partial weight-bearing or non-weight-bearing. **Partial weight-bearing (PWB)** means the resident is able to support some body weight on one or both legs. **Non-weight-bearing (NWB)** means the resident is unable to touch the floor or support any body weight on one or both legs. Once the person can bear full weight again, the order will be for full weight-bearing. **Full weight-bearing (FWB)** means the resident can bear full weight on both legs.

One of the goals of care for a post-operative hip replacement is to avoid dislocating the operated hip. To accomplish this, the affected hip may need to be kept in **abduction**, which means moving a body part away from the midline of the body. The hip that was replaced cannot be in **adduction**, which means moving a body part toward the midline of the body. If the hip is adducted, or moved toward the midline, it can dislocate, which can cause serious complications. A second surgery may be required, and each surgery an elderly person has to undergo can further weaken him.

An abduction pillow may be used to maintain proper position of the hip. This pillow will need to be in place whenever the resident moves or turns in the bed. For directions on the proper use of an abduction pillow, ask the nurse. You will learn more about abduction and adduction in Chapter 25.

Guidelines: Total Hip Replacement (THR)

G   Keep often-used items, such as call light, telephone, tissues, and water, within easy reach.

G   Follow the care plan exactly. If the resident wants to do more than is ordered, inform the nurse. Follow orders for weight-bearing.

G   Follow care plan regarding positioning and elevation of the head of the bed. Use abduction pillows as directed.

G   Assist with dressing the resident, starting with the weaker, or affected, side first.

G   Adaptive devices, such as a raised toilet seat, may be helpful for elimination (Fig. 21-7).

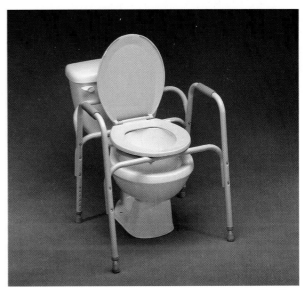

Fig. 21-7. *A raised toilet seat helps prevent excess hip flexion after a THR.* (PHOTO COURTESY OF NORTH COAST MEDICAL, INC., WWW.NCMEDICAL.COM, 800-821-9319)

G   Ask resident to use available handrails when moving into or out of a shower.

G   Encourage fluids to prevent complications of immobility, such as urinary tract infections and constipation. Using a fracture pan rather than a regular-sized bedpan may be easier for elimination.

G Assist with coughing and deep breathing exercises as ordered (see Chapter 20 for more information on these exercises).

G Apply anti-embolic stockings as ordered.

G Never rush the resident. Use praise and encouragement often.

G Do not perform range of motion exercises on a leg on the side of a hip replacement.

G Caution the resident not to cross legs in bed or in a chair or turn toes inward or outward. The hip cannot be bent or flexed more than 90 degrees (Fig. 21-8). It cannot be turned inward or outward.

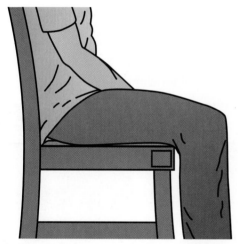

Fig. 21-8. *The hip cannot be bent or flexed more than 90 degrees.*

G Ask the nurse to give pain medication prior to moving and positioning if needed.

G If any of the following occur, notify the nurse:

- Incisions that are red, draining, bleeding, or warm to the touch

- Numbness or tingling

- Cyanosis or pale skin

- An increase in pain or a burning sensation, especially on the operated side or in the calves

- Edema (swelling) of the legs

- Fever or other change in vital signs

- Constipation

- Problems with appetite

- Resident is not following the doctor's orders for exercise and activity

Total Knee Replacement

Total knee replacement (TKR) is a surgical replacement of a knee with artificial materials. This may be necessary due to damage from injuries or arthritis or to help stabilize a knee that buckles repeatedly. The person may also need a knee replacement due to severe knee pain.

Care of a resident recovering from TKR is similar to that for the total hip replacement, but the recovery time is usually shorter. Residents may be better able to care for themselves. Promote self-care as much as possible.

Guidelines: Total Knee Replacement

G To prevent blood clots, apply special stockings or sleeves, such as anti-embolic stockings or sequential compression devices (SCD) as ordered (see Chapter 19).

G Special exercises may be ordered for the resident who has had a TKR. A physical therapist may perform these exercises. If you are asked to assist with these exercises, make sure you have been trained to perform them properly. Do not perform range of motion exercises unless ordered.

G Assist with coughing and deep breathing exercises as ordered.

G Encourage fluids to prevent complications of immobility, such as urinary tract infections and constipation.

G Ask the nurse to give pain medication prior to moving and positioning if needed.

G If any of the following occur, notify the nurse:

- Incisions that are red, draining, bleeding, or warm to the touch

- Numbness or tingling
- Cyanosis or pale skin
- An increase in pain or a burning sensation, especially on the operated side or in the calves
- Reduced mobility in the extremity
- Fever or other change in vital signs
- Constipation
- Problems with appetite
- Resident is not following the doctor's orders for exercise and activity

A device called a continuous passive motion (CPM) machine may be used for people who have had a TKR (Fig. 21-9). A CPM machine passively moves a specific joint repetitively through its normal range of motion. It helps to prevent stiffness and swelling that can occur postoperatively. It aids in increasing circulation. By continuously cycling through the knee's normal range of motion, it also helps prevent scar tissue and contractures from developing.

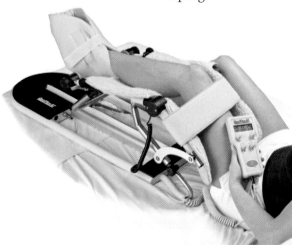

Fig. 21-9. *One type of CPM machine.* (PHOTO COURTESY OF THE MEDCOM GROUP, LTD., 800-231-4276, WWW.MEDCOMGROUP.COM)

A nurse or physical therapist will position the leg, set the machine rate, and turn on the machine. You may be asked to stay with the resident until the resident is comfortable with the movement of the machine. Notify the nurse if the resident complains of pain or discomfort or if the extremity moves out of proper position in the machine. The nurse or therapist will turn off the machine and remove the leg when the therapy has been completed.

Traction

Traction is a method of treating fractures by keeping bones in the proper position. Traction is also used to reduce pain and pressure or to relieve muscle spasms. Traction is used to treat a fracture by using weights and pulleys to keep the broken bones in proper position in order for the injury to heal. Careful observation of the resident is required to prevent complications.

Do not disconnect the traction assembly. Keep the resident in proper body alignment at all times. Make sure the weights are not touching the floor (Fig. 21-10). Do not adjust the weights on a traction unit.

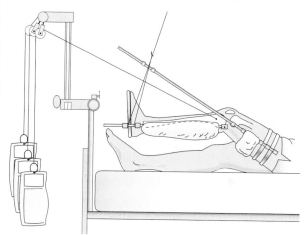

Fig. 21-10. *Make sure weights on a traction unit are not touching the floor, and do not adjust the weights.*

Observing and Reporting: Traction

If any of the following occur, notify the nurse:

- O/R Numbness or tingling
- O/R Cyanosis or pale skin
- O/R Wetness on sling
- O/R Odor around sling or boot
- O/R Sling or boot becomes loose or comes off or weights come off, touch the floor, or move
- O/R Pain, burning, pressure, swelling
- O/R Changes in skin temperature

O/R Redness, drainage, bleeding, or sores

O/R Resident moves to the side or slides down in bed

5. Describe elastic bandages

Elastic bandages, also called non-sterile or self-adhering bandages, are stretchy bandages that are wrapped around an injured body part. They are also referred to as "ACE® bandages," which is a common brand name for these bandages. Elastic bandages are used to keep dressings in place, hold splints in place, and provide protection, compression, and support for body parts (Fig. 21-11). These bandages are also used to decrease swelling from injuries and may be used to keep ice bags in place.

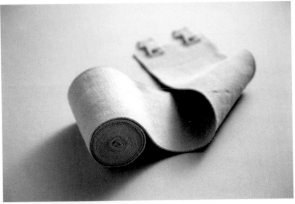

Fig. 21-11. *One type of elastic bandage.*

Elastic bandages must be wrapped snugly enough so that the proper amount of compression and support is provided. These bandages must be wrinkle-free and without twists to avoid too much compression to the area.

The bandage should not be applied too snugly, because it can interfere with circulation. Check on a resident 10 to 15 minutes after the bandage has been applied to make sure it is not interfering with circulation. After that, check on the resident periodically. Ask the resident to notify you if the bandage feels too tight or too loose. Report to the nurse if the bandage falls off.

Observing and Reporting: Elastic Bandages

If any of the following signs and symptoms of poor circulation occur, notify the nurse:

O/R Pale, gray, cyanotic, or white skin

O/R Skin that is cold to the touch

O/R Indentation marks on the skin

O/R Swelling

O/R Resident complains of the bandage feeling too tight

O/R Pain or discomfort

O/R Numbness or tingling

Applying elastic bandages

Equipment: elastic bandage in the correct size, clip, safety pin, or tape (if using self-adhering bandage, these are not needed)

1. Identify yourself by name. Identify the resident. Greet the resident by name.

2. Wash your hands.

3. Explain procedure to resident. Speak clearly, slowly, and directly. Maintain face-to-face contact whenever possible.

4. Provide for the resident's privacy with a curtain, screen, or door.

5. Adjust bed to safe working level, usually waist high. Lock bed wheels.

6. Avoid trauma or pain to the resident throughout the procedure.

7. Assist resident to get into the supine (flat on the back) position.

8. Expose only the part to be bandaged.

9. Hold the rolled bandage with one hand and, with the other hand, put the loose end on top of the extremity.

10. Wrap extremity, beginning at the spot furthest from the heart. Circulation returns toward the heart, and this allows extra fluid to flow to the heart and leave the area. (For the wrist, begin wrapping at the hand. For the ankle, begin at the foot.)

11. Wrap bandage once around the beginning spot, and turn over the tip so that an anchor is made (Fig. 21-12).

12. Wrap one more time around the spot where the anchor lies, and then begin slowly wrapping in overlapping spirals up the extremity.

13. Smooth out entire bandage, removing any wrinkles.

14. Secure bandage with self-closure, clip, safety pin, or tape. If using a pin, be careful not to pierce the resident's skin.

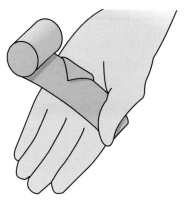

Fig. 21-12. Make an anchor at the beginning spot.

15. Straighten all of the linens.

16. Remove and re-apply bandage as directed. Wash and dry bandages as necessary.

17. Make resident comfortable.

18. Return bed to lowest position. Remove privacy measures.

19. Leave call light within resident's reach.

20. Wash your hands.

21. Be courteous and respectful at all times.

22. Report any changes in the resident to the nurse. Document procedure using facility guidelines.

Chapter Review

1. List the three types of muscles that are found in the human body (LO 2).

2. What are three functions of bones (LO 2)?

3. What are two functions of joints (LO 2)?

4. List five normal age-related changes of the musculoskeletal system (LO 3).

5. What happens when a muscle atrophies (LO 4)?

6. List three physical problems that muscular dystrophy can cause (LO 4).

7. List three causes of osteoporosis (LO 4).

8. What can happen to bones when they become brittle (LO 4)?

9. List three problems that arthritis can cause (LO 4).

10. List four treatments for arthritis (LO 4).

11. What are phantom sensation and phantom limb pain? Are they real (LO 4)?

12. List eight care guidelines for amputations and prostheses (LO 4).

13. What is a fracture (LO 4)?

14. Why is preventing falls so important for elderly residents (LO 4)?

15. Why should a sharp object never be placed inside a cast (LO 4)?

16. List three reasons why total hip replacement may be performed (LO 4).

17. What is the difference between partial weight-bearing (PWB) and non-weight-bearing (NWB) (LO 4)?

18. List ten guidelines for caring for a resident who has had a total hip replacement (LO 4).

19. List eight signs and symptoms about a resident who has had a total hip replacement to observe and report to the nurse (LO 4).

20. A person recovering from a total hip replacement should not bend or flex the hip more than ____ degrees (LO 4).

21. List two reasons why a total knee replacement is performed (LO 4).

22. Why should fluids be encouraged when a resident has had a total knee or total hip replacement (LO 4)?

23. List two reasons that traction is ordered (LO 4).

24. List eight signs and symptoms about a resident who is in traction to observe and report to the nurse (LO 4).

25. List six signs and symptoms about poor circulation due to elastic bandages to observe and report to the nurse (LO 5).

26. Regarding a muscle injury, what does the acronym "RICE" stand for (LO 5)?

22
The Nervous System

Galen and the Persian Patient

Galen was a physician who lived and worked in ancient Rome. He treated a man from Persia who had a loss of sensation only in certain parts of his hand. Galen determined the patient had fallen on his back and that caused the injury. He believed nerve damage caused the loss of sensation. Galen was amazed that the man could still move his hand. To him, this meant that different nerves controlled different parts of the body. In addition, Galen thought that an injury could affect feeling, but perhaps not always movement. This was a new and exciting idea at the time.

"The harvest of old age is the recollection and abundance of blessings previously secured."

Marcus Tullius Cicero, 106-43 B.C.

"He that wrestles with us strengthens our nerves and sharpens our skill . . ."

Edmund Burke, 1729-1797

1. Define important words in this chapter

age-related macular degeneration (AMD): a condition in which the macula degenerates, gradually causing central vision loss.

agitated: the state of being excited, restless, or troubled.

Alzheimer's disease (AD): a progressive, degenerative, and irreversible disease that is a form of dementia; there is no cure.

bipolar disorder: a type of depression that causes a person to have mood swings and changes in energy levels and the ability to function; also called manic depression.

brain: the part of the nervous system housed in the skull that is responsible for motor activity, memory, thought, speech, and intelligence, along with regulation of vital functions, such as heart rate, blood pressure, and breathing.

burnout: mental or physical exhaustion due to a prolonged period of stress and frustration.

cataract: a condition in which the lens of the eye becomes cloudy, causing vision loss.

catastrophic reaction: reacting to something in an unreasonable, exaggerated way.

central nervous system: part of the nervous system made up of the brain and spinal cord.

cerebrovascular accident (CVA): a condition caused when the blood supply to the brain is cut off suddenly by a clot or a ruptured blood vessel; also called a stroke.

cognition: the ability to think clearly and logically.

concussion: a head injury that occurs from a banging movement of the brain against the skull.

delirium: a sudden state of severe confusion due to a change in the body; also called acute confusional state or acute brain syndrome.

delusion: a belief in something that is not true or is out of touch with reality.

dementia: a serious, progressive loss of mental abilities such as thinking, remembering, reasoning, and communicating.

disruptive behavior: any behavior that disturbs others.

elopement: in medicine, when a person with Alzheimer's disease wanders away from a protected area and does not return on his own.

epilepsy: a disorder that causes recurring seizures.

farsightedness: the ability to see distant objects more clearly than objects that are near; also called hyperopia.

generalized anxiety disorder (GAD): an anxiety disorder characterized by chronic anxiety, excessive worrying, and tension, even when there is no cause for these feelings.

glaucoma: a condition in which the pressure in the eye increases, damaging the optic nerve and causing blindness.

hallucinations: seeing or hearing things that are not really there.

hearing aid: a battery-operated device that amplifies sound.

hemianopsia: loss of vision on one-half of the visual field, due to CVA, tumor, or trauma.

hoarding: collecting and putting things away in a guarded way.

intervention: a way to change an action or development.

irreversible: unable to be reversed or returned to the original state.

Meniere's disease: a disorder of the inner ear caused by a build-up of fluid, which causes vertigo (dizziness), hearing loss, tinnitus (ringing in the ear), and pain or pressure.

mental health: refers to the normal function of emotional and intellectual abilities.

mental illness: a disease that disrupts a person's ability to function at a normal level in the family, home, or community.

multiple sclerosis (MS): a progressive disease in which the protective covering of the nerves, spinal cord, and white matter of the brain breaks down over time; without this covering, nerves cannot send clear messages to and from the brain in a normal way.

nearsightedness: the ability to see objects that are near more clearly than distant objects; also called myopia.

neuron: the basic nerve cell of the nervous system.

obsessive-compulsive disorder (OCD): an anxiety disorder characterized by repetitive thoughts or behaviors.

otitis media: an infection in the middle ear that causes pain, pressure, fever, and reduced ability to hear.

pacing: walking back and forth in the same area.

panic disorder: an anxiety disorder that causes a person to have repeated episodes of intense fear that something bad will occur.

paranoid schizophrenia: a form of mental illness characterized by hallucinations and delusions.

paraplegia: a loss of function of the lower body and legs.

Parkinson's disease: a progressive disease that causes a portion of the brain to degenerate; causes rigid muscles, shuffling gait, pill-rolling, mask-like face, and tremors.

peripheral nervous system: part of the nervous system made up of the nerves that extend throughout the body and connect to the spinal cord.

perseveration: the repetition of words, phrases, questions, or actions.

pillaging: taking things that belong to someone else; not considered stealing.

post-traumatic stress disorder (PTSD): anxiety-related disorder caused by a traumatic experience.

progressive: something that continually gets worse or deteriorates.

psychotherapy: a method of treating mental illness that involves talking about one's problems with mental health professionals.

quadriplegia: loss of function of legs, trunk, and arms.

reality orientation: type of therapy that uses calendars, clocks, signs, and lists to help people with Alzheimer's disease remember who and where they are, along with the date and time.

reminiscence therapy: type of therapy that encourages people with Alzheimer's disease to remember and talk about the past.

remotivation therapy: type of group therapy that promotes self-esteem, self-awareness, and socialization for people with Alzheimer's disease.

rummaging: going through items that belong to other people.

schizophrenia: a form of chronic mental illness that may involve acute episodes; affects a person's ability to think, communicate, make decisions, and understand reality.

social anxiety disorder: a disorder in which a person has excessive anxiety about social situations; also called social phobia.

spinal cord: the part of the nervous system inside the vertebral canal that conducts messages between the brain and the body and controls spinal reflexes.

substance abuse: the use of legal or illegal substances in a way that is harmful to oneself or others.

sundowning: a condition in which a person gets restless and agitated in the late afternoon, evening, or night.

trigger: a situation that leads to agitation.

validating: giving value to or approving.

validation therapy: a type of therapy that lets people with Alzheimer's disease believe they are living in the past or in imaginary circumstances.

violent: word to describe actions that include attacking, hitting, or threatening someone.

wandering: walking around a facility without any known goal or purpose.

withdrawal: the physical and mental symptoms caused by ceasing to use a particular addictive substance.

2. Explain the structure and function of the nervous system

The nervous system controls and coordinates all body functions. It sends messages throughout the body and senses and interprets information from outside the body.

The **neuron**, or nerve cell, is the basic working unit of the nervous system. Neurons send and receive nerve impulses from the receptors through the spinal cord to the brain. Neurons are also involved in thought processes, directing the functioning of glands and the movement of muscles. The neuroglia hold together, support, and protect the neurons.

The nervous system is divided into two main parts: the central nervous system (CNS) and the peripheral nervous system (PNS). The brain and the spinal cord make up the **central nervous system**. The nerves connected to the spinal cord that extend throughout the body are classified as the **peripheral nervous system** (Fig. 22-1).

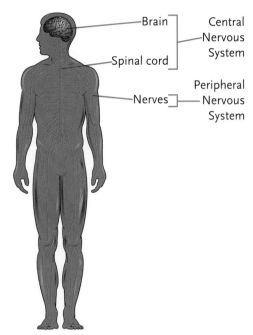

Fig. 22-1. The brain, spinal cord, and nerves throughout the body make up the nervous system.

The Central Nervous System (CNS)

The **brain** is housed within the cranium. It weighs approximately three pounds, which makes it one of the largest organs in the human body. The brain controls speech, motor and sensory activity, intelligence, reasoning, coordination, reflexes, breathing, emotions, and heart rate. It is responsible for memory and regulation of certain glands, such as the adrenal gland. The brain is divided into three main parts: the cerebrum, the cerebellum, and the brainstem (Fig. 22-2).

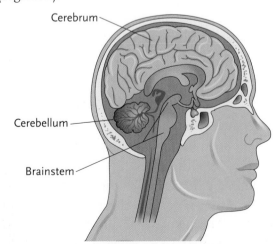

Fig. 22-2. The three main sections of the brain are the cerebrum, the brainstem, and the cerebellum.

The cerebrum is the largest section of the brain; it is the center of the brain where thought and intelligence exist. There are two sides, or cerebral hemispheres, in the brain. The right side of the brain, or right hemisphere, controls the motor activity on the left side of the body. The left side, or left cerebral hemisphere, controls the motor activity on the right side of the body (Fig. 22-3). The cerebellum is the center of coordination. It regulates the movements of the body and controls balance.

The cerebrum and cerebellum are connected to the spinal cord by the brainstem. The midbrain, pons, and the medulla oblongata rest within the brainstem. The medulla controls several major functions of the body, including breathing, opening and closing of blood vessels, and heart rate. The medulla controls swallowing, gagging, coughing, and vomiting.

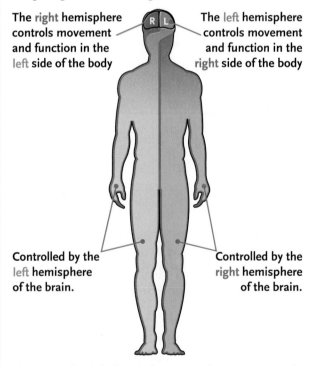

Fig. 22-3. The right hemisphere controls movement and function in the left side of the body. The left hemisphere controls movement and function in the right side of the body.

The **spinal cord** is located inside the vertebral canal in the spinal cavity of the body. It is about 18 inches long and is connected to the brain.

The spinal cord conducts messages between the brain and the body within its pathways. The spinal cord is also the center that controls the body's reflex activities. An example of a reflex activity is when you blink your eye because a particle of dirt has touched it.

The brain and the spinal cord are protected by bone. They are also surrounded by and suspended in cerebrospinal fluid (CSF). This fluid helps cushion the brain and the spinal cord from shocks, serves as a delivery system for certain types of nutrients, and eliminates waste products and toxins. Protective membranes called the meninges cover the brain and the spinal cord.

The Peripheral Nervous System (PNS)

The peripheral nervous system (PNS) consists of the cranial and spinal nerves. Nerves carry the messages to and from the brain from the rest of the body. There are 12 pairs of cranial nerves, and they have different functions. Cranial nerves direct aspects of the senses, such as taste, smell, and vision, deal with hearing and balance, and control certain muscles in the body.

There are 31 pairs of spinal nerves that emerge out of the spinal cord. Spinal nerves carry messages back and forth from the brain to the spinal cord. They also transmit messages to and from areas of the body to the spinal cord.

The peripheral nervous system is divided into the somatic nervous system (SNS) and the autonomic nervous system (ANS). The SNS helps with conscious movement of the skeletal muscles. The ANS has two parts: the parasympathetic and sympathetic nervous systems. The parasympathetic nervous system works to conserve the body's energy and provide for relaxation of the body. The parasympathetic nervous system is responsible for slowing body functions, such as heart rate and blood pressure.

The sympathetic nervous system activates the "fight-or-flight" response. This response occurs when a person faces excessive stress and must act quickly. The body prepares for "fight or flight," or fighting or running away, by increasing blood pressure and heart rate. This creates a surge in adrenaline (epinephrine), and increases the blood glucose (sugar) to be used for the needed energy.

The 3 Rs vs. Art

The left hemisphere of the brain is usually involved in a person's ability to do the "3 Rs," reading, writing and 'rithmetic, or mathematics. The right hemisphere of the brain is more involved in artistic and creative abilities.

The Sense Organs

The skin, tongue, nose, eyes, and ears are the body's sense organs. They receive impulses from the environment and relay these impulses to the brain.

Nerve endings within the dermis sense touch, temperature, pain, and pressure. Taste buds are found on papillae on the tongue. These papillae make the tongue bumpy. The nasal cavity is the receptacle of smell. Within the upper part of the nasal cavity, there is an area called the olfactory area. That area begins the process of sensing odors. It then sends messages to the brain where the odors are identified.

The eye is about an inch in diameter and is located in a bony socket in the skull (Fig. 22-4). The socket protects the eye and is surrounded by muscles that control eye movements. Within the eye are the receptors that function to allow the ability to see. The thickest layer and outer part of the eyeball is called the sclera, which is the white of the eye. The front part of the sclera is called the cornea, and it is transparent. It appears colored because it is positioned over the iris. The iris is the part of the eye that is genetically colored and gives the eyes their unique appearance. The pupil is the circular opening in the center of the iris, which dilates (opens) and constricts (closes) to adjust the amount of light coming into the eye. Inside the back of the eye is the retina. It contains cells that respond to light and send messages to the brain, where the picture is interpreted so you can "see."

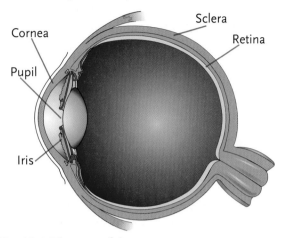

Fig. 22-4. *The parts of the eye.*

The ear is the sense organ that provides balance and hearing. It is divided into three sections: the outer, middle, and the inner ear (Fig. 22-5). The outer ear collects sound waves and directs them inward through the external auditory canal toward the middle ear. Hairs and earwax (cerumen) in the outer ear help protect the ear from foreign particles. The eardrum, or tympanic membrane, separates the outer ear from the middle ear. The middle ear amplifies and transfers sound waves to the inner ear. Tiny hair cells within the inner ear send nerve impulses to the brain.

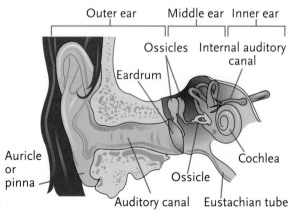

Fig. 22-5. *The outer ear, middle ear, and inner ear are the three main divisions of the ear.*

Hearing occurs when the sounds enter the ear canal. The structures of the middle ear trans-fer vibrations into the inner ear. This happens when the eardrum vibrates. The three tiny bones within the middle ear, known as the ossicles, pick up these vibrations and send impulses to the brain.

The functions of the nervous system are to:

- Control and coordinate mental processes and voluntary movements

- Provide reflex centers for heartbeat and respiration

- Sense and respond to changes occurring both inside and outside of the body

Destination: Homeostasis

To maintain homeostasis, the human body has to respond quickly to sudden changes in the environment. A reflex is a rapid, automatic response to a specific change in a person's environment. The body does not formally initiate its response; it is simply automatic. A reflex arc is the path that different types of neurons (nerve cells) travel in order to make the body respond to a sudden change or a stimulus. For example, if a finger touches a hot stove, the finger immediately withdraws from the intense heat. This is called a withdrawal reflex. Neurons send the message to the spinal cord that the surface is hot. Following the reflex, neurons return to their normal state until they are needed again. Homeostasis is restored.

3. Discuss changes in the nervous system due to aging

Normal age-related changes for the nervous system include the following:

- Responses and reflexes slow.

- Some memory loss occurs, especially short-term memory loss.

- Sensitivity of nerve endings in skin decreases, resulting in diminished sense of touch.

- Some hearing loss occurs.

- Senses of vision, smell, and taste weaken.

4. Discuss common disorders of the nervous system

Cerebrovascular Accident (CVA)

A **cerebrovascular accident (CVA)**, or stroke, occurs when blood supply to a part of the brain is blocked, or a blood vessel leaks or ruptures within the brain. An ischemic stroke is the most common type of stroke (Fig. 22-6). With this type of stroke, the blood supply is blocked. Without blood, part of the brain does not receive oxygen. Brain cells will begin to die, and additional damage can occur due to leaking blood, clots, and swelling of the tissues. Swelling can also cause pressure on other areas of the brain.

A hemorrhagic stroke, which is another type of stroke, occurs when there is leaking or a rupture of a blood vessel inside the brain.

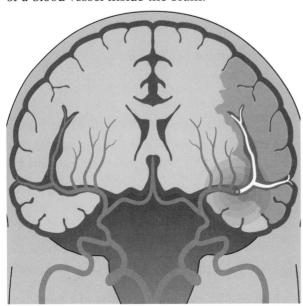

Fig. 22-6. *An ischemic stroke is caused by an obstruction of a blood vessel, which cuts off the blood supply to a part of the brain.*

A transient ischemic attack (TIA) is a warning sign of a CVA. It occurs when the brain loses a portion of its blood supply. The attack is usually quite sudden, and symptoms may last only a few minutes or up to 24 hours. Signs and symptoms that a TIA or CVA is occurring are listed in Chapter 8.

CVAs occur on either the right or left side of the brain. Blood flow is affected during a CVA and can cause brain damage and a variety of symptoms. Symptoms differ, depending on which side of the brain is affected. Strokes that occur on the right side of the brain affect functioning on the left side of the body. Strokes that occur on the left side of the brain affect functioning on the right side of the body. The following problems can result from right-sided or left-sided brain damage from a CVA:

- Hemiparesis (weakness on one side of the body)

- Hemiplegia (paralysis on one side of the body)

- One-sided neglect (tendency to ignore a weak or paralyzed side of the body)

- Loss of ability to tell where affected body parts are

- Expressive aphasia (inability to express needs to others through speech or writing)

- Receptive aphasia (inability to understand what others are communicating through speech or written words)

- Trouble understanding spoken or written words

- Emotional lability (inappropriate or unprovoked emotional responses, including crying, laughing, and anger)

- Loss of sensations, such as temperature or touch

- Loss of bowel or bladder control

- Cognitive impairments, such as poor judgment, memory loss, loss of problem-solving abilities, and confusion

- Changes in personality

- Loss of thinking and learning abilities

- Dysphagia (difficulty swallowing) or the total inability to swallow

- Vision impairments or blurred vision

- **Hemianopsia** (loss of vision in one-half of the visual field due to CVA, tumor, or trauma)

Tip

Left- and Right-Sided CVAs

Strokes can be documented in different ways. For example, a nurse might refer to a resident with a "right-sided CVA," but mean the person has a left-sided deficit (experiences symptoms on the left side of the body). A chart might identify a resident as having a "right-sided CVA" and mean that person has a right-sided deficit. Know how strokes are documented and referred to in your facility. This will help you provide better and safer care. If you are unsure which side of the body is affected, ask the nurse.

Guidelines: Residents Recovering from CVA

G Encourage independence and self-esteem. Use assistive devices when needed to promote self-care.

G Be patient with self-care and communication. Problems with speech and thinking abilities may make tasks take longer. Never rush residents.

G Encourage resting in between self-care tasks so as not to tire, confuse, or agitate residents who have had a recent CVA.

G Assist with range of motion exercises as ordered to prevent contractures and to strengthen muscles.

G Carefully assist with shaving, grooming, and bathing. Diminished sensation or one-sided paralysis causes a lack of awareness about such things as water temperature and sharpness of razors. Take care so that injury does not occur.

G Encourage fluids and proper nutrition to prevent unintended weight loss, constipation, and dehydration.

G Residents who have hemiplegia or hemiparesis will have a weaker, or affected, side of the body. Do not refer to weaker sides as "bad," such as the "bad leg" or "bad arm." When referring to a weaker side, use the terms "weaker," "affected," or "involved" instead.

G When assisting with eating, always place food in the unaffected, or stronger, side of the mouth.

G Assist with guidelines from the speech-language pathologist. Observe for swallowing problems. Thickening agents may be ordered to help with swallowing problems.

G Break instructions down into short, simple sentences. Use communication boards or cards to help make communication easier.

G Make sure a clock and calendar are visible to help remind residents regularly of the day and time.

G For one-sided neglect, remind residents often about the weaker side of the body.

G Assist with ambulation to prevent falls. When transferring, stand on and support the weaker side of the body. Lead with the stronger side. Use a gait or a transfer belt as needed (Fig. 22-7).

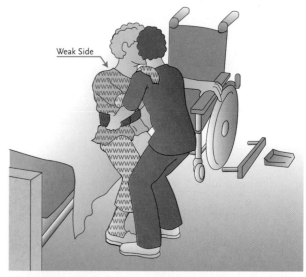

Weak Side

Fig. 22-7. When helping a resident transfer, support the weak side. Lead with the stronger side.

G Reposition often to help prevent pressure ulcers and contractures. Position in proper alignment using special positioning devices, when necessary.

G With emotional lability, a resident can cry for no apparent reason. Redirect the resident's attention, which will often stop the emotional outburst. Try asking a question or pointing out something in the room. Be patient and supportive.

G Use praise often, even for small successes. Encourage the resident's progress.

G Prevent withdrawal and feelings of isolation. Listen to resident if he/she wants to talk.

G Studies have shown benefits from speech, occupational, and physical therapy long after the stroke has occurred. Be positive and encouraging if residents have ongoing rehabilitation.

Many people have trouble with communication after having a stroke. The level of difficulty a person has depends on the severity of the stroke, as well as the resulting effects on speech and cognition. Use these guidelines to help communicate with a resident post-CVA:

G Speak clearly and face the resident when communicating.

G Do not rush the resident.

G Use signals, such as nodding the head and pointing, to assist with communication.

G Keep questions and directions simple.

G Use questions that can be answered with a "yes" or "no," such as "Would you like to eat your vegetables first?"

G Use special methods, such as communication boards, as directed (Fig. 22-8).

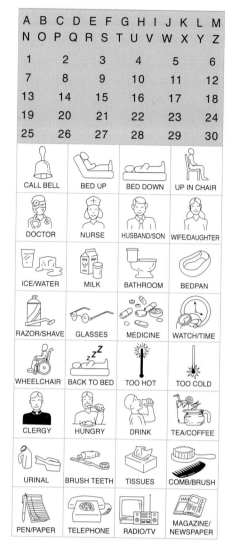

Fig. 22-8. *Communication boards can help make communication easier for residents who have had a CVA.*

Parkinson's Disease

Parkinson's disease is a progressive disorder that causes a part of the brain to degenerate. **Progressive** means that the disease gets worse with time. Neurons in the brain that produce the substance called dopamine, a neurotransmitter, begin to break down and die. This causes symptoms, such as tremors or shaking, that are uncontrollable. Tremors can make it difficult for a person to eat and perform other ADLs. This disease also causes a mask-like face, pill-rolling (moving the thumb and first finger together like rolling a pill), rigid muscles, and a shuffling gait, or walk. Speech may be affected, causing words to be slurred. Other symptoms are mood swings and gradual behavior changes.

Parkinson's disease usually begins after the age of 50. Drug therapy is one way to treat Parkinson's disease. Some people are candidates for surgery that can help reduce the need for medications.

Guidelines: Parkinson's Disease

G   Residents are at a high risk for falls. Assist with ambulation to prevent falls due to shuffling walk or gait.

G   Encourage resident to stand as straight as possible when ambulating.

G   Encourage self-care. Be patient with self-care and communication. Allow the resident time to do and say things. Listen.

G   Assist with ADLs as necessary.

G   Assist with range of motion exercises as ordered to prevent contractures and to strengthen muscles (Fig. 22-9).

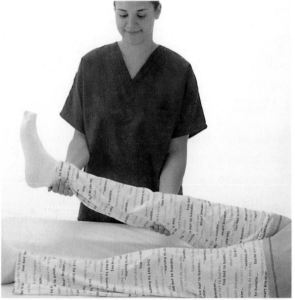

Fig. 22-9. *Range of motion exercises help prevent contractures, strengthen muscles and increase circulation.*

G   Encourage fluids and proper nutrition to prevent weight loss, constipation, and dehydration.

G   Help prevent depression. Listen to resident if he/she wants to talk.

G   If the following occur, notify the nurse:
- Severe trembling
- Severe muscle rigidity/contractures
- Mood swings
- Sudden incontinence
- Constipation
- Dehydration
- Weight loss
- Signs of depression

Multiple Sclerosis (MS)

Multiple sclerosis (MS) is a progressive nervous system disorder that affects the way impulses are transmitted to and from the brain. When a person has MS, there is a loss of myelin, the protective covering that covers the nerves and spinal cord. Without this covering, nerves cannot send clear messages to and from the brain in a normal way.

MS progresses in an unpredictable way. A person with MS will have varying abilities. Symptoms will vary as well, and may include the following (Fig. 22-10):

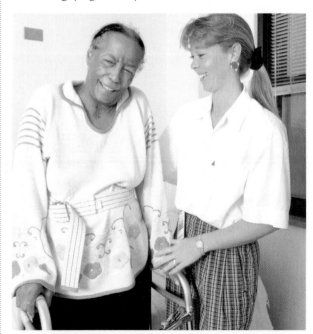

Fig. 22-10. *MS is an unpredictable disease that causes varying symptoms. MS can cause a range of problems, including fatigue, poor balance, and trouble walking.*

- Numbness and tingling
- Muscle weakness
- Extreme fatigue
- Tremors
- Vertigo (a spinning feeling)
- Reduced sensation
- Blurred or double vision, along with jerky eye movements
- Poor balance
- Difficulty walking
- Incontinence of bladder and bowel
- Paralysis in advanced cases

Multiple sclerosis is often diagnosed in young adulthood. The exact cause of multiple sclerosis is not known. It may be an autoimmune disease triggered by a type of virus. There is no cure for the disease at this time. Interferon is a substance that has shown some promise with people who have MS. New therapies are being tested all the time.

Guidelines: Multiple Sclerosis

G Assist with ambulation to prevent falls due to lack of coordination, fatigue, and vision impairments.

G Be patient with self-care and movement. Allow the resident time to do things. Assist with ADLs as needed.

G Offer rest periods as necessary.

G Give frequent skin care to help prevent pressure ulcers. Reposition residents at least every two hours.

G Assist with range of motion exercises as ordered to prevent contractures and to strengthen muscles.

G Do not rush the person regarding communication. People with MS may have difficulty communicating their thoughts.

G Stress can worsen the effects of MS. Be calm. Listen to residents, and try to provide a stress-free environment as much as possible.

G Encourage proper nutrition and fluid intake.

G Symptoms of MS sometimes change from day to day; offer support and encouragement.

G Prevent depression. Listen to resident if she wants to talk.

G If any of the following occurs, tell the nurse:
   - Red skin, pale skin, or the beginning of a pressure ulcer
   - The start of a contracture
   - Urinary tract infection symptoms, such as frequency or burning during urination, increased incontinence, or cloudy urine
   - Signs of depression

Head and Spinal Cord Injuries

Accidents, such as motor vehicle accidents, sporting injuries, gunshot wounds, stab wounds, or falls may cause head or spinal injuries. Head injuries are injuries that occur to the scalp, skull, or the brain. They can be open or closed injuries. A head injury that occurs from a banging movement of the brain against the cranium is classified as a **concussion**. A head injury that is a bruise on the brain is called a contusion.

A person can have a head injury and show few or no symptoms initially. Head injuries can cause confusion or disorientation, along with serious complications like coma and death. Other symptoms include headaches, drowsiness, loss of consciousness, seizures, noticeable fractures, drainage from the ears, nose or mouth, irritability, poor coordination, slurred speech, blurred vision, unequal pupil size, vomiting, a stiff neck, and a decreased sense of smell.

When a person sustains a spinal cord injury, it means that the spinal cord is cut or damaged in some way. Symptoms include paralysis and loss of function, depending on where the spine is injured. The higher the injury, the greater the loss of function. **Paraplegia** is the loss of function of the lower body and legs. It is caused by injuries in the thoracic or lumbar area of the spinal cord. **Quadriplegia** is the loss of function of the arms, trunk, and legs. It is caused by injuries in the cervical area of the spine (Fig. 22-11).

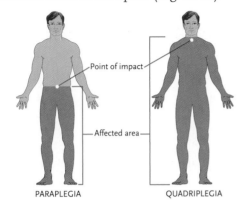

PARAPLEGIA   QUADRIPLEGIA

Fig. 22-11. *Loss of function depends on where the spine is injured.*

Spinal cord injuries are treated with some success if the cord is not completely cut or severed. The results of these injuries range from spasms, weakness, and difficulty coordinating movements to complete paralysis. Sometimes, rehabilitation helps a person regain some of his or her former abilities. In other cases, movement or sensation cannot be recovered. There is no current method to regenerate spinal cord tissue. However, research is being conducted that may prove successful in the future.

Guidelines: Head or Spinal Cord Injuries

G   Give frequent skin care to prevent pressure ulcers. A lack of sensation will prevent awareness that a pressure ulcer is developing. Change position every two hours or more often, if ordered.

G   Be gentle when turning and repositioning.

G   Perform passive range of motion exercises to prevent contractures and to strengthen muscles.

G   Allow as much independence as possible with ADLs.

G   Offer rest periods as necessary.

G   Help resident with bladder and bowel retraining as directed.

G   Immobility leads to constipation. Encourage fluids and a proper diet that is high in fiber.

G   Loss of control of urination can lead to the need for a catheter. Urinary tract infections are common. Give careful catheter care and encourage a high intake of fluids. Juices high in vitamin C, such as orange juice and cranberry juice, help prevent UTIs.

G   Protect residents from harm due to lack of sensation. Residents with paralysis are at a higher risk of injury from heat, cold, and sharp objects. Keep residents away from heaters, radiators, hot plates, or any other source of heat. Check for sharp edges or objects when repositioning residents.

G   Check water temperature carefully to prevent burns due to lack of sensation. Make sure hot drinks have cooled enough before offering.

G   Lack of activity can lead to poor circulation and fatigue. Use special stockings to help increase circulation as ordered.

G   Difficulty coughing and shallow breathing can lead to pneumonia. Encourage deep breathing exercises as ordered.

G   Male residents may have involuntary erections. Provide for privacy and be sensitive if this happens. Behaving professionally puts residents at ease.

G   Listen to the resident. Residents will need emotional support, as well as physical assistance. Anger, irritation, and frustration are some emotions they may experience while dealing with these injuries. Try not to take it personally, and be supportive.

G   If the following occur, notify the nurse:

•   Red skin, pale skin, or the beginning of a pressure ulcer

•   Start of a contracture

•   Urinary tract infection symptoms

•   Shortness of breath

•   Constipation

- Dehydration
- Weight loss
- Depression

Autonomic Hyperreflexia

People with spinal cord injuries can develop autonomic hyperreflexia. This is a reaction of the nervous system to overstimulation. While a healthy person can handle normal levels of stimulation, a person with a spinal cord injury may have an extreme nervous system response.

Increases in blood pressure, change in heart rate, fever, sweating, dizziness, muscle spasms, headache, and changes in skin color are symptoms that can occur.

When a person is experiencing this reaction, have him sit up and raise his head while you loosen any tight clothing. Medications may be needed for high blood pressure or changes in heart rate.

To help avoid this potential reaction, caregivers should control pain, prevent the bladder from becoming too full, avoid fecal impactions, and avoid pressure ulcers and infections of the skin.

Seizures (Convulsions)

Seizures are involuntary muscular contractions. They can involve a small area of the body or the entire body. Some causes of seizures are tumors, head injuries, medications, injuries to the brain during birth, high fevers, stroke, dementia, genetic factors, and alcohol and drug abuse.

Epilepsy is a disorder that causes people to have recurring seizures. With epilepsy, electrical signals within the brain are generated that cause seizures that recur.

Treatment for seizures, if the cause is known, includes medication. Surgery may be performed. For seizures caused by drug and alcohol abuse, rehabilitation can help. See Chapter 8 for more information on types of seizures and how to care for a resident who is having a seizure.

Vision Impairment

Vision changes can affect people of all ages. **Nearsightedness** (myopia) is the ability to see objects that are near more clearly than distant objects. **Farsightedness** (hyperopia) is the ability to see distant objects more clearly than objects that are near. Eyeglasses, contact lenses, or surgery can be used to correct these eye problems (Fig. 22-12).

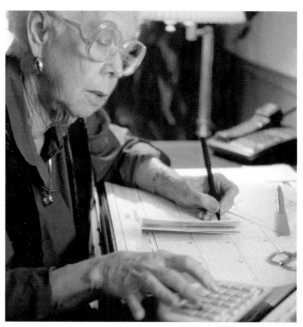

Fig. 22-12. Nearsightedness and farsightedness are often corrected by the use of eyeglasses.

Other vision problems include cataracts and glaucoma. A **cataract** develops when the lens of the eye, which is normally clear, becomes cloudy. Light is prevented from entering the eye, which causes decreased vision (Fig. 22-13). The first symptom is blurred vision. Other symptoms are glare when driving at night or a yellowing of vision. A cataract can eventually cause blindness in one or both eyes.

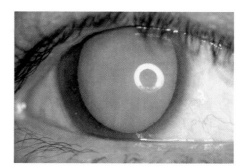

Fig. 22-13. When a cataract develops, the lens of the eye becomes cloudy, and light is prevented from entering the eye.

Cataracts may be inherited. They can be caused by diabetes or an eye injury, or they may just be a result of normal aging.

Treatment depends upon the level of maturity of the cataract. Surgery is usually performed to remove the cataract. The lens that has turned cloudy is removed, and an artificial lens, or lens implant, called an intraocular lens (IOL), is placed and remains there. The implanted lens is made of plastic or silicone. The eye must be carefully measured for the lens implant prior to the surgery. This implant is permanent; it rarely has to be removed. It is only removed when inflammation occurs or the implant moves out of place.

Glaucoma is an eye disorder which is the leading cause of blindness in the United States. The pressure inside the eye, called intraocular pressure, increases, causing damage to the optic nerve. This increase in the intraocular pressure can ultimately cause a loss of vision and blindness, if left untreated.

There are many forms of glaucoma. The majority of people have open-angle, or primary, glaucoma. Risk factors for open-angle glaucoma include elevated intraocular pressure, being over 45, family history of the disease, certain diseases and eye conditions, some medications, and ethnic background. All people with a family history of glaucoma should have their intraocular pressure checked regularly.

Symptoms of open-angle glaucoma may not be apparent. Over time, a person experiences a decrease in vision, especially in the peripheral vision.

Angle-closure glaucoma is a less common form of glaucoma. Angle-closure glaucoma can be chronic or acute. With acute angle-closure glaucoma, symptoms include pain, nausea, vomiting, seeing a halo around lights, reddening of the eye, and blurred vision. If not treated immediately, it can cause blindness very quickly.

Treatment of glaucoma includes eye drops and other medications. The correct dose of eye drops must be taken at the proper time. Report to the nurse if residents are not using their eye drops properly. Regular or laser surgery may also be used to treat glaucoma. The surgery does not work on every patient.

Age-related macular degeneration (AMD) is a condition in which the part of the retina that allows people to see detail, called the macula, degenerates. Central vision is gradually destroyed, which can affect a person's ability to drive, read, write, and do other tasks. Side vision, called peripheral vision, is not affected. AMD is the most common cause of vision loss in those 60 and older. There is no pain associated with this disorder, and it may evolve slowly. Vision problems may be different for each eye.

The two forms of this condition are wet and dry AMD; the dry form is more common. The exact cause of AMD is unknown. Risk factors include aging, smoking, sun exposure, heredity, gender, and race. Treatments for wet AMD include laser surgery and injections. Dry AMD may be treated with zinc and antioxidants to slow its progression. When dry AMD reaches the advanced stage, it cannot be treated, and vision loss results.

Guidelines: Vision Impairment

G   Encourage the use of eyeglasses, if worn.

G   Keep eyeglasses clean and in a safe place. If glasses are damaged or do not fit well, notify the nurse.

G   Encourage the use of contact lenses, also called "contacts," if used. Report to the nurse if the resident requires help handling contact lenses (Fig. 22-14).

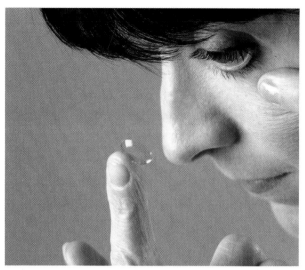

Fig. 22-14. Contact lenses are made of different types of plastic. Some can be worn and disposed of daily. Others are worn for longer periods. Residents usually insert contact lenses themselves.

G Always identify yourself as you enter the room. Do not touch the resident until you have done so. When leaving the room, let the resident know you are going.

G Keep doors completely open or closed, not partially open or closed.

G Leave furniture in place; never move furniture without the nurse's or the resident's permission.

G Use the face of an imaginary clock as a guide to explain the position of objects in a room.

G Make sure there is enough light in every room. Lighting should allow the resident to read in comfort without eye strain. Harsh, overly-bright lighting should not be used, however. It can put a strain on the eyes.

G Walk a little ahead of a visually-impaired resident while he touches your arm. This allows you to guide the person and warn him of steps, curbs, etc.

G Walk at the resident's pace, not yours.

G Assist residents who need help completing menus. Set up meal trays, cut meat and vegetables, and open beverage containers as needed. Use the imaginary clock face to explain the position of food and drink on the tray.

G Use special large-print books, audio books, and digital books, if available.

G Read to residents as often as time permits if they desire it. Volunteers and visitors can also help with this.

G Assist nurses or doctors with vision screenings as needed.

Tip

Using Braille

Braille is a system of touch reading for blind people that uses tiny, raised dots (Fig. 22-15). Braille was developed in the 1800s by Louis Braille when he was a teenager. It was based on a code used to help soldiers communicate in the dark. Braille is composed of an alphabet of "cells" that consists of dots. It takes time and special training to be able to read Braille.

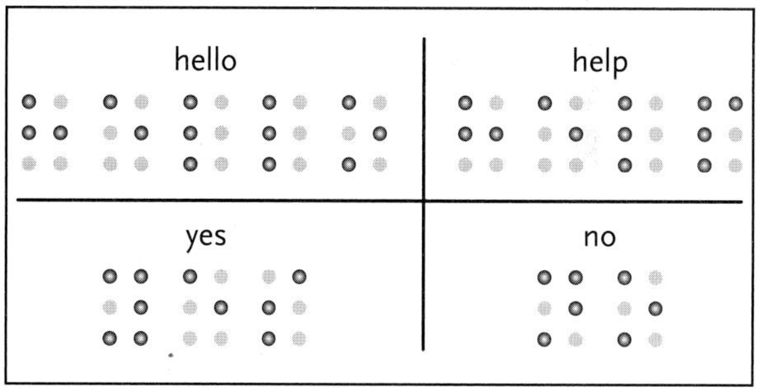

hello	help
yes	**no**

Fig. 22-15. Examples of words in Braille.

Tip

Print Disabilities and Digital Books

Residents who have print disabilities may require digital books. Bookshare is the largest online library of digital books in the world. You can download books for a Braille access device with a membership at bookshare.org.

For more information about visual impairment, see Chapter 4.

Caring for eyeglasses

Equipment: emesis basin, special cleaning fluid, 2 lens cloths, towel

1. Identify yourself by name. Identify the resident. Greet the resident by name.

2. Wash your hands.

3. Explain procedure to resident. Speak clearly, slowly, and directly. Maintain face-to-face contact whenever possible.

4. Provide for the resident's privacy with a curtain, screen, or door.

5. Gently remove eyeglasses and place in emesis basin.

6. Line sink with towel.

7. Clean eyeglasses over lined sink. Wash glass lenses in lukewarm water and rinse. Clean plastic lenses with cleaning fluid and a lens cloth. While cleaning, observe for loose screws or loose or broken lenses.

8. Dry with soft, 100% cotton cloth or special lens cloth. Do not dry with tissues, as they may scratch eyeglasses.

9. Gently assist resident to replace eyeglasses on face. Place over the ears and position comfortably. Observe for proper fit.

10. Make resident comfortable. Remove privacy measures.

11. Leave call light within resident's reach.

12. Wash your hands.

13. Be courteous and respectful at all times.

14. Report any changes in the resident to the nurse. Document procedure using facility guidelines.

The artificial eye is a type of prosthesis, sometimes called an ocular prosthetic. An artificial eye does not provide vision. It can, however, improve appearance. It may be used when a person has lost an eye due to disease or injury, such as cancer or a gunshot wound. Artificial eyes can be made of plastic or glass; however, most artificial eyes are made from a special kind of plastic. Plastic eyes can adapt to changes in the eye socket as a person ages, while a glass eye cannot be changed once it is produced. Plastic eyes do not require replacement very often, and they can be cleaned and polished repeatedly.

An artificial eye is held in place by suction. Some artificial eyes do not require frequent removal, unless the eye becomes uncomfortable. Others need daily removal and cleaning. Each eye specialist will give individual instructions to their patients. Carefully follow the instructions for your residents regarding care for their artificial eyes.

If the artificial eye has been removed, clean or rinse the resident's eye socket carefully using cotton balls and water or a special saline solution. Clean empty socket from the inner canthus (inner part of the eye) toward the outer canthus (outer part of the eye). Clean the eyelid.

If the artificial eye is in place in the eye socket, clean the area, moving in the opposite direction. Clean from the outer part of the eye toward the inner part of the eye. Cleaning in this direction helps prevent accidental movement and dislodging of the eye.

When removing and transporting an artificial eye, use an eyecup or a small basin. Follow manufacturer's instructions regarding cleaning and storing. Do not use rubbing alcohol to clean or soak the artificial eye. Do not use abrasives such as cleansers or toothpaste. The artificial eye can be permanently damaged by improper cleaning. It will usually be stored in water or saline solution. Always cover the eye completely with any solution used.

Be sure to be professional when caring for an artificial eye.

Hearing Impairment

There are many different kinds of hearing loss. A person may be born with a hearing impairment or it may happen gradually. Deafness is a partial or total hearing loss that occurs most often in people over the age of 65, but can occur in younger people.

Disorders can affect a person's hearing. **Otitis media** is an infection in the middle ear. Bacteria grow inside the middle ear, which causes symptoms such as pain, pressure, fever, and reduced ability to hear. Antibiotics may be ordered to treat the infection. Vital signs may be taken, especially to monitor temperature. You may be asked to change the resident's pillowcase often, especially if he or she has ear drainage. It is important that the person take all of the antibiotics.

Meniere's disease is a disorder of the inner ear caused by a build-up of fluid. It usually only affects one ear. The exact cause is unknown, but Meniere's disease may be caused by infections, allergies, or a genetic link. Symptoms include vertigo (dizziness), hearing loss, tinnitus (ringing in the ear), and pain or pressure. This disorder usually affects people between the ages of 40 and 60. Treatment includes medications, salt restriction and other dietary changes, cognitive therapy (a type of talk therapy), antibiotic or corticosteroid injections, and, in extreme cases, surgery.

A person who is hearing-impaired may read lips, use sign language to communicate, or use a hearing aid. A **hearing aid** is a battery-operated device that amplifies sound.

There are many different kinds of hearing aids (Fig. 22-16). Follow the manufacturer's or your facility's directions for cleaning them. In general, they need to be cleaned daily using a special cleaning solution or alcohol and a soft cloth. Do not submerge the hearing aid in water or allow the section that houses the battery to get wet. When cleaning a hearing aid, observe for wax buildup.

Hearing aids are expensive; handle them carefully. Turn the hearing aid off and keep it in a

safe place when it is not being worn. Turn the volume down before inserting a hearing aid. Be gentle when inserting it. Make sure it sits snugly in place before turning it on. The hearing aid should feel comfortable when in place. If you see any sores or abrasions in the ear, report it to the nurse.

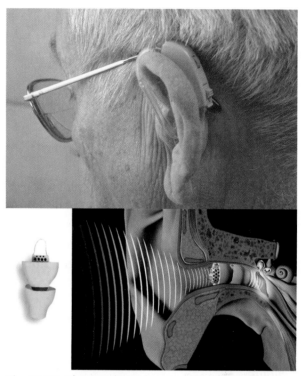

Fig. 22-16. *The top photo shows an older type of hearing aid. The bottom left photo shows a newer type of hearing aid, and the bottom right illustration shows this device placed inside the ear.* (BOTTOM PHOTOS COURTESY OF INSOUND MEDICAL, INC., WWW.LYRICHEARING.COM)

Guidelines: Hearing Aids

G   Handle hearing aids carefully; they are very expensive.

G   Turn off the hearing aid when not in use. This helps save the battery life. Store the hearing aid in a container labeled with the resident's full name, and room and bed number. It should be stored in a cool, dry area. Hot, sunny areas can damage the device.

G   Check the batteries often. Replace batteries as needed. Follow directions carefully when replacing batteries. Proper size batteries must be used, and they need to be firmly in place in the hearing aid.

G If the hearing aid does not work, check the batteries. If this does not solve the problem, ask the nurse to have the hearing aid checked for damage.

G Do not get the batteries wet. When cleaning a hearing aid earmold, carefully clean using a soft cloth and mild cleanser and water. Never place the hearing aid in water.

G Remove hearing aids before bathing, showering, or shampooing hair.

G Do not spray hair care products near a hearing aid.

G Check for hearing aids before removing bed linen and meal trays.

G Make sure that residents who use these devices have them inserted and turned on. If the hearing aid does not fit properly, notify the nurse.

For more information about hearing impairments, see Chapter 4.

Delirium

Confusion is a temporary or permanent state in which a person is unable to think clearly and logically. It interferes with the ability to make decisions and may change a person's personality. It may be due to a physical problem, such as a stroke or a seizure. It can also have many other causes, including medication and fever. See Chapter 4 for more information on confusion.

Delirium, also called acute confusional state or acute brain syndrome, is a sudden state of severe confusion due to a change in the body. Severe dehydration or malnutrition, fever, pain, poisons, alcohol and drug use, and prescribed medications can cause delirium. Other causes are hypoxia (low blood oxygen), head injuries, and illnesses such as cancer or diabetes. Infections such as pneumonia and urinary tract infections can also cause delirium.

Signs and symptoms of delirium include:

- Disorganized thinking

- Inability to concentrate

- Problems with speech

- Agitation

- Anger or irritability

- Drowsiness or sleep disturbances

- Decrease in short-term memory

- Lack of attention span, especially around familiar people

- Disorientation

- Changes in consciousness

- Decrease in the normal ability to move about

- Pulling out tubing, such as a nasogastric tube or a urinary catheter

- Hallucinations

Some effects of delirium are easily treatable with medication, which will reverse or control the delirium. Other causes require emergency care or a hospital stay. If you note any of these signs and symptoms, report them to the nurse immediately.

5. Discuss dementia and related terms

Cognition is the ability to think clearly and logically. A person with a cognitive impairment has a reduced ability to perform these mental tasks. Focus and memory, as well as self-awareness and judgment, may be impaired. Some loss of cognitive ability is a result of normal changes of aging in the brain.

Dementia is a general term for a more serious loss of mental abilities, such as thinking, remembering, reasoning, and communicating. It interferes with normal functioning, and a person may lose the ability to perform activities of daily living (ADLs). Social skills may be affected. Dementia is not a normal part of aging (Fig. 22-17).

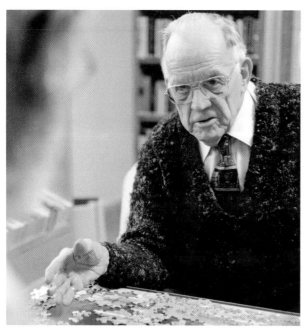

Fig. 22-17. *Some loss of cognitive ability is normal; however, dementia is not a normal part of aging.*

Alzheimer's disease is the most common form of dementia. You will learn more about Alzheimer's disease later in this chapter. Dementia may also be caused by these disorders:

- Vascular dementia, or multi-infarct dementia
- Lewy body dementia
- Parkinson's disease
- Acquired immunodeficiency syndrome (AIDS) (Chapter 24)
- Huntington's disease
- Excessive alcohol or drug use
- Head injuries
- Thyroid disorders
- Nutritional deficiencies, especially of the B vitamins

Some forms of dementia can be treated. Dementia caused by thyroid disorders or vitamin deficiencies can often be reversed with proper treatment. However, many forms of dementia are **irreversible**, meaning the disease cannot be cured. With those types of dementia, symptoms are managed with specific care techniques and different medications.

Diagnosing dementia is difficult. Physical and mental tests may be performed to rule out other causes. Testing may be started after a person develops two or more problems with brain functioning. Loss of speech or language ability, math skills, or memory skills are examples of problems that may occur.

Dementia and Delirium

Dementia is not the same thing as delirium. Delirium is a sudden state of severe confusion due to medical conditions and other causes. Dementia is a serious loss of cognitive abilities that is not a result of the aging process. However, people who have dementia may develop delirium.

6. Discuss Alzheimer's disease and identify its stages

Alzheimer's disease (AD) is a nervous system disorder that is both progressive and irreversible. Tangled nerve fibers and protein deposits form in the brain, eventually causing this disease. People with Alzheimer's disease lose memory and have behavioral changes. Most are eventually completely unable to care for themselves. There is no known cause of Alzheimer's disease.

Alzheimer's disease was first identified by Alois Alzheimer in 1907. The Alzheimer's Association estimates that as of 2011 there are more than 5.4 million people living in the U.S. with Alzheimer's disease. Most of these people are over the age of 65. The disease affects people from all races, backgrounds, socio-economic statuses, and cultures. By 2050, the Alzheimer's Association estimates that as many as 16 million Americans will have the disease.

Alzheimer's disease generally progresses in stages. In each stage, the symptoms become progressively worse. The majority of victims are eventually completely dependent on others for care.

Each person with AD may show different symptoms at different times. For example, one person may continue to read, but not be able to recognize a family member. Another can play a musical instrument, but does not know how to use the television controls. Skills a person has used over a lifetime are usually retained longer (Fig. 22-18).

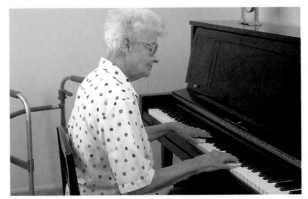

Fig. 22-18. *A person with AD may continue to have skills she has used her whole life.*

The Alzheimer's Association identifies seven general stages of Alzheimer's disease, based on a system developed by Barry Reisberg, M.D.:

Stage 1: No impairment

At this stage, the person does not show problems with memory loss or other symptoms. No signs of impairment are found during a medical examination.

Stage 2: Very mild decline

At this stage, the person has mild cognitive loss, which could be due to normal changes of aging or could be the earliest signs of Alzheimer's disease. There may be some memory loss, and the person forgets some words and the location of familiar objects. However, the person's medical examination does not show symptoms, and friends and family members do not notice any symptoms.

Stage 3: Mild decline

During this stage, people close to the person begin to notice some changes. A medical examination may show problems with memory and concentration. Other problems in this stage include the following:

- Difficulty with finding the right word or name
- Trouble remembering peoples' names
- Having a harder time functioning in social and work environments
- Forgetting material that one has just read
- Losing or misplacing objects
- Difficulty with planning or organizing

Stage 4: Moderate decline

At this stage, the person's medical examination shows clear problems, such as

- Forgetting recent events
- Problems doing more complex arithmetic
- Trouble performing more involved tasks, such as managing finances
- Forgetting some of one's own past experiences and background
- Being moody or withdrawn

Stage 5: Moderately severe decline

At this stage, cognitive impairment is noticeable. The person starts to need help with some daily activities. Symptoms include the following:

- Inability to recall one's own address, phone number, and other personal details
- Confusion about time and place
- Problems doing less complex arithmetic
- Needing help with some ADLs, such as choosing clothing appropriately

However, the person can often remember many important personal details and usually does not require help with other ADLs, like eating or toileting.

Stage 6: Severe decline

During this stage, memory loss and other problems worsen. More help is needed with daily activities. Symptoms include the following:

- Forgetting recent events, as well as not being aware of surroundings

- Forgetting one's own past experiences and background (may be able to remember name)

- Having trouble recalling the name of a family member or close friend or caregiver

- Needing more help with ADLs, such as dressing and toileting

- Trouble controlling bladder or bowels

- Having disruptions in sleep patterns

- Experiencing significant changes in personality and behavior (having delusions, being suspicious, showing compulsive behavior, wandering or becoming lost)

Stage 7: Very severe decline

In the final stage of AD, a person may be unable to communicate with others, control movement, or respond to his or her surroundings. The person needs significant help with ADLs, including eating and toileting. Muscles become rigid, and reflexes are abnormal. The person will have difficulty swallowing.

It is important to remember to encourage independence regardless of what symptoms a person with AD has. Helping residents keep their minds and bodies active may even help slow the progression of the disease (Fig. 22-19).

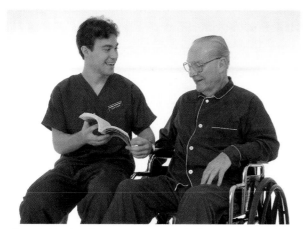

Fig. 22-19. Continue to encourage independence and activity for residents with AD.

Early Identification of Alzheimer's Disease

In April 2011, for the first time in 27 years, the Alzheimer's Association and the National Institute on Aging (NIA) of the National Institutes of Health published new guidelines for early diagnosis of Alzheimer's disease. Experts feel that diagnosing this disease before it progresses is important. They have identified three phases for diagnosing the disease:

1. Preclinical Alzheimer's disease occurs before obvious symptoms exist, such as memory loss, even though changes in the brain can be present. In the future, this phase may be diagnosed by the use of biomarkers (something in the body that can be measured).

2. Mild cognitive impairment due to Alzheimer's disease is a phase in which changes in memory and thinking are noted, but do not affect the person's ability to function from day to day.

3. Dementia due to Alzheimer's disease is the final phase in which symptoms regarding thinking, judgment, and memory are apparent. They may negatively affect a person's ability to function on a daily basis. However, some of these symptoms are not as severe as they used to be in order to have an Alzheimer's disease diagnosis.

The new guidelines define biomarkers and suggest that they may be a useful tool in the future for identifying or determining a person's risk of developing Alzheimer's disease. Testing of blood and cerebrospinal fluid (CSF), along with imaging of the brain, will be used to determine whether they might be biomarkers for Alzheimer's disease. More studies are needed; however, these new guidelines can assist doctors in an early diagnosis of Alzheimer's disease.

7. List strategies for better communication with residents with Alzheimer's disease

Many things can be done to improve communication with residents who have Alzheimer's disease. Some general communication guidelines follow:

Guidelines: General Tips for Communicating with Residents with Alzheimer's disease

G Always identify yourself and use the resident's name when greeting him. (Never touch first; this may upset the person.)

G Look at the resident the entire time you are speaking with him.

G Speak slowly and quietly. Be calm. Using a lower tone of voice than normal can be calming and easier to understand.

G Reduce background noise (Fig. 22-20).

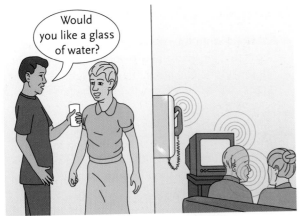

Fig. 22-20. *Try to find a room with little background noise and distraction when communicating with residents with AD.*

G Use touch and gestures if appropriate.

G Only talk about one subject at a time. Be patient. Use simple, short sentences.

G Repeat directions and answers as many times as needed.

G Use pictures.

G Praise often.

Communication with residents with AD can also be helped by following these specific techniques:

If the resident is frightened or anxious:

- Move and speak slowly.

- Speak in a quiet area with few distractions.

- Try to see and hear yourself as they might. Always describe what you are going to do.

- Use simple language and short sentences. If performing a procedure or assisting with self-care, simplify and list steps one at a time.

- Check your body language; make sure you are not tense or hurried.

If the resident forgets or shows memory loss:

- Repeat yourself. Use the same words if you need to repeat an instruction or question. However, you may be using a word the resident doesn't understand, such as "tired." Try other words like "nap" or "lie down."

- Repetition can also be soothing for a resident with AD. Alzheimer's disease may cause a resident to repeat words, phrases, questions, or actions. This is called **perseveration**, or repetitive phrasing. Do not try to stop a resident who is perseverating. Answer the questions each time in the same way. Even though responding over and over may frustrate you, it communicates comfort and security.

- Keep messages simple.

- Break complex tasks into smaller, simpler steps.

If the resident has trouble finding words or names:

- Suggest a word that sounds correct. If this upsets the resident, learn from it and try not to correct. As communicating with words (written and spoken) becomes more difficult, smiling, touching, and hugging can help show love and concern. But remember that some people find touch frightening or unwelcome.

If the resident seems not to understand basic instructions or questions:

- Ask the resident to repeat your statements. Use short words and sentences, allowing time to answer.

- Pay attention to the communication methods that are effective and use them.

- Watch for nonverbal cues as the ability to talk lessens. Observe body language—eyes, hands, facial expressions.

- Use signs, pictures, gestures, or written messages. For example, a picture of a toilet on the bathroom door can help remind a person where the bathroom is.

If the resident wants to say something but cannot:

- Encourage the resident to point, gesture, or act it out.

- If he is obviously upset but cannot explain why, offer comfort with a hug or a smile, or try to distract him.

If the resident is disoriented to time and place:

- Post reminders, such as calendars, activity boards, pictures, and signs on doors. Prior to the later stages of dementia, signs and labels can help with orientation. However, these techniques do not help and may only frustrate a person in the late stages of Alzheimer's disease.

If the resident does not remember how to perform basic tasks:

- Help by breaking each activity into simple steps. For instance, "Let's go for a walk. Stand up. Put on your sweater. First the right arm..." Always encourage residents to do what they can.

If the resident insists on doing something that is unsafe or not allowed:

- Try to limit saying "don't." Instead, redirect activities toward something else.

If the resident hallucinates (sees or hears things that are not really happening), is paranoid, or accusing:

- Do not take it personally.

- Try to redirect behavior or ignore it. Because attention span is limited, this behavior often passes quickly.

If the resident is depressed or lonely:

- Take time, one-on-one, to ask how the resident is feeling. Really listen.

- Try to involve the resident in activities. Always report signs of depression to the nurse.

If the resident is verbally abusive or uses bad language:

- Remember it is the dementia speaking and not the resident.

- Try to ignore the language. Redirect attention to something else.

If the resident has lost most verbal skills:

- Use nonverbal communication. As speaking abilities decline, people with AD will still understand touch, smiles, and laughter for much longer (Fig. 22-21). However, remember that some people do not like to be touched. Approach touching slowly. Be gentle, softly touching the hand or placing your arm around the resident. A hug can express affection and caring. A smile can say you want to help.

- Even after verbal abilities are lost, signs, labels, and gestures can reach people with dementia.

- Assume that residents with AD have insight and are aware of the losses in their abilities. Do not talk about them as though they were not there or treat them like children.

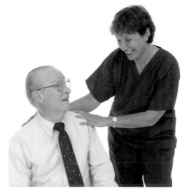

Fig. 22-21. *Touch, smiles, hugs, and laughter will be understood longer, even after a resident's speaking abilities decline.*

8. Identify personal attitudes helpful in caring for residents with Alzheimer's disease

The attitude of caregivers can make a big difference when caring for residents with AD. These attitudes will help you give the best care for your residents with Alzheimer's disease:

Do not take it personally. Alzheimer's disease is a devastating mental and physical disorder that affects everyone who surrounds and cares for the one with AD. People with AD do not always have control over their behavior. They may not be aware of what they say or do. If a resident with AD insults you, ignores you, or accuses you, remember that it is the disease causing the behavior. These actions are not within the person's control.

Put yourself in their shoes. Think about what it would be like to have Alzheimer's disease. Imagine being unable to perform your ADLs. Be understanding and compassionate. Assume that residents with AD have insight and are aware of the changes in their abilities. Provide security and comfort.

Work with the symptoms and behaviors you see (Fig. 22-22). Each person with Alzheimer's disease is an individual. AD does not progress the same way in everyone. Each resident will do some things that others will never do. Take an interest in each individual. Work with what you see each day. For example, a resident makes it to the bathroom one day, although the day before he could not walk to the door of his room. Notice changes in behavior, mood, and independence and report your observations to the nurse.

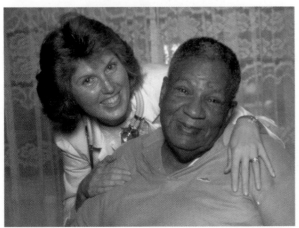

Fig. 22-22. *Treat each resident with AD as an individual and work with symptoms you see.*

Work as a team. Part of AD care is noticing changes in behavior, or physical and emotional health. When you work as a team, more subtle changes will be noticed. Share observations with the care team. Being with residents often allows you insights that others may not have. Make the most of this opportunity. People with AD may not distinguish between nursing assistants, nurses, or administrators, so be prepared to help when needed.

Take care of yourself. Caring for someone with dementia can be both emotionally and physically demanding. Take care of yourself in order to continue to give the best care (Fig. 22-23). Be aware of your body's signals to slow down, rest, or eat better. Remember that your feelings are real, and you have a right to them. Share your feelings with others, especially those experiencing similar situations. Do not worry about mistakes. Use them as learning experiences.

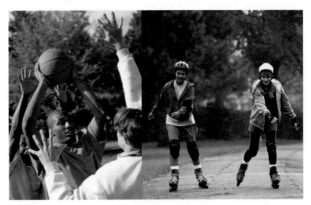

Fig. 22-23. *In order to give the best care, you need to take care of yourself. Regular exercise is an important part of taking care of yourself.*

Work with family members. Family members can be a great resource. They may know things you would have to learn by trial and error. Family can be of great comfort to victims of AD, helping you provide quality care.

Remember the goals of the care plan. Along with practical tasks, the care plan will call for maintaining residents' dignity and self-esteem. Provide security and comfort. Promote independence for as long as possible.

Burnout

Caregivers of residents with Alzheimer's disease tend to experience burnout. **Burnout** is mental or physical exhaustion due to a prolonged period of stress and frustration. Burnout can include feelings of failure about the work you do. If you feel this is happening to you, ask your supervisor for assistance. She can refer you to people or support groups who can help.

9. Describe guidelines for problems with common activities of daily living (ADLs)

The following guidelines are strategies for making care for a resident with AD easier. These are general tips and may not apply to every resident. Each resident with Alzheimer's disease is an individual. Remember to encourage as much independence as possible during care. Promote self-care. Help residents to care for themselves as much as possible. Residents with AD tend to do better if the staff follow a routine. Be consistent with routines if possible.

Bathing

- Schedule bathing when the resident is least agitated.

- Prepare the resident before bathing. Hand him the supplies, such as soap or towels, which can serve as a visual aid.

- Be organized so the bath can be quick. Give sponge baths if a shower or tub bath is resisted.

- Make sure the bathroom is well-lit.

- Provide for resident's privacy at all times.

- Check that the temperature of the room is comfortable.

- Confusion and frustration during bathing can be reduced by calmly explaining the procedure in the same way every time. Use simple words and short sentences (Fig. 22-24).

- Offer the resident a washcloth to hold, which can help distract him while you finish the bath.

- Ensure safety by using non-slip mats, tub seats, shower chairs and handholds.

- Do not try to force the resident to bathe. Be flexible and try again later in the day.

- Be relaxed during the bath and allow the resident to enjoy the bath.

- Be encouraging and positive. Offer praise and support.

- Observe the skin for any signs of breakdown or irritation during bathing.

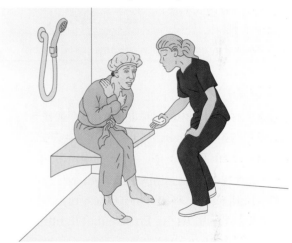

Fig. 22-24. A resident with AD may be frightened or not understand what you are going to do. Stay calm. Gently explain the procedure using simple words.

Grooming and Dressing

- Assist with grooming. Help residents you care for feel attractive and dignified.

- Choose clothing ahead of time. Mention that you are going to help the person get dressed. If resident is able, allow him to help with choice of clothing. Use clothing that is easy to put on.

- Lay out clothes in the order in which they should be put on (Fig. 22-25). Choose clothes that are simpler to put on. For example, use Velcro™ instead of buttons, slip-on instead of lace-up shoes, and pants or skirts instead of dresses.

- Provide for privacy at all times.

- Do not rush the resident.

- Praise and encourage the resident often.

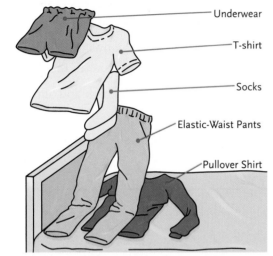

Fig. 22-25. *Lay out clothes in the order to be put on.*

Toileting

- Encourage fluids. Do not withhold or discourage fluids because a resident is incontinent.

- Mark the restroom with a sign as a reminder to residents of its location and that they should use it. Ensure that lighting is adequate.

- Check the resident often for episodes of incontinence. Be professional when cleaning a resident after an episode of incontinence. Show respect.

- Take the resident to the bathroom after drinking fluids; make sure resident actually urinates.

- Follow the toileting schedule carefully.

- Take resident to bathroom before meals and bedtime.

- If you know the resident's bathroom time, take him to the bathroom prior to and as near to this time as possible.

- If the resident has nighttime incontinence, take him to the bathroom as near to bedtime as possible. Use incontinence briefs as needed.

- Check skin regularly for signs of irritation.

- Cover garbage cans or waste baskets if the resident tries to urinate or defecate in them.

- Document bowel movements.

- Be supportive if family or friends are upset by incontinence.

Nutrition

Nutritional problems are common among people with AD. It is very important to offer nutritious snacks and encourage food and fluid intake. In addition, here are ideas for improving nutritional intake:

- Schedule meals at the same time each day and serve familiar foods.

- Remind the resident when it is mealtime.

- Encourage independence with eating and drinking.

- Make the dining area as pleasant and calm as possible. Use smaller dining areas and tables if needed to reduce distractions. The dining area should be well-lit.

- Make sure residents with AD are seated with other residents to encourage socialization. Adjust seating to allow for any eating problems.

- Foods should look and smell appealing.

- Food and drink should not be too hot.

- Plain plates without patterns or colors work best. Use a simple place setting with a single eating utensil (Fig. 22-26). Remove other items from the table.

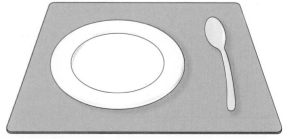

Fig. 22-26. *Simple place settings with white plates on a solid-colored place mat may help avoid confusion and distraction during eating.*

- Use a variety of foods that the resident enjoys to stimulate appetite; consider cultural preferences when choosing foods.

- Ask resident which food he would like to eat first, giving him a choice of two or three dishes. Residents in later stages of AD may not be able to make this choice.

- Finger foods may work well because they are easier to eat and allow residents to choose what they want (Fig. 22-27). Bite-sized pieces of food may also work well.

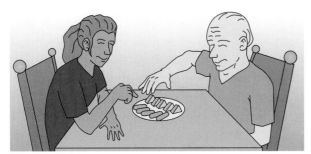

Fig. 22-27. Finger foods are often easier to eat and promote independence for residents with AD.

- During meals, offer one bite at a time.

- Offer fluids often. Have different types of fluids available, such as gelatin or popsicles.

- Obtain assistive devices for eating, if needed.

- Give resident simple instructions when eating. Ask the resident to open his mouth and place a spoon to the lips, if needed.

- Use the hand-over-hand method to help the resident eat.

- Allow plenty of time for eating and drinking.

- If your resident needs to be fed, do so slowly, offering small pieces of food.

- Sit directly in front of residents when helping with eating, and make simple conversation during the meal.

- Keep favorite nutritious snacks close by.

- If restlessness or wandering prevents getting through an entire meal, try smaller, more frequent meals.

- Observe and report changes or problems in eating habits. Observe for swallowing problems.

- Promptly report changes in intake or output. In addition, monitor weight accurately and frequently to discover potential problems.

See Chapter 14 for more information on nutrition.

Physical Health

- Prevent infections; they are the leading cause of death in people with Alzheimer's disease. Follow Standard Precautions.

- Help residents wash their hands frequently.

- Observe physical health and report any potential problems. People with dementia may not recognize their own health problems.

- Reduce the risk of falls; fractures can cause severe pain and a lengthy recovery.

- Provide careful skin care to reduce the risk of pressure ulcers.

- Take action to manage pain. Recognize nonverbal signs of pain, such as grimacing or clenching fists (Fig. 22-28). Promptly report possible signs of pain to the nurse. See Chapter 13 for symptoms of pain and ways to manage pain. Special pain management techniques will be used for residents with AD who are close to death. See Chapter 27 for more information.

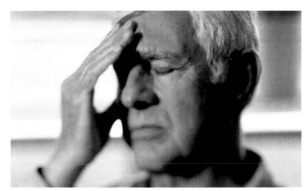

Fig. 22-28. Be aware of nonverbal signs of pain, such as holding or rubbing a body part. Report these signs to the nurse immediately.

Mental and Emotional Health

- Maintain self-esteem by encouraging independence in activities of daily living. Assistance with personal grooming will increase self-esteem.

- Provide a daily calendar to encourage activities.

- Share in enjoyable activities, looking at pictures, talking, etc.

- Reward positive and independent behavior with smiles, hugs, and warm touches.

Environmental Issues

Environmental changes can be made to make surroundings safer and more secure for residents with AD. They also can make the environment easier for the person to move around in. General tips for making the environment safer include the following:

- Use pictures or photos to identify each room, such as the dining room and the bathroom.

- Mark stairs and windows with brightly colored tape or signs.

- Use handrails in the bathroom, along with non-skid mats.

- Do not keep shampoos, cleaning agents, toxic substances, plants, or other potentially dangerous items within reach of confused or disoriented residents.

- Provide a safe area for pacing or wandering.

Residents' Rights

Residents' Rights and Alzheimer's Disease

Because people with Alzheimer's disease may not be aware of what they are doing, it is especially important to protect their dignity. For example, if a resident lifts up her skirt often, dress her in pants. If a resident is a messy eater, provide privacy when he is eating. Actively protect residents' privacy and promote their dignity and self-esteem, even if it seems that they are not aware of this.

10. Describe interventions for common difficult behaviors related to Alzheimer's disease

People with Alzheimer's disease can show different behaviors that may be difficult to deal with. By knowing interventions, you can give better responses to these behaviors. An **intervention** is a way to change an action or development.

Nursing assistants may receive special training on cognitive impairment. Sensitivity training can be included to help you understand the needs of residents with physical and/or cognitive impairment.

Agitation: A resident who is excited, restless, or troubled is said to be **agitated**. Feeling insecure or frustrated, encountering new people or places, and changes in routine can all trigger this behavior. A **trigger** is a situation that leads to agitation. Even watching television can cause agitation, as a person with AD may lose his ability to distinguish fiction from reality. Try to recognize the triggers and eliminate them. Keep a regular routine and avoid frustration. If a resident becomes agitated, a calm response and slow, soothing tone can help minimize the behavior. Reduce noise and distractions. Focusing on a familiar activity may help. Listen carefully and ask gentle questions. Reassure the resident that he is safe.

Catastrophic Reactions: When a person with AD reacts to something in an unreasonable, exaggerated way, it is called a **catastrophic reaction**. Many situations can cause this reaction, and they differ from person to person. It is most often triggered by these conditions:

- Fatigue

- Change of routine, environment, or caregiver

- Overstimulation, including noise, too much activity, difficult choices or tasks

- Physical pain or discomfort, including hunger or need for toileting

Respond to catastrophic reactions as you would to agitation. Try to eliminate triggers and help the resident focus on a soothing activity.

Violent Behavior: A resident who attacks, hits, or threatens someone is **violent**. Violent behavior also includes being violent to oneself. For example, a resident may bang his head repeatedly against a wall. Violence may be triggered by many situations. These include frustration, overstimulation, or a change in roommate, caregiver, or routine.

If any resident shows violent behavior, notify the nurse immediately. Block blows, but never hit back. Step out of reach and stay calm. Try to remove triggers if possible. Remove other residents or visitors from the area. Use the same techniques used for agitation to try to calm the resident. Do not try to restrain the resident. A care conference may be needed to discuss the behavior, especially if it is new behavior. For more information about aggressiveness, anger, and combativeness, see Chapter 4.

Hallucinations or Delusions: A resident who is having **hallucinations** is seeing things that are not there (Fig. 22-29). A resident who believes things that are not true is having **delusions** (Fig. 22-30). Most hallucinations and delusions are harmless and can be ignored. Reassure a resident who seems agitated or worried. Do not argue with a resident who is imagining things. Challenging serves no purpose and can make matters worse. Remember that the feelings are real to the resident with AD. Do not tell the resident that you can see or hear his hallucinations. Redirect the resident to other activities or thoughts.

Depression: People who become withdrawn, isolated, lack energy, and stop eating or doing things they used to enjoy may be depressed. Losing independence and facing the reality of an incurable disease can cause depression. Feelings of failure and fear are other causes. Chemical imbalances can cause depression. See informa-

tion in Learning Objective 13 for more information on depression and its symptoms.

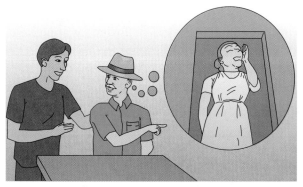

Fig. 22-29. *Hallucinating is seeing or hearing things that are not really there. For example, a resident may think he is hearing his mother calling him to dinner. You know that his mother died twenty years ago, but to him this is very real.*

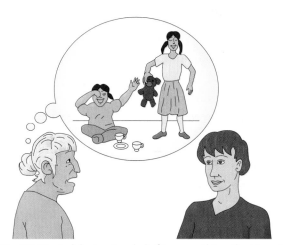

Fig. 22-30. *A delusion is a belief in something that is not true, or is out of touch with reality. For example, a resident thinks that her long-deceased sister is stealing from her room, like she did when they were young.*

Report signs of depression to the nurse immediately, as medications may help. Try to note the triggers or events that cause changes in mood. Encourage independence and self-care, and reward activities that improve moods. Find ways to help foster social relationships, such as group activities. Listen to residents if they want to share their feelings. Respect their right to feel sad; offer comfort and concern. Be as pleasant as possible. Use touch to communicate care if it does not bother the person.

Disruptiveness: **Disruptive behavior** is anything that bothers or disturbs others, such as yelling, banging on furniture, and slamming doors. Often this behavior is triggered by pain, constipation, frustration, or a wish for attention. When this behavior starts, get the resident's attention. It is important to stay calm and be friendly. Gently try to direct the resident to a quiet area. Ask the resident to tell you the problem, if possible. Try to find out why the behavior is occurring.

Inappropriate Sexual Behavior: Inappropriate sexual behavior, such as removing clothing, touching one's own genitals in public, or being sexually-aggressive can be disturbing to those who see it. When this happens, stay calm and be professional. Do not be judgmental or overreact. Try to determine if the cause is a simple problem, such as a rash, clothing that is too tight, or the need to urinate. Gently direct resident to a private area. Distract the resident if possible. Report this behavior to the nurse. Consider appropriate ways to provide physical stimulation, such as holding the resident's hand, giving a back rub, or offering a stuffed animal for him to hold. For more information about inappropriate sexual behavior, see Chapter 4.

Inappropriate Social Behavior: Residents can sometimes show inappropriate social behavior, such as cursing, name-calling, or yelling. As with violent or disruptive behavior, there may be a variety of causes. Do not take this behavior personally. When this behavior occurs, try to remove the resident from the area if he is disturbing others. Try to find out what caused the behavior (for example, stress, pain, noise, etc.). Stay calm. Report this behavior to the nurse.

Perseveration or Repetitive Phrasing: Residents with dementia may repeat words, phrases, or questions over and over again. This is called perseveration or repetitive phrasing. They may also repeat an action or task, such as tapping fingers and folding or cleaning things. Be patient with these repetitious behaviors. Remember that the resident is unaware of what he or she is doing. If questions are asked repeatedly, respond each time using the same words. Do not try to silence or stop the resident.

Pillaging, Rummaging, and Hoarding: **Pillaging** is taking things that belong to others. A person with AD may truly believe that something belongs to him, even when it clearly does not. **Hoarding** is collecting and putting items away in a guarded way. **Rummaging** is going through drawers, closets, or personal items that belong to oneself or to other people.

All of these behaviors are not within the control of a resident who has Alzheimer's disease. Pillaging and hoarding should not be considered stealing. These behaviors are not something that is deliberately or consciously planned. It is common for people with AD to wander around collecting items. They may pick up items that catch their attention and leave them somewhere else. This behavior is not intentional.

Take these steps to help this behavior: Label all of the resident's belongings. Note where missing items are located. Remember the hiding places so that you can look there if other things are missing in the future. Notify the family or friends so that they may be aware of this behavior. Enlist the family's help to notify you if they note this behavior. A special drawer for rummaging can be created. This drawer can hold items that are okay and safe for the resident to take with him.

Sundowning: When a resident with AD becomes restless and agitated in the late afternoon, evening, or night, it is called **sundowning**. Sundowning may be caused by hunger, fatigue, a change in routine or caregiver, or any new situation. The best ways to reduce this restlessness are to:

- Provide adequate lighting before it gets dark.

- Avoid stressful situations during this time. Limit activities, appointments, trips, and visits.

- Play soft music.

- Try to discourage residents from taking naps during the day.

- Set a bedtime routine and keep it.

- Recognize when sundowning occurs and plan a calming activity just before.

- Serve the evening meal long before bedtime.

- Eliminate caffeine from the diet.

- Give a soothing back rub.

- Try to redirect the behavior or distract the resident with a calm activity like looking at a magazine.

- Maintain a daily exercise routine.

Suspicion: As residents with AD begin to progress in their illness, they often become suspicious. They may accuse caregivers of lying to them or stealing from them. Suspicion may escalate to paranoia (having intense feelings of distrust and believing others are "out to get" them). When this occurs, do not argue with them. Arguing just increases defensiveness. Offer calm reassurance. Be understanding and supportive.

Pacing and Wandering: A resident who walks back and forth in the same area is **pacing**. A resident who walks around a facility without any known goal or purpose is **wandering**. Pacing and wandering can have many causes, including the following:
- Restlessness
- Hunger
- Disorientation
- The need to use the bathroom
- Constipation
- Pain
- Forgetting how or where to sit down
- Too much daytime napping

Responses to pacing and wandering include:
- Encourage an exercise routine.
- Minimize daytime napping.
- Let residents pace in a safe, locked area. Do

not restrain them (Fig. 22-31). Remove clutter and create clear paths. Use only non-skid rugs.

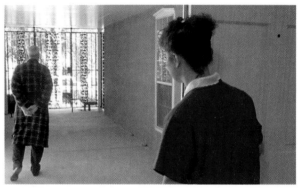

Fig. 22-31. *Do not restrain residents who pace. Let them pace or wander in a secure area.*

- Redirect attention to something the resident enjoys.

- Place stop signs or "closed" signs on doors to remind residents not to exit. Use alarms on exits to indicate the door has been opened. Locks placed either very high or very low may prevent exiting. Remember to keep a key nearby in case of emergency. Never leave a resident alone in a locked room.

- If residents wander away from a protected area in which they live and do not return on their own, it is called **elopement**. It is very important to keep doors locked when leaving an Alzheimer's unit or area. If a resident wanders away, notify the nurse in charge immediately. Follow all policies for emergency notification of the facility.

Tip

The Safe Return System
The Alzheimer's Association Safe Return® program can be used in the event a loved one with AD wanders away from home. The program is nationwide, and help is available 24 hours a day, 365 days a year. For a small fee, the family receives an ID bracelet, labels to sew on clothing, and a special wallet-sized card. The identification number matches the registration number with the association. For more information, contact the Alzheimer's Association at 800-272-3900 or at alz.org.

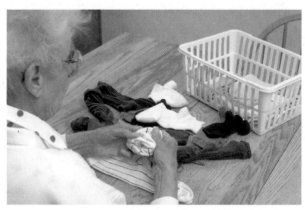

Fig. 22-32. *Activities that are not frustrating can help keep residents busy and engaged.*

11. Discuss ways to provide activities for residents with Alzheimer's disease

Activities are very important for residents with Alzheimer's disease. Activities that residents enjoy help them stay focused and prevent frustration and boredom.

When a person is first diagnosed with Alzheimer's disease or is admitted to the facility, staff should request a detailed biography from family or friends. Information that would be helpful includes likes, dislikes, cultural needs, work history, hobbies and interests, and a description of the person's personality. These can all be used to plan the most beneficial types of activities for residents with AD.

Meaningful activities help people with Alzheimer's disease maintain or improve their ability to function in daily life. They draw on past skills the resident has used throughout his life to help provide a focus. For example, if a resident was a person who filed medical records, giving her papers or folders to file can help her stay focused on a task.

Other activities—called "doing" activities—keep residents busy (Fig. 22-32). Folding towels can help the resident stay focused. Separating cards into groups can help with motor coordination and keep the resident focused.

Residents may only be able to stay focused for periods of about 20 to 30 minutes at a time for a given activity. Do not try to push them to continue the activity. Change from one activity to another if a specific activity is not working for a resident.

Some of the things staff can do to provide meaningful activities include the following:

- Encourage family participation in activities.
- Limit some activities to small groups.
- Use quiet areas for activities. Make sure the temperature in activity areas is comfortable.
- Set short time frames for activities to allow for limited attention spans.
- Help plan events that are of interest to residents, based on their interests and past experiences.
- Plan activities at times of the day when residents are feeling their best and are most engaged.
- Encourage residents to exercise in specially-designated areas.
- Plan activities that allow residents to make things that can be utilized by others.
- Encourage each resident's specific skills, such as playing a musical instrument.
- Immobile residents must not be forgotten; provide opportunities for them to participate in activities as well. Reading to them or playing music in their rooms are ways to provide activity for bed-bound residents.

In addition to encouraging residents to participate in activities, make sure residents are dressed and ready to go to activities at the designated time. They should be well-groomed, have had a meal or snack, and have been taken to the bathroom. Your responsibility may include taking the resident to the activity site.

12. Describe therapies for residents with Alzheimer's disease

There are different types of therapies that can improve the quality of life for people with Alzheimer's disease. These include the following:

Reality orientation uses calendars, clocks, signs, and lists to reorient the resident to person, place, and time. It can help reduce confusion or disorientation. It is useful in the early stages of Alzheimer's disease, before a person is totally disoriented. Later on, it may only frustrate the resident.

When using reality orientation, always identify yourself and call the resident by name. Ask about family, pictures, or personal items. Inquire about recent meals or activities. Use newspapers, magazines, TV, and radio to help residents know about current events. Point to clocks and calendars to show what time it is and what day of the week it is. Explain why you do things as you do them. For example, "We use your walker, Mrs. Martinez, to help make walking easier." Mention the season or month when selecting clothes or when looking out the window.

Validation therapy is letting residents believe they live in the past or in imaginary circumstances (Fig. 22-33). **Validating** means giving value to or approving and making no attempt to reorient the resident to actual circumstances. It is used for residents with advanced dementia.

For example, Mrs. Montego comes to you and says she is late for prom. Instead of telling her that prom happened many years ago, you quietly ask her about the color of her dress and ask her to describe it. You might ask her who her date is

and how late she can stay out. This allows her to work through the memory without forcing her back to reality.

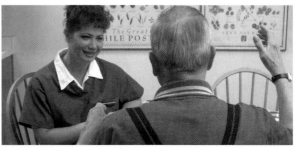

Fig. 22-33. *Validation therapy accepts a resident's fantasies. There is no attempt to reorient him to reality. By validating a resident's fantasies, you let him know that you take him seriously.*

Reminiscence therapy is a form of therapy that encourages the person to remember and talk about past experiences (Fig. 22-34). Explore memories by asking questions. Ask about details and work through feelings. If you trigger a painful past memory, do not hurry the resident through the memory. However, do not dwell on the painful memory. If the resident signals he wants to move on to other memories and thoughts, be ready to do this. Reminiscence therapy can help elderly people remember pleasant times in their past and allow caregivers to increase their understanding of their residents. This therapy can encourage staff to interact more with residents with Alzheimer's disease and other forms of dementia.

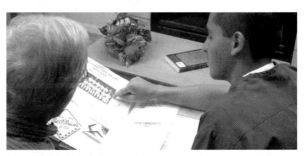

Fig. 22-34. *Reminiscence therapy encourages a resident to remember and talk about his past. It helps you show an interest in learning about him as a person who has had a wide range of experiences.*

Remotivation therapy promotes self-esteem, self-awareness, and socialization by having residents gather in small groups. Discussion focuses on facts rather than emotion. For example, a group discussion may have participants discuss their former professions in detail. This type of therapy discourages correcting residents, and it does not focus on personal problems. Discussion is based on the cognitive abilities of the people within the small group. Remotivation therapy can be used together with reality orientation and reminiscence therapy.

13. Discuss mental health, mental illness, and related disorders

Mental health is the ability of a person to use cognition and emotion appropriately throughout each day. A mentally healthy person will have successful relationships with family, friends, neighbors, and co-workers (Fig. 22-35). He will perform well in professional and home settings and will meet his responsibilities. He can control his desires and impulses properly. He will develop ways to deal with difficulties that occur throughout life.

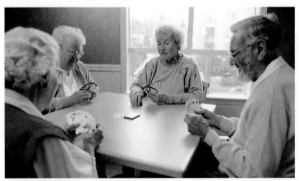

Fig. 22-35. Interacting well with others is a trait of mental health.

Mental illness is a disease, just like any physical disease. It affects a person's ability to function within family, home, work, or community settings. It often causes inappropriate behavior. Certain conditions can affect mental state and may worsen mental illness. Examples include various illnesses, substance abuse, physical abuse, unstable or traumatic relationships, genetic tendencies toward mental illness, and extreme stress.

Anxiety-Related Disorders

You first learned about anxiety in Chapter 4. For a mentally ill person, anxiety can exist all the time. If treatment is not sought, the anxiety can get worse. Types of anxiety disorders are as follows:

Generalized anxiety disorder (GAD) is an anxiety disorder characterized by chronic anxiety, excessive worrying, and tension, even when there is no cause for these feelings. Symptoms include headaches, muscle aches, sweating, shaking, difficulty swallowing and irritability. GAD is usually treated with medication and psychotherapy. **Psychotherapy** is a method of treating mental illness that involves talking about one's problems with mental health professionals.

Post-traumatic stress disorder (PTSD) is an anxiety disorder that may develop after a traumatic experience, such as a response to combat while in the military. PTSD can also develop after a crime, tornado, domestic violence, or a severe accident. Symptoms include flashbacks, withdrawal, and sleep disturbances. Flashbacks are experiences in which the person goes through the event again and again. PTSD is generally treated with medication and psychotherapy.

Obsessive-compulsive disorder (OCD) is an anxiety disorder characterized by repetitive thoughts or behavior. For example, a person with OCD may wash his hands over and over again, or check repeatedly to make sure the door is locked. A mentally healthy person will not exhibit this behavior, but a person with OCD cannot stop it. OCD is treated with medication and psychotherapy.

Social anxiety disorder, also called social phobia, is a disorder in which a person has excessive anxiety about social situations. It causes extreme self-consciousness in everyday situations, and the person may not want to be around other people at all. The person is unable to manage or control his fears. This phobia can interfere with the ability to attend school, work, social functions, and family events. Symptoms include sweating, shaking, and upset stomach. Medication and psychotherapy are used to treat this disorder.

Panic disorder is an anxiety disorder that causes a person to have repeated episodes of intense fear that something bad will occur. Symptoms include dizziness, rapid heartbeat, chest pain, difficulty breathing, and an upset stomach. The person may have a feeling of doom. Panic attacks may occur infrequently, or may be more frequent and interfere with the ability to function normally. Medication and psychotherapy are used to treat panic disorder.

Depression

Clinical depression is a serious mental illness in which feelings of overwhelming sadness make it difficult for a person to function normally. Other symptoms of depression are pain, fatigue, apathy (lack of interest), weight loss or gain, sleep problems, irritability, and feelings of worthlessness. A person who is depressed may not be able to perform normal tasks or participate in daily activities (Fig. 22-36).

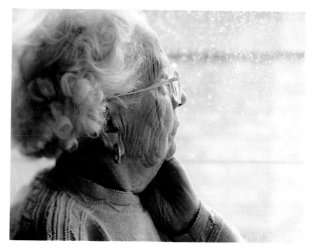

Fig. 22-36. Signs of depression, such as apathy, sleep problems, irritability, and being unable to perform normal tasks are important to report.

Depression is an illness and must be treated as such. A person cannot simply overcome depression through sheer will. Depression is more

common in the elderly population. It can happen due to the death of loved ones. It can occur along with other illnesses, such as cancer, Alzheimer's disease, HIV or AIDS, and after a heart attack.

Depression may be caused by abnormal levels of chemicals in the brain. Extreme depression can lead to thoughts of death and suicide. If you ever hear a resident make comments, even jokes, about hurting himself or others, report them immediately to the nurse. Depression is treated with medication and psychotherapy.

Bipolar disorder, or manic depression, is a type of depression that causes a person to have mood swings and changes in energy levels and the ability to function. The mood swings can go from extreme happiness to extreme sadness. The extreme "high" is called mania and the "low" is called depression. High energy, little sleep, high self-esteem, and poor judgment are other symptoms of this disorder. Suicide or thoughts of suicide can occur. Bipolar disorder requires long-term treatment with medication.

Schizophrenia

Schizophrenia is a form of chronic mental illness that may involve acute episodes. It is a brain disorder that affects a person's ability to think and communicate clearly. Problems with emotions, decision-making, and understanding reality may occur. A person may think she is hearing voices that tell her what to do. Symptoms include hallucinations, delusions, disorganized thinking and speech, and a lack of interest in life and planning activities. The person may have poor hygiene. Problems with memory may develop.

Paranoid schizophrenia is a form of mental illness characterized by hallucinations or delusions. For example, a person may believe that a neighbor is spying on her. She might be afraid that a co-worker is trying to poison her. These types of thoughts are called "delusions of persecution." Treatment of schizophrenia consists of long-term use of anti-psychotic medications.

Guidelines: Mentally Ill Residents

G   Encourage self-care.

G   Encourage independence with ADLs and activities. Watch for any change in a resident's ability to perform the ADLs.

G   Know your residents. Observe and watch for changes in behavior, such as episodes of mania in people with bipolar disorder.

G   Watch your body language when caring for the resident. He may be sensitive to this.

G   Do not treat mentally ill residents like children. Always treat residents like adults.

G   Do not yell or use a harsh tone of voice. Never argue with the resident.

G   Use eye contact when communicating.

G   Provide support for the resident and family and friends. Do not judge the behavior of the resident, friends, or family. Notify the nurse if you become concerned about any specific behavior.

G   If you observe any of the following, notify the nurse:

- Change in ability to perform ADLs

- Changes in mood, such as sadness, irritability, crying

- Change in behavior, such as the inability to make decisions, the inability to concentrate, or low self-esteem

- Behavior that seems extreme, dangerous, or frightening to others

- Excessive fatigue or insomnia

- Headaches

- Constipation

- Weight loss, lack of appetite, or anorexia

- Social withdrawal, or lack of participation in activities

- Hallucinations or delusions

- Any comments about suicide, even jokes

- Concerns that the resident is not properly taking a medication or is hiding medication

- Any person(s), activity, program, telephone call, specific date, object, article of clothing, or place that makes the person's behavior change in some way

14. Discuss substance abuse and list signs of substance abuse to report

Substance abuse is the use of legal or illegal substances in a way that is harmful to oneself or others. Many types of substances are abused, including alcohol, tobacco, legal and illegal drugs, glue, paint, and permanent markers (Fig. 22-37). These substances are also referred to as "mood-altering" substances. An abused substance creates a change in the person's perception or the control of his body. For example, alcohol is a depressant. It can cause slurred speech, slower reflex response, unsteadiness when walking, irritability, and unsafe driving.

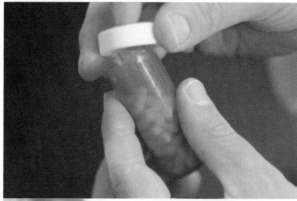

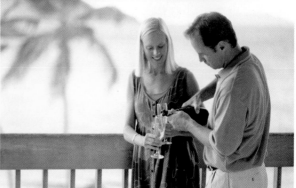

Fig. 22-37. *Prescription drugs, cigarettes, and alcohol are examples of legal substances that may be abused.*

Risk factors for substance abuse include difficult childhood, unstable home environment, and poor coping skills. Elderly people are more at risk for substance abuse when they have poor or absent relationships with family or friends. Because elderly people are often taking prescribed medication, substance abuse can cause even more problems due to possible drug interactions with their medications.

Observing and Reporting: Substance Abuse

If you observe any of the following signs, report them to the nurse. Simply report what you see, not what you think the cause may be.

- O/R Changes in physical appearance (torn clothing, red eyes, weight loss)

- O/R Changes in personality (moodiness, mood swings, odd behavior, lying)

- O/R Forgetfulness

- O/R Confusion

- O/R Loss of appetite

- O/R Stealing money or valuables

- O/R Smell of alcohol, cigarettes, or other substances in resident's room or on clothing

- O/R Strong smell of room fresheners

- O/R Increased use of breath fresheners

- O/R Hiding substances or alcohol

- O/R Blackouts or memory loss

- O/R Problems with other residents, staff, friends, or family

- O/R Constricted or dilated pupils

- O/R Slurred speech

- O/R Comments about thoughts of suicide

When a person stops using an addictive substance, withdrawal can occur. **Withdrawal** is the term used to describe physical and mental symptoms caused by ceasing to use a particular addictive substance. Without treatment, substance abuse can cause injury or even death. Treatment includes medication and behavioral health therapy.

Chapter Review

1. What is the basic working unit of the nervous system (LO 2)?

2. What makes up the central nervous system? What makes up the peripheral nervous system (LO 2)?

3. What part of the eye gives it its color (LO 2)?

4. What are two functions of the ear (LO 2)?

5. List three functions of the nervous system (LO 2).

6. List four normal age-related changes of the nervous system (LO 3).

7. List 13 problems that can result from a CVA (LO 4).

8. List 12 guidelines for caring for residents who are recovering from a CVA (LO 4).

9. List five care guidelines for residents who have Parkinson's disease (LO 4).

10. List eight care guidelines for residents who have multiple sclerosis (LO 4).

11. List 12 care guidelines for residents who have head or spinal cord injuries (LO 4).

12. What are four possible causes of seizures (LO 4)?

13. List 12 care guidelines for residents who have vision impairment (LO 4).

14. Why is it important not to use rubbing alcohol or abrasives to clean artificial eyes (LO 4)?

15. List seven care guidelines for hearing aids (LO 4).

16. List eight possible causes of delirium (LO 4).

17. What is dementia (LO 5)?

18. What is the most common cause of dementia (LO 5)?

19. Alzheimer's disease is a progressive, degenerative, and irreversible disease. What do each of these descriptions mean (LO 6)?

20. Why is it important for nursing assistants to encourage independence for as long as possible for residents who have AD (LO 6)?

21. Possible communication challenges for residents with AD are listed in Learning Objective 7. They include challenges with a resident who may:

- Be frightened or anxious
- Forget or show memory loss
- Have trouble finding words or names
- Seem not to understand basic instructions or questions
- Want to say something but cannot
- Be disoriented to time and place
- Not remember how to perform basic tasks
- Insist on doing something that is unsafe or not allowed
- Hallucinate, or be paranoid or accusing
- Be depressed or lonely
- Be verbally abusive, or use bad language
- Have lost most verbal skills

For each communication challenge, list one tip that may help.

22. Helpful personal attitudes when working with residents who have AD are in Learning Objective 8. They include the following:

- Do not take it personally.
- Put yourself in their shoes.
- Work with the symptoms and behaviors you see.
- Work as a team.
- Take care of yourself.
- Work with family members.
- Remember the goals of the care plan.

For each attitude, list one example of what nursing assistants can do to express that attitude.

23. List four guidelines for each of the following problems that may occur for a resident who has Alzheimer's disease: bathing, grooming and dressing, toileting, nutrition, physical health, mental and emotional health, and environmental issues (LO 9).

24. List one intervention for each of these problem behaviors related to Alzheimer's disease as described in Learning Objective 10: agitation; catastrophic reactions; violent behavior; hallucinations and delusions; depression; disruptiveness; inappropriate sexual behavior; inappropriate social behavior; perseveration; pillaging, rummaging, and hoarding; sundowning; suspicion; and pacing and wandering.

25. What is the difference between "meaningful" activities and "doing" activities (LO 11)?

26. Briefly describe each of the four creative therapies for AD (LO 12).

27. What are three characteristics of mental health (LO 13)?

28. What conditions can cause or worsen mental illness (LO 13)?

29. Briefly define each of these anxiety disorders: generalized anxiety disorder, post-traumatic stress disorder, obsessive-compulsive disorder, social anxiety disorder, and panic disorder (LO 13).

30. Does a person usually overcome depression through sheer will (LO 13)?

31. What should a nursing assistant do if a resident makes comments or jokes about suicide (LO 13)?

32. List four symptoms of schizophrenia (LO 13).

33. List six care guidelines for mental illness (LO 13).

34. List 13 possible signs of substance abuse that must be reported to the nurse (LO 14).

23
The Endocrine System

Brown-Sequard: The Father of Endocrinology?

Charles-Edouard Brown-Sequard (1817-1894) has been called the "Father of Endocrinology." He was the son of an American sea captain and a French mother, and he traveled and lectured widely. Brown-Sequard noted that organs like the thyroid, liver, spleen, and kidneys secreted substances that traveled into the blood. These substances were ultimately called hormones.

" . . . Who dodges life's stress and its strains . . . "
Donald Robert Perry, 1878-1937

" . . . Complaints is many and various, And my feet are cold . . . "
Robert Graves, 1895-1985

1. Define important words in this chapter

diabetes: a condition in which the pancreas does not produce insulin or does not produce enough insulin; causes problems with circulation and can damage vital organs.

hyperthyroidism: a condition in which the thyroid gland produces too much thyroid hormone, which causes body processes to speed up and metabolism to increase.

hypothyroidism: a condition in which the body lacks thyroid hormone, which causes body processes to slow down.

pre-diabetes: a condition in which a person's blood glucose levels are above normal but not high enough for a diagnosis of type 2 diabetes.

2. Explain the structure and function of the endocrine system

The endocrine system regulates many important body functions. The endocrine system is made up of glands in different areas of the body (Fig. 23-1). The glands are organs that produce and secrete chemicals called hormones. Hormones are chemical substances created by the body that control numerous body functions. They are vital to survival. Hormones are carried in the blood for delivery to target tissues or organs.

The pituitary gland, also called the "master gland," is located at the base of the brain, and is attached to the hypothalamus. It is called the master gland due to its ability to control the hormone production of other glands. There are two parts, or lobes, of the pituitary gland: the anterior (front) and the posterior (back). The anterior lobe releases the hormones, while the posterior lobe stores hormones for release when needed.

The thyroid gland is located in the neck below the larynx, or voice box. Thyroid hormones primarily regulate metabolism and growth. Metabolism is the process of breaking down and transforming all nutrients that enter the body to provide energy, growth, and maintenance.

Thyroid hormones also stimulate the growth of nervous tissue.

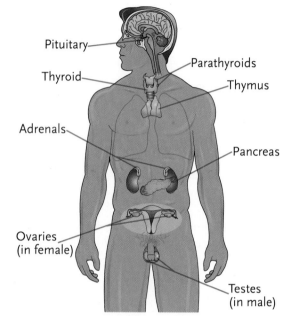

Fig. 23-1. *The endocrine system includes glands that produce hormones that regulate body processes.*

Four tiny parathyroid glands are embedded in the thyroid gland. They are responsible for the production of parathyroid hormone. This hormone regulates the levels of calcium and phosphate in the bloodstream.

Two adrenal glands are located on top of the kidneys. They secrete adrenaline (epinephrine) and noradrenaline (norepinephrine), aldosterone, and cortisol. During stressful situations, adrenaline, and the less-potent noradrenaline, increase the efficiency of muscle contractions, increase heart rate and blood pressure, and also increase blood glucose levels to provide extra energy. This is called the "fight-or-flight response." It enhances body performance during stressful or threatening situations. Aldosterone regulates the balance of sodium, potassium, and water. Cortisol (hydrocortisone) maintains the metabolism by regulating the amount of glucose (natural sugar) in the blood.

The pancreas is a gland located in the back of the abdomen and behind the stomach. The pancreas produces the hormone insulin. Insulin regulates the amount of glucose available to the cells for metabolism. Cells cannot absorb sugar without insulin.

Male and female sex glands, called the gonads, are endocrine glands. The ovaries in the female secrete estrogen and progesterone. The testes in the male secrete testosterone.

The functions of the endocrine system are to:

* Maintain homeostasis through hormone secretion
* Influence growth and development
* Regulate levels of calcium and phosphate in the body
* Maintain blood sugar levels
* Regulate the body's ability to reproduce
* Determine how quickly cells burn food for energy

Destination: Homeostasis

The parathyroid glands work to maintain calcium levels in the body. If the blood calcium gets too low—for example, due to surgery or cancer—the parathyroid glands increase production of parathyroid hormone (PTH). When the blood calcium reaches the proper level, the parathyroid glands stop the production of PTH. This quick response of the parathyroid glands helps the body return to homeostasis.

Tip

Iodine Allergy and Dye

Iodine is very important for the thyroid gland to function normally. Most people get their daily intake of iodine from common table salt. If a person is allergic to iodine, his or her doctor must be informed. This allergy needs to be listed in a person's medical record. Any test that requires dye to be injected into the body can cause a life-threatening allergic reaction for a person who is allergic to iodine.

3. Discuss changes in the endocrine system due to aging

Normal age-related changes for the endocrine system include the following:

* Levels of estrogen and progesterone decrease, which signal the onset of menopause in women.

- Testosterone levels in males usually decrease but production does not stop.

- Insulin production decreases.

- Body is less able to handle stress.

4. Discuss common disorders of the endocrine system

Diabetes

Diabetes mellitus, commonly called diabetes, is a disease that can affect people of any age. **Diabetes** is a condition in which the pancreas does not produce insulin or does not produce enough insulin. Without insulin to process glucose, or natural sugar, glucose builds up in the blood. This causes hyperglycemia, or high blood sugar. Because the body is unable to get energy from the sugar in the blood, it has to find energy another way. Usually the energy is obtained by burning fat. Diabetes is common in people with a family history of the illness, in the elderly, and in people who are obese.

Diabetes can cause many complications, including the following:

- Hypoglycemia (insulin reaction) and diabetic ketoacidosis (DKA) are complications of diabetes that can be life-threatening (Chapter 8).

- Decreased blood flow can cause problems with circulation, such as CAD or PVD (Chapter 19). These problems increase the risk of heart attack, stroke, or impaired circulation in the legs. Poor circulation in the legs can increase the risk of infection and the loss of toes, feet, or legs to gangrene.

- Diabetic retinopathy, or damage to blood vessels in the retina, can cause blindness.

- Damage to vital organs, such as the kidneys being unable to properly filter the blood, is another complication of diabetes.

- Diabetic peripheral neuropathy can result from diabetes. It causes numbness, pain, or tingling of the legs and/or feet and causes nerve damage over time.

There are a few different types of diabetes:

Pre-diabetes is a condition in which glucose levels are elevated, but not high enough to establish a diagnosis of diabetes. Many millions of people in the United States have pre-diabetes. They may already have some damage to their vital organs.

In order to be diagnosed with pre-diabetes, a fasting blood sugar level must be above 99 mg/dl. Pre-diabetes can be delayed or prevented with certain lifestyle changes. A change in the diet, along with daily exercise, can reduce weight and lower the risk of pre-diabetes or diabetes.

Type 1 diabetes is a condition that is usually diagnosed in children and young adults. It was formerly known as juvenile diabetes. In type 1 diabetes, the pancreas does not produce any insulin. This condition will continue throughout a person's life. Daily injections of insulin are needed, but these injections do not always prevent complications of diabetes. Special diets help treat this disorder and must be followed carefully. Blood glucose testing must also be done to monitor the diabetes.

Type 2 diabetes is the most common form of diabetes; it can occur at any age. It was formerly known as adult-onset diabetes. In type 2 diabetes, either the body does not produce enough insulin or the body fails to properly use insulin. This is known as "insulin resistance."

Type 2 diabetes is the milder form of diabetes. It usually develops after age 35. However, the number of children with type 2 diabetes is growing rapidly. This form of diabetes often occurs in obese people or those with a family history of the disease.

Treatment for type 2 diabetes includes careful monitoring of blood glucose levels. It can often be controlled with diet, including weight loss, and medication. Oral medications or injections of insulin will be used to control blood glucose. Smoking will be discouraged. Exercise may be ordered by a doctor to help with weight loss.

People with diabetes may have many different signs and symptoms, including the following:

- Excessive thirst
- Excessive hunger
- Excessive urination
- High blood sugar levels
- Glucose in the urine
- Very dry skin
- Fatigue
- Blurred vision or visual changes
- Slow-healing sores, cuts, or bruises
- Tingling or numbness in hands or feet
- Unexplained weight loss
- Increased number of infections

Tip

What is your risk for diabetes?

The American Diabetes Association (ADA) has developed a test to see whether or not a person is at risk for developing pre-diabetes or type 2 diabetes. It is called the "Diabetes Risk Test." You will answer a few questions and your score determines if you are at risk for developing these conditions. For more information, visit diabetes.org.

Hypothyroidism (Underactive Thyroid Gland)

Hypothyroidism is a condition in which the body lacks thyroid hormone, which causes body processes to slow down. It is an autoimmune disorder in which the body produces antibodies that attack the thyroid. The antibodies cause the gland to be unable to produce sufficient thyroid hormone.

Hypothyroidism is often caused by Hashimoto's disease, also known as Hashimoto's thyroiditis. Other causes include surgical removal of the thyroid gland, radioactive iodine therapy, and

thyroiditis (inflammation of the thyroid). Symptoms of hypothyroidism include:

- Fatigue and weakness
- Weight gain
- Constipation
- Intolerance to cold
- Dry skin
- Thinning hair or hair loss
- Brittle hair or fingernails
- Slow heart rate
- Low blood pressure
- Abnormally low body temperature
- Enlarged thyroid (goiter)
- Hoarseness
- Heavier than normal menstrual periods or absent menses
- Depression

Blood tests and neck examinations diagnose this condition. Treatment is thyroid hormone replacement therapy.

Hyperthyroidism (Overactive Thyroid Gland)

Hyperthyroidism is a condition in which the thyroid gland produces too much thyroid hormone. Body processes speed up, and metabolism increases, causing weight loss, a rapid heartbeat, and sweating. Nervousness and irritability may result.

Hyperthyroidism is primarily caused by Graves' disease, an autoimmune disorder in which antibodies cause the thyroid gland to produce excessive thyroid hormone. Lumps in the gland, called nodules, thyroiditis, or taking too much thyroid medication can also cause hyperthyroidism. Symptoms of hyperthyroidism include:

- Nervousness
- Restlessness
- Fatigue

- Visual problems or eye irritation

- Bulging or protruding eyes (exophthalmos)

- Trembling, especially of the hands

- Intolerance to heat

- Excessive perspiration

- Rapid heartbeat

- High blood pressure

- Increase in appetite

- Weight loss

- Changes in bowel movements

- Irregular or absent menstrual periods

- Enlarged thyroid (goiter)

Blood tests and physical examinations help diagnose this condition. Treatment includes anti-thyroid drugs, other medications called beta-blockers, or radioactive iodine to destroy the thyroid gland. If a goiter is large, surgery may be done. If the thyroid is removed, medication will need to be taken for the rest of the person's life.

5. Describe care guidelines for diabetes

Care of the person with diabetes includes a plan of care associated with every system in the body. Diabetes must be carefully controlled to prevent complications and serious illness. Follow the care plan closely.

Guidelines: Diabetes

G Give frequent skin care. The skin should always be clean and dry.

G Observe the skin carefully for sores, blisters, cuts, or any other breaks in the skin. Report any of these signs immediately to the nurse (Fig. 23-2). Wounds, skin breaks, and pressure ulcers must be prevented. A small sore can grow into a large wound that may not heal, which can require amputation.

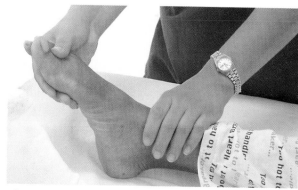

Fig. 23-2. *Observe the legs and feet carefully when giving care. Poor circulation can increase the risk of infection and the loss of toes, feet, or legs to gangrene.*

G Encourage diabetic residents to follow their exercise plans (Fig. 23-3). Exercise will be ordered to help with circulation and maintaining a healthy weight. Ambulation, range of motion exercises, frequent position changes, or other activity may be ordered. Report muscle weakness, change in gait, and any change in the ability to ambulate.

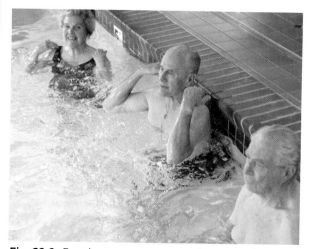

Fig. 23-3. *Exercise programs are very important for diabetic residents. They need to increase circulation and maintain a healthy weight.*

G Report complaints of pain, numbness, or tingling in the arms or legs immediately.

G Perform foot care carefully and as directed. Report any changes in the feet. Never clip or trim toenails, especially a diabetic's toenails. A nurse or doctor will do this.

G Encourage diabetics to wear proper shoes. Shoes should fit well and not hurt the feet.

Shoes made of material that breathes, such as leather or cotton, help prevent moisture build-up. All-cotton socks are best for absorbing sweat. Residents with diabetes should not go barefoot or wear tight-fitting clothing on the legs and feet.

G   Carefully following diet instructions is very important to help manage diabetes. Meals must be served at the same time every day. Meals and snacks must be completely eaten in order to keep blood sugar stable. Always report to the nurse if meals and snacks are not being eaten. Report if visitors bring snacks or treats to residents.

G   The ADA recommends that people with diabetes work with a registered dietitian (RDT) or a certified diabetes educator (CDE) to help develop individualized meal plans. The ADA's website, diabetes.org, contains many ideas for planning meals.

G   Keep track of any special tests the resident may have. Tests can affect diet and insulin dosage. If a resident is fasting for a blood test, for example, food and insulin may need to be withheld until after the test is completed. Notify the nurse immediately when the test has been completed.

G   Insulin dosage is based upon a variety of factors. Balancing factors like caloric intake, metabolism, exercise levels, stress levels, and the relative condition of the resident is important. Report if the resident is not following the care plan exactly.

G   Perform blood glucose tests only as directed and if trained. Not all states allow nursing assistants to perform this testing. Follow facility policy.

G   If any of the following occur, notify the nurse:

   • Any sign of skin breakdown anywhere on the body, especially on the feet and toes

   • Visual changes, especially blurred vision

   • Changes in mobility

   • Nervousness or anxiety

   • Dizziness or loss of coordination

   • Numbness or tingling in the arms or legs

   • Irritability or confusion

   • Changes in appetite or increased thirst

   • Fruity or sweet-smelling breath

   • Weight change

   • Nausea or vomiting

   • Change in urine output, any signs of urinary tract infection, fruity or sweet-smelling urine

Blood Glucose Monitoring

You may assist the nurse with blood glucose monitoring or have special training on how to do this yourself. Monitoring equipment measures the level of glucose in the blood throughout the day. Normal blood glucose is from 70 to 99 mg/dl. Strips are used, along with a blood glucose meter, a special glucose monitoring machine (Fig. 23-4). Make sure that strips have not expired. Always wear gloves when assisting with or performing this procedure. Handle and dispose of sharps properly.

The blood glucose meter tells people with diabetes what their blood sugar level is at any one time. Estimated average glucose (eAG) and A1C are two tests used to help track and regulate glucose levels over time. These tests show average blood glucose levels over the past few months. A1C, also known as glycated hemoglobin or HbA1C, is reported as a percent. Estimated average glucose (eAG) is a newer test that uses the same numbers (in units) as glucose testing meters.

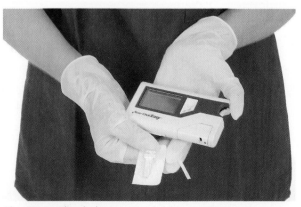

Fig. 23-4. *Blood glucose monitoring equipment.*

6. Discuss foot care guidelines for diabetes

Quality foot care is vital for people with diabetes. Diabetes weakens the immune system, which reduces resistance to infections. Poor circulation due to the narrowing of the blood vessels also increases the risk of infection. Infections of the feet, when noted in the early stages, can be treated successfully. However, when foot infections are not caught early, they can take months to heal. If wounds do not heal, amputation of a toe, an entire foot, or a leg may be necessary.

Foot care to prevent infection should be a part of daily care of residents. Keeping the feet clean and dry is a way to help prevent complications. It is important to observe the feet carefully during care.

Guidelines: Safe Diabetic Foot Care

G   Inspect and clean resident's feet every day during bathing. Make sure to check the entire foot and between the toes for rashes, cuts, sores, blisters, bruises, or fungus.

G   Avoid harsh soaps and hot water when bathing feet. Use only warm water and mild soaps.

G   Always dry feet thoroughly, especially between toes. Do not rub the skin; pat it dry.

G   Never cut toenails, corns, or calluses for any reason.

G   Do not use any object, such as a nail stick, to try to remove dirt from a toenail.

G   Use a doctor-recommended cream or lotion on the feet, but do not apply anything between the toes. Do not use powders. Make sure feet are completely dry after applying lotion or cream.

G   Check shoes for rocks or other objects before putting them on residents.

G   Remind residents not to walk around barefoot. Always use clean cotton socks with comfortable shoes or non-skid slippers. Do not turn socks over at the top, as this can decrease circulation. Make sure shoes fit properly.

G   If any of the following occur, notify the nurse:

   • Excessive dryness of the skin of the feet

   • Breaks or tears in the skin

   • Ingrown toenails

   • Reddened areas on the feet

   • Drainage or bleeding

   • Change in color of the skin or nails, especially blackening

   • Change in the temperature of the skin

   • Corns, blisters, calluses, or warts

   • Blood or drainage on the feet or toes

   • Painful, tender, soft, or fragile areas, or burning in the feet

Providing foot care

Equipment: basin, bath mat, soap, lotion, gloves, washcloth, 2 towels, bath thermometer, clean socks

1. Identify yourself by name. Identify the resident. Greet the resident by name.

2. Wash your hands.

3. Explain procedure to resident. Speak clearly, slowly, and directly. Maintain face-to-face contact whenever possible.

4. Provide for the resident's privacy with a curtain, screen, or door.

5. If the resident is in bed, adjust bed to lowest position. Lock bed wheels.

6. Fill the basin halfway with warm water. Test water temperature with thermometer or your wrist. Ensure it is safe. Water temperature should be 105°F. Have resident check water temperature. Adjust if necessary.

7. Place basin on the bath mat. Support the foot and ankle throughout the procedure.

8. Remove resident's socks. Completely submerge resident's feet in water. Soak the feet for five to ten minutes.

9. Put on gloves.

10. Remove one foot from water. Wash entire foot, including between the toes and around nail beds, with a soapy washcloth (Fig. 23-5).

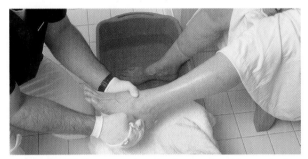

Fig. 23-5. *While supporting the foot and ankle, wash the entire foot with a soapy washcloth.*

11. Rinse entire foot, including between the toes.

12. Using a towel, pat dry entire foot, including between the toes.

13. Repeat steps 10 through 12 for the other foot.

14. Put lotion in hand. Warm lotion by rubbing hands together.

15. Massage lotion into feet (top and bottom), except between the toes, removing excess (if any) with a towel. Make sure lotion has been absorbed and feet are completely dry.

16. Empty, rinse, and wipe basin. Return to proper storage.

17. Dispose of soiled linen in the proper container.

18. Remove and discard gloves. Wash your hands.

19. Assist resident to put on clean socks. Make resident comfortable.

20. Remove privacy measures.

21. Leave call light within resident's reach.

22. Wash your hands.

23. Be courteous and respectful at all times.

24. Report any changes in the resident to the nurse. Document procedure using facility guidelines.

Chapter Review

1. Which gland is known as the "master gland" (LO 2)?

2. Where is insulin produced (LO 2)?

3. List four functions of the endocrine system (LO 2).

4. List three normal age-related changes of the endocrine system (LO 3).

5. What are three conditions that make it more likely for a person to have diabetes (LO 4)?

6. List four complications that can result from diabetes (LO 4).

7. What are two ways to delay or prevent pre-diabetes (LO 4)?

8. Which form of diabetes is more common—type 1 or type 2 (LO 4)?

9. List ten symptoms of diabetes (LO 4).

10. List ten symptoms of hypothyroidism (LO 4).

11. List ten symptoms of hyperthyroidism (LO 4).

12. Briefly discuss ten care guidelines for a person with diabetes (LO 5).

13. List seven foot care guidelines for a person with diabetes (LO 6).

14. List ten signs and symptoms to report to the nurse about a resident's feet (LO 6).

24
The Immune and Lymphatic Systems and Cancer

The Amazing Phagocytes

Elie Metchnikoff (1845-1916), a Russian zoologist and microbiologist, discovered that bacteria could be destroyed by certain cells that seemed to consume or "eat" them. He called these cells phagocytes (from Greek meaning "devouring cells") and named the process "phagocytosis." This process is an important part of the immune system's response to harmful bacteria. He won the Nobel Prize in 1908 for this discovery.

"Healing is a matter of time, but it is sometimes also a matter of opportunity."

Hippocrates, 460-377 B.C.

"There are some remedies worse than the disease."

Publilius Syrus, circa 42 B.C.

1. Define important words in this chapter

acquired immune deficiency syndrome (AIDS): the final stage of HIV infection, in which infections, tumors, and central nervous system symptoms appear due to a weakened immune system that is unable to fight infection.

autoimmune disease: a disease in which the body is unable to recognize its own tissue and begins to attack these tissues.

benign: non-cancerous.

biopsy: a removal of a sample of tissue for examination and diagnosis.

breakthrough pain: a type of severe pain that happens unexpectedly in people who have cancer.

cancer: a general term used to describe a disease in which abnormal cells grow in an uncontrolled way.

homophobia: a fear of homosexuality.

human immunodeficiency virus (HIV): a virus that attacks the body's immune system and gradually disables it; eventually causes AIDS.

lymph: a clear yellowish fluid that carries disease-fighting cells called lymphocytes.

malignant: cancerous.

metastasize: to spread from one part of the body to another.

opportunistic infection: an illness caused by microorganisms due to a person's inability to fight infection.

remission: the disappearance of signs and symptoms of cancer or other diseases; can be temporary or permanent.

tumor: a group of abnormally-growing cells.

2. Explain the structure and function of the immune and lymphatic systems

The Immune System

The immune system protects the body from harmful substances, such as disease-causing bacteria, viruses, and microorganisms. There are two types of immunity: nonspecific immunity and specific immunity.

Nonspecific Immunity

Nonspecific immunity is present at birth. It protects the body from disease in general. Nonspecific immunity is the first line of defense against invading bacteria or organisms. When foreign materials try to enter the body, it produces a response in which additional white blood cells begin fighting against the disease-causing organisms. Examples of things within the body that help nonspecific immunity are intact (unbroken) skin, saliva, mucous membranes, and tears. The inflammatory response, including redness, swelling, heat and pain is another defense. This response removes foreign toxins and other materials and begins tissue repair. Fever can also help fight infection.

Specific Immunity

Specific immunity is a type of immunity that is acquired by the body. Specific immunity is either active or passive. In active immunity, the body manufactures antibodies as a response to an antigen, or foreign substance, in the body. For example, when a person gets chickenpox (varicella-zoster virus), antibodies are created. The body will then "remember" the pathogen each time it is exposed to it in the future. The second time the virus tries to invade the body, the antibodies that had formed during the first illness work to prevent a second infection.

Active immunity is also acquired by a vaccine. Vaccines cause the body to produce antibodies to protect against a particular disease. These antibodies will usually protect the person from getting the disease in the future. Vaccines help people develop immunity to diseases without first having the disease. Vaccines can be made with live organisms or with organisms killed by heat or chemicals.

With passive immunity, a person is given the antibodies needed to defend against the antigen. The antibodies can be passed from mother to baby or via an injection. Passive immunity is temporary because the antibodies have a limited life span.

The Lymphatic System

The lymphatic system is composed of the lymph, lymph vessels, lymph nodes, spleen, and the thymus gland. The lymphatic system produces and moves lymph fluid from the body's tissues to the circulatory system. The lymphatic system works to remove excess fluids and waste products from the tissues. It transports fat and vitamins from the gastrointestinal tract to the circulatory system. The lymphatic system also helps the immune system fight infection.

Lymph is a clear yellowish fluid that moves into the lymph system from the tiny capillaries in the circulatory system. Lymph carries disease-fighting cells called lymphocytes. The lymph fluid flows in only one direction.

Lymphatic vessels, or capillaries, are tiny vessels found all over the body. They carry the lymph from the tissues into larger lymphatic vessels. While in the vessels, the lymph travels through and is filtered by the lymph nodes. The larger lymphatic vessels transport lymph into the lymph ducts, from which the lymph drains back into the blood.

The lymph nodes are clumps of lymphatic tissue found in groups along the lymph vessels. These nodes work as filters to clean the lymph fluid of microorganisms, such as bacteria, along with other foreign substances. Lymph nodes are strategically located in places where pathogens can be trapped and prevented from harming the body (Fig. 24-1). Tonsils are large clumps of lymphatic tissue at the back of the oral cavity at the entrance to the throat (pharynx). Tonsils work to prevent microorganisms from entering the body, especially through the mouth or nose.

The spleen, an organ, is the biggest cluster of lymph tissue in the human body. One of its main functions is to work as a type of storage shed for blood. The spleen works as a filter to clean old red blood cells and bacteria from the blood.

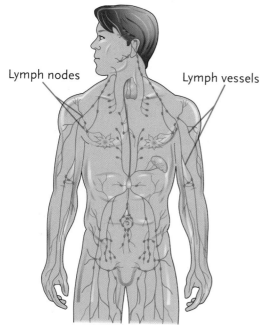

Fig. 24-1. *Lymph nodes work as filters and are located throughout the body.*

Lymph nodes

Lymph vessels

The thymus gland is located in the upper chest, just behind the sternum. Its duty is to make T-cells, or CD4+ lymphocytes, which attack and destroy specific types of pathogens. The thymus reaches its greatest size at puberty and shrinks as we become adults. Once its work is completed, the gland turns into fat and other tissue.

The functions of the immune and lymphatic systems are to:

* Protect against the invasion of foreign substances and pathogens

* Return extra fluid to the circulatory system

3. Discuss changes in the immune and lymphatic systems due to aging

Normal age-related changes for the immune and lymphatic systems include the following:

* Immune system weakens, causing increased risk of all types of infections.

* Antibody response slows.

* T-cells decrease in number.

* Response to vaccines decreases.

4. Describe a common disorder of the immune system

Acquired Immunodeficiency Syndrome (AIDS)

Acquired immune deficiency syndrome (AIDS) is a disease caused by the **human immunodeficiency virus (HIV)**. HIV attacks the body's immune system and damages or destroys its cells. HIV gradually weakens and disables the immune system. AIDS is caused by acquiring the HIV virus through blood or body fluids from an infected person. AIDS is the final stage of HIV infection in which infections, tumors, and central nervous system symptoms appear, due to a weakened immune system that is unable to fight infection. It can take years for HIV to develop into AIDS.

Approximately 11% of HIV cases in the United States are in people over the age of 50. Specific behaviors put people at high risk for acquiring HIV/AIDS. These are the most common methods of transmission of HIV:

- Having unprotected or poorly-protected oral, vaginal, or anal sex with an infected person

- Sharing drug needles or syringes

- Transmission from an infected mother to her newborn during pregnancy or birth, or by breastfeeding

In the healthcare setting, infections can be spread through accidental contact with contaminated blood or body fluids, needles or other sharp objects, or contaminated supplies or equipment (Fig. 24-2).

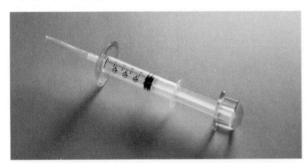

Fig. 24-2. *In health care, contact with contaminated needles or sharps is the most common way for HIV to be transmitted. Handle sharps carefully and dispose of them properly.*

Common Misconceptions About HIV Transmission

The HIV virus cannot survive outside the body for very long. According to the CDC, HIV is not spread in any of these ways:

- Through air or water

- By insects, including mosquitoes

- In saliva, tears, or sweat

- Through casual contact, such as hugging, shaking hands, or sharing dishes

- Through closed-mouth or "social" kissing, such as kissing someone's cheek

Ways to protect against the spread of HIV/AIDS include the following:

- Practice Standard Precautions on every person in your care.

- Be careful when handling any type of sharps and dispose of sharps properly.

- Cover any cuts, sores, tears, breaks, or rashes before caring for residents.

- Never share needles or syringes.

- Do not have unprotected sex. Use condoms if you have sex.

- Stay in a monogamous relationship. Monogamous means having only one sexual partner. You and your partner can be tested for bloodborne diseases like AIDS and hepatitis before having sex.

- Practice abstinence. Abstinence means not having sexual contact with anyone.

- Get tested for HIV and re-tested if necessary. HIV is able to be detected in most people within two to eight weeks. However, it may take up to three months for HIV to be able to be detected and up to six months in rare cases.

The beginning stages of HIV show flu-like symptoms along with swollen glands. Symptoms like headache, fever, fatigue, and swollen lymph glands can appear, last for a few months, and then disappear. Additional symptoms may appear soon after, or they can take many years to develop.

Over time, the HIV virus destroys T-cells, or CD4+ lymphocytes, which are a type of white blood cell. Specifically, the virus reduces the number of T-cells that work to fight infections in the body. This weakens the immune system and makes the person more susceptible to illness. The diagnosis of AIDS is made when the CD4+ cell count falls to 200 or below. The infected person will generally begin to show symptoms, conditions, and diseases that are commonly seen with AIDS.

Signs and symptoms of HIV infection and AIDS include the following:

- Flu-like symptoms, including fever, cough, and severe or constant fatigue
- Headaches
- Loss of appetite
- Weight loss
- Night sweats
- Shaking, chills
- Dry cough
- Shortness of breath
- Swollen lymph nodes
- Sore throat
- Cold sores or fever blisters on the lips
- Mouth sores
- White patches in the mouth or on the tongue
- Cauliflower-like warts on the skin and in the mouth
- Bleeding, inflamed gums
- Yeast infections
- Skin rashes or sores
- Bruising that does not go away
- Dry skin
- Nausea and vomiting
- Blurred vision
- Memory loss

Other diseases can develop in people who have AIDS. Due to the weakened immune system,

opportunistic infections can occur and may be fatal. An **opportunistic infection** is an illness caused by microorganisms due to a person's inability to fight infection. Some of these infections do not cause disease in people who have healthy immune systems. Lack of treatment for HIV/AIDS can increase the risk of serious complications and death from these diseases.

Other diseases that can develop in people with AIDS are pneumocystis carinii pneumonia (PCP), a lung infection, and cryptococcal meningitis, a nervous system disorder. Tuberculosis, herpes, bacterial infections, and hepatitis can also result.

People with AIDS can also develop certain types of cancers. Cervical cancer and a form of cancer called Kaposi's sarcoma are examples. Kaposi's sarcoma is a form of skin cancer that appears as purple, red, or brown skin lesions (Fig. 24-3). The lesions may be painful.

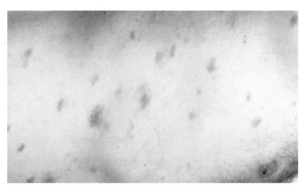

Fig. 24-3. *A purple, red, or brown skin lesion called Kaposi's sarcoma can develop when a person has AIDS.*

In the late stages of AIDS, a form of dementia called AIDS dementia complex (ADC) can develop due to damage to the central nervous system. Symptoms of ADC include memory loss, limited attention span, irritability, poor coordination, lack of judgment, withdrawal from social situations, and depression.

There is no cure for this disease, and there is no vaccine to prevent the disease. Without medication, the HIV-infected person's weakened resistance to infections may lead to AIDS and eventually to death. Many people are living longer with HIV by taking combinations of medications every day. HAART, or highly active antiretroviral therapy, has been shown to control the HIV virus. Three or more medications are used for this therapy.

Treatments used for HIV must generally be taken at specific times throughout the day. They are very expensive and can produce many unpleasant side effects. Gastrointestinal symptoms like nausea, vomiting, and diarrhea, as well as fever and skin rashes, are some of the side effects. Certain medications can be effective, but the length of time they will continue to work for each infected person varies.

Autoimmune Diseases

The immune system protects the body from microorganisms and toxic substances. With an **autoimmune disease**, the body is unable to recognize its own tissue. The immune mechanism sees the normal body tissues as foreign and begins to attack these tissues.

Types of organs and tissues that may be affected by this disease are blood cells, the pancreas, the joints, and the skin. Examples of autoimmune diseases are systemic lupus erythematosis (SLE) and rheumatoid arthritis (RA) (Chapter 21).

Autoimmune disorders have no known cause. Some causes may be genetic links, specific microorganisms, or medications that trigger these disorders.

Signs and symptoms vary and depend upon the disease and the organ(s) or tissues affected. Fever, fatigue, and dizziness are commonly seen with many disorders.

Specific blood tests help diagnose certain autoimmune disorders. Treatment and outlook will depend upon the disorder. The person may require hormone supplements, medications, blood transfusions, or insulin.

---

5. Discuss infection prevention guidelines for a resident with HIV/AIDS

Overall care of a resident with HIV/AIDS involves protecting from infections, providing a safe environment, offering emotional support, and managing symptoms. Follow all infection prevention precautions. The most important reason to always follow Standard Precautions is that you cannot tell by looking at people whether or not they have a bloodborne disease, such as HIV/AIDS. Follow Transmission-Based Precautions if they are ordered in addition to Standard Precautions. See Chapter 6 for more information on Standard and Transmission-Based Precautions.

If you are practicing all infection prevention precautions correctly, there should be no differences in how you care for a resident who has a diagnosis of AIDS and how you provide care for other residents. Casual contact cannot spread HIV/AIDS.

Guidelines: Infection Prevention for HIV/AIDS

G   Always follow proper infection prevention procedures and Standard Precautions with all residents.

G   Wear gloves and other PPE, such as goggles, if you anticipate having contact with blood or other body fluids that might contain blood, like urine and feces (Fig. 24-4). Wear goggles, masks, and/or face shields when splashes or spills may occur.

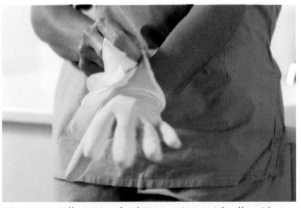

Fig. 24-4. *Follow Standard Precautions with all residents in your care. Wear gloves if you may come into contact with blood, body fluids, non-intact skin, or mucous membranes.*

G   Cover all open sores, cuts, abrasions, rashes, or skin breaks or tears with appropriate bandages or dressings before performing care.

Notify the nurse if you have cuts, sores, or breaks in the skin before beginning care.

G Wash hands and any other areas of the body immediately after contact with blood or other body fluids.

G Handle sharps carefully. Dispose of all sharps properly and safely. Never attempt to re-cap sharps.

G Remind residents and visitors to wash their hands frequently to avoid infection.

G Do not share residents' personal items, such as toothbrushes, hair brushes, razors, etc., with other residents. Put equipment away in its proper place after it has been used.

G Properly disinfect surfaces soiled with blood or body fluids according to facility policy.

Residents' Rights

HIV Testing and Confidentiality

The right to confidentiality is especially important to people with HIV/AIDS because others may pass judgment on people with this disease. A person with HIV/AIDS cannot be fired from a job because of the disease; however, a healthcare worker with HIV/AIDS may be reassigned to job duties with a lower risk of transmitting the disease and a reduced risk of acquiring certain infections from patients.

HIV testing requires consent. That means no one can force you to be tested for HIV unless you agree. HIV test results are confidential and should not be shared with a person's family, friends, or employer without his or her consent. If you are HIV-positive, consider confiding in your supervisor so your assignments can be adjusted to avoid putting you at high risk for exposure to infections. Everyone has a right to privacy regarding his health status. Do not discuss a resident's status with anyone except care team members during reports and rounds.

6. Discuss care guidelines for a resident with HIV/AIDS

Helping residents with HIV or AIDS avoid infection and live safely and comfortably is important. Your quality care and attention may go a long way in helping residents with HIV/AIDS.

Guidelines: HIV/AIDS

G Wash your hands often and help residents to wash their hands.

G Disinfect surfaces in the resident's room and bathroom often.

G Protect the resident from people who have known contagious diseases, including the common cold virus.

G Change linen whenever it is soiled. Linen should be clean and dry and should lie flat, without wrinkles (Fig. 24-5).

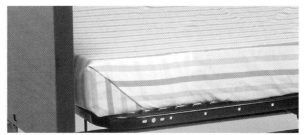

Fig. 24-5. Hospital corners help keep the flat sheet wrinkle-free, which helps promote comfort and prevent pressure ulcers.

G Observe the skin closely for skin changes. Keeping skin clean and dry will help prevent skin breakdown. Follow the care plan on the use of soaps and other cleansers.

G Change position every two hours or as directed. Take great care when moving and positioning residents to prevent bruising.

G Give back rubs for comfort.

G Monitor vital signs often, especially temperature. Fever can occur with infections.

G Residents with HIV/AIDS may have fatigue and severe weakness. Allow enough rest and recognize limitations.

G Ambulate carefully. Provide assistance as needed.

G Allow plenty of time to perform ADLs and help as needed.

G Perform range of motion exercises as ordered (Chapter 25).

G Give quality mouth care frequently. Special mouth rinses may be ordered for mouth sores.

G Use special soft toothbrushes or swabs when cleaning the mouth and performing oral care.

G Because weight loss is a problem for people with HIV/AIDS, special diets may be ordered to assist with maintaining or gaining weight. For example, a high-calorie diet can help maintain weight. Special liquid drinks fortified with extra protein can be used. Report to the nurse if a resident does not seem to be eating or enjoying his food.

G Special diets may also be ordered to help prevent complications. For example, a high-fiber diet may aggravate diarrhea, so it will be avoided. Soft or pureed foods may be easier to swallow for residents who have mouth infections. Cool or warm, rather than hot, food may be easier to eat. Eliminating spices and foods high in acids may be ordered. Encourage residents to follow their special diets.

G Encourage fluids. Filtered water may be ordered by the doctor. If so, make sure the resident does not drink regular water or fluids made with regular water, such as tea. Do not use ice made from regular water.

G Small meals given throughout the day can help nausea, vomiting, and diarrhea. Extra fluids may be ordered to help replace fluid lost. A BRAT (bananas, rice, applesauce, and toast) diet can also help diarrhea. Other diets that help with an upset stomach are the BRATY (bananas, rice, applesauce, toast, and yogurt) and BRATT (bananas, rice, applesauce, tea, and toast) diets.

G Carefully measure weight and intake and output.

G People with AIDS are prone to having diarrhea. Offer a trip to the bathroom or bedpan as often as needed.

G Encourage residents to be as independent as possible.

G Give emotional support, as well as physical care. A resident with AIDS may have been abandoned by family or friends due to the fear of the disease itself. Some people avoid a person with AIDS due to **homophobia**, or a fear of homosexuality. They may also have lost friends who have died from AIDS. Emotions the resident may be experiencing include anxiety, stress, fear, guilt, sadness, depression, and loneliness. It is important to treat residents with respect and help provide the emotional support they need. Listen if the resident wants to talk.

G Other support systems include family, friends, and the person's clergyperson, along with various HIV/AIDS support groups. Special religious or community groups may be of assistance. Depending on your community, many resources and services may be available for people with HIV/AIDS. These include counseling, meal services, access to experimental drugs, and other services. Look online for resources available in your area, or speak to your supervisor if you feel a resident with HIV/AIDS needs more help. Report any comments about suicide immediately to the nurse.

G Notify the nurse if any of the following occur:
- Loss of appetite, nausea, vomiting, or diarrhea
- Weight loss
- Reduced intake of fluids
- Mouth sores or discomfort
- Dysphagia (difficulty swallowing)
- Bleeding from anywhere on the body
- Bruising of the skin
- Pressure ulcers
- Cracks, breaks, rashes, lumps, or sores anywhere on the skin
- Blood in the stool
- Changes in vital signs, especially fever

- Nervousness, withdrawal, severe mood swings, or depression
- Any behavior that puts the resident or others at risk; suicidal thoughts or comments

Residents' Rights

Residents' Rights and HIV/AIDS

Spend quality time with residents who have HIV or AIDS. This may mean sitting and listening quietly to their concerns. It can mean reading to them if they wish. Encouraging participation in activities of their choice may be helpful. Do not avoid residents who have this disease. HIV/AIDS is not transmitted by breathing the same air as someone who is infected. These residents need the same attentive and thoughtful care you give all of your residents.

Tip

Pets and People with HIV/AIDS

Some facilities have one or more cats and/or dogs living on the premises. Due to their weakened immune systems, people who are infected with HIV or AIDS may not be able to be around pets due to the risk of different types of infection. Follow facility policy. Always wash your hands with soap and water after touching a pet, and before touching any resident. Ask visitors to do the same.

For more information about HIV/AIDS and other bloodborne pathogens, see Chapter 6.

7. Describe cancer

Cancer is a general term used to describe a disease in which abnormal cells grow in an uncontrolled way. These cancerous cells do not die like normal cells do. They live longer than normal cells and can continue to increase in number.

Cancer usually occurs in the form of a tumor that grows on or within the human body. A **tumor** is a group of abnormally-growing cells. Tumors are either **benign** (non-cancerous) or **malignant** (cancerous). Benign tumors grow slowly and do not spread to other parts of the body. Malignant tumors grow rapidly and invade surrounding tissue.

Cancer can act in different ways. It can **metastasize**, or spread, to other areas of the body. Oncology is the branch of medicine that deals with the study of and treatment of cancer.

Risk factors for cancer include the following:

- Age
- Race
- Gender
- Family history
- Tobacco use
- Alcohol use
- Poor diet/obesity
- Lack of exercise
- Chemicals and food additives
- Radiation
- Sun exposure (Fig. 24-6)

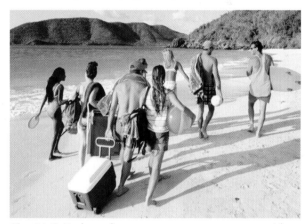

Fig. 24-6. *Prolonged sun exposure puts a person at risk for skin cancer.*

There is no known cure for cancer. However, when cancer is caught early, it can be treated effectively and controlled. The American Cancer Society (ACS) has identified these signs of cancer:

- Fever
- Fatigue
- Unexplained weight loss
- Pain
- Skin changes, such as change in skin color (e.g. jaundice)
- New mole or a change in the appearance of an existing mole, wart, or spot

- Change in bowel/bladder function
- A sore that does not heal
- Unusual bleeding/discharge
- Any thickening in breast, scrotum, or other areas
- Indigestion or difficulty swallowing
- Nagging cough or hoarseness

A diagnosis of cancer is made after various tests, such as a biopsy, have been performed. A **biopsy** is the removal of a sample of tissue for examination and diagnosis (Fig. 24-7). After the diagnosis of cancer is made, the treatment plan is developed. Treatment is based on whether or not the cancer has spread to other parts of the body. The choice of therapy is determined by the person's prognosis, or outlook. Common treatments for cancer, which may be used in combination, are as follows:

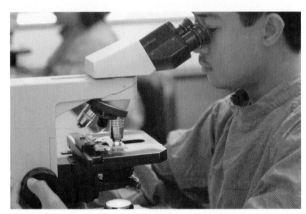

Fig. 24-7. Tissue that is biopsied is checked for malignant cells.

Surgery to remove malignant tumors is performed for some types of cancer. The goal of the operation(s) is to try to remove as much of the cancer as possible. Surgery is generally performed for cancers of the breast, skin, and colon.

Radiation therapy (radiotherapy) uses high-energy rays to attempt to destroy cancer cells in a specific area (Fig. 24-8). It can also be used to control cancerous growths. Radiation treatments do not cause pain. However, side effects of radiation therapy include skin irritation and burns, which may cause pain. Radiation therapy may also cause an increased risk of infection.

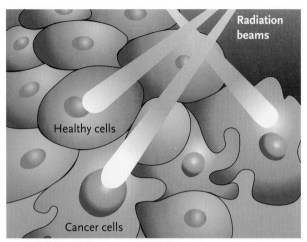

Fig. 24-8. Radiation is targeted at cancer cells, but it also destroys some healthy cells in its path.

Chemotherapy involves chemical agents or medications being administered, usually intravenously, to kill malignant cells and tissues. Chemotherapy is chosen for cancers that have spread. It can also be used to slow growth of a cancer or to prevent the cancer in a certain area from spreading. There are many severe side effects of this treatment, including bone or joint pain, temporary hair loss, nausea and vomiting, diarrhea, fatigue, mouth sores, peripheral neuropathy (Chapter 23), and a higher risk of infections. Chemotherapeutic agents are generally given into a vein through an IV, but some are given by mouth or by injection.

Hormone therapy uses medications to alter the hormones in the body. This can be effective when the tumors rely on specific hormones to survive and grow. Hormone therapy reduces certain hormones in the body. It also changes the ability of the tumors to use the hormones. Side effects include hot flashes, weight gain, and fluid retention.

Immunotherapy is another form of cancer treatment. This therapy uses the body's immune system to fight the malignant tumors. Cancer vaccines are a form of immunotherapy. Another form of immunotherapy is through the administration of antibodies.

There are two forms of cancer vaccines. Cancer preventive vaccines are given to try to prevent healthy people from developing cancer. Two types have been approved by the FDA: a vaccine for types of the human papillomavirus, which can cause cervical cancer, and a vaccine for the hepatitis B virus, which can cause liver cancer.

Cancer treatment vaccines are the other type of cancer vaccine. They are given to treat a cancer that already exists by trying to make the body's immune system fight the disease. One vaccine in this category has been approved for some men with prostate cancer.

Immunotherapy works in different ways. One way it works is to interfere with the growth of cancer cells. Side effects depend upon the specific treatment used. They include fever, weakness, nausea, vomiting, and diarrhea. This form of therapy is often combined with chemotherapy or other cancer therapies.

Remission is the disappearance of signs and symptoms of cancer or other diseases. It can be partial or complete. A remission can be temporary or permanent.

Palliative care will be provided for someone with advanced cancer. This type of care works to relieve the symptoms and to reduce pain and suffering caused by the disease. Complications are treated early, which helps reduce discomfort. Care conferences include family and friends, along with a large palliative care team. This team is devoted to providing the resident with the best quality of life possible. See Chapter 27 for more information on palliative care.

8. Discuss care guidelines for a resident with cancer

The resident with cancer will require careful and attentive physical and emotional care.

Guidelines: Cancer

G **Skin care**. Observe the skin carefully to help prevent pressure ulcers. Change position every two hours or as directed. Be careful when moving and positioning residents to reduce bruising. Follow any special skin care orders exactly (for example: no hot or cold packs, no soap, lotion, or other cosmetics, no garters or tight stockings). Special mattresses or pads used in beds and chairs can help reduce the risk of pressure ulcers. Keep skin clean and dry. Apply lotion to dry skin if ordered. Do not use lotion on areas having radiation therapy. Do not remove any markings that are used with radiation therapy. If skin problems or infections occur, they can cause odors. Notify the nurse if you observe any signs of infection, such as swelling, warmth, redness, or draining wounds.

G **Self-image**. Hair loss, weakness, changed appearance, and dependency on caregivers can change a person's self-image. Help residents stay clean and well-groomed. Offer wigs, scarves, or hats for hair loss. Assist with application of make-up, as requested.

G **Oral care**. Give oral care often and help as needed. Be gentle when brushing teeth; soft brushes or special swabs can help with mouth pain or sores or lip sores. Mild mouth rinses (avoid mouthwashes) can reduce bad taste in the mouth due to medication or vomiting.

G **Pain**. Cancer can cause severe pain. It can affect the ability to sleep, eat, and move about. Medications and other measures are used to treat pain. Be alert for signs of pain and notify the nurse as soon as pain occurs. Provide comfort measures to reduce pain. Give back rubs and help residents change positions in bed or in a chair. Other measures include playing soft music, reading, or talking quietly with residents.

Pain medications can cause side effects, including constipation, upset stomach, and fatigue. Notify the nurse if these side effects occur. If a resident has a transdermal patch on the skin to help with pain, report any redness, swelling, or irritation. The nurse is responsible for applying and removing these patches. Notify the nurse if you see more than one patch on the resident's body.

The resident may be using a PCA pump for pain relief. A PCA pump, or patient-controlled analgesia, allows the person to press a button which releases pain medication. Observe and report redness, swelling, and warmth around the insertion site.

Cancer may cause **breakthrough pain**, which is a type of severe pain that happens unexpectedly. Even though the person is regularly taking pain medication, this pain is not helped by this medication. The pain periodically "breaks through" the medication. Report signs of pain to the nurse. Guided imagery and relaxation techniques can help with breakthrough pain.

G **Vital signs**. Changes in vital signs can occur with cancer and with cancer therapy. Monitor all vital signs, especially temperature. Fever can occur with some forms of cancer therapy. Report changes in vital signs to the nurse.

G **Mobility**. People with cancer may have fatigue and weakness, which can make movement difficult. Allow plenty of time for rest and recognize limitations. Gently assist with ambulation, if needed.

G **Nutrition**. Good nutrition is important for people with cancer. They need to eat and drink enough to maintain their energy levels. Unintended weight loss can occur with cancer or with cancer treatment. Provide small, frequent meals to reduce nausea and help prevent weight loss. Serve favorite foods and keep nutritious snacks available. Liquid nutrition supplements may be used in addition to, not in place of, meals. Provide food whenever hunger occurs, as allowed. Try cool or cold foods if hot foods increase nausea. Cut food into small pieces if necessary. Use plastic utensils if silver utensils cause a bitter taste in the mouth. Weigh residents as ordered,

and report weight loss or gain. Encourage fluids as allowed. Fortified liquid supplements may be ordered. Carefully monitor intake and output and report changes.

G **Bladder and bowel changes**. Bladder and bowel habits can be affected in those with cancer. Urine may have blood in it, and output may decrease. Urine can become more concentrated and have an odor. Diarrhea can occur, along with blood in the stool. Assist residents to the bathroom or offer the bedpan often. Give catheter care as needed. Carefully measure output. Give proper perineal care, as needed. Test stool as ordered for hidden (occult) blood.

G **Mental status and emotional needs**. Some people with cancer want to talk about their diagnosis and treatment; others withdraw and avoid discussing their disease. Be sensitive to this, and follow residents' wishes. Listen and allow them to express their feelings. Spend as much time with residents as possible (Fig. 24-9). Encourage involvement in activities, if possible. There are many support groups available for people with cancer. The nurse can ask the social worker to help the resident contact a support group. When talking with residents, do not use clichés such as, "You will be just fine." Provide support during painful episodes and difficult times. Remind residents that there can still be good days and special times ahead. Observe and report signs of depression, including comments about suicide.

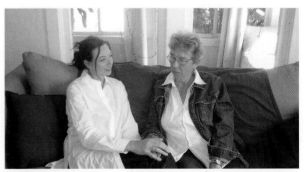

Fig. 24-9. *Give residents with cancer as much emotional support as possible.*

G Notify the nurse if any of the following occur:

- Pain or increased pain
- Changes in vital signs, especially fever
- Signs of any new bumps or lumps or any other changes in the skin
- Rashes, cracks, sores, breaks, or reddened areas on the skin
- Odors
- Burns or skin irritation
- Bruising of the skin
- Difficulty with ambulation
- Fainting
- Increased fatigue or weakness
- Chest pain or tightness
- Shortness of breath
- Appetite changes or weight loss
- Difficulty chewing or swallowing
- Dry, sore mouth and mouth or lip sores
- Inflammation or irritation of the mucous membranes in the mouth
- Bleeding from gums or anywhere inside the mouth
- Nausea or vomiting
- Flatus, diarrhea, or constipation
- Blood in the stool
- Change in output
- Any change in urine or blood in the urine
- Urinary tract infection
- Change in mental status or confusion
- Anxiety, fear, or angry feelings
- Signs of depression

Residents' Rights

Cancer

The term "cancer" may frighten you. However, understanding the facts may help lessen your fears. Cancer is not a contagious disease. It cannot be transmitted through touch or hugs or by being close to a person who has it. Do not avoid residents who have cancer. Spend as much time as possible with them. It is the caring and right thing to do.

Chapter Review

1. Briefly describe nonspecific immunity and specific immunity (LO 2).

2. Give one example of active immunity and one example of passive immunity (LO 2).

3. What is the function of lymph (LO 2)?

4. List four normal age-related changes of the immune and lymphatic systems (LO 3).

5. How is HIV transmitted (LO 4)?

6. List four risk factors for acquiring HIV (LO 4).

7. List five common misconceptions about how HIV is transmitted (LO 4).

8. Is there a cure for HIV or AIDS (LO 4)?

9. What is an autoimmune disease (LO 4)?

10. List six infection prevention guidelines for HIV/AIDS (LO 5).

11. Can a person be forced to be tested for HIV without agreeing to the test (LO 5)?

12. Can an HIV test result be shared with anyone requesting information (LO 5)?

13. List 15 care guidelines for a resident with HIV/AIDS (LO 6).

14. What is the difference between benign and malignant tumors (LO 7)?

15. List nine signs of cancer identified by the ACS (LO 7).

16. Briefly describe five treatments for cancer: surgery, radiation therapy, chemotherapy, hormone therapy, immunotherapy (LO 7).

17. For each of these topics—skin care, self-image, oral care, pain management, vital signs, mobility, nutrition, bladder and bowel changes, mental status and emotional needs—list one way a nursing assistant can help a resident with cancer (LO 8).

25
Rehabilitation and Restorative Care

A View from the Past: Rehabilitation

In 1918 there were so many injured veterans returning from World War I that doctors in the United States developed an idea about how to bring an injured person to the point where he would be able to return to work. Following WWI, the idea of rehabilitation grew. Facilities and programs were created, and when the thousands of victims of the war returned to the U.S. (many without arms or legs), they were able to begin their rehabilitation.

"You cannot run away from a weakness. You must some time fight it out or perish . . ."

Robert Louis Stevenson, 1850-1894

"The best of healers is good cheer."

Pindar, 522-438 B.C.

1. Define important words in this chapter

abduction: moving a body part away from the midline of the body.

active assisted range of motion (AAROM): exercises to put a joint through its full arc of motion that are done by a resident with some help from a staff member.

active range of motion (AROM): exercises to put a joint through its full arc of motion that are done by a resident alone, without help.

adaptive devices: special equipment that helps a person who is ill or disabled perform ADLs; also called assistive devices.

adduction: moving a body part toward the midline of the body.

assistive devices: special equipment that helps a person who is ill or disabled perform ADLs; also called adaptive devices.

dorsiflexion: bending backward.

extension: straightening a body part.

flexion: bending a body part.

foot drop: weakness of muscles in the feet and ankles that interferes with the ability to flex the ankles and walk normally.

hyperextension: extending a joint beyond its normal range of motion.

opposition: touching the thumb to any other finger.

orthotic devices: devices applied externally to limbs to support, protect, improve function, and prevent complications.

passive range of motion (PROM): exercises to put a joint through its full arc of motion that are done by staff without the resident's help.

physiatrists: doctors who specialize in rehabilitation.

pronation: turning downward.

range of motion (ROM): exercises that put a joint through its full arc of motion.

rehabilitation: care that is managed by professionals to restore a person to the highest possible level of functioning after an illness or injury.

restorative care: care used after rehabilitation to maintain a person's function and increase independence.

rotation: turning the joint.

supination: turning upward.

2. Discuss rehabilitation and restorative care

A disability results from physical, personal, and environmental factors that, when combined, limit a person's ability to function properly. When a person develops a change in his ability to function, rehabilitation may be necessary. **Rehabilitation** is care used to restore a person to his highest level of functioning possible after an accident, illness, or injury. Rehabilitation revolves around holistic care, or treating the whole person. All of the person's needs are assessed, including his psychological needs. The type of rehabilitation ordered and how much progress is made depend upon many factors. Some of these factors include the following:

- How soon rehabilitation began

- Any pre-existing diseases or injuries that the person may have

- Overall motivation of the person

- Type of facility where the person is living

- Combined efforts of the staff and the person's family and friends

- Attitude of the rehabilitation team

- Consistency in following the care plan

For rehabilitation to succeed, all staff members must work together to return the person to his highest level of functioning. The rehabilitation team is made up of highly skilled and trained professionals, including (Fig. 25-1):

- **Physiatrists** (doctors who specialize in rehabilitation) and other doctors

- Speech-language pathologists and physical and occupational therapists

- Nurses

- Social workers

- Discharge planners

- Nursing assistants

- Resident

- Resident's family and friends

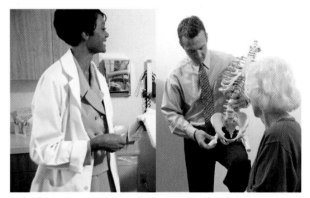

Fig. 25-1. *A team of specialists, including doctors and physical therapists, helps assist residents with rehabilitation.*

The nursing staff will develop a care plan based on goals for restoring and maintaining the resident's function. Each body system will be considered when creating the care plan. For example, the team will work to prevent contractures, a musculoskeletal condition and a serious complication of immobility.

Goal-setting is done with the participation of all departments. For each task requiring improvement, the team will develop specific steps to meet the goals. The rehabilitation team will carefully follow the goals listed in each resident's care plan. The goals of rehabilitative care include the following:

- Assist the resident in maintaining and/or regaining the ability to perform activities of daily living (ADLs)

- Promote resident's independence and help resident adapt to the new disability

- Prevent complications of immobility

Nursing assistants are vital members of the rehabilitation team. OBRA states that NAs must be properly trained to work with residents who are in a rehabilitative setting. Not only will they provide quality physical care, they will also help with the resident's emotional needs. Nursing assistants should work to make the environment as safe and secure for the resident as possible.

When the goals of rehabilitation have been met, restorative care may be ordered. **Restorative care** works to maintain a person's functioning and to increase independence.

During rehabilitation and restorative care, the team must work together to prevent complications. The attitude of staff has a great impact on the success of the program. Follow these guidelines to help give quality care to residents in these programs:

Guidelines: Rehabilitation and Restorative Care

G   Understand the diagnosis and the disability. Know any limitations the resident may have. Be familiar with the resident's ability to perform ADLs. OBRA requires that residents must receive all of the therapy listed in the care plan each day.

G   Be patient with the resident and his family and friends. Offer praise frequently, even if the improvement is small. For example, a resident can hold a spoon on Monday. On Tuesday, he is able to lift the spoon. Praise each success.

G   Maintain a positive attitude at all times. Be empathetic. An optimistic and positive attitude is a key to success (Fig. 25-2). Never become frustrated or angry with the resident or his family or friends. The nursing staff will set the stage for the care.

G   Spend as much time as possible listening to the resident's thoughts and feelings about the process. Sitting quietly and listening can be very helpful.

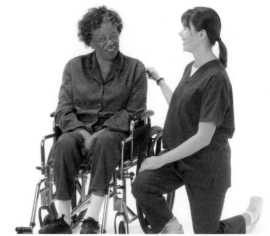

Fig. 25-2. *Be optimistic and encouraging. Your good attitude has a positive effect on residents.*

G   Provide plenty of privacy while working with residents. It helps to avoid distractions and potential embarrassment.

G   Encourage residents' independence, along with personal choice. They must do as much for themselves as possible. Ask family and friends to encourage residents' independence, too. See Learning Objective 3 of this chapter for more on independence.

G   Encourage as much daily activity as possible. Inactivity causes complications and can cause setbacks in rehabilitation, along with other problems.

G   Accept that the resident may have setbacks. Each person is different. Focus on the things that the resident can do, and not what he or she cannot do.

G   Nursing assistants are often the first staff members who observe a potential problem or complication with the rehabilitative process. Report any of the following signs and symptoms to the nurse:

- Lack of motivation

- Signs of withdrawal or depression

- Any change in ability, positive or negative

- Decreased strength

- Change in ability to perform range of motion

Residents' Rights

The Restorative Environment

A resident's surroundings are very important to the success of rehabilitation. The environment should be set up to encourage a positive outcome. The rehabilitation team should:

- Create a secure, quiet, and pleasant rehabilitative environment.
- Encourage residents to make decisions.
- Ensure that residents are bathed, dressed, and well-groomed every day.
- Maintain privacy and allow for private visits from family and friends.
- Encourage friendly relationships between residents.
- Spend time with residents as often as possible.
- Encourage participation in appropriate activities.

3. Describe the importance of promoting independence

An injury or illness that results in a loss of function can cause dependence on others for help with daily activities. Residents may never have needed help before with bathing, dressing, eating, or other tasks during their entire adult lives. Being required to accept help with ADLs can cause anger, frustration, depression, and embarrassment, along with an increase in dependence.

As you have learned, promoting each resident's independence is an important duty of the care team. Encouraging independence has positive effects on self-image, attitude, and abilities. Sometimes it will appear easier for you to do things for residents, rather than allowing them to accomplish tasks independently. However, let residents do as much as they can for themselves, regardless of how long it takes or how poorly they are able to do it. Even if you think you could do a task better or faster, be patient. Encourage each resident to perform as much self-care as possible (Fig. 25-3). Independence helps self-esteem, along with speeding recovery. Self-care also helps the body stay active and prevents complications of immobility.

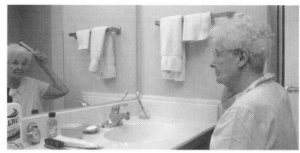

Fig. 25-3. *Encourage residents to perform self-care no matter how long it takes them to do it.*

Cues

A common approach to promoting independence with rehabilitative care is to try cues. Cues can be verbal or physical. A verbal cue is a short sequence of words that directs the person to complete a specific step. For example, you say, "Take a sip of water." A physical cue is showing the person how to do the activity. For example, you place your hand over the resident's hand around the cup, helping him bring it to his mouth for a drink. Cues may be used with residents during rehabilitation and also for residents with other conditions, such as Alzheimer's disease. See Chapters 14 and 22 for more information on cues.

Residents' Rights

The Right To Make Choices

Residents should make as many choices as possible. They have the right to choose their food, clothing, doctors, visitors, and how to spend their time. This is not just their legal right; it also helps to encourage independence.

4. Explain the complications of immobility and describe how exercise helps maintain health

Activity is an essential part of a person's life. When a person becomes immobile and inactive, the body does not respond well. Complications that result from a lack of exercise and activity, organized by body system, include the following:

- Gastrointestinal: constipation
- Urinary: urinary tract infection (UTI)
- Integumentary: pressure ulcers and slow-healing wounds

- Circulatory: blood clots, especially in the legs
- Respiratory: pneumonia
- Musculoskeletal: muscle atrophy and contractures
- Nervous: depression or insomnia
- Endocrine: weight gain

Just as inactivity and immobility have negative effects, regular activity and exercise have many benefits for the body:

- Gastrointestinal: promotes appetite and aids regular elimination
- Urinary: improves elimination, helping to decrease infection
- Integumentary: improves the quality and health of the skin
- Circulatory: improves circulation
- Respiratory: reduces the chance of infections, such as pneumonia, and improves oxygen level
- Musculoskeletal: increases blood flow to the muscles and improves strength
- Nervous: improves relaxation and sleep
- Endocrine: increases metabolism, helping to maintain healthy weight

5. Describe canes, walkers, and crutches

Residents may require temporary or permanent walking aids. Canes, walkers, and crutches are assistive devices that help a person with ambulation. You first learned about how to assist with ambulation in Chapter 11.

A cane is used to help a person with balance. It is not meant to completely support a person's weight. Residents who use a cane should be able to bear some weight on both legs, even if one leg is weaker. If one leg is weaker, the cane should be held on the stronger side. The proper height of the cane will be determined by the physical therapy department.

Types of canes include the C cane, the functional grip cane, and the quad cane. The C cane is very common and is shaped like a curved candy cane.

It usually has a rubber-tipped bottom to prevent slipping. A functional grip cane is like a C cane, except that it has a straight grip handle, rather than the curved one. This helps the person grip the handle better. A quad cane has four rubber-tipped feet and a rectangular base. Quad canes are able to bear more weight than other canes.

Walkers are walking aids that offer additional support (Fig. 25-4). The walker gives more stability when a person is unsteady or has some weakness. The feet may be rubber-tipped or the walker may have wheels. Walkers are used when a resident can bear some weight on his legs. When using a walker, the walker is moved first, then the weak leg, then the strong leg.

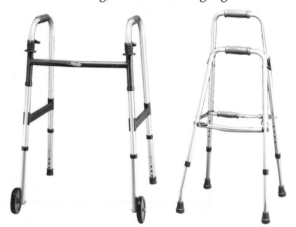

Fig. 25-4. *The photo on the left shows a standard walker and the photo on the right shows a "Hemi Walker," which is a walker that is designed for people who have difficulty using an arm or a hand.* (PHOTO COURTESY OF INVACARE CONTINUING CARE, 1-800-668-2337, WWW.INVACARE-CC.COM)

Crutches are used when a person can only bear limited weight or cannot bear any weight at all on one leg. Crutches have rubber-tipped feet to prevent sliding. One or two crutches may be used. When a resident uses crutches, stay on his weaker side.

Canes, walkers, and crutches are specially fitted to each resident. A physical therapist or a nurse will take measurements for walking aids and will give instructions to residents about how to use this equipment. When helping residents, know how to assist with each device. If you are unsure about anything or have any questions, notify the nurse.

Guidelines: Canes, Walkers, and Crutches

G   Carefully check cane, walker, or crutches for any damage before using these devices. Make sure there are no cracks and that the device is not bent. Make sure any rubber pieces are snugly in place and are in good condition.

G   Make sure resident is wearing non-skid shoes with the laces tied or straps fastened. Clothing should not be so loose or long that it catches in the equipment when moving.

G   Watch for and avoid unsafe environmental situations, such as wet floors or clutter in the hallways. Wipe up spills and keep walkways clear.

G   Encourage residents to use good posture when walking, if possible.

G   Do not rush the resident.

G   Do not hang heavy items on a walker.

G   Have the resident hold the cane on his stronger side.

G   While the resident is ambulating, stay near on the weaker side.

G   If the resident has pain while ambulating, move him to a chair or back to the bed, if near, then notify the nurse.

G   Return the resident safely back to the bed or chair after activity is completed.

Assisting with ambulation for a resident using a cane, walker or crutches

Equipment: gait belt, non-skid shoes for resident, cane, walker, or crutches

1.   Identify yourself by name. Identify the resident. Greet the resident by name.

2.   Wash your hands.

3.   Explain procedure to resident. Speak clearly, slowly, and directly. Maintain face-to-face contact whenever possible.

4.   Provide for the resident's privacy with a curtain, screen, or door.

5.   Adjust bed to a low position so that the resident's feet are flat on the floor. Lock bed wheels.

6.   Put non-skid footwear on resident and securely fasten.

7.   Stand in front of and face resident.

8.   Place gait belt below the rib cage and above the waist. Do not put it over bare skin. Check to make sure that breasts are not caught under the belt. Grasp belt securely on both sides.

9.   Brace resident's lower legs with your legs to prevent slipping. This can be done by placing both of your knees in front of the resident's knees.

10. On the count of three, slowly help resident to stand.

11. Help as needed with ambulation.

a.   ***Cane.*** Resident places cane about six inches, or a comfortable distance, in front of his stronger leg (Fig. 25-5). He brings weaker leg even with cane. He then brings stronger leg forward slightly ahead of cane. Repeat.

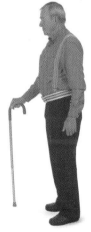

Fig. 25-5. *The cane moves in front of the stronger leg first.*

b.   ***Walker.*** Resident picks up or rolls the walker. He places it about six inches, or a comfortable distance, in front of him. All four feet or wheels of the walker should be on the ground before resident steps forward to the walker. The walker should not be moved again until the resident has moved both feet forward and is steady (Fig. 25-6). The resident should never put his feet ahead of the walker.

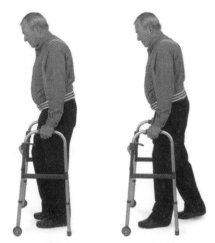

Fig. 25-6. The walker can be moved after the resident is steady and both feet are forward.

c. **Crutches**. Resident should be fitted for crutches and taught to use them correctly by a physical therapist or nurse. The resident may use the crutches several different ways. It depends on the weakness. No matter how they are used, weight should be on the resident's hands and arms. Weight should never be on the underarm area (Fig. 25-7).

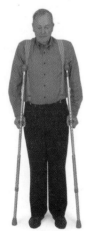

Fig. 25-7. When using crutches, weight should be on the hands and arms, not the underarms.

12. Walk slightly behind and on the weaker side of resident. Hold the gait belt, if one is used.

13. Watch for obstacles in the resident's path. Ask the resident to look ahead, not down at his feet.

14. Encourage resident to rest if he is tired. When a person is tired, it increases the risk of a fall. Let resident set the pace. Discuss how far he plans to go based on the care plan.

15. After ambulation, remove gait belt. Make resident comfortable.

16. If leaving the resident in bed, return bed to lowest position. Remove privacy measures.

17. Leave call light within resident's reach.

18. Wash your hands.

19. Be courteous and respectful at all times.

20. Report any changes in the resident to the nurse. Document procedure using facility guidelines.

6. Discuss other assistive devices and orthotics

People in rehabilitation may struggle to perform their activities of daily living (ADLs), such as dressing, eating, bathing, oral care, hair care, moving, nail care, toileting, and eating and drinking. The rehabilitation team works to help restore a resident's ability to do ADLs. **Assistive** or **adaptive devices** can help people who are recovering from an illness or adapting to a physical disability. They also help promote a person's independence. Examples are special combs, plate guards, and prostheses (Chapter 21). There are many types of assistive devices available to help with ADLs. Examples are shown in Figure 25-8.

Positioning devices are used to help prevent complications from inactivity and immobility. These devices aid in proper body alignment and positioning. They include the following:

• Backrests can be regular pillows or special wedge-shaped foam pillows. They provide

Rehabilitation and Restorative Care

support and comfort and maintain proper body alignment.

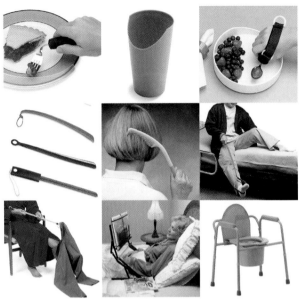

Fig. 25-8. *Many assistive devices are available. They help make it easier for residents to adapt to physical changes.* (PHOTOS COURTESY OF NORTH COAST MEDICAL, INC., WWW.NCMEDICAL.COM, 800-821-9319)

• Footboards are padded boards or pillow-like devices placed against the resident's feet to keep them properly aligned. They help prevent foot drop. **Foot drop** is a weakness of muscles in the feet and ankles that interferes with the ability to flex the ankles and walk normally. Footboards are also used to keep linens off the feet.

• Bed cradles or foot cradles are used to keep bed covers from resting on the resident's legs and feet (Fig. 25-9).

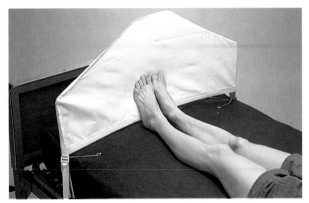

Fig. 25-9. *Bed cradles help prevent bed covers from resting on the legs and feet.* (REPRINTED WITH PERMISSION OF BRIGGS CORPORATION, WWW.BRIGGSCORP.COM, 800-247-2343)

• Heel protectors are padded protectors wrapped around feet and heels to help keep feet properly aligned, which helps prevent foot drop (Fig. 25-10).

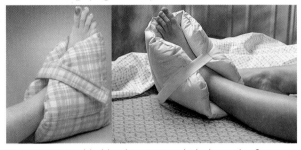

Fig. 25-10. *Padded heel protectors help keep the feet properly aligned.* (REPRINTED WITH PERMISSION OF BRIGGS CORPORATION, WWW.BRIGGSCORP.COM, 800-247-2343)

• Abduction wedges/splints/pads (hip wedges) keep hips in proper position after hip surgery.

• Trochanter rolls are rolled-up bath blankets or towels that prevent the hip and leg from turning outward (Fig. 25-11).

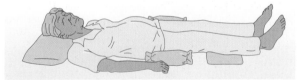

Fig. 25-11. *Trochanter rolls prevent the hip and leg from turning outward.*

• Handrolls are cloth-covered or rubber grips that keep the hand and/or fingers in a normal and natural position. Handrolls help prevent finger, hand, or wrist contractures (Fig. 25-12).

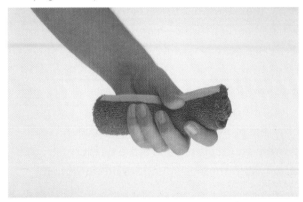

Fig. 25-12. *Handrolls keep the hand and/or fingers in a natural position, helping to prevent contractures.* (REPRINTED WITH PERMISSION OF BRIGGS CORPORATION, WWW.BRIGGSCORP.COM, 800-247-2343)

- Finger cushions are stuffed devices made of terry cloth or a similar material that keep the fingers separated. They help prevent contractures of the thumb or fingers.

- Elbow protectors are padded protectors wrapped around elbows to help prevent rubbing, irritation, and pressure ulcers.

- **Orthotic devices** are devices applied externally to a limb for support and protection (Fig. 25-13). They keep the joints in the correct position and are used to improve function and prevent complications, such as contractures. Other names for orthotic devices are splints or braces.

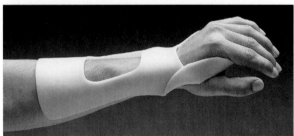

Fig. 25-13. *Two types of splints.* (PHOTO COURTESY OF NORTH COAST MEDICAL, INC., WWW.NCMEDICAL.COM, 800-821-9319)

7. Discuss range of motion exercises

When a resident is immobile for a period of time, many complications can result, as you learned earlier in the chapter. Range of motion exercises are often ordered to prevent complications from inactivity and immobility. **Range of motion (ROM)** exercises are exercises that put a joint through its full arc of motion. The goals of range of motion exercises are to decrease or prevent contractures and atrophy, increase circulation, and improve strength and movement.

ROM exercises may be ordered at various times during a resident's day. There will also be guidelines for how many times a ROM exercise for a

particular joint should be performed each session. The procedure below states that these exercises should be performed at least three times for each joint per session. Follow the care plan and your facility's specific policies, which may require more exercises to be completed.

Three types of range of motion exercises are:

Active range of motion (AROM) exercises put a joint through its full arc of motion and are done by a resident alone, without help.

Active-assisted range of motion (AAROM) exercises put a joint through its full arc of motion and are done by a resident with some help from a staff member.

Passive range of motion (PROM) exercises put a joint through its full arc of motion and are done by staff, without the resident's help. These are ordered when a resident cannot move on his own.

Range of motion exercises are specific for each area of the body. Be familiar with the following body movements (Fig. 25-14):

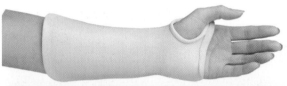
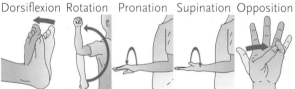

Fig. 25-14. *The different range of motion body movements.*

- **Abduction**: moving a body part away from the midline of the body

- **Adduction**: moving a body part toward the midline of the body

- **Extension**: straightening a body part

- **Flexion**: bending a body part

- **Dorsiflexion**: bending backward

- **Rotation**: turning the joint
- **Pronation**: turning downward
- **Supination**: turning upward
- **Opposition**: touching the thumb to any other finger

Guidelines: ROM Exercises

G   Follow the care plan carefully. A doctor or physical therapist will give the order for ROM exercises to be performed. The head and neck are usually not exercised by NAs without specific instructions from a nurse or doctor.

G   Use proper body mechanics when performing ROM exercises.

G   You will work on both sides of the body, unless instructed otherwise. Begin at the head and work down the body.

G   Support the joint, both above and below, while giving ROM exercises.

G   Follow instructions for limiting ROM exercises. Do not exercise a joint that is bandaged or has a dressing, cast, or special tubing. Never exercise a joint that has reddened areas, rashes, bruises, sores, or one that is draining fluid.

G   Maintain privacy at all times when doing ROM exercises. Expose only the area being exercised at one time.

G   Never push the resident to move further than what is comfortable. **Hyperextension**, extending a joint beyond its normal range of motion, can cause injury. Promptly stop and report any complaints of pain or any other problem, such as difficulty breathing, to the nurse.

G   Keep the resident's body in good alignment. Use pillows as needed (see Chapter 11).

G   Use ROM exercises as an opportunity to provide holistic care to residents. For example, listen to and talk with the resident while performing these exercises. Let the resident voice any problems or concerns he may have. Give praise often.

Assisting with passive range of motion exercises

1. Identify yourself by name. Identify the resident. Greet the resident by name.

2. Wash your hands.

3. Explain procedure to resident. Speak clearly, slowly, and directly. Maintain face-to-face contact whenever possible.

4. Provide for the resident's privacy with a curtain, screen, or door.

5. Adjust the bed to a safe level, usually waist high. Lock the bed wheels.

6. Position the resident lying supine—flat on his or her back—on the bed. Position body in good alignment.

7. Repeat each exercise at least three times.

8. *Shoulder*. Support resident's arm at elbow and wrist while performing ROM for shoulder. Place one hand under the elbow and the other hand under the wrist. Raise the straightened arm from the side position upward toward head to ear level and return arm down to side of the body (extension/flexion) (Fig. 25-15).

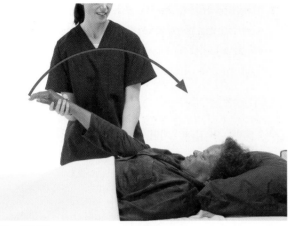

Fig. 25-15.

Move straightened arm away from side of body to shoulder level and return arm to side of body (abduction/adduction) (Fig. 25-16).

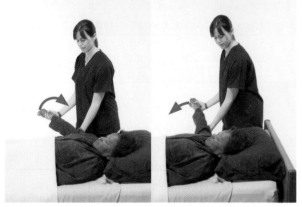

Fig. 25-16.

9. **Elbow.** Hold the wrist with one hand. Hold the elbow with the other hand. Bend elbow so that the hand touches the shoulder on that same side (flexion). Straighten arm (extension) (Fig. 25-17).

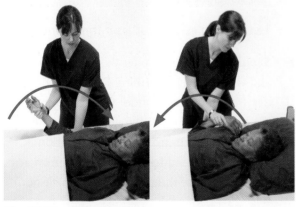

Fig. 25-17.

Exercise forearm by moving it so palm is facing downward (pronation) and then upward (supination) (Fig. 25-18).

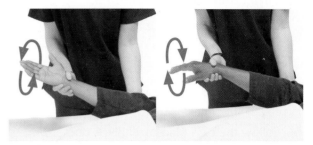

Fig. 25-18.

10. **Wrist.** Hold the wrist with one hand. Use the fingers of your other hand to help the joint through the motions. Bend the hand down (flexion). Bend the hand backward (dorsiflexion) (Fig. 25-19).

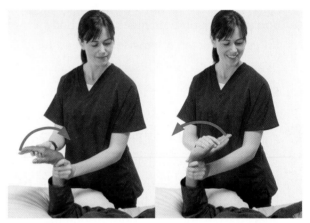

Fig. 25-19.

Turn the hand in the direction of the thumb (radial flexion). Then turn the hand in the direction of the little finger (ulnar flexion) (Fig. 25-20).

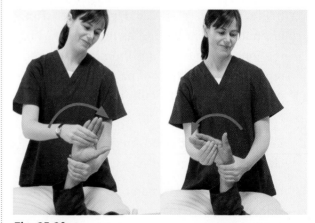

Fig. 25-20.

11. **Thumb**. Move the thumb away from the index finger (abduction). Move the thumb back next to the index finger (adduction) (Fig. 25-21).

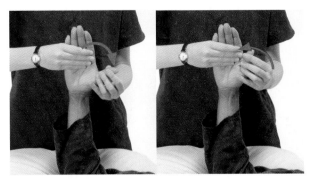

Fig. 25-21.

Touch each fingertip with the thumb (opposition) (Fig. 25-22).

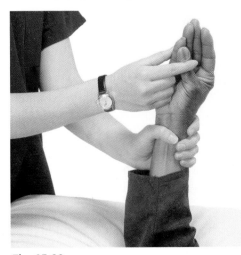

Fig. 25-22.

Bend thumb into the palm (flexion) and out to the side (extension) (Fig. 25-23).

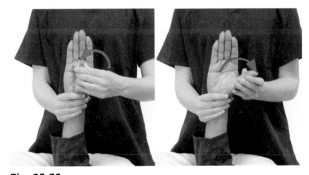

Fig. 25-23.

12. **Fingers**. Make the hand into a fist (flexion). Gently straighten out the fist (extension) (Fig. 25-24).

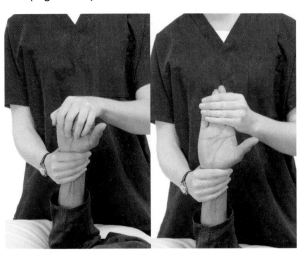

Fig. 25-24.

Spread the fingers and the thumb far apart from each other (abduction). Bring the fingers back next to each other (adduction) (Fig. 25-25).

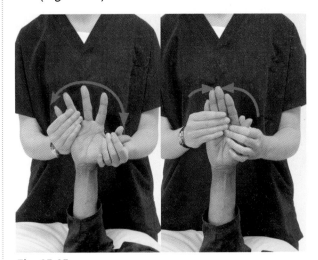

Fig. 25-25.

13. **Hip**. Support the leg by placing one hand under the knee and one under the ankle. Straighten the leg. Raise it gently upward. Move the leg away from the other leg (abduction). Move the leg toward the other leg (adduction) (Fig. 25-26).

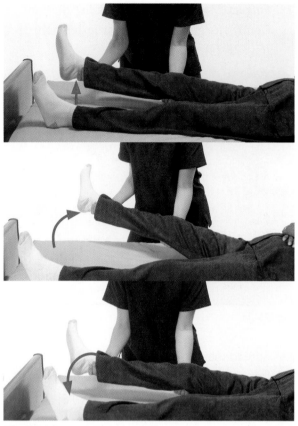

Fig. 25-26.

Gently turn the leg inward (internal rotation). Turn the leg outward (external rotation) (Fig. 25-27).

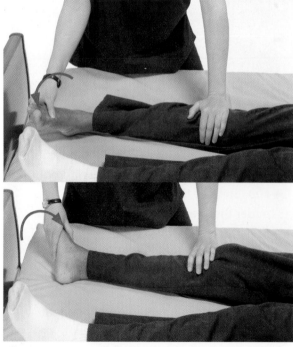

Fig. 25-27.

14. **Knees**. Support resident's leg under the knee and ankle while performing ROM for knee. Bend the knee to the point of resistance (flexion). Return leg to resident's normal position. (extension) (Fig. 25-28).

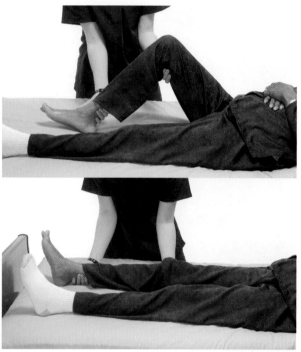

Fig. 25-28.

15. **Ankles**. Support the foot and ankle close to the bed while performing ROM for the ankle. Push/pull foot up toward head (dorsiflexion). Push/pull foot down, with the toes pointed down (plantar flexion) (Fig. 25-29).

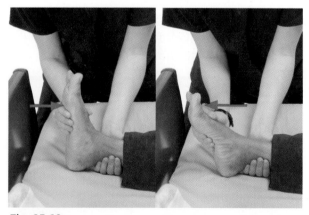

Fig. 25-29.

Turn inside of the foot inward toward the body (supination). Bend the sole of the foot away from the body (pronation) (Fig. 25-30).

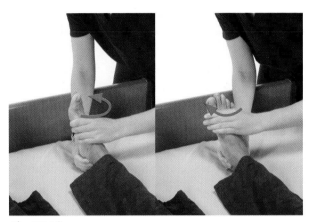

Fig. 25-30.

16. **Toes**. Curl and straighten the toes (flexion and extension) (Fig. 25-31).

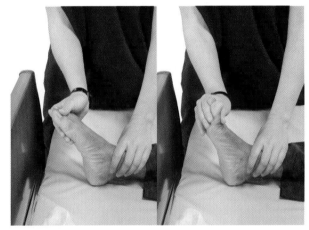

Fig. 25-31.

Gently spread the toes apart (abduction) (Fig. 25-32).

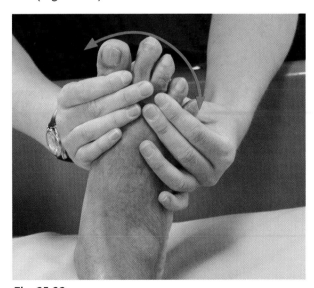

Fig. 25-32.

17. While supporting the limbs, move all joints gently, slowly, and smoothly through the range of motion to the point of resistance. Stop exercises if any pain occurs.

18. Return bed to lowest position. Remove privacy measures.

19. Leave call light within resident's reach.

20. Wash your hands.

21. Be courteous and respectful at all times.

22. Report any changes in the resident to the nurse. Document procedure using facility guidelines.

Tip

No ROM With Osteoporosis

Range of motion exercises may not be recommended for residents who have osteoporosis or other conditions that cause brittle bones or weak joints. Never perform ROM exercises without a doctor's order.

Chapter Review

1. What factors influence the type of rehabilitation ordered and how much progress is made (LO 2)?

2. List three goals of rehabilitation (LO 2).

3. List seven guidelines for rehabilitation and restorative care (LO 2).

4. How can being dependent on others for help with ADLs affect emotions (LO 3)?

5. List three positive effects that encouraging independence and self-care can have on a resident (LO 3).

6. List one complication for each body system listed that results from a lack of exercise and activity (LO 4).

7. List one benefit for each body system listed that results from regular activity and exercise (LO 4).

8. Briefly describe three types of canes (LO 5).

9. When a resident has one weaker leg, should a cane be held on the resident's weaker or stronger side (LO 5)?

10. After a resident moves a walker, should the weaker or stronger leg follow first (LO 5)?

11. When a resident uses a cane, walker, or crutches, on which side should the nursing assistant stay—the weaker or stronger (LO 5)?

12. List three purposes of assistive, or adaptive, devices (LO 6).

13. What are orthotic devices, and what do they do (LO 6)?

14. Look at the adaptive devices in Figure 25-8. Choose one and describe how it might help a resident recovering from or adapting to a physical condition (LO 6).

15. What are the goals of ROM exercises (LO 7)?

16. List and define three types of ROM exercises (LO 7).

17. Define each of the following body movements: abduction, adduction, extension, flexion, dorsiflexion, pronation, rotation, supination, and opposition (LO 7).

18. When performing ROM exercises, where on the body should the nursing assistant begin? In which direction should the nursing assistant work (LO 7)?

26
Subacute Care

1. Define important words in this chapter

central venous line: a type of intravenous line
(IV) that is inserted into a large vein in the body.

chest tubes: hollow drainage tubes that are inserted into the chest to drain air, blood, pus, or
fluid that has collected inside the pleural space/
cavity.

gastrostomy: an opening in the stomach and
abdomen.

intubation: the method used to insert an artificial airway; involves passing a plastic tube
through the mouth or nose and into the trachea
or windpipe.

mechanical ventilator: a machine used to inflate and deflate the lungs when a person cannot
breathe on his own.

nasogastric tube: a feeding tube that is inserted through the nose and into the stomach.

**percutaneous endoscopic gastrostomy (PEG)
tube:** a tube placed through the skin directly
into the stomach to assist with eating.

pulse oximeter: device that measures a person's
blood oxygen level and pulse rate.

sedation: the use of medication to calm a
person.

sepsis: a serious illness caused by an infection,
usually bacterial, that requires immediate care.

telemetry: application of a cardiac monitoring
device that transmits information about the heart
rhythm and heart rate to a central monitoring
station for assessment.

total parenteral nutrition (TPN): the intravenous infusion of nutrients in a basic form that
is absorbed directly by the cells, bypassing the
digestive tract.

2. Discuss the types of residents who are in a subacute setting

A subacute setting is a special unit or facility
that is for people who need more care than most
long-term care facilities can provide. Hospitals

and long-term care facilities may offer subacute care. Residents in subacute care settings need a higher level of care than other residents. They will require more direct care and close observation by staff. The cost for subacute care is usually less than care received in a hospital, but more expensive than what long-term care costs.

Recent surgery or chronic illnesses, such as AIDS or cancer, may require subacute care (Fig. 26-1). Other conditions that warrant subacute care are serious burns or dialysis. Dialysis cleans the body of wastes that the kidneys cannot remove due to chronic renal failure (CRF) (Chapter 16). Residents in subacute care units may also be on a **mechanical ventilator**, a machine used to inflate and deflate the lungs when a person cannot breathe on his own.

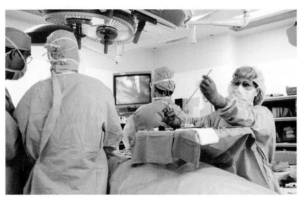

Fig. 26-1. *Subacute care provides a higher level of care. Subacute care may be necessary for surgery, illness, serious burns, and dialysis.*

3. List care guidelines for pulse oximetry

When residents are on oxygen, require surgery, or have bleeding or breathing problems, a pulse oximeter may be used. A **pulse oximeter** measures a person's blood oxygen level and pulse rate. Blood oxygen is the oxygen level inside the arteries and is also called oxygen saturation. A sensor is clipped on a finger, ear lobe, or toe (Fig. 26-2). Adhesive probes may be used on fingers, the forehead, or the nose. The sensor warns of a low blood oxygen level before any observable signs or symptoms develop. It works by moving red and infrared light through the skin.

The sensor measures the amount of each type of light absorbed by the hemoglobin in the blood. Blood with oxygen absorbs more of the infrared light, while blood without oxygen absorbs more red light.

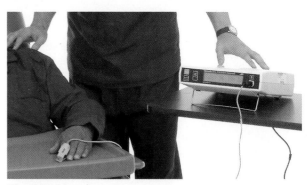

Fig. 26-2. *A pulse oximeter.*

Normal blood oxygen levels measure between 95% and 100%. However, normal ranges may differ from person to person. Diseases such as COPD (Chapter 20) can lower a person's blood oxygen levels. Other factors that affect pulse oximetry readings include the following:

- Reduced circulation to the extremities
- Smoking
- Recent exposure to various dyes for healthcare testing
- Oxygen therapy
- Exposure to a fire or carbon monoxide
- Exposure of the probe to bright light
- Nail polish or artificial nails
- Skin tones (people with darker skin tones may have inaccurate readings due to increased pigmentation of their skin on fingers and toes)

Report any increase or decrease in residents' oxygen levels promptly to the nurse.

Guidelines: Pulse Oximeter

G   The nurse will set the alarm so it will alert staff to a resident's low oxygen saturation. If the alarm on the pulse oximeter sounds, report it to the nurse immediately.

G Be careful when moving and positioning residents to make sure the oximeter does not come off or move.

G Report dyspnea (difficulty breathing) or shortness of breath.

G Report cyanotic, pale, grayish, or darkening skin or mucous membranes.

G Observe and report any signs of skin breakdown from the device, such as irritation, rash, breaks, cracking, sores, bleeding, or drainage. Check the skin around and under the oximeter.

G Carefully monitor all vital signs and report changes to the nurse. Pulse oximetry readings between 95% and 100% are generally considered normal. Promptly report readings that are considered abnormal for the resident.

Applying a pulse oximetry device

Equipment: pulse oximetry clip-on sensor probe, nail polish remover, if needed

1. Identify yourself by name. Identify the resident. Greet the resident by name.

2. Wash your hands.

3. Explain procedure to resident. Speak clearly, slowly, and directly. Maintain face-to-face contact whenever possible.

4. Provide for the resident's privacy with a curtain, screen, or door.

5. Remove nail polish from digits to be used for pulse oximetry, if necessary.

6. Remove sensor probe from package and place clip-on probe on finger, toe, or earlobe. The index finger is usually preferable. The probe must be placed fully onto the finger or toe; it should not be placed just on the tip of the finger or toe.

7. Blood pressure and pulse measurements may be needed prior to placing the device. If

device does not seem to be working, make sure wires on pulse oximetry device are in place and that device is plugged in. Turn on the device. The pulse oximetry reading should appear on the screen quickly.

8. Ask resident to not remove or adjust pulse oximetry device. Ask resident to press call signal if the device comes off or dislodges.

9. Make resident comfortable.

10. Remove privacy measures.

11. Leave call light within resident's reach.

12. Wash your hands.

13. Be courteous and respectful at all times.

14. Report any changes in the resident to the nurse. Document procedure using facility guidelines.

4. Describe telemetry and list care guidelines

Telemetry is the application of a cardiac monitoring device that transmits information about the heart's rhythm and rate to a central monitoring station. Monitoring screens are watched constantly by trained staff. A specially-trained team member then assesses the data.

A portable telemetry unit attaches to a resident's chest and is carried in a pack that allows for movement. There are different methods of connecting the device to a person's chest. One type uses sponge-like adhesive pads or patches (also called leads or electrodes) that stick to different parts of the chest. The pad attaches to a wire that is connected to the telemetry battery pack.

Guidelines: Telemetry

G Do not get the unit, wires, pads, or electrodes wet during bathing. Report to the nurse if they become wet.

G   If the alarm sounds, notify the nurse. The alarm may sound with movement, a disconnected lead, or a low battery.

G   Monitor vital signs carefully as ordered.

G   Check pads for loosening. Report if they become loose.

G   Check the skin under and around the pads for irritation, rashes, broken skin, or cracking. Report these signs to the nurse.

G   Remind the resident not to leave the range of the monitoring area during ambulation.

G   Notify the nurse if any of the following occur:

   •   Change in vital signs

   •   Chest pain or discomfort

   •   Rapid pulse (tachycardia)

   •   Sweating

   •   Shortness of breath

   •   Dyspnea

   •   Dizziness

5. Explain artificial airways and list care guidelines

An artificial airway is any plastic, metal, or rubber device inserted into the respiratory tract for the purpose of maintaining an airway and facilitating ventilation. Artificial airways keep the airway open. A clear airway is needed for the lungs to perform air exchange.

An artificial airway is needed when the airway is obstructed from illness, injury, secretions, or aspiration, and sometimes is needed when a person has surgery. Some residents who are unconscious will need an artificial airway.

An artificial airway is inserted during a procedure called **intubation**. It involves a doctor passing a tube through the mouth, nose, or opening in the neck and into the trachea (windpipe). There are different types of artificial airways (Fig. 26-3).

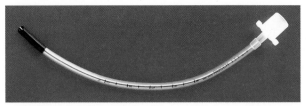

Fig. 26-3. *An endotracheal tube is a type of artificial airway that is inserted through the mouth and then into the trachea.* (PHOTO COURTESY OF TELEFLEX)

A common type of artificial airway is a tracheostomy. A tracheostomy is a surgically-created opening through the neck into the trachea. A tracheostomy tube is inserted through this opening, or stoma, into the trachea. It is also called a "trach tube." More information on tracheostomies is in the next Learning Objective.

Guidelines: Artificial Airways

G   Observe resident closely. If tubing falls out, use the call light to notify the nurse immediately. Do not leave the resident.

G   Proper positioning helps reduce the risk of aspiration; orders will depend upon the type of airway, the need for mechanical ventilation, and the level of consciousness. A semi-reclined (semi-Fowler's) or an upright position (Fowler's) may be ordered. Follow orders for positioning of the head and neck; maintain the proper position at all times.

G   Check vital signs as ordered and report any changes.

G   Perform oral care as directed at least every two hours.

G   Watch for biting or tugging on the tube. Report this to the nurse.

G   Use other methods of communication if the resident cannot speak. Communication boards, writing notes, and drawing pictures can be helpful. Observe for hand or eye signals.

G   Be supportive and encouraging. Having an artificial airway can be frightening and uncomfortable. It can cause choking and gagging. Be empathetic; try to imagine how you might feel if you had a tube in your nose, mouth, or throat.

G   Notify the nurse if any of the following occur:

- Drainage

- Change in vital signs

- Wheezing or other unusual breathing sounds or difficulty breathing

- Secretions in tubing

- Cyanosis, pale, gray, or darkening skin or mucous membranes

- Nervousness or anxiety

6. Discuss care for a resident with a tracheostomy

A tracheostomy is a common type of artificial airway (Fig. 26-4). It may be necessary due to an obstruction, cancer, infection, severe injuries, serious allergic reactions, or coma. It may also be used for a person recovering from facial burns or gunshot wounds and to prevent aspiration in an unconscious person. The tracheostomy tube is held in place by a cuff that attaches to the end of the device in the trachea. The cuff prevents the accidental aspiration of food or fluids.

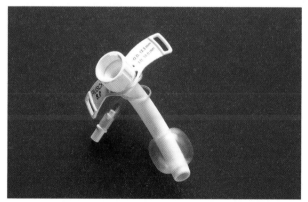

Fig. 26-4. *A tracheostomy tube is inserted into the trachea through a surgically-created opening in the neck.* (PHOTO COURTESY OF TELEFLEX)

While the tracheostomy is in place, the resident may not be able to speak. He or she may also have a reduced sense of taste and/or smell.

Being unable to speak can cause fear and anxiety. Be supportive and responsive. Carefully observe residents who have a tracheostomy. Use other methods of communication if the resident cannot speak, such as notepads, communication boards, or hand signals. Answer call lights promptly.

General tracheostomy care includes keeping the skin around the opening, or stoma, clean, assisting with dressing changes, and helping with the cleaning of the inner part of the device. Suctioning may be needed frequently. Gurgling sounds during breathing are one sign that suctioning is needed.

Nursing assistants do not perform tracheostomy care or suctioning. However, careful observation and reporting is vital. In addition, follow these guidelines:

Guidelines: Tracheostomies

G   Answer call lights promptly.

G   Use alternate methods of communication when needed.

G   Assist resident into the ordered position. A semi-Fowler's or Fowler's position may be ordered for a conscious resident with a tracheostomy. If the resident is unconscious, a side-lying position (lateral) may be ordered in order to help drain secretions. Gently move and position residents; always get enough help.

G   Inspect tape or ties often. Do not untie or unfasten the tracheostomy tape or ties.

G   Report kinks or disconnected tubing.

G   Do not get the tracheostomy dressing wet.

G   Do not cover the tracheostomy opening.

G   Provide careful skin care to the site around the tracheostomy. Assist with dressing changes as requested.

G   Be careful to prevent aspiration when cleaning the mouth. Use special swabs as needed. Perform oral care at least every two hours.

G   Observe for mouth sores and cracks, breaks, or sores on the skin. Apply lubricant to lips as needed.

G   Observe skin carefully for pale, bluish, or darkening skin or mucous membranes.

G   Carefully monitor vital signs, if not measured by machine.

G   Do not tire resident when performing care.

G   Do not move or remove spare tracheostomy tubes or spare bag valve mask (device used to provide ventilation to a person who is not breathing, not breathing adequately, or during power failures to a person on a mechanical ventilator). A special bag valve mask with a removable mask is needed for use with a tracheostomy.

G   Notify the nurse if any of the following occur:

  • Cyanosis, pale, gray, or darkening skin or mucous membranes

  • Mouth sores or discomfort

  • Cracks, breaks, or sores on the skin

  • Gurgling sounds during breathing

  • Dyspnea or shortness of breath

  • Change in vital signs, especially respiratory rate

  • Disconnected tubing

  • Loose or wet tape or dressings

7. Describe mechanical ventilation and explain care guidelines

A resident in a subacute unit may be on a mechanical ventilator (Fig. 26-5). A ventilator performs the process of breathing for a person who cannot breathe on his own. Many conditions can cause a person to require mechanical ventilation. Injuries that affect the ability to breathe, such as a spinal cord injury, or diseases such as cancer, are examples.

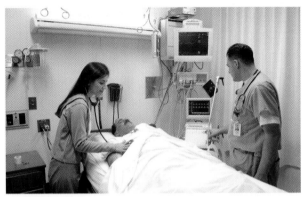

Fig. 26-5. *A mechanical ventilator.* (PHOTO COURTESY OF PULMO-NETIC SYSTEMS)

Residents on a ventilator will not be able to speak. This is because air will no longer reach the larynx (vocal cords). This can cause intense anxiety. The resident may think that no one will know if he has trouble breathing. Being on a ventilator has been compared to breathing through a straw. Residents will need a lot of support while being connected to the ventilator. Spend as much time as you can with the person. Enter the room often so that the resident can see you. This provides reassurance. Clipboards, pads, and communication boards help with communication.

Residents on a ventilator are often heavily sedated. **Sedation** is the use of medication to calm a person. Sedation helps reduce anxiety and discomfort that can occur with mechanical ventilation. Whether alert or unconscious, continue to speak to the person when providing care. Assume that he is able to understand everything going on around him.

People on ventilators are at a higher risk of getting a type of pneumonia called "ventilator-acquired pneumonia," or VAP. Nursing assistants play a role in preventing this complication. Carefully follow the doctor's orders regarding positioning of the person on a ventilator. For example, the person may need the head of the bed elevated 30 degrees at all times. The resident may need to be turned from side to side at specific times. Frequent mouth care may be ordered. Wash your hands often when working with residents on ventilators. Follow the care plan and the nurse's instructions.

Guidelines: Mechanical Ventilator

G Report to the nurse right away if the alarm sounds.

G Watch for kinks or disconnected tubing; report them immediately.

G Watch for biting on the tube if orally intubated. Report this to the nurse.

G Answer the call light promptly.

G Give frequent oral care as directed. Observe and report mouth sores or discomfort.

G Reposition at least every two hours. Follow instructions carefully when moving and positioning. Keep the resident's head properly elevated in the ordered position, usually semi-Fowler's. Always get enough help when moving a resident. Have the nurse check the resident after repositioning.

G Give regular skin care to prevent pressure ulcers. Observe for cracks, breaks, or sores in the skin, especially at the intubation site.

G Allow time for rest.

G Be patient during communication. Offer communication aids to assist. Watch for hand or eye signals.

G Provide support during difficult times. Being dependent can cause feelings of despair.

G Do not move or remove spare artificial airway tubes or bag valve masks from the bedside.

G Residents on ventilators will require one-on-one care during a power failure. A bag valve mask and a portable oxygen tank will need to be used by the caregiver until the power is restored.

G Notify the nurse if any of the following occur:

- The alarm sounds

- Secretions collect in the tubing

- Mouth sores or discomfort

- Cracks, breaks, or sores anywhere on the skin, especially at the site of intubation

- Change in vital signs

- Nervousness or anxiety

- Depression

Sepsis

Sepsis is a life-threatening illness caused by an infection, usually bacterial, that requires immediate care. Early, subtle symptoms of sepsis include elevated heart rate, elevated respiratory rate, a slightly-elevated temperature or, in some cases, a low body temperature. Being familiar with residents' normal vital signs will help you better recognize changes. Other symptoms are chills, excessive sweating, a general feeling of sickness, weakness, low blood pressure, decreased urine output, headache, skin rash, shortness of breath, and confusion or a change in mental status. If you notice any of these symptoms, report them immediately.

Some of the risks for sepsis are being over the age of 65, chronic diseases like diabetes, heart disease, liver or kidney disease, infections, HIV, having a transplanted organ, pressure ulcers, cancer, burns, having a surgical drain, having an indwelling catheter, and recent hospitalization.

Treatment for sepsis depends on the type of infection, but includes antibiotics, other medications, IV fluids, oxygen, and careful monitoring of blood glucose. The person may require a ventilator.

8. Describe suctioning and list signs of respiratory distress

Subacute care units include residents who require suctioning. Suctioning is needed when a person has increased secretions that they cannot expel themselves. Suctioning can be performed through the mouth (oropharyngeal), the nasal passages (nasopharyngeal), the trachea and the bronchi (endotracheal). A person with a tracheostomy may also need suctioning. Nurses or respiratory therapists will perform the suctioning; nursing assistants do not perform suctioning.

Suction comes from a wall hook-up or a portable pump. A container collects the suctioned material from the airway (Fig. 26-6). Sterile water or sterile saline is normally used to rinse the suction catheter after suctioning. Nurses will change the tubing at least once daily.

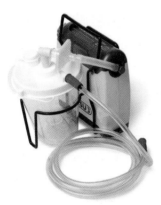

Fig. 26-6. *A suctioning pump. Nursing assistants do not perform suctioning. They help by reporting signs of respiratory distress and monitoring vital signs.* (PHOTO COURTESY OF LAERDAL MEDICAL CORPORATION)

A resident who needs frequent suctioning may show signs of respiratory distress. Signs of respiratory distress include gurgling, an elevated respiratory rate, shortness of breath, difficulty breathing (dyspnea), pallor, or cyanosis.

Guidelines: Assisting with Suctioning

G   Follow Standard Precautions. Wear gloves, gown, mask, or goggles as directed.

G   Place resident in position as directed by nurse, normally semi-Fowler's or lateral.

G   Place pad or towel under the chin before the nurse begins suctioning; have a wet wash- cloth ready.

G   Give oral and nasal care after suctioning as directed. Apply ordered lubricant to the lips as needed.

G   If you note any signs of respiratory distress, report them immediately. An inability to breathe freely causes great anxiety. It is dan- gerous to remain in respiratory distress for any length of time.

G   Answer call lights promptly.

G   Observe skin color carefully for pale, bluish, or darkening skin or mucous membranes.

G   Monitor vital signs closely, especially respira- tory rate. Report changes.

G   Be supportive during periods of difficult breathing. Use touch if appropriate.

G   Notify the nurse if any of the following occur:

•   Change in vital signs, especially respira- tory rate

•   Gurgling sounds or unusual sounds dur- ing breathing

•   Change in the color, amount, or qual- ity (thickness/thinness) of secretions coughed up

•   Dyspnea or shortness of breath

•   Cyanosis, pale, gray or darkening skin or mucous membranes

•   Nervousness or anxiety

9. Describe chest tubes and explain related care

Chest tubes are hollow drainage tubes that are inserted into the chest during a sterile proce- dure. They can be inserted at the bedside or dur- ing surgery. Chest tubes are placed between the ribs into the pleural cavity or space to drain air, blood, pus, or fluid that has collected inside the cavity. The pleural cavity is the space between the two layers of the pleura, the thin tissue lay- ers covering the lungs. Chest tubes are also inserted to allow full expansion of the lungs. Conditions that require chest tubes include:

•   Pneumothorax: air or gas in the pleural cavity

•   Hemothorax: blood in the pleural cavity

•   Empyema: pus in the pleural cavity

•   Certain types of surgery

•   Chest trauma or injuries

A doctor normally inserts chest tubes. The chest tube is connected to a container of sterile water. Drainage systems include those using grav- ity drainage and suction. This system must be sealed so that air cannot enter the pleural cavity. The system must be airtight.

When X-rays show that the air, blood, or fluid has been drained, the tube is removed. Medications may be used to prevent or treat infection.

Guidelines: Chest Tubes

G Be aware of the number and location of chest tubes. Tubes may be in the front, back, or side of the body.

G Check vital signs as directed. Report any changes immediately to the nurse.

G Report signs of respiratory distress to the nurse immediately. Report complaints of pain.

G Always keep the drainage system below the level of the resident's chest.

G Make sure the drainage containers remain upright and level at all times. Inform the nurse right away if containers are not upright.

G Make sure tubing is not kinked. Report kinks in tubing to the nurse.

G Watch for disconnected tubing. If this happens, report it immediately.

G Certain equipment is kept nearby in case the tube is pulled out. This includes special gauze, clamps, and containers of sterile fluid. Do not remove these items from the area.

G Observe chest tube drainage for color, amount, and consistency of drainage, and report any changes.

G Report if there are clots in the tubing.

G Observe the dressings for drainage, saturation, or bleeding.

G Follow the repositioning schedule. Be very gentle with turning and repositioning. Move the resident and the tubes at the same time to prevent pulling the tubes out. Always get enough help when moving and positioning.

G Provide rest periods as needed.

G Follow fluid intake orders carefully. Measure intake and output carefully as ordered.

G If asked to assist with coughing and deep-breathing exercises, be encouraging and patient. These exercises can cause pain.

G Notify the nurse if any of the following occur:

- Complaints of pain
- Any signs of respiratory distress
- Changes in vital signs
- Change in oxygen level or if pulse oximetry alarm sounds
- An increase or decrease in bubbling in the drainage system
- Disconnected tubing
- Kinks in the tubing
- Clots in the tubing
- Any change in the amount, color, or consistency of chest drainage
- Wet or loose dressings
- Odor in the chest tube area

10. Describe alternative feeding methods and related care

When a person is unable to consume food normally due to disease or injury, other methods are used. When a person has difficulty swallowing or is unable to swallow, he may be fed through a tube. One tube is called a nasogastric tube (N/G). A **nasogastric tube** is inserted into the nose, down the back of the throat through the esophagus and into the stomach. The tube is secured to the nose with dressing tape and to the gown with tape or a clip. An orogastric tube (O/G) is used for people who are intubated. It is inserted into the mouth and down the throat, through the esophagus and into the stomach.

Another type of tube that is placed through the skin directly into the abdomen is called a **percutaneous endoscopic gastrostomy (PEG) tube**. The opening in the abdomen and the stomach is called a **gastrostomy** (Fig. 26-7).

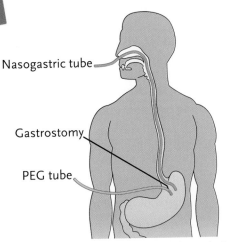

Nasogastric tube

Gastrostomy

PEG tube

Fig. 26-7. *Nasogastric tubes are inserted through the nose, and PEG tubes are inserted through the skin directly into the stomach.*

Tube feedings are used when residents have swallowing difficulties, but are able to digest food. Other conditions that may require tube feedings are coma, cancer, stroke, birth defects, or extreme weakness.

Nursing assistants do not insert tubes, give the feedings, or clean or suction the tubes. However, you may assist the nurse by assembling equipment, positioning the resident, observing the tube site for signs of infection, and cleaning the tube site. Your duties may also include discarding used equipment and cleaning and storing supplies.

Guidelines: Tube Feedings

G Observe carefully for any signs of aspiration during and after a tube feeding (Chapter 14).

G Follow instructions for positioning residents. They will need to sit upright during the feeding and for at least 30 minutes following the feeding to help prevent aspiration.

G Follow fluid orders. The resident may have an order for nothing by mouth (NPO).

G Give frequent nose and mouth care to prevent dryness and irritation. Apply lubricant as ordered.

G Do not pull or tug tubing. Make sure that tubing is not kinked.

G Observe for tape or clip falling off gown.

G Feeding pumps may be used to administer tube feedings. Pumps help regulate the amount of fluid given. Notify the nurse if an alarm sounds.

G Make conversation or read to residents during tube feedings to help make this time more social.

G Notify the nurse if any of the following occur:

- Irritation or sores around the nose or mouth

- Plugged tubing

- Kinked, cracked, broken, or disconnected tubing

- Tube comes out of abdomen

- Leaking or empty bag or container

- Loose tape

- Dyspnea or shortness of breath

- Cyanosis, pale, gray, or darkening skin or mucous membranes

- Nausea, vomiting, or cramping

- Fluid gathering in the mouth

- Signs of infection at the tube site, such as warm skin, reddened skin, sores, swelling, or pus

- Bleeding or drainage at the gastrostomy site

- Signs of aspiration such as choking, gagging, or clutching the throat

- Resident pulling on the tube (increases risk of aspiration)

- Feeding pump alarm sounds

If a person's digestive system does not function properly, he is unable to eat, or his nutritional needs cannot be met by tube feedings, **total parenteral nutrition (TPN)**, or hyperalimentation, may be ordered. With TPN, a resident receives nutrients intravenously, bypassing the digestive tract. The nutrients are in their most basic forms of carbohydrates, proteins, and fats and are absorbed directly by the cells. Total parenteral nutrition may be also necessary due to surgery, disease, significant weight loss, and coma.

When the need for TPN is expected to continue for a while, a central venous line is usually inserted. A **central venous line** is a type of intravenous line (IV) that is placed in one of the larger veins in the body, usually in the upper chest or neck.

When caring for a resident on TPN, observe and report fever, headache, swelling, redness, bleeding, or leaking at the insertion site. Residents on TPN can have fluctuations in their blood sugar. Caregivers will need to watch for signs of hyperglycemia which can occur at the initiation of TPN, and hypoglycemia, which can occur upon discontinuation of TPN. (See Chapter 8 for signs of hyperglycemia and hypoglycemia.) Report any change in condition right away. Residents on TPN may find it difficult to be on a restricted diet. Be supportive and positive.

Tip

Gastric Suctioning

Tubes can be inserted into the stomach for reasons other than feeding. Tubes may be used post-operatively for nausea, vomiting, bloating, and to remove materials from the body via suctioning. In addition, poisons can be removed from the stomach with a special wash that is done via a tube.

11. Discuss care guidelines for dialysis

As you learned in Chapter 16, kidney dialysis is a process that cleans the body of wastes that the kidneys cannot remove due to chronic renal failure (CRF). Dialysis can be done via a site in the person's arm (access arm or vascular access), or a catheter, which is usually inserted into the neck. Central lines in the neck are generally used for temporary dialysis.

When providing care, follow the care plan and the nurse's instructions. Make sure residents avoid putting pressure on the access arm. Keep the access arm area clean. Residents should not sleep on their access arm/vascular access or lift heavy things with that arm.

Loose sleeves may need to be worn. Specific dietary and fluid restrictions will be ordered for a resident on dialysis. Follow instructions for intake and output (I&O) measurement carefully. You may be asked to check vital signs and measure weight daily. Do not take a blood pressure reading on the access arm.

Report difficulty breathing, shortness of breath, changes in vital signs, pain, drainage or bleeding from the insertion site, change in I&O, and any swelling of extremities (edema) to the nurse.

Chapter Review

1. What kinds of conditions require subacute care (LO 2)?

2. What does a pulse oximeter measure (LO 3)?

3. List five care guidelines for telemetry (LO 4).

4. What is the purpose of artificial airways (LO 5)?

5. What kinds of alternate methods of communication can be used for residents who have an artificial airway (LO 5)?

6. What does general tracheostomy care involve (LO 6)?

7. List 10 care guidelines for tracheostomies (LO 6).

8. Why is it important to enter the room often when a resident is using a mechanical ventilator (LO 7)?

9. List eight care guidelines for mechanical ventilators (LO 7).

10. List eight symptoms of sepsis (LO 7).

11. List five symptoms of respiratory distress (LO 8).

12. What types of materials are drained by chest tubes (LO 9)?

13. What observations should nursing assistants make about chest drainage (LO 9)?

14. Briefly define "nasogastric tube" and "PEG tube" (LO 10).

15. What are generally NOT nursing assistant responsibilities with feeding tubes (LO 10)?

16. How does TPN deliver nutrients (LO 10)?

17. List six signs and symptoms to report about a resident who is on dialysis (LO 11).

27
End-of-Life Care

The Ancient Egyptian Art of Embalming the Dead

Many people in ancient Egypt focused on preparing for the afterlife. Their hope was that the afterlife would be a joyful paradise. The art of embalming dead bodies was common, especially for people of "high birth." Embalming consisted of removing and preserving organs, such as the liver and the lungs. They were placed inside jars and then covered. Body cavities were washed out with spices, and then the body was soaked for 70 days with a substance called natron. Natron was made of clay mixed with certain salts. The body was then coated with various gums and wrapped with pieces of fine linen. People who were of "lower birth" were destined to be buried in the sand without any of these preparations.

"As a well-spent day brings happy sleep, so life well used brings happy death."

Leonardo Da Vinci, 1452-1519

"Men fear death as children fear to go in the dark; and as that natural fear in children is increased with tales, so is the other."

Publilius Syrus, circa 42 B.C.

1. Define important words in this chapter

anticipatory grief: a period of mourning when the dying person or his family is expecting the death.

autopsy: an examination of a body by a pathologist to try to determine the cause of death.

bereavement: the period following a loss in which mourning occurs.

complicated grief: grief complicated by disorders or conditions, such as depression and substance abuse.

cremation: the process of burning a dead body until it turns to ash.

death: the end of life; the cessation of all body functions.

grief: a deeply emotional process that is a response to loss.

grief process: the varying emotional responses to grief.

grief therapy: therapy to try to resolve problems due to separation from the deceased.

mourning: the period in which people work to adapt to a loss; influenced by culture, tradition, and society.

palliative care: care given to people who have serious, life-threatening diseases; goals are to control symptoms, reduce suffering, prevent side effects and complications, and maintain quality of life.

pathologist: a doctor with advanced training in the examination of organs and tissues.

postmortem care: care of the body after death.

rigor mortis: Latin for "stiffness of death;" refers to the stiffness that occurs after death due to muscles becoming rigid.

terminal illness: a disease or condition that will eventually cause death.

unresolved grief: grief that continues beyond what is considered a reasonable period of time; may affect the person's ability to function.

2. Describe palliative care

Palliative care is care given to people who have serious, life-threatening diseases, such as cancer, AIDS, and congestive heart failure. The goals of palliative care are to control symptoms, reduce suffering, prevent side effects and complications, and maintain the best quality of life possible. Palliative care emphasizes a holistic approach. Both physical and psychosocial needs are considered in palliative care.

It is important to understand that palliative care works to manage symptoms, not to cure the disease. The care plan will include instructions about how to recognize and treat complications early and how to relieve chronic pain and discomfort. This helps to maintain a person's quality of life. Palliative care involves residents' families and friends. Regular care conferences that include the resident, his family and friends, and various palliative care team members will take place. Doctors, nurses, clergy, social workers, dietitians, physical therapists, and nursing assistants are some of the members of the palliative care team. The team will provide access to other specialists. Counseling is made available to residents, families, and friends to help them deal with the stress that accompanies a loved one's serious illness.

3. Discuss hospice care

When a serious illness is classified as a "**terminal illness**," or a disease or condition that will eventually cause **death**, hospice care is often the next step. Hospice care is ordered by a doctor when a person has approximately six months or less to live. This type of care is a compassionate way to care for dying people and their families. Hospice care uses a holistic approach, giving physical and emotional care and comfort. The focus is on pain and symptom management, meeting psychosocial needs, and involving family and friends.

Hospice care can be given in a hospital, at a care facility, or in the home (Fig. 27-1). It is available seven days a week, 24 hours a day. There is always a nurse on call to answer questions, make an additional visit, or solve a problem. Members of the hospice care team include doctors, nurses, social workers, counselors, nursing assistants, therapists, clergy, dietitians, and volunteers. Goals of hospice care include the following:

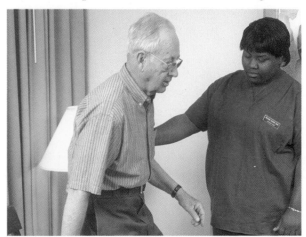

Fig. 27-1. *Hospice care can be given anywhere, including in a person's home. The focus of hospice care is on relieving pain and managing symptoms, rather than on curing an illness.*

- Using a holistic approach to care

- Providing an alternative to traditional hospital care

- Offering medically-directed, team-managed care

- Focusing on the resident and family as a unit of care

- Offering compassionate care for a person with a terminal illness

- Focusing on soothing and comfort care, rather than curative care

- Emphasizing pain and symptom management

- Offering assistance in meeting psychosocial needs for the family

- Helping the family obtain financial counseling and legal assistance as needed

Hospice care strives to meet all of the needs of the dying person. The resident and his family and friends are directly involved in care decisions. The resident is encouraged to participate in decision-making as long as possible.

Hospice care focuses on pain relief by monitoring the administration and effectiveness of medications, which are prescribed by a doctor. Report complaints of pain or signs of pain to the nurse immediately. These observations are communicated to the doctor, and adjustments are made as needed.

Hospice care encourages the involvement of the resident's spiritual or religious leader, if the resident has one. Hospice also supports both the family and the dying resident in their continued involvement in social activities. Reading, listening to music, visiting with friends, and learning new skills are encouraged. Residents who are dying need to feel independent for as long as possible. They need to have control over their lives for as long as they are able.

Tip

Hospice cares.

According to the National Hospice and Palliative Care Organization, over 1.5 million people received hospice services in 2009. An estimated 468,000 volunteers provided hospice care in the United States in 2009. Volunteers gave more than 22 million hours of their time to help people who were dying. Hospice volunteers attend a special training program to prepare them for hospice work. Visit nhpco.org for more information on hospice care.

4. Discuss the grief process and related terms

Grief is a deeply emotional response to loss. It is an adaptive, or changing, process, and usually involves healing in some way. Grief includes physical, psychological, emotional, social, and spiritual reactions to the loss.

Dr. Elisabeth Kubler-Ross wrote the book *On Death and Dying* in 1969. She developed a theory that dying people experience a common grief process. Her model includes five different emotional stages that a person may experience prior to death. The five stages of grief are denial, anger, bargaining, depression, and acceptance. Not all people go through all of the stages. Some may stay in one stage until death, while others may move back and forth between stages during the process.

Stage 1. Denial: People in the denial stage may refuse to believe they are dying. They may think a mistake has been made and demand that lab work be repeated. They may avoid discussion about their illnesses and simply act like it is not happening. This is the "No, not me" stage.

Stage 2. Anger: Once people start to face the possibility of death, they may become angry. They may be angry because they think they are too young to die or because they have always taken care of themselves. Anger may be directed at staff, visitors, roommates, family, or friends. Anger is a normal reaction. Even though it may be upsetting, do not take anger personally. This is the "Why me?" stage.

Stage 3. Bargaining: Once people have begun to believe that they really are dying, they may start trying to bargain with God or a higher power in hopes of recovery. They may make promises and try to bargain for the ability to attend an important function, such as a wedding. This is the "Yes me, but..." stage.

Stage 4. Depression: As dying people become weaker and their symptoms get worse, they may become deeply sad or depressed. They may cry or become withdrawn (Fig. 27-2). They may be unable to do simple tasks. They need additional physical and emotional support. It is important for you to listen and be understanding.

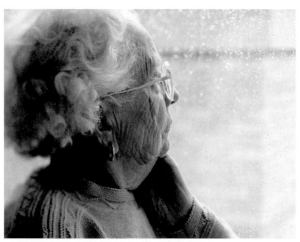

Fig. 27-2. *A dying person may become depressed and withdrawn.*

Stage 5. Acceptance: Peace or acceptance may or may not come to a person before he dies. Some people who are dying are eventually able to accept death and prepare for it. They may make arrangements with attorneys, accountants, and loved ones for the care of important people, pets, and belongings. They may prepare for ceremonies before and/or after death and plan for their last days. At this stage, people who are dying may seem detached.

These stages of dying may not be possible for someone who dies suddenly, unexpectedly, or quickly. You cannot force anyone to move from stage to stage. You can only listen and be ready to offer any help the person needs.

Terms Associated with Death and Dying

Some terms you may hear that are associated with death and dying include the following:

anticipatory grief: a period of mourning when the dying person or his family is expecting the death.

bereavement: the period following a loss in which mourning occurs.

complicated grief: grief complicated by disorders or conditions, such as depression and substance abuse.

grief process: the varying emotional responses to grief; many models have been developed to explain this process.

grief therapy: therapy to try to resolve problems due to separation from the deceased.

mourning: the period in which people work to adapt to a loss; heavily influenced by culture, tradition, and society.

unresolved grief: grief that continues beyond what is considered a reasonable period of time; may affect the person's ability to function normally.

5. Explain the dying person's rights

When a person is dying, there are legal rights that must be respected. Remembering these rights will help you provide proper care, as well as promote the dying person's dignity. Some legal rights to remember when caring for the terminally ill include the following:

The right to have visitors: Residents who are dying have the right to have visitors of their choosing. They can have visits from family, friends, pets, healthcare providers, clergy, members of the community, and others. Visitors must not be prevented from entering the resident's room unless the resident asks them to leave. Normal visiting hours are generally suspended during this difficult time. You may see visitors throughout the night. Only report a problem with a visitor if he is upsetting the resident, if he is purposely disruptive to the unit, or if he becomes a threat to other residents, visitors, or staff.

The right to privacy: Dying residents have the right to privacy. Dying individuals may ask one or more people to leave their room. They may ask a spouse to leave during an examination or a procedure. You must honor these requests. If any problem results with a visitor, promptly report this to the nurse.

The right to be free from pain: Dying residents have the right to be free of pain. Pain must be carefully monitored, and medication and pain relief measures must be given to keep the resident as pain-free as possible.

The right to honest and accurate information: Residents who are dying have the right to know the truth about their diagnosis. Information about treatment, possible risks or complications, and side effects must be presented honestly. If residents have questions about their condition, notify the nurse. Avoid answering questions beyond your scope of practice.

The right to refuse treatment: Dying residents have the right to make choices about their care, including refusing treatment for their illness. Do not judge these decisions, even if you do not agree with them. The choice belongs to the resident and/or his family. See Chapter 2 for more information on living wills and advance directives.

Other rights of a dying person are listed below in "The Dying Person's Bill of Rights." This was created at a workshop entitled "The Terminally Ill Patient and the Helping Person," sponsored by Southwestern Michigan In-Service Education Council, and appeared in the *American Journal of Nursing*, Vol. 75, January 1975, p. 99.

I have the right to:

- Be treated as a living human being until I die.

- Maintain a sense of hopefulness, however changing its focus may be.

- Be cared for by those who can maintain a sense of hopefulness, however changing this might be.

- Express my feelings and emotions about my approaching death in my own way.

- Participate in decisions concerning my care.

- Expect continuing medical and nursing attentions even though "cure" goals must be changed to "comfort" goals.

- Not die alone.

- Be free from pain.

- Have my questions answered honestly.

- Not be deceived.

- Have help from and for my family in accepting my death.

- Die in peace and dignity.

- Retain my individuality and not be judged for my decisions, which may be contrary to the beliefs of others.

- Discuss and enlarge my religious and/or spiritual experiences, whatever these may mean to others.

- Expect that the sanctity of the human body will be respected after death.

- Be cared for by caring, sensitive, knowledgeable people who will attempt to understand my needs and will be able to gain some satisfaction in helping me face my death.

6. Explain how to care for a dying resident

The focus of care for a dying resident is to meet all physical needs, as well as to provide comfort and emotional support. Promoting independence is emphasized in end-of-life care. The dying resident needs to have as much control over his life as possible. When a person's ability to perform his ADLs decreases, staff will meet additional responsibilities as needed. Family and friends may assist with this care.

Guidelines: Dying Resident

G **Skin, Nose, and Mouth Care**: Give frequent skin care. Bathe residents often if they are perspiring heavily. Change gowns and sheets for comfort. Give incontinence care promptly. Keep resident clean and dry. Turn and reposition resident often to prevent pressure ulcers. More help may be needed when moving the resident due to fatigue and a decrease in muscle strength. Give oral care frequently to rinse secretions. Offer ice chips to help keep the mouth moist. Use light lubricant on the nose and mouth to prevent cracking. A room humidifier can help with dryness in the nose and mouth.

G **Pain Control and Comfort**: Dying residents may be in pain. Pain relief is critical; observe and report signs of pain to the nurse immediately. Residents may be connected to a patient-controlled analgesia (PCA) device (Chapter 24) that they control themselves. They press a button to give themselves a dose of pain medication. Some residents will not be able to communicate that they are in pain. Watch for body language and other signs that they are in pain (Chapter 13). Excessive drowsiness can result from pain medication. Report this to the nurse.

If body temperature rises, and the resident is perspiring, remove heavier blankets. Fever can cause chills; use extra blankets if resident needs more warmth.

G **Diminished Senses**: Vision may begin to fail as death nears. Keep the room softly lit without glare (Fig. 27-3). Verbal communication may become difficult. Try using communication boards, pictures, or hand or eye signals. The sense of hearing is usually the last sense to leave the body. Speak in a normal tone of voice and tell the resident about care that is being performed. Describe what is happening around the resident, but do not expect an answer.

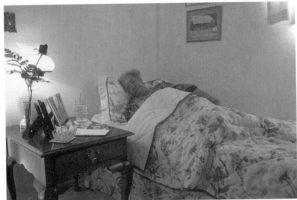

Fig. 27-3. Keep a dying resident's room softly lit without glare.

G **Breathing Problems**: Dying residents may have difficulty breathing. They may have alternating slow, irregular respirations followed by rapid, shallow respirations, called Cheyne-Stokes respirations. They may also have gurgling or rattling sounds as they breathe. This is caused by a build-up of secretions in the throat. Notify the nurse if any of these conditions occur. If coughing becomes severe, notify the nurse. Suctioning may be needed. To ease problems with breathing, elevate the head of the bed and help the resident change positions, as ordered. Oxygen therapy and/or a humidifier may be used.

G **Food and Fluid Issues**: Remember that residents have the right to refuse food or fluids. Do not force residents to eat or drink. Feed residents slowly to help prevent choking and aspiration. Small, frequent meals can help. Encourage fluids as desired. Report nausea, vomiting, and diarrhea to the nurse. A clear liquid diet may be ordered. Elevation of the head of the bed can help reduce burping and acid reflux.

If the resident is constipated, the nurse can provide a stool softener or other medication to help. Bowel obstructions can occur in people who are dying. Report any signs and symptoms of a bowel obstruction to the nurse (see Chapter 15).

Residents' Rights

Remember that hearing is usually the last sense to disappear.

Do not say anything inappropriate around dying residents or their families. The sense of hearing is usually the last sense to leave a person. Be professional. Explain procedures and talk to the resident as you normally would. Never act like the resident is not there or cannot understand you.

7. Discuss factors that influence feelings about death and list ways to meet residents' individual needs

Feelings and attitudes about death differ greatly and are influenced by many factors. These factors include the person's previous experience with death, personality type, religious beliefs, and cultural background (Fig. 27-4).

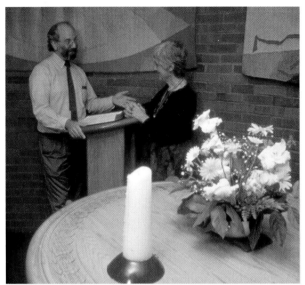

Fig. 27-4. *Spiritual beliefs affect a person's feelings about death and dying.*

Cultural groups may have different practices to deal with grieving. For example, some groups grieve openly when a loved one is dying, while others show little or no emotion. Some may want to talk and share stories about the person who is ill (Fig. 27-5). Others will not want to discuss their feelings.

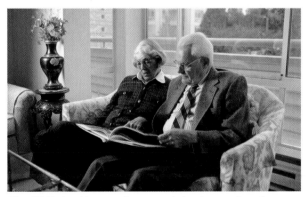

Fig. 27-5. *Looking at photos and sharing stories about a person who is dying is one way family and friends may grieve.*

After death, cultural and spiritual beliefs play an important part. Some groups share food, play music, and talk about the person who has died. Customs may include burying personal items with the body or having specific rules on wash-ing the body after a person has died. Some bury their dead in a coffin, while others prefer to be cremated. **Cremation** is the process of burning a dead body until it turns to ash. Cultural groups may request spiritual or religious leaders, or specific people, to be involved in a ceremony after a person has died.

It is important to understand that no matter how residents and their families deal with dying and death, staff members must respect their wishes, preferences, and behavior. Honoring cultural traditions whenever possible is important. The care team must always respond in a culturally-sensitive way to different practices and individual beliefs. In addition, follow these guidelines to help meet a dying resident's psychosocial and spiritual needs:

Guidelines: Psychosocial and Spiritual Needs of a Dying Resident

G   Do not isolate or avoid a dying resident; spend as much time as you can with a resident who is dying.

G   Listen more; talk less. When dealing with a resident who will die soon, listening is often one of the most important things you can do (Fig. 27-6).

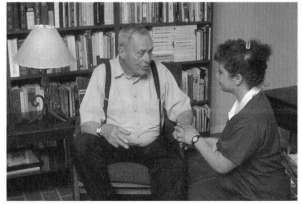

Fig. 27-6. *A good listener can be a great comfort for a resident who is dying.*

G   Do not judge anything the resident tells you about his past.

G   Do not bring your religious beliefs into the conversation. Do not try to change or influence the resident's religious or spiritual beliefs or lack of beliefs.

G   Notify the nurse immediately if resident requests a visit from a clergy person or any spiritual leader.

G   Provide privacy for visits from family, friends, or clergy. Let residents and visitors know you will be there if you are needed.

G   Never share anything private that is said to you by the resident with anyone other than the nurse.

G   Never share anything about the resident, including conversations, appearance, or anything else with any other person. This includes other staff members, volunteers, your own family and friends, or the media.

G   If a resident discusses a serious fear of dying with you, tell the nurse immediately. Therapists and other professionals can try to help the resident work through these fears.

8. Identify common signs of approaching death

When a person is dying, all body systems are affected. Common signs of approaching death include the following:

- Cyanotic, pale, or darkening skin or mucous membranes
- Cold skin
- Skin that looks bruised (mottling)
- Heavy perspiration
- Fever
- Extreme weakness and exhaustion
- Loss of muscle tone
- Fallen jaw, causing the mouth to stay open
- Decreased sense of touch

- Loss of feeling, beginning in the legs and feet
- Loss of vision
- Dilated pupils and staring eyes
- Inability to speak
- Extreme drowsiness
- Disorientation or confusion
- Hallucinations
- Low blood pressure
- Increased pulse
- Cheyne-Stokes breathing
- Gurgling and rattling sound when breathing
- Difficulty swallowing
- Decreased appetite and sense of thirst
- Dry mouth
- Nausea, vomiting, and diarrhea
- Urinary and fecal incontinence
- Decreased urinary output
- Loss of hearing

9. List changes that may occur in the human body after death

When death occurs, the body will not have a pulse, respiration, or blood pressure. Other physical signs you may see include the following:

- A dropped jaw, which causes the mouth to stay open
- Eyelids that are partially open, with eyes in a fixed stare
- Urinary and fecal incontinence
- Fixed and dilated pupils (this means there is no blood flow inside the brain)

Though these things are a normal part of death, they can be unsettling. If you see any of these signs, tell the nurse immediately so that she can confirm the death.

Tip

Terms to Describe the Body after Death

These Latin terms describe changes in the body after death:

- *Algor mortis* is the cooling of the body after death and the decrease in elasticity of the skin.
- *Livor mortis* is skin discoloration after death in the dependent areas of the body, such as the feet and legs.
- **Rigor mortis** is the stiffness that occurs after death due to a biochemical change that causes muscles to become rigid.

10. Describe ways to help family and friends deal with a resident's death

When a loved one dies, there is a range of emotions that family and friends may experience. These feelings include the following:

- Feeling numb or being in shock

- Physical reactions or symptoms, such as pain, especially chest pain, nausea, or difficulty breathing (report these to the nurse immediately)

- Feelings of guilt, especially if there were any unresolved problems or issues with the relationship

- Disbelief or denial of the death

- Feelings of relief

- Intense sadness and crying

- Anxiety or fear

- Anger

Family may direct anger at staff members. They may just be reacting to the loss of a loved one. They may blame staff for a problem that they feel was not addressed. Whatever the reason, refer any family complaints to the nurse. Do not try to calm a family member or friend who is upset with staff.

Allowing the family and friends to show their feelings is one of the first steps in the grieving process. Do not ask them to stop crying or to not be upset about their loss. Do not use clichés or

tell them that it is for the best. Treat family and friends with respect and compassion.

Nursing assistants can help families and friends after a loved one dies. Here are some guidelines to follow:

Guidelines: Helping the Family Deal with a Resident's Death

G   Be available for the family and friends. Talking is an important part of the grieving process. Listen to them if they want to talk (Fig. 27-7). Let them talk, and only respond if needed. Remaining silent can be beneficial.

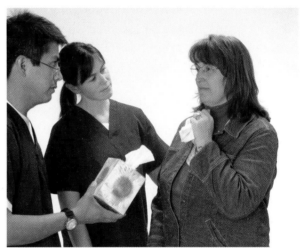

Fig. 27-7. *Be available for family and friends if they want to talk. Allow them to express their feelings.*

G   Do not be afraid to show your feelings for a resident who has died. Family and friends may feel better knowing that their loved one was valued by staff.

G   Do not make inappropriate comments or use cliches, such as, "This will pass," or "You will get over it." These are painful comments and are not helpful.

G   If family or friends make a request to see a spiritual leader or clergyperson, report this to the nurse immediately.

Some facilities have designated staff members available to help families after a resident has died. These people may be social workers, therapists, hospice workers, or spiritual leaders.

11. Describe ways to help staff members cope with a resident's death

Staff members and other residents may be very upset by the death of a beloved resident. Being able to grieve is important. Some facilities offer bereavement therapy to help staff with grieving. This is also called grief counseling. Identifying feelings in a formal setting can help staff work through their loss. Many facilities also allow caregivers and residents to participate in memorial or religious services following a death. Some may be held in the facility.

If you are grieving, it is important not to underestimate your feelings. Do not hesitate to seek out counseling or bereavement therapy to help you work through this difficult time. Do not be ashamed because you feel grief about a resident's death. This grief is a testament to the kind of person you are and the kind of person your resident was. Grieve at your own pace.

Ways that staff can cope with the death of a resident include the following:

- Do not hesitate to express your feelings. Sadness and crying are normal responses to grieving.

- Share important memories about the resident with others.

- Spend quality time with the people you love (Fig. 27-8).

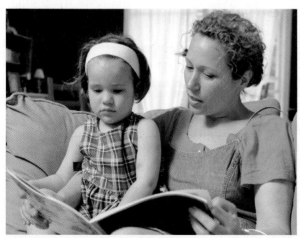

Fig. 27-8. *To help cope with your grief, spend time with people you love doing activities you enjoy.*

- Do things that make you happy. Be active and exercise regularly. Spend time outside. Take your dog for a walk.

- Talk to a counselor if the need arises.

- Join a special support group for grieving.

- Take care of yourself. Get enough sleep and eat nutritious foods. Do not smoke. Drink only in moderation.

12. Describe postmortem care

Postmortem care is care of the body after death. Be sensitive to the needs of family and friends after death occurs. They may wish to stay with the body for a while. Allow them time to do so. Be aware of any religious and cultural practices that the family wants to observe. Facilities will have different policies on postmortem care. Ask the nurse for instructions before beginning this type of care. A shroud kit containing a large white piece of material for covering the body may be used. It may include special pads, a chin strap, and ID tags. Follow your facility's policies and procedures. Do only assigned tasks.

An **autopsy** is an examination of a body by a pathologist to try to determine the cause of death. A **pathologist** is a doctor with advanced training in the examination of organs and tissues. If the body is to be autopsied, the person may need to be transferred to another facility.

> **Tip**
>
> **Care of the Belongings after Death**
> Your facility will have a policy for handling residents' personal items after death, such as jewelry, pictures, and other personal belongings. Carefully follow your facility's policy.

Postmortem care

Equipment: two pairs of gloves, drainage pads, shroud kit or sheets, clean gown, toilet tissue, washcloth or wipes, wash basin of warm water, towel, plastic bags for clothing and belongings

1.   Identify the resident.

2. Wash your hands.

3. Explain procedure to resident's family and ask them to step outside. Be courteous, respectful, and compassionate at all times.

4. Provide for privacy with a curtain, screen, or door.

5. Adjust bed to safe working level, usually waist high. Lock bed wheels.

6. Avoid trauma to the resident's body throughout the procedure. Treat the body with the utmost respect.

7. Put on gloves.

8. Turn off any oxygen, suction, or other equipment, if directed by the nurse. Do not remove any tubes or other equipment. A nurse or the funeral home will perform these tasks.

9. Gently close eyes without pressure.

10. Position the body in good alignment, on the back with legs straight. Fold arms across the abdomen. It is important to position the body before *rigor mortis* occurs, as it will make positioning difficult. The period from two to four hours after death is most common for the development of *rigor mortis*.

11. Close the mouth. Place rolled towel under the chin.

12. Gently bathe the body. Be careful to avoid bruising. Replace any dressings only if directed to do so.

13. Comb or brush hair gently without tugging.

14. Place drainage pads where needed. Most often this is under the head and/or under the perineal area and buttocks.

15. Put a clean gown on the body.

16. Cover body to just over the shoulders with sheet. Do not cover face or head.

17. Tidy room so family may visit.

18. Remove all used supplies and linen.

19. Follow your facility's policy for handling or removing personal items. Always have a witness if personal items are removed or given to a family member.

20. Remove and discard gloves.

21. Wash your hands.

22. Return bed to low position if raised. Turn lights down and allow family to enter and spend private time with resident.

23. Return after family departs and put on clean gloves.

24. Place shroud on resident and follow instructions on completing ID tags.

25. Remove and discard gloves.

26. Wash your hands.

27. Report and record observations. Document procedure using facility guidelines.

The body will be transported to a morgue or the funeral home. Your responsibilities may include transferring the body on a stretcher to the pick-up area. Ask a co-worker to assist you with the transfer. Use the designated elevator and cover the body with a sheet or shroud during transport. Be careful during the transfer to avoid any bumping or bruising. Behave professionally. Be courteous and respectful at all times.

After the body has been transported, return to the room. Put on gloves. Strip the bed and remove all linen and trash. Open windows to air the room as needed. See Chapter 10 for information on unit cleaning.

Tip

Unexpected Sounds or Movements after Death

After a person dies, the body may make sounds or movements. Breathing sounds, movement of the hands or legs, eyes opening, jaws opening, and bouts of incontinence may occur. It is common for this to happen; try not to be frightened. If you notice anything that concerns you, report promptly to the nurse.

Trivia

Two Early Autopsies

Julius Caesar, the well-known Roman leader, was killed on March 15th, known as the "Ides of March," in 44 B.C. The first recorded autopsy was done on Julius Caesar by a physician named Antistius. Antistius noted 23 stab wounds, and is thought to have determined that the chest wound was the fatal blow.

An early autopsy was also performed in 1302 when the nobleman Azzolino died under suspicious circumstances. Bartolomeo da Varignana, a doctor, performed an autopsy to determine the cause of death. He found Azzolino had not died of poisoning, as had been suspected, but from internal bleeding.

Chapter Review

1. What are the goals of palliative care (LO 2)?

2. When is hospice care usually ordered by a doctor (LO 3)?

3. List seven goals of hospice care (LO 3).

4. Briefly describe each of the five stages of grief (denial, anger, bargaining, depression, and acceptance) as defined by Elisabeth Kubler-Ross. (LO 4).

5. List five legal rights to remember when caring for the terminally ill (LO 5).

6. For each of the guidelines for caring for a dying person (skin, nose, and mouth care; pain control and comfort; diminished senses; breathing problems; food and fluid issues), list one way that the nursing assistant can help (LO 6).

7. Which sense is usually the last sense to leave the person (LO 6)?

8. List eight ways that nursing assistants can meet a dying resident's psychosocial and spiritual needs (LO 7).

9. List 20 physical signs that a person is approaching death (LO 8).

10. List six physical signs that may occur in the body after death (LO 9).

11. List four ways that nursing assistants can help families and friends after a loved one has died (LO 10).

12. What is bereavement therapy (LO 11)?

13. What are six methods that can help staff members cope with a resident's death (LO 11)?

14. Define "postmortem" (LO 12).

15. What is the goal of an autopsy (LO 12)?

28
Your New Position

The Good Old Days?

Job descriptions of the distant past included things that seem strange and even laughable today. Nurses had to act as wardens to prevent patients from playing cards, stealing from one another, drinking, or fighting. Nurses spent long hours washing and waxing floors. They even had to carry coal and fill lamps with oil. Sometimes they acted as chimney sweeps, too. Nurses were not allowed to openly smoke, drink, or go out socially. In some places, nursing staff were forbidden to meet or see anyone of the opposite sex. So if you ever find yourself upset about a current challenge, consider the harsh circumstances of the past!

"When men are employed, they are best contented; for on the days they worked they were good-natured and cheerful, and, with the consciousness of having done a good day's work, they spent the evening jollily."

Benjamin Franklin, 1706-1790

"The superior man is the providence of the inferior. He is eyes for the blind, strength for the weak, and a shield for the defenseless. He stands erect by bending above the fallen. He rises by lifting others."

Robert Green Ingersoll, 1833-1899

1. Define important words in this chapter

conflict resolution: the process of resolving conflicts in a positive way so that everyone is satisfied.

constructive criticism: feedback that involves giving opinions about the work of others in a non-aggressive way.

job description: an outline of what will be expected in a job.

résumé: a summary of a person's education and experience.

stress: a mentally or emotionally disruptive or upsetting condition that occurs due to changes in the environment.

stressor: internal or external factors or stimuli that cause stress.

2. Describe how to write a résumé and cover letter

Before you begin a new position as a nursing assistant, you have to look for a job. The first step in any job search is preparing a well-written résumé. A **résumé** is a summary of your education and experience. You will need to include information on these topics when preparing a résumé:

- **Objective**: State your main goals in the field in which you wish to work.

- **Education**: List schools or G.E.D. courses completed, starting from high school and including any college courses. List any certifications you have received, such as CNA, CPR, or first aid certification.

- **Experience**: Identify the work experience you have had to this point, placing your current job first and moving backwards. A general rule is to list positions you have held for more than six months.

- **Volunteer Work**: Describe all volunteer work, emphasizing any work related to the health-care field.

- **Skills**: List all of your special skills, including things like typing, computer skills, and languages that you speak.

- **References**: State that your references are available upon request.

The following are general rules for writing a résumé:

- Limit your résumé to one page. Use short, precise sentences.

- Do not add borders or color. Use high quality, white paper.

- Use a basic, 12-point, plain font. Boldface your name (you can even make it larger than a 12-point font), and include your address, phone number, and e-mail address at the top of the page.

- If using a computer, do not rely on a spell-check program. Use it first, check spelling yourself, then have a friend check the spelling. Read the résumé out loud to make sure you have not made any errors.

- Do not staple anything to your résumé.

An example of a well-written nursing assistant résumé is shown in Figure 28-1. Take time to make your résumé the best it can be.

A cover letter is a letter that will be included with your résumé. A sample cover letter is shown in Figure 28-2. This letter should be brief and serves as your introduction to the interviewer. It should include information about why you are seeking the job and why you are qualified for the position.

After a résumé and cover letter have been created, you will need to identify potential employers. Use the Internet, newspaper, the telephone book, and personal contacts to find employers. Ask your instructor, too; he or she may have some recommendations.

3. Identify information that may be required for filling out a job application

Completing a job application can be stressful. Being prepared will help you present yourself well (Fig. 28-3). To save time and avoid mistakes, take a piece of paper and write down information that you may need for the application. You will take this paper with you, along with a new copy of your résumé, when you go to complete the application. Include the following general information:

- Your address and phone number

- Your e-mail address

- Your social security number

- Salary information from your past and present positions

- Names, addresses, and telephone numbers of the schools or programs where you were trained and the date you completed training

- Certification numbers and expiration dates from your nursing assistant certification card, CPR card, and first aid cards

- Former and present supervisors' and employers' names, titles, addresses, and phone numbers

- Exact dates of past and current employment and your reasons for leaving each of your former jobs

- Complete names, addresses, and phone numbers of personal and professional references

- Names of other people you know who work at the facility

- The days and hours you can work (for example, weekdays, nights, or weekends)

Sarah Harris
1234 Sandia Court
Albuquerque, NM 87126
505-555-1274
sarah@hartmanonline.com

OBJECTIVE: To secure an entry-level nursing assistant job in a long-term care facility.

EDUCATION: Hobbs High School, Hobbs, NM, Diploma 2008
Hartman Medical Institute, Albuquerque, NM 2009
Certified Nursing Assistant

EXPERIENCE: Sunnyvale Nursing Home 2010 - present
Albuquerque, NM
Nursing Assistant
• Performed personal care duties and assisted with ADLs.
• Worked mostly with residents who have dementia.

Happy Home Nursing Center 2009-2010
Austin, Texas
Receptionist
• Managed multi-line phone system.
• Made appointments for staff.
• Visited residents and read to them.
• Made arrangements for resident activities outside of the facility.

SKILLS: Microsoft Word, Microsoft Excel, Adobe Acrobat, and ACT! database.

VOLUNTEER WORK: National Diabetes Foundation, Hospice Foundation

REFERENCES: Available upon request.

Fig. 28-1. A sample résumé.

November 10, 2012
Sarah Harris
1234 Sandia Court
Albuquerque, NM 87126
505-555-1274
sarah@hartmanonline.com

Mr. David Pomazal
Human Resources Manager
Nursing Assistant Finders
PO Box 555
Albuquerque, NM 87102

Dear Mr. Pomazal:

Please consider this letter and the enclosed résumé and application for the nursing assistant position advertised in last Sunday's edition of the *Albuquerque Journal*.

I am an energetic, detail-oriented person who has strong organizational skills, experience, and the ability to work well with people from all walks of life. In addition, I have held positions of responsibility in four community organizations over the last eight years and was chosen the 2010 National Diabetes Foundation Volunteer of the Year.

As you can see from my résumé, I thrive in a busy atmosphere that involves many different tasks, and I value the opportunity to work with residents. I would appreciate an interview to discuss the possibility of joining your staff. I will call you next week to request an appointment, or you may call or e-mail me at your convenience at 555-1274 or sarah@hartmanonline.com.

Thank you for your consideration of my application. I look forward to meeting you soon.

Sincerely,

Sarah Louise Harris
Enclosure

Fig. 28-2. *A sample cover letter.*

Employment Application

Personal Information

Name: Rosie Ferguson Date: 12/15/2012

Social Security Number: 555-99-9999

Home Address: 8529 Indian School Rd. NE

City, State, Zip: Albuquerque, NM 87112

| Home Phone: 505-291-1274 | Business Phone: N/A |
| US Citizen? Yes | If Not, Give Visa No. & Expiration: |

Position Applying For

| Title Nursing Assistant | Salary Desired: $8.50/hr |
| Referred By: Ms. McClain Instructor, NA Training Center | Date Available: 12/15/2012 |

Education

High School (Name, City, State): Laguna High School Albuquerque, NM

Graduation Date: November 2012

Technical or Undergraduate School: NA Training Center Albuquerque, NM

| Dates Attended: June-November 2012 | Degree Major: |

References

Mr. Robert Castro, Instructor, NA Training Center, 505-291-1284

Ms. Scott, Health Occupations, Laguna HS, 505-555-6255

Kate Crawford, Instructor, NA Training Center, 505-291-1294

Fig. 28-3. *A sample job application.*

Before going to the facility, think about any potential problems in your job application. For example, if you have a time when you did not work at all, an interviewer may ask for the reason for the gap in employment. Imagine being the interviewer and consider the questions you might ask yourself.

When you actually fill out the job application, here are a few steps that can make the process run smoothly:

- Fill out the application carefully and neatly. Use a pen to complete it. If you are filling it out at home, use a dictionary to check spelling.

- Never lie on a job application. Tell the truth. Be honest if you have a criminal record. By law the employer is required to do a complete criminal background check. This law is in place to protect residents at facilities. If you do have a record, write a complete explanation in the appropriate section so that they will have your side of the story.

- Do not leave anything blank on the application. You may write N/A (not applicable) if the question does not apply to you. If you do not understand something on the application, ask about it before filling in the space.

4. Discuss proper grooming guidelines for a job interview

In Chapter 1, professional grooming guidelines were described. Good grooming is equally important when applying for a job. Creating a good first impression can increase your chance of success, so you should look and dress appropriately. Follow these guidelines:

Guidelines: Proper Grooming for a Job Interview

G   Bathe and use deodorant.

G   Wear clean, nice clothes. Make sure that skirts, dresses, and pants are wrinkle-free and without stains or holes. Dresses and skirts should not be shorter than knee-length. Do not wear jeans or shorts.

G   Wash your hands and clean and file your nails. Nails should be medium length or shorter. Do not wear artificial nails.

G   Wear simple makeup and jewelry or none at all.

G   Wear your hair in a simple style.

G   Make sure your shoes are polished. Do not wear sneakers or open-toed sandals.

G   Men should shave right before the interview.

G   Brush your teeth. Check your teeth right before the interview begins.

G   Do not smoke. You will smell like smoke during the interview.

G   Do not wear perfume or cologne. Many people dislike or are allergic to scents.

5. List techniques for interviewing successfully

Use these guidelines to make the best impression at a job interview:

Guidelines: Interviewing Successfully

G   Practice for the interview with a friend or family member. There are books that have commonly-asked job interview questions. Practice answering these questions.

G   Tests may be given during the interview to see how skilled you are for the job. Find out if there will be a test, and if so, study beforehand to feel better prepared.

G   Get directions to the interview site. If you are taking the bus, make sure you have bus fare the night before. If you are driving, get gas the day before.

G   Arrive 10 or 15 minutes early.

G   Turn off your cell phone.

G   Be courteous to other staff members you meet.

G   Introduce yourself to the interviewer. Smile and offer to shake hands. Your handshake should be firm and confident (Fig. 28-4).

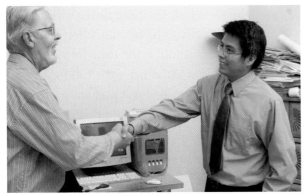

Fig. 28-4. Smile and shake hands confidently when you arrive at a job interview.

G   Answer questions clearly and completely.

G   Do not exaggerate your accomplishments.

G   Make eye contact during the interview (Fig. 28-5). Do not look up or down or left or right during the interview. The interviewer may think that you are not telling the truth or are not interested in the conversation. Maintain eye contact to show that you are sincere.

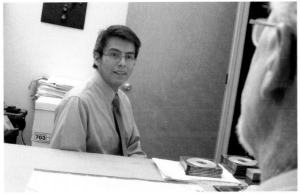

Fig. 28-5. Be polite and make eye contact while interviewing.

G   Do not use slang or curse words.

G   Do not eat or chew gum during the interview.

G   Be positive and look happy to be there.

G   Do not bring children, other family members, friends, or pets with you.

G   Relax. You have worked hard to get this far. You understand the work and what is expected of you. Be confident!

During the interview, emphasize what you think you will enjoy about your work as a nursing assistant. Do not speak negatively about a former employer. Ask questions if you are unsure about anything. Take notes if needed. You may want to write questions down before the interview so that you do not forget.

After the interview is over, stand up, smile, and shake hands again. You will probably be told when you can expect to hear from the person. Thank him for taking the time to meet with you.

Tip

It pays to say thank you!

Always write a thank-you letter after every job interview. This shows your continued interest in a job and helps to remind the interviewer who you are. If you haven't heard from a potential employer within the time frame you discussed with the interviewer, call and politely ask if the job has been filled.

6. Describe a standard job description and list steps for following the scope of practice

A **job description** is an outline of what will be expected of you in your job. It can be a long, complex form, and you should read it before you sign it. Ask questions if you do not understand anything in the job description.

Nursing assistants have to follow their scope of practice. You learned about this in Chapter 2. A scope of practice lists the tasks that nursing assistants are permitted to perform, as allowed by state or federal law. Follow these tips when deciding whether or not to perform a procedure:

•   Do not perform a procedure if it is not listed in your job description. Doing things that are beyond your scope of practice could injure a resident, you, or another staff member.

- Do not perform a procedure if you have not been trained to do it.

- Do not perform the procedure if you have forgotten how to do all or part of it. Ask the nurse for a reminder about how to perform the procedure before you do it.

- If you have been trained to perform a procedure that is within your scope of practice, but you believe it may not be appropriate for a certain resident, ask the nurse.

Tip

Organizing Your Days

When you start a new job, you will want to be as organized as possible during your workday. You can purchase an inexpensive pocket organizer. These can be found at uniform stores, as well as in many uniform catalogs. These are available ready-to-be-filled or as a complete filled package, with bandage scissors, penlight, pen, and a small notebook. Some organizers even have room for a stethoscope.

7. Identify guidelines for maintaining certification and explain the state's registry

In order to meet OBRA requirements (Chapter 2), several organizations, including the National Council of State Boards of Nursing, created nurse aide training and competency evaluation (testing) programs (NATCEP). These programs serve as a guide for each state's development of its NA testing program. OBRA requires that nursing assistants complete at least 75 hours of training before being employed. Many states' requirements exceed the minimum 75 hours.

After completing a state's required number of hours of training, NAs may then take the test in that state. A fee may be charged to take this test. Once a nursing assistant has passed both the written and manual skills test, a certificate is issued and mailed to the recipient.

Each state has different requirements for maintaining certification. Know and follow your state's specific requirements. General guidelines on obtaining and keeping nursing assistant certification include the following:

- A nursing assistant has a certain amount of time from the date he or she is employed to take the state test. Your employer will supply you with that information when you are hired. Pay attention to the time frame. If you do not take the test during the time given, you will not be able to work as a nursing assistant until you have passed the tests.

- A nursing assistant usually must take the state test within 24 months of completing the nursing assisting course. If the test is not taken during that time period, he or she will have to complete a new training course and state examination.

- A nursing assistant must work for pay during the 24-month certification period. If the nursing assistant does not, a new training program and examination must be completed.

- In most states, a nursing assistant has three chances to pass the state test.

- A nursing assistant must keep his or her certification current, if the state requires certification. File a change-of-address with your state agency if you move to make sure you receive your certification renewal. Some states require that you file a change-of-address form within 30 days.

Your employer will require that you show proof of renewal of your certificate each time it expires. Do not allow your certificate to expire. Respond immediately to your state's request to renew your certification. There may be a renewal fee.

In the United States, each state keeps a registry for certified nursing assistants (CNAs). This registry keeps track of every nursing assistant working in that state. Information kept in this registry includes the following:

- A nursing assistant's full name, along with any other names the person may have used

- A nursing assistant's home address and other information, such as date of birth and social security number

- The date that the nursing assistant was placed in the registry and results from the state test

- Expiration dates of each nursing assistant's certificates

- Information about investigations and hearings regarding abuse, neglect, or theft, which becomes a part of a nursing assistant's permanent record

Nursing assistants can ask for a written statement to be added to the file. This includes information explaining events in the nursing assistant's own words. NAs have the right to correct any errors in a registry file.

It is possible for a nursing assistant's certification to be suspended, revoked, or denied. Reasons for this vary. Be familiar with your state's guidelines. A nursing assistant can also voluntarily surrender her certification. If a nursing assistant surrenders her certification or has her certification revoked, she will not be able to practice in that state.

8. Describe continuing education for nursing assistants

The OBRA law requires that nursing assistants have 12 hours of continuing education each year in order to keep their certification current. Some states require more hours. These classes help keep your knowledge and skills up to date. Your facility is required to provide and document this continuing education, sometimes called in-services.

Some of the subjects covered in continuing education classes include the following:

- Residents' Rights

- Fire safety

- Safety

- CPR

- Infection prevention

- Confidentiality

- Bloodborne pathogens

- Tuberculosis

Make sure you attend all of the required in-services. Pay attention in class and participate in discussions (Fig. 28-6). Do any required homework or projects. After the in-service is over, keep copies of any certificates and records that show you have successfully completed the class.

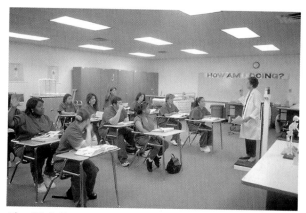

Fig. 28-6. *Pay attention and participate during in-service courses.*

Tip

Hepatitis B Vaccine and TB Tests

Employers are required to provide free hepatitis B vaccines to all employees after hire. It is one way to prevent the spread of hepatitis.

At least once per year, employers are required to test all employees for tuberculosis. You will receive a notice when it is time to have a TB skin test. Make sure you promptly take this test and return for follow-up as instructed. For more information on hepatitis and tuberculosis, see Chapters 6 and 20.

9. Describe employee evaluations and discuss criticism

An annual evaluation, sometimes called a performance appraisal or review, is used to evaluate the performance of each employee. Some of the things you will be evaluated on are overall knowledge, conflict resolution, and team effort. Flexibility, friendliness, trustworthiness, and customer service skills are other qualities considered in an evaluation. A performance review or appraisal may be done after a three-month probationary period and then annually thereafter. As long as you demonstrate consistent professionalism, excellent customer service, dependability, and ethical behavior, you will usually receive a satisfactory or better evaluation.

Employee evaluations include constructive criticism. **Constructive criticism** is feedback that involves giving opinions about the work of others, which includes helpful suggestions for change. It may involve both positive and negative feedback, but it is done in a non-aggressive way. Constructive criticism should be given in a private setting. It should be work-related; it should not include personal attacks. It is not the same as hostile criticism. Hostile criticism is angry and negative. Constructive criticism is meant to help you improve in your job.

When receiving constructive criticism, be open to suggestions, as they will help you grow and be more successful in your work. Try to listen without becoming upset or angry. Consider how you can address or fix the problem; offer ideas during the session (Fig. 28-7). If you are not sure how to avoid a mistake you have made, always ask for suggestions. A person who readily accepts constructive criticism can do well in the workplace.

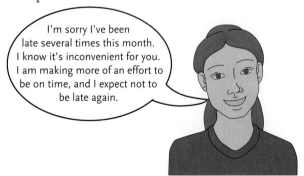

I'm sorry I've been late several times this month. I know it's inconvenient for you. I am making more of an effort to be on time, and I expect not to be late again.

Fig. 28-7. *Be open to suggestions when receiving constructive criticism.*

It is important for an employee to try each year to improve his or her performance appraisal score. Performance reviews are frequently the basis for salary increases. In addition, a satisfactory review can increase your chances of advancing within the facility. Ask for and keep a copy of every evaluation you receive.

10. Discuss conflict resolution

When you work with a group of people, conflicts can arise. **Conflict resolution** is the process of resolving conflicts in a positive way so that everyone is satisfied with the result. Most people do not like to disagree; however, sometimes it cannot be avoided. Before reacting, think about possible reasons why someone is behaving in an undesirable way. For example, a co-worker may have had a fight with a family member, or an angry resident may be in pain or may be lonely.

When you disagree with a policy at your facility, know that the management makes the best and most informed decisions that they can make. If you have a conflict with your boss or supervisor, understand that this person really wants to help you. However, policy cannot be changed for you at the expense of other staff. In short, conflict resolution works best when you are reasonable with your requests.

Sometimes resolving a conflict means you have to compromise. In order to compromise, think about how important the problem is. What is the worst that could happen if it is not solved your way? Making a list of pros and cons may help clarify your options. Identify the benefits of working with others to solve the issue. Think about whether another person, such as an arbitrator or a mediator, could help resolve the conflict.

Conflicts will occur in the workplace. The key to conflict resolution is to think about the issue before reacting. Think about how to best solve the problem. Know when to stand firm, when to walk away, and when it is time to compromise.

11. Define "stress" and explain ways to manage stress

Many things, both personal and professional, cause stress. **Stress** is a mentally or emotionally disruptive or upsetting condition that occurs due to changes in the environment. Internal factors like worry can also cause stress. Stress causes physical changes in the body. When a person is frightened, anxious, excited, confused, or in danger, stress can occur.

Stress happens because of a stressor. A **stressor** is an internal or external factor or stimulus that causes stress. Anything can be a stressor. Finding out you have a new supervisor can create stress. Being asked to speak in front of fellow employees at a staff meeting can cause stress. A visit from a relative can be stressful.

Stress is linked to many diseases, including hypertension, depression, ulcers, and migraines. It also increases the risk of developing other chronic diseases. Severe stress that does not go away may be linked to premature death.

If stress is unrelieved, burnout can occur. As you learned in Chapter 22, burnout is mental or physical exhaustion due to a prolonged period of stress and frustration.

Signs of burnout include arguing frequently, losing patience, being angry, wanting too much control in situations, and obsessing over small, unimportant things. A person who is experiencing burnout may also be rude, irritated, and frustrated. He or she may have trouble focusing on residents and procedures.

It is important to find ways to manage stress. Learning how to recognize stress and its causes

is helpful. Avoid things that you know cause stress. People, situations, places, or things can all cause stress.

Guidelines: Managing Stress

G   Increase your level of exercise (Fig. 28-8).

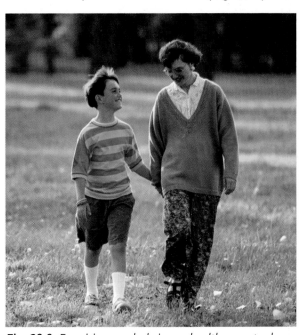

Fig. 28-8. *Exercising regularly is one healthy way to decrease stress.*

G   Get enough sleep.

G   Eat a healthy diet. Eliminate or reduce caffeine in your diet. Caffeine can cause nervousness and irritability, along with increasing anxiety.

G   Do not smoke or take illegal drugs. Drink only in moderation.

G Do one task at a time, then move on to the next task. Multi-tasking tends to increase anxiety.

G Develop new hobbies. Riding a bike, dancing, or taking classes can reduce stress. Listening to music can be calming for some people.

G Seek help from others with managing stress (Fig. 28-9). Appropriate people to turn to for help include your supervisor, your doctor, your clergyperson or spiritual leader, your friends, your family, or a local mental health agency. Do not talk to residents or their families about your stress. That is inappropriate.

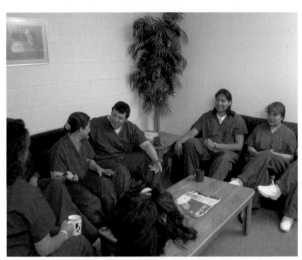

Fig. 28-9. *Support groups can help you deal with different types of stress.*

G Seek counseling if needed. Do not feel embarrassed if you need help. It takes courage to seek help for a problem. Counselors can suggest a variety of methods to reduce stress.

G Set realistic goals. People can set both short-term and long-term goals for themselves and their families.

G Use a personal reward system. When you accomplish something that makes you happy, do something nice for yourself. See a movie, go out to dinner with friends, or visit a loved one.

Goal-Setting

Setting goals can help manage stress. The key is to make the goals reachable. Do not set only long-term goals. Identify short-term, reachable goals that you can meet in a reasonable time period. The course you are taking right now is an example of a short-term goal, and you are close to meeting this important goal. If you create long-term goals, do not set a time frame of over three to five years. Set only long-term goals that you believe you can meet.

Relaxation Techniques

Abdominal Breathing:

• Stop, sit down, and breathe.

• Rest your hands on your abdomen and close your eyes.

• Breathe slowly and regularly, pushing your hands out with each breath.

• Do this a few times until you feel yourself begin to relax.

Muscle Relaxation:

• Starting with your head and jaw, relax as many muscles as you can.

• Do this one muscle at a time, from top to bottom, until you reach your feet and toes.

Holding Hands

Holding hands with someone special in your life may decrease stress. Try it and see if it makes you feel calmer and more relaxed.

12. Describe how to be a valued member of the healthcare community

You have now reached the end of your nursing assistant course. Very soon you will be a practicing nursing assistant. Remember what you have accomplished and know the importance of the work you have chosen to do. You are going to be a valuable member of a care team, a team that literally saves lives every day. It is a noble profession, and one that provides a tremendous service to the community. Be very proud of yourself. As you graduate, make sure you thank your family, friends, instructors, and classmates for everything they have done to help you during your course.

As you move forward in your new profession, never stop learning. Learn new things every day. Stay current in your field. Collect reading materials about health care and other topics. Create your own medical library at home.

Value your profession and treat your new position with all of the respect that it deserves. You worked so hard to get where you are—now it is time to reward yourself!

Chapter Review

1. List six topics you should include when preparing a résumé (LO 2).

2. How long should a résumé be (LO 2)?

3. What are two items that should be included in a cover letter (LO 2)?

4. List six examples of information that you may need in order to complete a job application (LO 3).

5. Why do you think employers are required to do a criminal background check on nursing assistants (LO 3)?

6. List eight grooming guidelines for job interviews (LO 4).

7. List nine guidelines for successful job interviewing (LO 5).

8. List four ways a nursing assistant can make sure she is following her scope of practice before accepting a task (LO 6).

9. How many hours of training does OBRA require a nursing assistant to complete before being employed (LO 7)?

10. Within how many months of training is a nursing assistant usually required to take the state test (LO 7)?

11. List the information about nursing assistants that is kept in the state registry (LO 7).

12. How many hours of continuing education does the federal government require for nursing assistants each year (LO 8)?

13. List four areas on which a nursing assistant may be evaluated in an annual employee performance appraisal (LO 9).

14. What is constructive criticism (LO 9)?

15. Before reacting to a conflict, what should a nursing assistant do (LO 10)?

16. What is stress (LO 11)?

17. List three signs of burnout (LO 11).

18. List ten ways to manage stress (LO 11).

Abbreviations

abd	abdomen
ABR	absolute bedrest
ac, a.c.	before meals
AD	Alzheimer's disease
ad lib	as desired
ADLs	activities of daily living
adm.	admission
AIDS	acquired immune deficiency syndrome
AMA	against medical advice, American Medical Association
amb	ambulate, ambulatory
as tol	as tolerated
ax.	axillary (armpit)
BID, b.i.d.	two times a day
BM	bowel movement
BP, B/P	blood pressure
BPM	beats per minute
BR	bedrest
BRP	bathroom privileges
BSC	bedside commode
c̄	with
cath.	catheter
CBR	complete bedrest
C. diff	*clostridium difficile*
CHF	congestive heart failure
ck ✓	check
cl liq	clear liquid

CNA	certified nursing assistant
c/o	complains of, in care of
COPD	chronic obstructive pulmonary disease
CPR	cardiopulmonary resuscitation
CS	Central Supply
CVA	cerebrovascular accident, stroke
CVP	central venous pressure
CXR	chest X-ray
DAT	diet as tolerated
DM	diabetes mellitus
DNR	do not resuscitate
DON	director of nursing
Dr., DR	doctor
drsg	dressing
Dx/dx	diagnosis
EMS	emergency medical services
exam	examination
FF	force fluids
ft	foot
F/U, f/u	follow-up
geri-chair	geriatric chair
H_2O	water
h, hr, hr.	hour
HBV	hepatitis B virus
HIPAA	Health Insurance Portability and Accountability Act
HIV	human immunodeficiency virus

HOB	head of bed
HS/hs	hours of sleep
ht	height
HTN	hypertension
hyper	above normal, too fast, rapid
hypo	low, less than normal
inc	incontinent
I&O	intake and output
isol	isolation
IV, I.V.	intravenous (within a vein)
L, lt	left
lab	laboratory
lb.	pound
lg	large
LPN	licensed practical nurse
LTC	long-term care
LVN	licensed vocational nurse
M.D.	medical doctor
MDS	minimum data set
meds	medications
MI	myocardial infarction
min	minute
mm HG	millimeters of mercury
mL	milliliter
mod	moderate
MRSA	methicillin-resistant *staphylococcus aureus*
MSDS	material safety data sheet

NA	nursing assistant
N/C	no complaints, no call
NG, ng	nasogastric
NKA	no known allergies
NPO	nothing by mouth
NVD	nausea, vomiting and diarrhea
OBRA	Omnibus Budget Reconciliation Act
OOB	out of bed
OSHA	Occupational Safety and Health Administration
oz.	ounce
p̄	after
pc, p.c.	after meals
peri care	perineal care
per os	by mouth
PHI	protected health information
PO	by mouth
PPE	personal protective equipment
p.r.n., prn	when necessary
q2h	every two hours
q3h	every three hours
q4h	every four hours
q̄	every
qh, qhr	every hour
qhs	every night at bedtime
q.i.d., qid	four times a day
R	respirations, rectal
R, rt.	right

rehab	rehabilitation
res.	resident
resp.	respiration
RF	restrict fluids
RN	registered nurse
R/O	rule out
ROM	range of motion
RR	respiratory rate
s̄	without
SOB	shortness of breath
SP	Standard Precautions
spec.	specimen
ss	one-half
S&S, S/S	signs and symptoms
stat, STAT	immediately
std. prec.	Standard Precautions
T., temp	temperature
TB	tuberculosis
t.i.d., tid	three times a day
TLC	tender loving care
TPR	temperature, pulse and respiration
U/A, u/a	urinalysis
UTI	urinary tract infection
VRE	vancomycin-resistant *enterococcus*
VS, vs	vital signs
w/c, W/C	wheelchair
wt.	weight

Symbols

©	copyright
&	and
☣	biohazard
△	change, heat
°	degree
♀	female
♂	male
%	percent
☢	radiation

Appendix

In life, it is important to continue to improve oneself and to strive to learn something new each day. This section includes a brief review of many basic skills; you may or may not already be familiar with this material. Feel free to refer to it any time you need a refresher on writing, studying, note-taking or math.

Grammar, Punctuation, and Capitalization

It is important to speak well and to use grammar correctly. Grammar is the correct use of the rules of a language. Here are some basic grammatical terms and their definitions:

- A noun is a person, place, or thing. Examples: car, home, lipstick, school.

- An adjective is a word that describes a noun. Examples: *blonde* hair, *gray* sweater.

- A pronoun is a word that takes the place of a noun. Examples: I, he, him, she, them, we.

- A verb is a word that expresses an action or the condition of a person. Examples: jumps, drives, lifts.

- An adverb is a word that describes a verb, adjective, or adverb. Examples: He smiled *happily*. She skated *quickly*.

- A conjunction is a connecting word. Examples: and, but, neither, nor, or.

- A sentence is a group of words with a subject and verb that expresses a complete thought. Example: The fireman rescued the cat from the tree.

Punctuation is the use of marks in writing to separate words and ideas. Here are some common punctuation marks and their definitions:

- A period (.) is the punctuation mark placed at the end of sentences and other statements that are considered complete. Examples: Hello. Welcome to the nursing assistant training class.

Periods are also placed after many abbreviations. For example, "Dr." is an abbreviation for the word "Doctor."

- A comma (,) separates thoughts or items in a list, such as a list of adjectives. Example: The hospital sat on top of a tall, grassy hill.

- A semicolon (;) connects two sentences with closely related ideas. Example: John has great patience; we appreciate him.

- A colon (:) introduces a list or indicates that an addition is coming. Examples: Kelley picked up these items: a comb, a razor, and soap. There was only one thing they needed to make their family complete: a pet.

- An apostrophe (') shows possession (ownership). It also shows where letters are missing in contractions. Examples: Susan took Sarah's toy. Elizabeth wasn't trained to do that task (contraction of "was not").

- Quotation marks ("") identify what someone has said or written. Example: The resident said, "I am having pain in my shoulder."

Capitalization is the writing of a word with its first letter as an upper case letter and the remaining letters in lowercase letters. Capitalize the following:

- The first word of a sentence, question, or quote. Example: The gate is open.

- Proper names and titles. Example: "Hello, Mr. Dickens. How are you and Margaret today?"

- Names of peoples. Example: Asian

- Names of religious groups and of sacred texts. Examples: Catholic, Buddhist, the Bible, the Koran

- Names of countries, states, cities, or areas. Examples: Italy, Massachusetts, Dallas, the Pacific Northwest

- Names of streets or roads. Example: Thatcher Road

- Names of buildings, organizations, colleges, and schools. Examples: Yale University, the

United Nations, Roosevelt High School, the White House

- Holidays, historical and special events, and holy days. Examples: Labor Day, Passover, the Civil War

- Days of the week and months of the year. Examples: Tuesday, May

- Trade names. Examples: Arby's, Target, Nike

Reading Skills

Reading well is an important part of being a nursing assistant. In the healthcare field, you must be able to read assignments, care plans, menus, activity schedules, and many other documents. Improving your reading skills can help in these situations, and reading well will also help with doing homework and studying for exams.

Choose a place to read in your home where you can concentrate. If one is not available, try a library. When you read your textbook, follow these guidelines:

- Know yourself. Choose the site where you can read best.

- Use eyeglasses or contact lenses if you need them.

- Have enough light to read.

- Sit comfortably so that you do not hurt your back or neck. Use supportive pillows if needed.

- Take notes if you need to.

- Practice saying words you do not know. Do not be embarrassed to ask for help pronouncing a word.

- Refer to a dictionary when you need help.

When reading textbooks, make sure to separate and organize important information. First, look at the objectives for the chapter or unit; this will help you understand its primary goals. Complete each chapter section or learning objective before moving on to the next one. After all notes are taken and the sections for that chapter are finished, complete the chapter review. If you can successfully answer the questions asked in the review, move on to the next chapter.

Note-Taking

People take notes all the time. You may take notes while in class or while reading this textbook. There are many ways to take notes. Here are three methods that can make this process easier:

1. **Outline Method**: Write down the subject. Then put all sentences about that subject under it in outline form (see the box below). Use a highlighting marker to highlight the subjects and words or points you need to remember.

Menus

I. Positioning of Residents
   a. Purpose
   b. Preparation

2. Types of Positions
   a. Supine
   b. Lateral
   c. Dorsal recumbent
   d. Knee-chest
   e. Prone
   f. Sims'
   g. Fowler's/semi-Fowler's
   h. Lithotomy

3. Positions Requiring Doctor's Order
   a. Trendelenburg
   b. Reverse Trendelenburg

2. **Index Card Method**: Write down all of your notes neatly on large index cards. Use one card for each topic. To keep cards together, use rubber bands or punch a hole in the corner and use rings (one ring for every chapter).

3. **Rewrite Method**: Rewrite your notes neatly in a spiral notebook to keep them together. Rewriting them may help you remember more material.

Studying Effectively

It is not enough to simply sit down and start studying; having the proper tools will help. The following tips may help you study more effectively:

- Keep a large pad of paper to write down questions or notes.
- Use pens and highlighters. After making notes, highlight all important words and main subjects in your notes.
- Record your thoughts and ideas about each chapter. This may help you to remember them. Some people replay their thoughts while resting.
- Take regular breaks, such as every 30 minutes or once per hour. Get a drink of water, take a walk, etc.
- Keep a regular dictionary and a medical dictionary nearby. Write new words down in a notepad or on index cards. Look up any terms you do not know and write down their meanings. Review these words each time you study.

Taking Exams

Sometimes so much effort is put into mental preparation for a test that people forget to prepare their bodies as well. Physical condition affects mental abilities.

Before taking a test, get plenty of rest and watch what you eat and drink. On the day of the exam, eat a good breakfast. It is hard to think if you are hungry. Eat foods such as whole grain breads, cereals, and proteins. Avoid simple sugars like candy, doughnuts, and soda.

Being in good physical shape allows more blood to get to your brain. A person who gets regular physical exercise will have a body that uses oxygen more effectively than someone who is completely out of shape. Even exercising for a few days in a row before a test can make a noticeable difference in your thinking abilities.

Decrease your stress level before an exam. Fill up the car with gas or get correct bus fare the day before. Make lunch the night before. In short, try to avoid stress on the day of an exam. Stress may affect your grade.

When taking the exam, listen carefully to any instructions given. Be sure to read the directions. When taking a multiple-choice test, first eliminate answers you know are wrong. Since your first choice is usually correct, do not change your answers unless you are sure of the correction.

Do not spend too much time on any one question. If you do not understand it, move on and go back if time allows. Remember to leave that question blank on your answer sheet. Be careful to answer the next question in the proper space.

When you are finished with a test, go over the entire answer sheet. Check to make sure you have circled an answer for each question. Make sure you have placed an answer for each question on the answer sheet in the correct space.

Basic Math Skills

Some people have been out of school for a while and begin to overuse calculators. They start to rely on them too much. Nursing assistants need math skills when doing certain tasks, such as recording how much a resident eats and drinks. A basic math review is listed below.

Addition

	3,457		11,999
+	398	+	7,657
	3,855		19,656

Subtraction

	27,785		179,746
−	9,358	−	37,437
	18,427		142,309

Multiplication

```
      3,754              92
  x     129          x    37
  ─────────          ─────────
     33,786              644
     75,080          +  2,760
  + 375,400          ─────────
  ─────────            3,404
    484,266
  ─────────
```

Division

```
         49                 33
  26 │ 1,274         16 │  528
     - 1,040            -  480
     ───────            ───────
        234                 48
      - 234              -  48
      ───────            ───────
          0                  0
```

Converting Decimals, Fractions, and Percentages

Decimals, fractions, and percentages are all related. A decimal is a fraction whose denominator is a power of 10. A percentage is a way of expressing a fraction as a whole number, by using 100 as the denominator. To express one-half (½) as a decimal, we would say 0.5. To express one-half (½) as a percentage, we would say 50% or 50/100.

Here are some examples:

Example: ½=0.5=50%

To get the decimal 0.5 from ½, divide the denominator (2) into the numerator (1).

To change 0.5 into a percent, move the decimal sign two places to the right and add the percent sign.

0.5 = 50%

Example: ¼ = 0.25 = 25%

To change 0.25 into a percent, move the decimal sign two places to the right and add the percent sign.

0.25 = 25%

Example: ¾ = 0.75 = 75%

To change 0.75 into a percent, move the decimal sign two places to the right and add the percent sign.

0.75 = 75%

Other Useful Information

Multiplication Table

1	2	3	4	5	6	7	8	9	10	11	12
2	4	6	8	10	12	14	16	18	20	22	24
3	6	9	12	15	18	21	24	27	30	33	36
4	8	12	16	20	24	28	32	36	40	44	48
5	10	15	20	25	30	35	40	45	50	55	60
6	12	18	24	30	36	42	48	54	60	66	72
7	14	21	28	35	42	49	56	63	70	77	84
8	16	24	32	40	48	56	64	72	80	88	96
9	18	27	36	45	54	63	72	81	90	99	108
10	20	30	40	50	60	70	80	90	100	110	120
11	22	33	44	55	66	77	88	99	110	121	132
12	24	36	48	60	72	84	96	108	120	132	144

Conversions: Volume

1 milliliter (mL) = 1 cubic centimeter (cc)

1 ounce (oz.) = 30 mL (cc)

¼ cup = 2 oz. = 60 mL (cc)

½ cup = 4 oz. = 120 mL (cc)

1 cup = 8 oz. = 240 mL (cc)

1 Liter = 1000 mL (cc)

Conversions: Weight

2 pints = 1 quart (qt.) = 960 mL (cc)

2 quarts = ½ gallon (gal.) = 1920 cc = 2 liters (L)

4 quarts = 1 gallon (gal.)

2.2 pounds (lbs.) = 1 Kilogram (kg)

1 gram (g) = 1000 milligrams (mg)

Conversions: Length

1 inch (in.) = 2.54 centimeters (cm)
(or round off to 2.5)

12 inches = 1 foot

3 feet = 1 yard

10 millimeters (mm) = 1 centimeter (cm)

100 centimeters (cm) = 1 meter

Glossary

24-hour urine specimen: a urine specimen consisting of all urine voided in a 24-hour period.

abdominal girth: a measurement of the circumference around the abdomen at the umbilicus (navel).

abdominal thrusts: a method of attempting to remove an object from the airway of someone who is choking.

abduction: moving a body part away from the midline of the body.

absorption: the digestive process in which digestive juices and enzymes break down food into materials the body can use.

abuse: purposely causing physical, mental, emotional, or financial pain or injury to someone.

accountable: answerable for one's actions.

acquired immune deficiency syndrome (AIDS): the final stage of HIV infection, in which infections, tumors, and central nervous system symptoms appear due to a weakened immune system that is unable to fight infection.

active assisted range of motion (AAROM): exercises to put a joint through its full arc of motion that are done by a resident with some help from a staff member.

active listening: a way of communicating that involves giving a person your full attention while he is speaking and encouraging him to give information and clarify ideas; includes nonverbal communication.

active neglect: purposely harming a person physically, mentally, or emotionally by failing to provide needed care.

active range of motion (AROM): exercises to put a joint through its full arc of motion that are done by a resident alone, without help.

activities of daily living (ADLs): personal daily care tasks, including bathing, skin, nail, and hair care, walking, eating and drinking, mouth care, dressing, transferring, and toileting.

acute care: 24-hour skilled care for short-term illnesses or injuries; generally given in hospitals and ambulatory surgical centers.

adaptive devices: special equipment that helps a person who is ill or disabled perform ADLs; also called assistive devices.

additive: a substance added to another substance, changing its effect.

adduction: moving a body part toward the midline of the body.

admission pack: personal care items supplied upon a resident's admission.

adult daycare: care given to adults at a facility during daytime work hours.

advance directives: legal documents that allow people to decide what kind of medical care they wish to have if they are unable to make those decisions themselves.

ageism: stereotyping of, prejudice toward, and/or discrimination against the elderly.

age-related macular degeneration (AMD): a condition in which the macula degenerates, gradually causing central vision loss.

agitated: the state of being excited, restless, or troubled.

agnostic: a person who claims that he does not know or cannot know if God exists.

airway: the natural passageway for air to enter into the lungs.

alveoli: tiny, grape-like sacs in the lungs where the exchange of oxygen and carbon dioxide occurs.

Alzheimer's disease (AD): a progressive, degenerative, and irreversible disease that is a form of dementia; there is no cure.

ambulation: walking.

amputation: the surgical removal of an extremity.

anatomy: the study of body structure.

anemia: a condition in which the amount of red blood cells or hemoglobin in the body is less than normal.

angina pectoris: chest pain, pressure, or discomfort.

anticipatory grief: a period of mourning when the dying person or his family is expecting the death.

anti-embolic stockings: special stockings used to help prevent swelling and blood clots and aid circulation; also called elastic stockings.

antimicrobial: an agent that destroys, resists, or prevents the development of pathogens.

anxiety: uneasiness or fear, often about a situation or condition.

apathy: a lack of interest.

apical pulse: the pulse on the left side of the chest, just below the nipple.

apnea: the absence of breathing.

artery: vessel that carries blood away from the heart.

arthritis: a general term that refers to inflammation of the joints.

artificial airway: any plastic, metal, or rubber device inserted into the respiratory tract for the purpose of maintaining an airway and facilitating ventilation.

aspiration: the inhalation of food, fluid, or foreign material into the lungs.

assault: the act of threatening to touch a person without his or her consent.

assisted living: a residence for people who require some help with daily care, but who need less care than a long-term care facility offers.

assistive devices: special equipment that helps a person who is ill or disabled perform ADLs; also called adaptive devices.

asthma: a chronic and episodic inflammatory disease that makes it difficult to breathe and causes coughing and wheezing.

atheist: a person who claims that there is no God.

atria: the upper two chambers of the heart.

atrophy: weakening or wasting of muscles.

autoclave: an appliance used to sterilize medical instruments or other objects by using steam under pressure.

autoimmune disease: a disease in which the body is unable to recognize its own tissue and begins to attack the tissues.

autopsy: an examination of a body by a pathologist to try to determine the cause of death.

axilla: underarm or armpit area.

barrier: a block or an obstacle.

baseline: initial value that can be compared to future measurements.

battery: touching a person without his or her consent.

bedridden: confined to bed.

benign: non-cancerous.

benign prostatic hypertrophy: a disorder that can occur in men as they age, in which the prostate becomes enlarged and causes problems with urination and/or emptying the bladder.

bereavement: the period following a loss in which mourning occurs.

biology: the study of all life forms.

biopsy: a removal of a sample of tissue for examination and diagnosis.

biorhythms: natural rhythms or cycles related to bodily functions.

bipolar disorder: a type of depression that causes a person to have mood swings and changes in energy levels and the ability to function; also called manic depression.

bloodborne pathogens: microorganisms found in human blood that can cause infection and disease.

Bloodborne Pathogen Standard: federal law requiring that healthcare facilities protect employees from bloodborne health hazards.

body fluids: tears, saliva, sputum (mucus coughed up), urine, feces, semen, vaginal secretions, pus or other wound drainage and vomit.

body language: all of the conscious or unconscious messages your body sends as you communicate, such as facial expressions, shrugging your shoulders, and wringing your hands.

body mechanics: the way the parts of the body work together when a person moves.

body systems: groups of organs that perform specific functions in the human body.

bones: rigid connective tissues that make up the skeleton, lend support to body structures, allow the body to move, and protect the organs.

bony prominences: areas of the body where the bone lies close to the skin.

bowel elimination: the physical process of releasing or emptying the colon or large intestine of solid waste, called stool or feces.

BPM: the medical abbreviation for "beats per minute."

brachial pulse: the pulse inside the elbow; about 1 to 1½ inches above the elbow.

bradycardia: a slow heart rate—under 60 beats per minute.

brain: the part of the nervous system housed in the skull that is responsible for motor activity, memory, thought, speech, and intelligence, along with regulation of vital functions, such as heart rate, blood pressure, and breathing.

breakthrough pain: a type of severe pain that happens unexpectedly in people who have cancer.

bridge: a type of dental appliance that replaces missing or pulled teeth.

bronchi: branches of the passages of the respiratory system that lead from the trachea into the lungs.

bronchiectasis: a condition in which the bronchi become permanently dilated (widened) and damaged.

bronchitis: an irritation and inflammation of the lining of the bronchi.

bruise: a purple, black, or blue discoloration on the skin caused by the leakage of blood from broken blood vessels into the surrounding tissues; also called a contusion.

Buddhism: a religion that follows the teachings of Buddha.

burnout: mental or physical exhaustion due to a prolonged period of stress and frustration.

bursae: tiny sacs of fluid that are located near joints and help reduce friction.

bursitis: a condition in which the bursae become inflamed and painful.

calculi: kidney stones.

cancer: a general term used to describe a disease in which abnormal cells grow in an uncontrolled way.

capillaries: tiny blood vessels in which the exchange of gases, nutrients, and waste products occurs between blood and cells.

cardiac arrest: the medical term for the stopping of the heartbeat.

cardiomyopathy: a weakening of the heart muscle due to enlargement or thickening, which reduces the heart's ability to pump blood effectively.

care conference: a meeting to share and gather information about residents in order to develop a care plan.

care plan: a written plan for each resident created by the nurse; outlines the steps taken by the staff to help the resident reach his or her goals.

care team: the group of people with different kinds of education and experience who provide resident care.

carrier: person who carries a pathogen usually without signs or symptoms of disease but who can spread the disease.

cartilage: the protective substance that covers the ends of bones and makes up the discs that are found between vertebrae.

cataract: a condition in which the lens of the eye becomes cloudy, causing vision loss.

catastrophic reaction: reacting to something in an unreasonable, exaggerated way.

catheter: tube inserted through the skin or into a body opening that is used to add or drain fluid.

C. difficile (C. diff, clostridium difficile): a bacterial illness that can cause diarrhea and colitis; spread by spores in feces that are difficult to kill.

cells: the basic structural unit of all organisms.

Celsius: the centigrade temperature scale in which the boiling point of water is 100 degrees and the freezing point of water is 0 degrees.

Centers for Disease Control and Prevention (CDC): federal government agency responsible for improving the overall health and safety of the people of the United States.

central nervous system: part of the nervous system made up of the brain and spinal cord.

central venous line: a type of intravenous line (IV) that is inserted into a large vein in the body.

cerebrovascular accident (CVA): a condition caused when the blood supply to the brain is cut off suddenly by a clot or a ruptured blood vessel; also called a stroke.

cervical cancer: a form of female reproductive cancer that begins in the cervix; can occur at any age and has few symptoms.

chain of command: the order of authority within a facility.

charge nurse (nurse-in-charge): a nurse responsible for a team of healthcare workers.

charting: the act of noting care and observations; documenting.

chemical restraint: medications used to control a person's behavior.

chest percussion: clapping the chest to help lungs drain with the force of gravity.

chest tubes: hollow drainage tubes that are inserted into the chest to drain air, blood, pus or fluid that has collected inside the pleural space/cavity.

Cheyne-Stokes respiration: type of respiration with periods of apnea lasting at least 10 seconds, along with alternating periods of slow, irregular respirations and rapid, shallow respirations.

chlamydia: a sexually-transmitted infection caused by bacteria.

Christianity: a religion that follows the teachings of Jesus Christ.

chronic: the term for an illness or condition that is long-term or long-lasting.

chronic obstructive pulmonary disease (COPD): a chronic, progressive, and incurable lung disease that causes difficulty breathing.

chronic renal failure (CRF): progressive condition in which the kidneys cannot filter certain waste products; also called chronic kidney failure.

chyme: semi-liquid substance made as a result of the chemical breakdown of food in the stomach.

circadian rhythm: the 24-hour day-night cycle.

cite: in a long-term care facility, to find a problem through a survey.

civil law: private law; law between individuals.

clean: a condition in which an object has not been contaminated with pathogens.

clean-catch specimen: a urine specimen that does not include the first and last urine that is voided; also called mid-stream.

closed bed: bed completely made with the bedspread and blankets in place.

closed wound: a type of wound in which the skin's surface is not broken.

code: in health care, an emergent medical situation in which specially-trained responders provide resuscitative measures to a person.

code status: formally written status of the type and scope of care that should be provided in the event of a cardiac arrest, other catastrophic failure, or terminal illness; terms and acronyms are used to identify the care desired by the person, such as "DNR" (do not resuscitate) and "no code."

code team: group of people chosen for a particular shift to respond to resident emergencies.

cognition: the ability to think clearly and logically.

colon: the large intestine.

colostomy: surgically-created opening through the abdominal wall into the large intestine to allow feces to be expelled.

coma: state of unconsciousness in which a person is unable to respond to any change in the environment, including pain.

combative: violent or hostile.

combustion: the process of burning.

communicable disease: an infectious disease transmissible by direct contact or by indirect contact.

complicated grief: grief complicated by disorders or conditions, such as depression and substance abuse.

concussion: a head injury that occurs from a banging movement of the brain against the skull.

condom catheter: a catheter that has an attachment on the end that fits onto the penis; also called an external or Texas catheter.

conflict resolution: the process of resolving conflicts in a positive way so that everyone is satisfied.

confusion: the inability to think clearly and logically.

congestive heart failure (CHF): a condition in which the heart muscle is damaged and fails to pump effectively.

conscientious: guided by a sense of right and wrong; principled.

conscious: the state of being mentally alert and having awareness of surroundings, sensations, and thoughts.

constipation: the inability to eliminate stool, or the infrequent, difficult and often painful elimination of a hard, dry stool.

constructive criticism: the process of giving opinions about the work of others in a non-aggressive way.

contagious disease: a type of communicable disease that spreads quickly from person to person.

contaminated: soiled, unclean; having disease-causing organisms or infectious material on it.

continuity of care: coordination of care for a resident over time, during which the care team is always exchanging information about the resident and working toward shared goals.

contracture: the permanent and often painful shortening of a muscle, usually due to a lack of activity.

coronary artery disease (CAD): a condition in which the coronary arteries become damaged and narrow over time, causing chest pain and other symptoms.

courteous: polite, kind, considerate.

CPR (cardiopulmonary resuscitation): refers to medical procedures used when a person's heart and lungs have stopped working.

cremation: the process of burning a dead body until it turns to ash.

criminal law: public law; related to committing a crime against the community.

critical thinking: the process of reasoning and analyzing in order to solve problems; for the nursing assistant, critical thinking means making good observations and promptly reporting all potential problems.

Crohn's disease: a disease that causes the wall of the intestines (large or small) to become inflamed (red, sore, and swollen).

cross-infection: the physical movement or transfer of harmful bacteria from one person, object, or place to another, or from one part of the body to another.

cultural diversity: the variety of people living and working together in the world.

culture: a set of learned beliefs, values, traditions, and behaviors shared by a social, ethnic, or age group.

cyanosis: blue or pale skin and/or mucous membranes due to decreased oxygen in the blood.

dandruff: excessive shedding of dead skin cells from the scalp.

dangle: to sit up with the legs over the side of the bed in order to regain balance.

death: the end of life; the cessation of all body functions.

defecation: the process of eliminating feces from the rectum through the anus.

defense mechanisms: unconscious behaviors used to release tension and/or help a person cope with stress.

dehydration: an excessive loss of water from the body; a condition that occurs when fluid loss is greater than fluid intake.

delegation: transferring authority to a person for a specific task.

delirium: a sudden state of severe confusion due to a change in the body; also called acute confusional state or acute brain syndrome.

delusion: a belief in something that is not true, or is out of touch with reality.

dementia: a serious, progressive loss of mental abilities such as thinking, remembering, reasoning, and communicating.

dentures: artificial teeth.

depressant: a substance that causes calmness and drowsiness.

depression: an illness that causes social withdrawal, lack of energy, and loss of interest in activities, as well as other symptoms.

dermis: the inner layer of the two main layers of tissue that make up the skin.

developmental disability: a chronic condition that restricts physical and/or mental abilities.

diabetes: a condition in which the pancreas does not produce insulin or does not produce enough insulin; causes problems with circulation and can damage vital organs.

diabetic ketoacidosis: a life-threatening complication of diabetes that can result from undiagnosed diabetes, not enough insulin, eating too much, not getting enough exercise, and stress; also known as ketoacidosis or hyperglycemia.

diagnosis: the identification of a disease by its signs and symptoms and from the results of different tests.

dialysis: a process that cleans the body of wastes that the kidneys cannot remove due to kidney failure.

diarrhea: frequent elimination of liquid or semi-liquid feces.

diastole: phase when the heart muscle relaxes.

diastolic: second measurement of blood pressure; phase when the heart relaxes.

diet cards: cards that list residents' names and information about special diets, allergies, likes and dislikes, and any other dietary instructions.

digestion: the process of breaking down food so that it can be absorbed into the cells.

dilate: to widen.

direct contact: way to transmit pathogens through touching the infected person or his or her secretions.

direct spread: method of transmission of disease from one person to another.

dirty: a condition in which an object has been contaminated with pathogens.

disinfection: a measure used to decrease the spread of pathogens and disease by destroying pathogens.

disorientation: confusion about person, place, or time; may be permanent or temporary.

disposable: only to be used once and then discarded.

disruptive behavior: any behavior that disturbs others.

diuretics: medications that reduce fluid volume in the body.

diverticulitis: inflammation of sacs that develop in the wall of the large intestine due to diverticulosis.

diverticulosis: a disorder in which sac-like pouchings develop in weakened areas of the wall of the large intestine (colon).

DNR (do-not-resuscitate): an order that tells medical professionals not to perform CPR.

doff: to remove.

domestic violence: physical, sexual, or emotional abuse by spouses, intimate partners, or family members.

don: to put on.

dorsal recumbent: position with the person flat on her back with knees flexed and slightly separated and her feet flat on the bed.

dorsiflexion: bending backward.

drainage: flow of fluids from a wound or cavity.

draw sheet: an extra sheet placed on top of the bottom sheet; used for moving residents.

duodenum: the first part of the small intestine, where the common bile duct enters the small intestine.

durable power of attorney for health care: a signed and dated legal document that appoints someone to make the medical decisions for a person in the event he or she becomes unable to do so.

dysphagia: difficulty in swallowing.

dyspnea: difficulty breathing.

eczema: a temporary or chronic skin disorder that results in redness, itching, burning, swelling, cracking, weeping, and lesions; also called dermatitis.

edema: swelling in body tissues caused by excess fluid.

edentulous: lacking teeth; toothless.

electrolytes: chemical substances that are essential to maintaining fluid balance and homeostasis in the body.

elimination: the process of expelling wastes.

elopement: in medicine, when a person with Alzheimer's disease wanders away from a protected area and does not return on his own.

emesis: the act of vomiting, or ejecting stomach contents through the mouth and/or nose.

empathetic: identifying with and understanding another's feelings.

emphysema: a chronic, incurable lung disease in which the alveoli in lungs become filled with trapped air; usually results from smoking and chronic bronchitis.

endometrial cancer: a form of female reproductive cancer that begins in the uterus; symptoms include vaginal bleeding and pelvic pain.

end-stage renal disease (ESRD): condition in which kidneys have failed and dialysis or transplantation is required to sustain life.

enema: a specific amount of water, with or without an additive, introduced into the colon to eliminate stool.

epidermis: the outer layer of the two main layers of tissue that make up the skin.

epilepsy: a disorder that causes recurring seizures.

epistaxis: a nosebleed.

ergonomics: the science of designing equipment, areas, and tasks to make them safer and to suit the worker's abilities.

ethics: the knowledge of right and wrong; standards of conduct.

etiquette: the code of proper behavior and courtesy in a certain setting.

eupnea: normal respirations.

expiration: the process of exhaling air out of the lungs.

exposure control plan: plan that outlines specific work practices to prevent exposure to infectious material and identifies step-by-step procedures to follow when exposures do occur.

exposure incident: specific eye, mouth, other mucous membrane, non-intact skin, or parenteral contact with blood or other potentially infectious materials that results from the performance of an employee's duties.

expressive aphasia: inability to express oneself to others through speech or written words.

extension: straightening a body part.

Fahrenheit: a temperature scale in which the boiling point of water is 212 degrees and the freezing point of water is 32 degrees.

fainting: loss of consciousness; also called syncope.

false imprisonment: the unlawful restraint of someone which affects the person's freedom of movement; includes both the threat of being physically restrained and actually being physically restrained.

farsightedness: the ability to see distant objects more clearly than objects that are near; also called hyperopia.

fasting: a period of time during which food is given up voluntarily.

fecal impaction: a mass of dry, hard stool that remains packed in the rectum and cannot be expelled.

fecal incontinence: an inability to control the muscles of the bowels, which leads to an involuntary passage of stool or gas; also called anal incontinence.

feces: solid body waste excreted through the anus from the large intestine; also called stool.

financial abuse: the act of stealing, taking advantage of, or improperly using the money, property, or other assets of another.

first aid: care given by the first people to respond to an emergency.

first impression: a way of classifying or categorizing people at the first meeting.

flammable: easily ignited and capable of burning quickly.

flatulence: air in the intestine that is passed through the rectum; also called gas or flatus.

flexion: bending a body part.

fluid balance: taking in and eliminating equal amounts of fluid.

fluid overload: a condition in which the body cannot eliminate the fluid consumed.

fomite: an object that is contaminated with a pathogen and can spread the pathogen to another person.

foot drop: weakness of muscles in the feet and ankles that interferes with the ability to flex the ankles and walk normally.

force fluids: a medical order for a person to drink more fluids.

Fowler's: position in which a person is in a semi-sitting position (45 to 60 degrees).

fracture: a broken bone.

fracture pan: a bedpan that is flatter than a regular bedpan; used for small or thin people or those who cannot lift their buttocks onto a standard bedpan.

full weight-bearing (FWB): a doctor's order stating that a person has the ability to support full body weight on both legs and has no weight-bearing limitations.

functional nursing: method of care assigning specific tasks to each team member.

gait belt: a belt made of canvas or other heavy material used to help people who are weak, unsteady, or uncoordinated to stand, sit, or walk; also called a transfer belt.

gangrene: death of tissue caused by infection or lack of blood flow.

gastroesophageal reflux disease (GERD): a chronic condition in which the liquid contents of the stomach back up into the esophagus.

gastrointestinal tract: a continuous tube from the opening of the mouth all the way to the anus, where solid wastes are eliminated from the body.

gastrostomy: an opening in the stomach and abdomen.

generalized anxiety disorder (GAD): an anxiety disorder characterized by chronic anxiety, excessive worrying, and tension, even when there is no cause for these feelings.

genital herpes: a sexually-transmitted, incurable infection caused by herpes simplex viruses type 1 (HSV-1) or type 2 (HSV-2).

genital HPV infection: a sexually-transmitted infection caused by human papillomavirus (HPV).

gingivitis: an inflammation of the gums.

glands: structures in the body that produce substances.

glaucoma: a condition in which the pressure in the eye increases, damaging the optic nerve and causing blindness.

glucose: natural sugar.

gonads: the male and female sexual reproductive glands.

gonorrhea: a sexually-transmitted infection caused by bacteria.

graduate: a measuring container for measuring fluid volume.

grief: a deeply emotional process that is a response to loss.

grief process: the varying emotional responses to grief.

grief therapy: therapy to try to resolve problems due to separation from the deceased.

grooming: practices to care for oneself, such as caring for fingernails and hair.

halitosis: bad-smelling breath.

hallucinations: seeing or hearing things that are not really there.

hand hygiene: washing hands with either plain or antiseptic soap and water and using alcohol-based hand rubs.

hand rubs: an alcohol-containing preparation designed for application to the hands for reducing the number of microorganisms on the hands.

health: state of physical, mental, and social well-being.

healthcare-associated infection (HAI): an infection associated with healthcare delivery in any setting (e.g., hospitals, long-term care facilities, ambulatory settings, or home care).

hearing aid: a battery-operated device that amplifies sound.

heart: four-chambered pump that is responsible for the flow of blood in the body.

heartburn: a condition that results from a weakening of the sphincter muscle which joins the esophagus and the stomach; also known as acid reflux.

hemianopsia: loss of vision on one-half of the visual field due to CVA, tumor or trauma.

hemiparesis: weakness on one side of the body.

hemiplegia: paralysis of one side of the body.

hemoptysis: the coughing up of blood from the respiratory tract.

hemorrhoids: enlarged veins in the rectum that can cause itching, burning, pain, and bleeding.

hepatitis: inflammation of the liver caused by certain viruses and other factors, such as alcohol abuse, some medications, and trauma.

Hinduism: a religion that believes in the unity of everything and that all are a part of God.

HIPAA (Health Insurance Portability and Accountability Act): a federal law that sets standards for protecting the privacy of patients' health information.

hoarding: collecting and putting things away in a guarded manner.

holistic: care that involves the whole person; this includes his or her physical, social, emotional, and spiritual needs.

home health care: care that takes place in a person's home.

homeostasis: the condition in which all of the body's systems are balanced and are working at their best.

homophobia: a fear of homosexuality.

hormones: chemical substances produced by the body that control numerous body functions.

hospice care: care for people who have approximately six months or less to live; care is available until the person dies.

human immunodeficiency virus (HIV): a virus that attacks the body's immune system and gradually disables it; eventually causes AIDS.

hygiene: methods of keeping the body clean.

hyperextension: extending a joint beyond its normal range of motion.

hyperglycemia: a life-threatening complication of diabetes that can result from undiagnosed diabetes, not enough insulin, eating too much, not getting enough exercise, and stress; also known as diabetic ketoacidosis (DKA) or ketoacidosis.

hypertension: high blood pressure, measuring 140/90 or higher.

hyperthyroidism: a condition in which the thyroid gland produces too much thyroid hormone, which causes body processes to speed up and metabolism to increase.

hypoglycemia: a life-threatening complication of diabetes that can result from either too much insulin or too little food; also known as insulin reaction and insulin shock.

hypotension: low blood pressure, measuring 100/60 or lower.

hypothermia: a condition in which body temperature drops below the level required for normal functioning; severe sub-normal body temperature.

hypothyroidism: a condition in which the body lacks thyroid hormone, which causes body processes to slow down.

hypoxia: a condition in which the body does not receive enough oxygen.

ileostomy: surgically-created opening into the end of the small intestine, the ileum, to allow feces to be expelled.

immunity: resistance to infection by a specific pathogen.

impairment: a partial or complete loss of function or ability.

impotence: the inability to have or maintain a penile erection.

incident: an accident, problem, or unexpected event during the course of care.

incident report: a report documenting an incident and the response to the incident; also known as an occurrence report or event report.

incontinence: the inability to control the bladder or bowels, which leads to an involuntary loss of urine or feces.

incubation period: the period of time between the time a pathogen enters the body and the time it causes visible signs and symptoms of disease.

indirect contact: a way to transmit pathogens from touching something contaminated by the infected person.

indirect spread: method of transmission of disease from an object, insect, or animal to a person.

indwelling catheter: a catheter that stays inside the bladder for a period of time; urine drains into a bag.

infection: the state resulting from pathogens invading and growing within the human body.

infection prevention: set of methods used to control and prevent the spread of disease; formerly known as "infection control."

infectious disease: any disease caused by growth of a pathogen.

ingestion: the process of taking food or fluids into the body.

input: the fluid a person consumes; also called intake.

insomnia: the inability to fall asleep or remain asleep.

inspiration: the process of breathing air into the lungs.

insulin reaction: a life-threatening complication of diabetes that can result from either too much insulin or too little food; also known as hypoglycemia or insulin shock.

intake: the fluid a person consumes; also called input.

integument: natural protective covering.

inter-generational care: mixing children and the elderly in the same care setting.

intervention: a way to change an action or development.

intubation: the method used to insert an artificial airway; involves passing a plastic tube through the mouth or nose and into the trachea or windpipe.

invasion of privacy: a violation of the right to be left alone and the right to control personal information.

involuntary seclusion: separating or confining a person from others against the person's will.

irreversible: unable to be reversed or returned to the original state.

irritable bowel syndrome (IBS): a chronic condition of the gastrointestinal tract that is worsened by stress.

ischemia: a lack of blood supply to an area.

Islam: a religion that follows the prophet Muhammad and the Five Pillars of Islam.

isolate: to keep something separate, or by itself.

job description: an outline of what will be expected in a job.

Joint Commission: a not-for-profit organization that evaluates and accredits different types of healthcare facilities.

joints: the points where two bones meet; provide movement and flexibility.

Judaism: a religion that follows the teachings of God as given to Moses in laws and commandments.

ketones: chemical substances that the body produces when it does not have enough insulin in the blood.

kilogram: a unit of mass equal to 1000 grams; one kilogram equals 2.2 pounds.

knee-chest: position in which a person is lying on his abdomen with knees pulled up towards the abdomen and with legs separated; arms are pulled up and flexed and the head is turned to one side.

lactose intolerance: the inability to digest lactose, a type of sugar in milk and other dairy products.

lateral: position in which a person is lying on either side.

laws: rules set by the government to help protect the public.

length of stay: the number of days a person stays in a healthcare facility.

lesion: an area of abnormal tissue or an injury or wound.

liability: a legal term that means a person can be held legally responsible for harming someone else.

licensed practical nurse (LPN) or licensed vocational nurse (LVN): licensed nurse who has completed one to two years of education; LPN/LVN administers medications, gives treatments, and may supervise daily care of residents.

ligaments: strong bands of fibrous connective tissue that connect bones or cartilage and support the joints and joint movement.

lithotomy: position in which a person is on her back with her hips at the edge of the exam table; legs are flexed and feet are in padded stirrups.

living will: a document that states the medical care a person wants, or does not want, in case he or she becomes unable to make those decisions.

localized infection: infection limited to a specific part of the body; has local symptoms.

logrolling: moving a person as a unit, without disturbing the alignment of the body.

long-term care: 24-hour care provided for people with ongoing conditions who are generally unable to manage their ADLs.

lungs: main organs of respiration responsible for the exchange of oxygen and carbon dioxide.

lymph: a clear yellowish fluid that carries disease-fighting cells called lymphocytes.

malabsorption: a condition in which the body cannot absorb or digest a particular nutrient properly.

malignant: cancerous.

malnutrition: a serious condition in which a person is not getting proper nutrition.

malpractice: a negligent or improper act by a professional that results in damage or injury to a person.

mandated reporters: people who are required to report suspected or observed abuse or neglect due to their regular contact with vulnerable populations, such as the elderly in long-term care facilities.

masturbation: to touch or rub sexual organs in order to give oneself or another person sexual pleasure.

Material Safety Data Sheet (MSDS): sheet that provides information on the safe use of and hazards of chemicals, as well as emergency steps to take in the event chemicals are splashed, sprayed, or ingested.

mechanical lift: special equipment used to lift and move or lift and weigh a person; also called hydraulic lift.

mechanical ventilator: a machine used to inflate and deflate the lungs when a person cannot breathe on his own.

medical asepsis: refers to practices used to reduce and control the spread of microorganisms, such as handwashing.

medical chart: written legal record of all medical care a patient, resident, or client receives.

melanin: the pigment that gives skin its color.

melanocyte: cell in the skin that produces and contains the pigment called melanin.

Meniere's disease: a disorder of the inner ear caused by a build-up of fluid, which causes vertigo (dizziness), hearing loss, tinnitus (ringing in the ear), and pain or pressure.

menopause: the end of menstruation.

menstruation: the shedding of the lining of the uterus that occurs approximately every 28 days; also known as the menstrual cycle or period.

mental health: refers to the normal function of emotional and intellectual abilities.

mental illness: a disease that disrupts a person's ability to function at a normal level in the family, home, or community.

metabolism: the process of breaking down and transforming all nutrients that enter the body to provide energy, growth, and maintenance.

metastasize: to spread from one part of the body to another.

metric: system of weights and measures based upon the meter.

microbe: a tiny living thing visible only by microscope; also called a microorganism.

microorganism (MO): a tiny living thing not visible to the eye without a microscope; also called a microbe.

micturition: the process of emptying the bladder of urine; also called urination or voiding.

Minimum Data Set (MDS): a detailed form with guidelines for assessing residents in long-term care facilities; also details what to do if resident problems are identified.

misappropriation: the act of taking what belongs to someone else and using it illegally for one's own gain.

mores: the accepted traditional customs of a particular social group.

mourning: the period in which people work to adapt to a loss; influenced by culture, tradition, and society.

MRSA (methicillin-resistant *Staphylococcus aureus*) infection: an infection caused by specific bacteria that has become resistant to many antibiotics.

MSDs: acronym that stands for work-related musculoskeletal disorders.

mucous membranes: the membranes that line body cavities that open to the outside of the body, such as the linings of the mouth, nose, eyes, rectum, and genitals.

multidrug-resistant organisms (MDROs): microorganisms, mostly bacteria, that are resistant to one or more antimicrobial agents.

multidrug-resistant TB (MDR-TB): disease that occurs when the full course of medication is not taken for tuberculosis (TB).

multiple sclerosis (MS): a progressive disease in which the protective covering for the nerves, spinal cord, and white matter of the brain breaks down over time; without this covering, nerves cannot send messages to and from the brain in a normal way.

muscles: groups of tissues that contract and relax, allowing motion, supporting the body, protecting organs, and creating heat.

muscular dystrophy: an inherited, progressive disease that causes a gradual wasting of muscle, weakness, and deformity.

myocardial infarction (MI): a condition in which blood flow to the heart is blocked and muscle cells die; also called a heart attack.

myocardial ischemia: a condition in which the heart muscle does not receive enough blood and lacks oxygen; can cause angina pectoris.

nasogastric tube: a feeding tube that is inserted through the nose into the stomach.

NATCEP (Nurse Aide Training and Competency Evaluation Program): part of OBRA that sets minimum requirements for nursing assistants for training and testing.

nearsightedness: the ability to see objects that are near more clearly than distant objects; also called myopia.

necrosis: the death of living cells or tissues caused by disease or injury.

need: something necessary or required.

negligence: actions, or a failure to act or give proper care, that results in injury to a person.

neuron: the basic nerve cell of the nervous system.

nitroglycerin: medication that relaxes the walls of the coronary arteries.

non-communicable disease: a disease not capable of being spread from one person to another.

non-intact skin: skin that is broken by abrasions, cuts, rashes, acne, pimples, lesions, surgical incisions, or boils.

nonverbal communication: communication without using words, such as making gestures and facial expressions.

non-weight-bearing (NWB): a doctor's order stating that a person is unable to touch the floor or support any weight on one or both legs.

normal flora: the microorganisms that normally live in and on the body and do not cause harm in a healthy person, as long as the flora remain in or at that particular area.

nursing assistant: person who performs assigned nursing tasks and gives personal care.

nursing process: an organized method used by nurses to determine residents' needs, plan the appropriate care to meet those needs, and evaluate how well the plan of care is working; five steps are assessment, diagnosis, planning, implementation, and evaluation.

nutrient: substance in food that enables the body to use energy for metabolism.

nutrition: the taking in and using of food by the body to maintain health.

objective information: factual information collected using the senses of sight, hearing, smell, and touch; also called signs.

OBRA (Omnibus Budget Reconciliation Act): federal law that includes minimum standards for nursing assistant training, staffing requirements, resident assessment instructions, and information on rights for residents.

obsessive-compulsive disorder (OCD): an anxiety disorder characterized by repetitive thoughts or behavior.

obstructed airway: a condition in which the tube through which air enters the lungs is blocked.

occlusion: a complete obstruction of a blood vessel.

occult: hidden.

Occupational Safety and Health Administration (OSHA): a federal government agency that makes and enforces rules to protect workers from hazards on the job.

occupied bed: a bed made while the person is in the bed.

ombudsman: person assigned by law as the legal advocate for residents.

open bed: bed made with linen folded down to the foot of the bed.

open wound: a type of wound in which the skin's surface is not intact.

opportunistic infection: an illness caused by microorganisms due to a person's inability to fight infection.

opposition: touching the thumb to any other finger.

organ: a structural unit in the human body that performs a specific function.

orientation: a person's awareness of person, place, and time.

orthopnea: shortness of breath when lying down that is relieved by sitting up.

orthostatic hypotension: a sudden drop in blood pressure that occurs when a person stands up; also called postural hypotension.

orthotic devices: devices applied externally to limbs to support, protect, improve function, and prevent complications.

osteoarthritis: a type of arthritis that usually affects weight-bearing joints, especially the hips and knees; also called degenerative joint disease.

osteoporosis: a condition in which the bones become brittle and weak; may be due to age, lack of hormones, not enough calcium in bones, or lack of exercise.

ostomy: surgical creation of an opening from an area inside the body to the outside.

otitis media: an infection in the middle ear that causes pain, pressure, fever, and reduced ability to hear.

outpatient care: care usually given for less than 24 hours to people who have had treatments, procedures, or surgery.

output: fluid that is eliminated each day through urine, feces, and vomitus, as well as perspiration; also includes suction material and wound drainage.

ovarian cancer: a form of female reproductive cancer that begins in the ovaries; can occur at any age and has few symptoms.

ovum: female sex cell or egg.

oxygen therapy: the administration of oxygen to increase the supply of oxygen to the lungs.

pacing: walking back and forth in the same area.

palliative care: care given to people who have serious, life-threatening diseases; goals are to control symptoms, reduce suffering, prevent side effects and complications, and maintain quality of life.

panic disorder: an anxiety disorder that causes a person to have repeated episodes of intense fear that something bad will occur.

paranoid schizophrenia: a form of mental illness characterized by hallucinations and delusions.

paraplegia: a loss of function of lower body and legs.

parasomnias: sleep disorders.

Parkinson's disease: a progressive disease that causes a portion of the brain to degenerate; causes rigid muscles, shuffling gait, pill-rolling, mask-like face, and tremors.

partial bath: bath that includes washing the face, underarms, hands, and perineal area.

partial weight-bearing (PWB): a doctor's order stating that a person is able to support some body weight on one or both legs.

PASS: acronym for use of a fire extinguisher; stands for Pull-Aim-Squeeze-Sweep.

passive neglect: unintentionally harming a person physically, mentally, or emotionally by failing to provide needed care.

passive range of motion (PROM): exercises to put a joint through its full arc of motion that are done by staff, without the resident's help.

pathogen: microorganisms that are capable of causing infection and disease.

pathologist: a doctor with advanced training in the examination of organs and tissues.

pathophysiology: the study of the disorders that occur in the body.

pediculosis: an infestation of lice.

percutaneous endoscopic gastrostomy (PEG) tube: a tube placed through the skin directly into the stomach to assist with eating.

perineal care: care of the genitals and anal area by cleaning.

peripheral nervous system: part of the nervous system made up of the nerves that extend throughout the body and connect to the spinal cord.

peripheral vascular disease (PVD): a condition in which the legs, feet, arms, or hands do not have enough blood circulation.

peristalsis: muscular contractions that push food through the gastrointestinal tract.

perseveration: the repetition of words, phrases, questions, or actions.

pet therapy: the practice of bringing pets into a facility or home to provide stimulation and companionship.

phantom limb pain: pain in a limb (or extremity) that has been amputated.

phantom sensation: warmth, itching, or tingling from a body part that has been amputated.

phlebitis: inflammation of the veins in the lower extremities.

physiatrists: doctors who specialize in rehabilitation.

physical abuse: intentional or unintentional treatment that causes harm or injury to a person's body.

physiology: the study of how body parts function.

pillaging: taking things that belong to someone else; not considered stealing.

plaque: a substance that accumulates on the teeth from food and bacteria.

pneumonia: acute inflammation in the lung tissue caused by a bacterial, viral, or fungal infection and/or chemical irritants.

policy: a course of action to be followed.

portable commode: a chair with a toilet seat and a removable container underneath; used for elimination; also called a bedside commode.

positioning: the act of helping people into positions that will be comfortable and healthy for them.

postmortem care: care of the body after death.

post-traumatic stress disorder (PTSD): anxiety-related disorder caused by a traumatic experience.

posture: the way a person holds and positions his body.

pound: a unit of weight equal to 16 ounces.

PPE (personal protective equipment): a barrier between a person and pathogens; includes gloves, gowns, masks, goggles, and face shields.

pre-diabetes: a condition in which a person's blood glucose levels are above normal but not high enough for a diagnosis of type 2 diabetes.

prefix: a word part added to the beginning of a root to create a new meaning.

prehypertension: a condition in which a person has a systolic measurement of 120–139 mm Hg and a diastolic measurement of 80–89 mm Hg; indicator that even though the person does not have high blood pressure now, he or she is likely to have it in the future.

pressure points: areas of the body that bear much of its weight.

pressure ulcer: a serious wound resulting from skin breakdown; also known as pressure sore, decubitus ulcer, or bed sore.

primary nursing: method of care in which the registered nurse gives much of the daily care to residents.

prioritize: to place things in order of importance.

procedure: a method, or way, of doing something.

professionalism: the act of behaving properly for a certain job.

progressive: something that continually gets worse or deteriorates.

pronation: turning downward.

prone: position in which a person is lying on his or her stomach.

prostate cancer: a form of male reproductive cancer that begins in the prostate gland; usually occurs in older men, and symptoms include urinating during the night, a weak flow of urine, painful urination, blood in urine, and problems with maintaining an erection.

prosthesis: an artificial device that replaces a body part, such as an eye, hip, arm, leg, tooth, or heart valve; helps improve function and/or appearance.

protected health information (PHI): information that can be used to identify a person and relates to the patient's past, present, or future physical or mental condition, including any health care that patient has had, or payment for that health care.

psoriasis: a chronic skin condition caused by skin cells growing too quickly which results in red, white, or silver patches, itching and discomfort.

psychological abuse: any behavior that causes a person to feel threatened, fearful, intimidated, or humiliated in any way.

psychosocial needs: needs that involve social interaction, emotions, intellect, and spirituality.

psychotherapy: a method of treating mental illness that involves talking about one's problems with mental health professionals.

puberty: the period at which a person develops secondary sex characteristics.

pulmonary edema: a condition in which there is an accumulation of fluid in the lungs; usually due to heart failure.

pulse oximeter: device that measures a person's blood oxygen level and pulse rate.

puree: to chop, blend, or grind food into a thick paste of baby food consistency.

quadriplegia: loss of function of legs, trunk, and arms.

RACE: acronym for steps taken during a fire; stands for Remove-Activate-Contain-Extinguish.

radial pulse: the pulse on the inside of the wrist, where the radial artery runs just beneath the skin.

range of motion (ROM): exercises that put a joint through its full arc of motion.

reality orientation: type of therapy that uses calendars, clocks, signs, and lists to help people with Alzheimer's disease remember who and where they are, along with the date and time.

receptive aphasia: inability to understand what others are communicating through speech or written words.

registered nurse (RN): a licensed nurse who has completed two to four years of education; RNs assess residents, create the care plan, monitor progress, provide skilled nursing care, give treatments, and supervise the care given by nursing assistants and other members of the care team.

rehabilitation: a program of care given by a specialist or a team of specialists to restore or improve function after an illness or injury.

reinfection: being infected again with the same pathogen.

religion: a set of beliefs and practices followed by a group of people.

reminiscence therapy: type of therapy that encourages people with Alzheimer's disease to remember and talk about the past.

remission: the disappearance of signs and symptoms of cancer or other diseases; can be temporary or permanent.

remotivation therapy: type of group therapy that promotes self-esteem, self-awareness, and socialization for people with Alzheimer's disease.

resident: a person living in a long-term care facility.

resident-focused care: method of care in which the resident is the primary focus; residents and their families actively participate in care, and their choices are honored by caregivers whenever possible.

Residents' Council: a group of residents who meet regularly to discuss issues related to the long-term care facility.

Residents' Rights: rights identified in OBRA that relate to how residents must be treated while living in a long-term care facility; they provide an ethical code of conduct for healthcare workers.

resistance: the body's ability to prevent infection and disease.

respiration: the process of inhaling air into the lungs and exhaling air out of the lungs.

respiratory arrest: the medical term for the stopping of breathing.

restorative care: care used after rehabilitation to maintain a person's function and increase independence.

restraint: a physical or chemical way to restrict voluntary movement or behavior.

restraint alternatives: measures used instead of physical or chemical restraints.

restraint-free care: an environment in which restraints are not kept or used for any reason.

restrict fluids: a medical order that limits the amount of fluids a person takes in.

résumé: a summary of a person's education and experience.

rheumatoid arthritis: a type of arthritis in which joints become red, swollen, and very painful; movement is restricted, and deformities of the hands are common.

rigor mortis: Latin for "stiffness of death;" refers to the stiffness that occurs after death due to muscles becoming rigid.

root: the main part of a word that gives it meaning.

rotation: turning the joint.

rounds: physical movement of staff from room to room to discuss each resident and his or her care plan.

routine urine specimen: a urine specimen that can be collected any time a person voids.

rummaging: going through items that belong to other people.

sandwich generation: people responsible for the care of both their children and aging relatives.

sanitation: ways individuals and communities maintain clean, hygienic conditions that help prevent disease, such as the disposal of sewage and solid waste.

scabies: a contagious skin infection caused by mites burrowing into the skin that results in pimple-like irritations, rashes, intense itching, and sores.

scalds: burns caused by very hot liquids.

schizophrenia: a form of chronic mental illness that may have acute episodes; affects a person's ability to think, communicate, make decisions, and understand reality.

scope of practice: defines the tasks that healthcare providers are legally permitted to perform as allowed by state or federal law.

sedation: the use of medication to calm a person.

sentinel event: an unexpected occurrence involving death or serious physical or psychological injury.

sepsis: a serious illness caused by an infection, usually bacterial, that requires immediate care.

sequential compression device (SCD): a machine used to help improve circulation, reduce fluid build-up, and prevent blood clots; compression sleeves are placed around the legs and are inflated and deflated regularly.

sexual abuse: forcing a person to perform or participate in sexual acts against his or her will.

sexual harassment: any unwelcome sexual advance or behavior that creates an intimidating, hostile, or offensive working environment.

sexually-transmitted infections (STIs): infections caused by sexual contact with infected people; signs and symptoms are not always apparent.

shearing: rubbing or friction resulting from the skin moving one way and the bone underneath it remaining fixed or moving in the opposite direction.

shingles: a viral infection caused by the same virus that causes chickenpox; results in pain, itching, rashes, and possibly fever and chills.

shock: a condition in which there is decreased blood flow to organs and tissues.

Sims': position in which a person is in a left side-lying position with the upper knee flexed and raised toward the chest.

sitz bath: a warm soak of the perineal area to clean perineal wounds and reduce inflammation and pain.

skilled care: medically-necessary care given by a skilled nurse or therapist.

skin cancer: the growth of abnormal skin cells; symptoms include changes in mole, wart, or spot on the skin, sores that do not heal, itching, pain, and skin that is oozing or bleeding.

sleep: natural period of rest for the mind and body during which energy is restored.

sling: a bandage or piece of material that is suspended from the neck for the purpose of holding and supporting a forearm.

slip knot: a quick-release knot used to tie restraints.

social anxiety disorder: a disorder in which a person has excessive anxiety about social situations; also called social phobia.

special diet: a diet for people who have certain illnesses or conditions; also called therapeutic or modified diet.

specific gravity: a test performed to measure the density of urine.

specimen: a sample, such as tissue, blood, urine, stool, or sputum, used for analysis and diagnosis.

sperm: male sex cells.

sphincter: a ring-like muscle that opens and closes an opening in the body.

sphygmomanometer: a device that measures blood pressure.

spinal cord: the part of the nervous system inside the vertebral canal that conducts messages between the brain and the body and controls spinal reflexes.

spirituality: of or relating to the concerns of the spirit, the sacred, or the soul.

sputum: mucus coughed up from the lungs.

stable angina: chest pain that occurs when a person is active or under severe stress.

Standard Precautions: a method of infection prevention in which all blood, body fluids, non-intact skin (like abrasions, pimples, or open sores), and mucous membranes (lining of mouth, nose, eyes, rectum, or genitals) are treated as if they were infected with a disease.

stereotype: a biased generalization about a group that is usually based on opinions and distorted ideas.

sterilization: a measure used to decrease the spread of pathogens and disease by destroying all microorganisms, including those that form spores.

stethoscope: an instrument used to hear sounds in the human body, such as the heartbeat or pulse, breathing sounds, or bowel sounds.

stimulant: a drug that increases or quickens actions of the body.

stoma: an artificial opening in the body.

straight catheter: a catheter that does not stay inside the person; it is removed immediately after urine is drained or collected.

stress: a mentally or emotionally disruptive or upsetting condition that occurs due to changes in the environment.

stressor: internal or external factors or stimuli that cause stress.

subacute care: care for an illness or condition given to people who need less care than for an acute (sudden onset, short-term) illness or injury but more than for a chronic (long-term) illness.

subjective information: information collected from residents, their family members and friends; information may or may not be true but is what the person reported; also called symptoms.

substance abuse: the use of legal or illegal substances in a way that is harmful to oneself or others.

suffix: a word part added to the end of a root or a prefix to create a new meaning.

suffocation: the stoppage of breathing from a lack of oxygen or excess of carbon dioxide in the body that may result in unconsciousness or death; also known as asphyxia.

sundowning: a condition in which a person gets restless and agitated in the late afternoon, evening, or night.

supination: turning upward.

supine: position in which a person is lying flat on his or her back.

suppository: a medication given rectally to cause a bowel movement.

surgical asepsis: method that makes an area or an object completely free of microorganisms; also called sterile technique.

surgical bed: bed made so that a person can easily move onto it from a stretcher.

syncope: loss of consciousness; also called fainting.

syphilis: a sexually-transmitted infection caused by bacteria.

systemic infection: an infection that occurs when pathogens enter the bloodstream and move throughout the body; causes general symptoms, such as chills and fever.

systole: phase where the heart is at work, contracting and pushing blood out of the left ventricle.

systolic: first measurement of blood pressure; phase when the heart is at work, contracting and pushing blood out of the left ventricle.

tachycardia: a fast heartbeat, over 100 beats per minute.

tachypnea: rapid respirations—over 20 breaths per minute.

tartar: hard deposits on the teeth that are filled with bacteria; may cause gum disease and loose teeth if they are not removed.

team leader: a nurse in charge of a group of residents for one shift of duty.

team nursing: method of care in which a nurse acts as a leader of a group of people giving care.

telemetry: application of a cardiac monitoring device that transmits information about the heart rhythm and heart rate to a central monitoring station for assessment.

tendons: tough fibrous bands that connect muscle to bone.

terminal illness: a disease or condition that will eventually cause death.

testicular cancer: a form of male reproductive cancer that begins in the testes.

thermometer: a device used for measuring the degree of heat or cold.

tinea: a fungal infection that causes red, scaly patches to appear in a ring shape, generally on the upper body, or the hands and feet.

tissues: a group of cells that performs similar tasks.

total hip replacement (THR): a surgical replacement of the head of the femur (long bone of the leg) and the socket it fits into where it joins the hip with artificial materials.

total knee replacement (TKR): a surgical replacement of a damaged or painful knee with artificial materials.

total parenteral nutrition (TPN): the intravenous infusion of nutrients in a basic form that is absorbed directly by the cells, bypassing the digestive tract.

trachea: an air passage that goes from the throat (pharynx) to the bronchi; also called the windpipe.

tracheostomy: a surgically-created opening through the neck into the trachea.

transcultural nursing: the study of various cultures with the goal of providing care specific to each culture.

transfer belt: a belt made of canvas or other heavy material used to assist residents who are weak, unsteady, or uncoordinated to stand, sit, or walk; also called a gait belt.

transmission: the way and means by which a disease is spread.

trichomoniasis: a sexually-transmitted infection caused by protozoa (single-celled animals).

trigger: a situation that leads to agitation.

trustworthy: deserving the trust of others.

tuberculosis (TB): a contagious lung disease caused by a bacterium that is transmitted through the air; causes coughing, difficulty breathing, fever, and fatigue.

tumor: a group of abnormally-growing cells.

ulcerative colitis: a chronic inflammatory disease of the large intestine.

unoccupied bed: a bed made while no person is in the bed.

unresolved grief: grief that continues beyond what is considered a reasonable period of time; may affect the person's ability to function.

unstable angina: chest pain that occurs while a person is at rest and not exerting himself.

ureterostomy: a type of urostomy in which a surgical creation of an opening from the ureter through the abdomen is made for urine to be eliminated.

urinary incontinence: the inability to control the bladder, which leads to an involuntary loss of urine.

urinary tract infection (UTI): a disorder that causes inflammation of the bladder; also called cystitis.

urostomy: the general term used for any surgical procedure that diverts the passage of urine by redirecting the ureters.

vaccine: a substance prepared from weakened or killed microorganisms that is used to give immunity to disease.

vaginal irrigation: a rinsing of the vagina in order to clean the vaginal tract or to introduce medication into the vagina; also called a douche.

vaginitis: an inflammation of the vagina; symptoms include vaginal discharge, itching, and pain.

validating: giving value to or approving.

validation therapy: a type of therapy that lets people with Alzheimer's disease believe they are living in the past or in imaginary circumstances.

vegans: vegetarians who do not eat any animal products, including milk, cheese, other dairy items, or eggs; vegans may also not use or wear any animal products, including wool, silk, and leather.

vegetarians: people who do not eat meat, fish, or poultry for religious, moral, personal, or health reasons; they may or may not eat eggs and dairy products.

vein: vessel that carries blood to the heart.

ventilation: in medicine, the exchange of air between the lungs and the environment.

ventricles: the lower two chambers of the heart.

verbal abuse: the use of language—spoken or written—that threatens, embarrasses, or insults a person.

verbal communication: communication involving the use of spoken or written words or sounds.

violent: word to describe actions that include attacking, hitting, or threatening someone.

vital signs: measurements—temperature, pulse, respirations, blood pressure, pain level—

that monitor the functioning of the vital organs of the body.

voiding: the process of emptying the bladder of urine; also called urination or micturition.

VRE (vancomycin-resistant *enterococcus*): a strain of the bacterium *enterococcus* that is resistant to the powerful antibiotic vancomycin; infections occur when the bacteria enter the bloodstream, urinary tract, or surgical wounds.

wandering: walking around a facility without any known goal or purpose.

wart: contagious hard bump caused by a virus.

wellness: successfully balancing things that happen in everyday life; includes five different types: physical, social, emotional, intellectual, and spiritual.

withdrawal: the physical and mental symptoms caused by ceasing to use a particular addictive substance.

workplace violence: verbal, physical, or sexual abuse of staff by residents, other staff members, or visitors.

Index